THERAPEUTIC MODALITIES
in
Rehabilitation

THERAPEUTIC MODALITIES
in
Rehabilitation

Third Edition

WILLIAM E. PRENTICE, PhD, PT, ATC

Professor, Coordinator of Sports Medicine Program
Department of Exercise and Sport Science
University of North Carolina
Chapel Hill, North Carolina

With Case Studies and Lab Activities Contributed by:

WILLIAM S. QUILLEN, PhD, PT, SCS

Professor and Director
School of Physical Therapy
University of South Florida
College of Medicine
Tampa, Florida

FRANK UNDERWOOD, PhD, MPT, ECS

Associate Professor
Department of Physical Therapy
University of Evansville
Evansville, Indiana

Clinical Electrophysiologist
Rehabilitation Service
Orthopaedic Associates, Inc.
Evansville, Indiana

McGraw-Hill
Medical Publishing Division

New York / Chicago / San Francisco / Lisbon / London / Madrid / Mexico City
Milan / New Delhi / San Juan / Seoul / Singapore / Sydney / Toronto

The McGraw-Hill Companies

Therapeutic Modalities in Rehabilitation, Third Edition

Previous editions published as *Therapeutic Modalities for Physical Therapists*, copyright © 2002 by The McGraw-Hill Companies, Inc.; and as *Therapeutic Modalities for Allied Health Professionals*, copyright © 1998 by The McGraw-Hill Companies, Inc.

2 3 4 5 6 7 8 9 0   KGP/KGP   0 9 8 7 6 5

ISBN 0-07-144123-9

This book was set in Caslon by International Typesetting and Composition.
The editors were Michael Brown and Michelle Watt.
The production supervisor was Richard Ruzycka.
Project management was provided by International Typesetting and Composition.
The cover designer was Janice Bielawa.
The indexer was Susan G. Hunter.
Quebecor World Kingsport was printer and binder.

This book is printed on acid-free paper.

Library of Congress Cataloging-in-Publication Data

Therapeutic modalities in rehabilitation / [edited by] William E. Prentice.—3rd ed.
    p. ; cm.
    Rev. ed. of: Therapeutic modalities for physical therapists / William E. Prentice. 2nd ed. ©2002.
    Includes bibliographical references and index.
    ISBN 0-07-144123-9 (alk. paper)
    1. Physical therapy. 2. Therapeutics, Physiological. I. Prentice, William E. II. Prentice, William E. Therapeutic modalities for physical therapists.
    [DNLM: 1. Physical Therapy Techniques. 2. Rehabilitation—methods. WB 460 T3984 2005]
RM700.P78   2005
615.8′2—dc22
                          2004061005

CONTENTS

CONTRIBUTORS   xvii

PREFACE   xix

PART ONE
FOUNDATIONS OF THERAPEUTIC MODALITIES

≋1. THE SCIENCE OF THERAPEUTIC MODALITIES   3
    WILLIAM E. PRENTICE

RADIANT ENERGY   3

ELECTROMAGNETIC RADIATIONS   4

WAVELENGTH AND FREQUENCY   6

LAWS GOVERNING THE EFFECTS OF ELECTROMAGNETIC RADIATIONS   6
    ARNDT-SCHULTZ PRINCIPLE   6
    LAW OF GROTTHUS-DRAPER   7
    COSINE LAW   7
    INVERSE SQUARE LAW   8

THE APPLICATION OF THE ELECTROMAGNETIC SPECTRUM TO
    THERAPEUTIC MODALITIES   8
    ELECTRICAL STIMULATING CURRENTS   9
    ELECTROMYOGRAPHIC BIOFEEDBACK   9
    SHORTWAVE AND MICROWAVE DIATHERMY   9
    INFRARED MODALITIES   9
    LASER   10
    ULTRAVIOLET LIGHT   10

THE ACOUSTIC SPECTRUM AND ULTRASOUND   11
    EXTRACORPOREAL SHOCK WAVE THERAPY (ESWT)   11

        Summary   12

≋2. THE HEALING PROCESS AND GUIDELINES FOR USING
    THERAPEUTIC MODALITIES   14
    WILLIAM E. PRENTICE

UNDERSTANDING THE HEALING PROCESS   15
    INFLAMMATORY-RESPONSE PHASE   15
    FIBROBLASTIC-REPAIR PHASE   17
    MATURATION-REMODELING PHASE   18
    FACTORS THAT IMPEDE HEALING   20

INJURY MANAGEMENT USING MODALITIES   21
    INITIAL ACUTE INJURY PHASE   21
    INFLAMMATORY-RESPONSE PHASE   23

FIBROBLASTIC-REPAIR PHASE 23
MATURATION-REMODELING PHASE 24

OTHER CONSIDERATIONS IN TREATING INJURY 24

INDICATIONS AND CONTRAINDICATIONS 25

Summary 26

≋3. THE ROLE OF THERAPEUTIC MODALITIES IN WOUND HEALING 28
PAMELA E. HOUGHTON

SUPERFICIAL HOT AND COLD 28

HYDROTHERAPY 29

ELECTRICAL STIMULATION 30

ULTRASOUND 37

LASER 40

ULTRAVIOLET LIGHT 42

PNEUMATIC COMPRESSION THERAPY 45

CHOOSING THE BEST MODALITY FOR THE TREATMENT OF DELAYED
OR NONHEALING WOUNDS 45
INDICATIONS, CONTRAINDICATIONS 45

REVIEW OF CLINICAL RESEARCH EVIDENCE 48

ALGORITHM FOR CHOOSING THE APPROPRIATE
THERAPEUTIC MODALITY 51

Summary 53

≋4. MANAGING PAIN WITH THERAPEUTIC MODALITIES 60
CRAIG R. DENEGAR and PHILLIP B. DONLEY

UNDERSTANDING PAIN 60

TYPES OF PAIN 61

PAIN ASSESSMENT 61
PAIN ASSESSMENT SCALES 62

TISSUE SENSITIVITY 65

GOALS IN MANAGING PAIN 65

PAIN PERCEPTION AND NEURAL TRANSMISSION 65
SENSORY RECEPTORS 65

NEURAL TRANSMISSION 66
FACILITATORS AND INHIBITORS OF SYNAPTIC TRANSMISSION 67
NOCICEPTION 69

NEUROPHYSIOLOGIC EXPLANATIONS OF PAIN CONTROL 70
BLOCKING PAIN IMPULSES WITH ASCENDING A-BETA INPUT 71
DESCENDING PAIN CONTROL MECHANISMS 72
BETA-ENDORPHIN AND DYNORPHIN 73

Summary of Pain Control Mechanisms 74

Cognitive Influences 74

Pain Management 75

Summary 77

Part Two
Electrical Modalities

5. Basic Principles of Electricity 83

William E. Prentice

Components of Electrical Currents 84

Electrotherapeutic Currents 85

Generators of Electrotherapeutic Currents 86

Waveforms 87

Waveform Shape 87

Pulses versus Phases and Direction of Current Flow 87

Pulse Amplitude 89

Pulse Charge 90

Pulse Rate of Rise and Decay Times 90

Pulse Duration 91

Pulse Frequency 91

Current Modulation 92

Electrical Circuits 94

Series and Parallel Circuits 94

Current Flow Through Biologic Tissues 96

Physiologic Responses to Electrical Current 96

Safety in the Use of Electrical Equipment 97

Summary 99

6. Electrical Stimulating Currents 104

Daniel N. Hooker

Physiologic Response to Electrical Currents 105

Muscle and Nerve Responses to Electrical Currents 106

The Effects of Electrical Stimulation on Nonexcitable Tissues and Cells 111

Electrical Concepts: Effects of Changes in Current
Parameters and Their Effect on Treatment Protocols 121

Biphasic versus Monophasic Current 121

Tissue Impedance 122

Current Density 122

Frequency 123

Intensity 124

Duration 124

Polarity 125

Electrode Placement 126

THERAPEUTIC USES OF ELECTRICALLY INDUCED
MUSCLE CONTRACTION 127
   MUSCLE REEDUCATION 128
   MUSCLE PUMP CONTRACTIONS 129
   RETARDATION OF ATROPHY 129
   MUSCLE STRENGTHENING 131
   INCREASING RANGE OF MOTION 131
   THE EFFECT OF NONCONTRACTILE STIMULATION ON EDEMA 132

STIMULATION OF DENERVATED MUSCLE 134
   TREATMENT PARAMETERS FOR STIMULATING DENERVATED MUSCLE 135

THERAPEUTIC USES OF ELECTRICAL STIMULATION OF
SENSORY NERVES 135
   GATE CONTROL THEORY 135
   DESCENDING PAIN CONTROL THEORY (CENTRAL BIASING THEORY) 136
   OPIATE PAIN CONTROL THEORY 136
   PLACEBO EFFECT OF ELECTRICAL STIMULATION 138

CLINICAL USES OF LOW-VOLTAGE CONTINUOUS
MONOPHASIC CURRENT 138
   MEDICAL GALVANISM 138
   IONTOPHORESIS 139
   TREATMENT PRECAUTIONS WITH CONTINUOUS MONOPHASIC CURRENTS 139

FUNCTIONAL ELECTRICAL STIMULATION (FES) 139
   CLINICAL USES OF FES 140

SPECIALIZED ELECTRICAL CURRENTS 140
   LOW-INTENSITY STIMULATORS (LIS) 140
   RUSSIAN CURRENTS (MEDIUM-FREQUENCY CURRENT GENERATORS) 143
   INTERFERENTIAL CURRENTS 145

CONCLUSION 147
   Summary 147

7.   IONTOPHORESIS 165
       WILLIAM E. PRENTICE

IONTOPHORESIS VERSUS PHONOPHORESIS 165

BASIC MECHANISMS OF ION TRANSFER 166
   PHARMACOKINETICS OF IONTOPHORESIS 166
   MOVEMENT OF IONS IN SOLUTION 166
   MOVEMENT OF IONS THROUGH TISSUE 166

IONTOPHORESIS EQUIPMENT AND TREATMENT TECHNIQUES 168
   TYPE OF CURRENT REQUIRED 168
   IONTOPHORESIS GENERATORS 169
   CURRENT INTENSITY 169
   TREATMENT DURATION 170
   DOSAGE OF MEDICATION 170
   ELECTRODES 170
   SELECTING THE APPROPRIATE ION 171

CLINICAL APPLICATIONS FOR IONTOPHORESIS 172

TREATMENT PRECAUTIONS AND CONTRAINDICATIONS 174

TREATMENT OF BURNS 175

SENSITIVITY REACTIONS TO IONS 175

Summary 175

8. BIOFEEDBACK 182
WILLIAM E. PRENTICE

ELECTROMYOGRAPHY AND BIOFEEDBACK 182

THE ROLE OF BIOFEEDBACK 183

BIOFEEDBACK INSTRUMENTATION 183

PERIPHERAL SKIN TEMPERATURE 183

FINGER PHOTOTRANSMISSION 184

SKIN CONDUCTANCE ACTIVITY 185

ELECTROMYOGRAPHIC BIOFEEDBACK 185

MOTOR UNIT RECRUITMENT 185

MEASURING ELECTRICAL ACTIVITY 186

CONVERTING ELECTROMYOGRAPHIC ACTIVITY TO
MEANINGFUL INFORMATION 188

BIOFEEDBACK EQUIPMENT AND TREATMENT TECHNIQUES 189

ELECTRODES 189

DISPLAYING THE INFORMATION 191

CLINICAL APPLICATIONS FOR BIOFEEDBACK 192

MUSCLE REEDUCATION 192

RELAXATION OF MUSCLE GUARDING 193

PAIN REDUCTION 193

Summary 194

9. PRINCIPLES OF ELECTROPHYSIOLOGIC EVALUATION
AND TESTING 201
JOHN HALLE and DAVID GREATHOUSE

INTRODUCTION 202

ELECTROPHYSIOLOGIC TESTING EQUIPMENT AND SETUP 203

EVALUATION OF THE PERIPHERAL NERVOUS SYSTEM 211

ANATOMY OF THE SPINAL NERVE AND NEUROMUSCULAR JUNCTION 213

THE ELEMENTS OF THE SPINAL NERVE 215

TESTING PROCEDURES 215

LIMB TEMPERATURE AND AGE CONSIDERATIONS 216

NERVE CONDUCTION STUDY 216

THE ELECTROMYOGRAPHIC EXAMINATION 231

SOMATOSENSORY EVOKED POTENTIALS 242

OTHER ELECTROPHYSIOLOGIC TESTING PROCEDURES 243

REQUESTING NCS/EMG EXAMINATIONS 244

CONCLUSION 244

Summary 245

PART THREE
THERMAL MODALITIES

≋10. SHORTWAVE AND MICROWAVE DIATHERMY 259
WILLIAM E. PRENTICE and DAVID O. DRAPER

PHYSIOLOGIC RESPONSES TO DIATHERMY 260
THERMAL EFFECTS 260
NONTHERMAL EFFECTS 261

SHORTWAVE DIATHERMY EQUIPMENT AND TREATMENT TECHNIQUES 261
SHORTWAVE DIATHERMY GENERATORS 261
SHORTWAVE DIATHERMY ELECTRODES 263
PULSED SHORTWAVE DIATHERMY 269
TREATMENT TIME 271

MICROWAVE DIATHERMY 272
MICROWAVE DIATHERMY GENERATORS 273
MICROWAVE DIATHERMY APPLICATORS 273
MICROWAVE TREATMENT TECHNIQUE 274

CLINICAL APPLICATIONS FOR DIATHERMY 275

DIATHERMY TREATMENT PRECAUTIONS AND CONSIDERATIONS 276

COMPARING SHORTWAVE DIATHERMY AND ULTRASOUND AS THERMAL MODALITIES 278

GUIDELINES FOR THE SAFE USE OF DIATHERMY 280

Summary 280

≋11. INFRARED MODALITIES 290
GERALD W. BELL and WILLIAM E. PRENTICE

MECHANISMS OF HEAT TRANSFER 290

APPROPRIATE USE OF THE INFRARED MODALITIES 291

CLINICAL USE OF THE INFRARED MODALITIES 292
EFFECTS OF TISSUE TEMPERATURE CHANGE ON CIRCULATION 292
EFFECTS OF TISSUE TEMPERATURE CHANGE ON MUSCLE SPASM 293
EFFECTS OF TEMPERATURE CHANGE ON PERFORMANCE 294

CRYOTHERAPY 295
PHYSIOLOGIC EFFECTS OF TISSUE COOLING 295
CRYOTHERAPY TREATMENT TECHNIQUES 297

THERMOTHERAPY 313
PHYSIOLOGIC EFFECTS OF TISSUE HEATING 313
THERMOTHERAPY TREATMENT TECHNIQUES 314

COUNTERIRRITANTS 325

CONCLUSIONS 325

Summary 326

≋12. THERAPEUTIC ULTRASOUND 360

DAVID O. DRAPER and WILLIAM E. PRENTICE

ULTRASOUND AS A THERMAL MODALITY 361

TRANSMISSION OF ACOUSTIC ENERGY IN BIOLOGIC TISSUES 361

TRANSVERSE VERSUS LONGITUDINAL WAVES 361
FREQUENCY OF WAVE TRANSMISSION 361
VELOCITY 362
ATTENUATION 362

BASIC PHYSICS OF THERAPEUTIC ULTRASOUND 363

TRANSDUCER 365
FREQUENCY OF THERAPEUTIC ULTRASOUND 367
THE ULTRASOUND BEAM 369
PULSED VERSUS CONTINUOUS WAVE ULTRASOUND 371
AMPLITUDE, POWER, AND INTENSITY 372

PHYSIOLOGIC EFFECTS OF ULTRASOUND 374

THERMAL EFFECTS 374
NONTHERMAL EFFECTS 375

ULTRASOUND TREATMENT TECHNIQUES 376

FREQUENCY OF TREATMENT 377
DURATION OF TREATMENT 377
COUPLING METHODS 378
EXPOSURE TECHNIQUES 379
MOVING THE TRANSDUCER 381
RECORDING ULTRASOUND TREATMENTS 383

CLINICAL APPLICATIONS FOR THERAPEUTIC ULTRASOUND 383

SOFT-TISSUE HEALING AND REPAIR 383
SCAR TISSUE AND JOINT CONTRACTURE 385
STRETCHING OF CONNECTIVE TISSUE 385
CHRONIC INFLAMMATION 387
BONE HEALING 387
PAIN REDUCTION 388
PLANTAR WARTS 388
PLACEBO EFFECTS 388

PHONOPHORESIS 389

USING ULTRASOUND IN COMBINATION WITH OTHER MODALITIES 391

ULTRASOUND AND HOT PACKS 391
ULTRASOUND AND COLD PACKS 391
ULTRASOUND AND ELECTRICAL STIMULATION 392

TREATMENT PRECAUTIONS 393

GUIDELINES FOR THE SAFE USE OF ULTRASOUND EQUIPMENT 393

Summary 394

PART FOUR
LIGHT THERAPY

13. LOW-LEVEL LASER THERAPY   409
ETHAN SALIBA and SUSAN FOREMAN-SALIBA

PHYSICS   410
STIMULATED EMISSIONS   410

TYPES OF LASERS   412

LASER GENERATORS   413
HELIUM NEON LASERS   413
GALLIUM ARSENIDE LASERS   414

LASER TREATMENT TECHNIQUES   415
LASING TECHNIQUES   416
DOSAGE   417
DEPTH OF PENETRATION   419

CLINICAL APPLICATIONS FOR LASERS   419
WOUND HEALING   420
PAIN   422
BONE RESPONSE   423

SUGGESTED TREATMENT PROTOCOLS   423
PAIN   424
WOUND HEALING   424
SCAR TISSUE   425
EDEMA AND INFLAMMATION   425

SAFETY   425
PRECAUTIONS AND CONTRAINDICATIONS   426

CONCLUSION   426
Summary   426

14. ULTRAVIOLET THERAPY   433
J. MARC DAVIS

ULTRAVIOLET RADIATION   433

EFFECT ON CELLS   434

EFFECT ON NORMAL HUMAN TISSUE   434
SHORT-TERM EFFECT ON SKIN   434
TANNING   436
LONG-TERM EFFECT ON SKIN   437

EFFECT ON EYES   437

SYSTEMIC EFFECTS   438

ULTRAVIOLET GENERATORS   438

ULTRAVIOLET TREATMENT TECHNIQUES   440
   DETERMINING THE MINIMAL ERYTHEMAL DOSE   440
   POSITIONING THE LAMP   441

CLINICAL APPLICATIONS FOR ULTRAVIOLET   442
   PSORIASIS   442
   DISTURBANCES OF CALCIUM AND PHOSPHORUS ABSORPTION   443
   PRESSURE SORES   444
   STERILIZATION   444
   DIAGNOSIS   444

CONCLUSION   444
   Summary   444

PART FIVE
MECHANICAL MODALITIES

15. SPINAL TRACTION   453
   DANIEL N. HOOKER

THE PHYSICAL EFFECTS OF TRACTION   453
   EFFECTS ON SPINAL MOVEMENT   453
   EFFECTS ON BONE   454
   EFFECTS ON LIGAMENTS   454
   EFFECTS ON THE DISK   455
   EFFECTS ON ARTICULAR FACET JOINTS   456
   EFFECTS ON THE MUSCULAR SYSTEM   456
   EFFECTS ON THE NERVES   456
   EFFECTS ON THE ENTIRE BODY PART   457

TRACTION TREATMENT TECHNIQUES   458

LUMBAR POSITIONAL TRACTION   458

INVERSION TRACTION   461

MANUAL LUMBAR TRACTION   462
   LEVEL-SPECIFIC MANUAL TRACTION   462
   UNILATERAL LEG PULL MANUAL TRACTION   463

MECHANICAL LUMBAR TRACTION   465
   PATIENT SETUP AND EQUIPMENT   465
   BODY POSITION   468
   TRACTION FORCE   471
   INTERMITTENT VERSUS SUSTAINED TRACTION   472
   DURATION OF TREATMENT   473
   PROGRESSIVE AND REGRESSIVE STEPS   473

MANUAL CERVICAL TRACTION   475

MECHANICAL CERVICAL TRACTION   476

INDICATIONS AND CONTRAINDICATIONS 478
   Summary 479

16. INTERMITTENT COMPRESSION DEVICES 484
   DANIEL N. HOOKER

THE LYMPHATIC SYSTEM 485
   PURPOSES OF THE LYMPHATIC SYSTEM 485
   STRUCTURE OF THE LYMPHATIC SYSTEM 485
   PERIPHERAL LYMPHATIC STRUCTURE AND FUNCTION 485

INJURY EDEMA 486
   FORMATION OF PITTING EDEMA 487
   FORMATION OF LYMPHEDEMA 487
   THE NEGATIVE EFFECTS OF EDEMA ACCUMULATION 489

TREATMENT OF EDEMA 489

INTERMITTENT COMPRESSION TREATMENT TECHNIQUES 490
   INFLATION PRESSURES 491
   ON-OFF SEQUENCE 491
   TOTAL TREATMENT TIME 491
   PATIENT SETUP AND INSTRUCTIONS 492

COLD AND COMPRESSION COMBINATION 494

SEQUENTIAL COMPRESSION PUMPS 494

INDICATIONS AND CONTRAINDICATIONS FOR USE 496
   Summary 496

PART SIX
OTHER MODALITIES

17. THERAPEUTIC MASSAGE 503
   WILLIAM E. PRENTICE and CLAIRBETH LEHN

THE VALUE OF MANUAL THERAPY TECHNIQUES 503

THE EVOLUTION OF MASSAGE AS A TREATMENT MODALITY 503

PHYSIOLOGIC EFFECTS OF MASSAGE 504
   REFLEXIVE EFFECTS 504
   MECHANICAL EFFECTS 505

PSYCHOLOGIC EFFECTS OF MASSAGE 507

MASSAGE TREATMENT CONSIDERATIONS AND GUIDELINES 507
   EQUIPMENT 509
   PREPARATION OF THE PATIENT 510

MASSAGE TREATMENT TECHNIQUES 512
   HOFFA MASSAGE 512
   FRICTION MASSAGE 518
   CONNECTIVE TISSUE MASSAGE 518
   ACUPRESSURE AND TRIGGER POINT MASSAGE 520

MYOFASCIAL RELEASE 524

STRAIN/COUNTERSTRAIN 525

POSITIONAL RELEASE THERAPY 526

ACTIVE RELEASE TECHNIQUE 526

ROLFING 528

TRAGER 528

THE CURRENT ROLE OF MASSAGE IN PHYSICAL THERAPY 529

Summary 529

18. EXTRACORPOREAL SHOCK WAVE THERAPY 537
CHARLES THIGPEN

HISTORY OF ESWT 537

PHYSICAL CHARACTERISTICS OF EXTRACORPOREAL SHOCK WAVE 538

SHOCK WAVE GENERATION 540

PHYSICAL PARAMETERS OF SHOCK WAVES 540

BIOLOGIC EFFECTS 541

BONE 542

TENDON 542

CLINICAL APPLICATIONS 543

PLANTAR FASCIITIS 543

MEDIAL/LATERAL EPICONDYLITIS 544

CALCIFIC TENDINITIS OF THE SHOULDER 544

EVALUATION OF ESWT LITERATURE FOR
EVIDENCE-BASED PRACTICE 545

Summary 545

PART SEVEN
SUMMARY

19. THE PHYSIOLOGIC EFFECTS OF THERAPEUTIC MODALITY
INTERVENTION ON THE BODY SYSTEMS 551
ERIC SHAMUS and STANLEY H. WILSON

SYSTEMS APPROACH 552

ELECTRICAL STIMULATING CURRENTS 552

INTERFERENTIAL CURRENT (IFC) 552

NEUROMUSCULAR ELECTRICAL STIMULATION (NMES) 553

TRANSCUTANEOUS ELECTRICAL NERVE STIMULATION (TENS) 554

IONTOPHORESIS 555

BIOFEEDBACK 556

CRYOTHERAPY TECHNIQUES 557

THERMOTHERAPY TECHNIQUES 558

WARM WHIRLPOOL HOT PACKS 558

PARAFFIN 560

INFRARED LAMPS   560

FLUIDOTHERAPY   561

THERAPEUTIC ULTRASOUND (US)   561

ULTRAVIOLET THERAPY (UV)   562

TRACTION (MANUAL AND MECHANICAL)   563

COMPRESSION DEVICES   564

MASSAGE   565

APPENDIX A-1. LOCATIONS OF THE MOTOR POINTS   570

APPENDIX A-2. UNITS OF MEASURE   573

INDEX   575

CONTRIBUTORS

Gerald W. Bell, EdD, PT, ATC
Professor
Department of Kinesiology
University of Illinois at Urbana-Champaign
Urbana, Illinois

J. Marc Davis, PT, ATC
Physical Therapist/Athletic Trainer
Division of Sports Medicine
Student Health Service
University of North Carolina
Chapel Hill, North Carolina

Craig R. Denegar, PhD, PT, ATC
Professor of Athletic Training
Department of Kinesiology
Pennsylvania State University
State College, Pennsylvania

Phillip B. Donley, MS, PT, ATC
Director, Chester County Orthopaedic and Sports
Physical Therapy
West Chester, Pennsylvania

David O. Draper, EdD, ATC
Professor
Department of Physical Education
Brigham Young University
Provo, Utah

David Greathouse, PhD, PT, ECS
Professor and Chair
School of Physical Therapy
Belmont University
Adjunct Professor
School of Physical Therapy
Vanderbilt University
Nashville, Tennessee

John Halle, PhD, PT, ECS
Professor
School of Physical Therapy
Belmont University
Adjunct Professor
School of Physical Therapy
Vanderbilt University
Nashville, Tennessee

Daniel N. Hooker, PhD, PT, SCS, ATC
Coordinator of Athletic Training and Physical Therapy
Division of Sports Medicine
Student Health Service
University of North Carolina
Chapel Hill, North Carolina

Pamela E. Houghton, BSc PT, PhD
Chair, MSc Program
Associate Professor
School of Physical Therapy
University of Western Ontario
London, Ontario

Clairbeth Lehn, PT, ATC
Physical Therapist/Athletic Trainer
Division of Sports Medicine
Student Health Service
University of North Carolina
Chapel Hill, North Carolina

William E. Prentice, PhD, PT, ATC
Professor, Coordinator of Sports Medicine Program
Department of Exercise and Sport Science
University of North Carolina
Chapel Hill, North Carolina

William S. Quillen, PhD, PT, SCS
Professor and Director
School of Physical Therapy
University of South Florida
College of Medicine
Tampa, Florida

Ethan N. Saliba, PhD, PT, ATC
Head Athletic Trainer
Department of Athletics
Assistant Professor
Department of Kinesiology
University of Virginia
Charlottesville, Virginia

Susan Foreman-Saliba, PhD, PT, ATC
Head Associate Athletic Trainer
McCue Sports Medicine Center
Sports Medicine Instructor
Department of Kinesiology
University of Virginia
Charlottesville, Virginia

Eric Shamus, PhD, PT, CSCS
Assistant Professor
Department of Physical Therapy
College of Osteopathic Medicine
Nova Southeastern University
Ft. Lauderdale, Florida

Charles Thigpen, MS, PT, ATC-L
Interdisciplinary Program in Human
　Movement Science
Sports Medicine Research Lab
University of North Carolina
Chapel Hill, North Carolina

Frank Underwood, PhD, MPT, ECS
Associate Professor, Department of Physical Therapy
University of Evansville
Clinical Electrophysiologist
Rehabilitation Service
Orthopaedic Associates, Inc.
Evansville, Indiana

Stanley Wilson, EdD, PT
Chair, Associate Professor
Department of Physical Therapy
Nova Southeastern University
Ft. Lauderdale, Florida

PREFACE

Physical therapists, occupational therapists, physical therapy assistants, and physical therapy aides use a wide variety of therapeutic techniques in the treatment and rehabilitation of their patients. A thorough treatment regimen often involves the use of therapeutic modalities. At one time or another, virtually all therapists make use of some type of modality. This may involve a relatively simple technique such as using an ice pack for an acute injury or more complex techniques such as the stimulation of nerve and muscle tissue by electrical currents. There is no question that therapeutic modalities are useful tools in injury rehabilitation. When used appropriately, these modalities can greatly enhance the patient's chances for complete recovery. Unfortunately, the therapists' rationale for using a particular modality is too often based on habit rather than on logic or analysis of effectiveness. For the therapist, it is essential to possess knowledge regarding the scientific basis and the physiologic effects of the various modalities on a specific injury. When this theoretical basis is applied to practical experience, it has the potential to become an extremely effective clinical method.

It must be emphasized that the use of therapeutic modalities in any treatment program is an inexact science. If you were to ask 10 different therapists what combination of modalities and therapeutic exercise they use in a given treatment program, you would likely get 10 different responses. There is no way to "cookbook" a treatment plan that involves the use of modalities. Thus, what this book will attempt to do is to present the basis for use of each different type of modality and allow the therapist to make his or her own decision as to which will be most effective in a given situation. Some recommended protocols developed through the experiences of the contributing authors will be presented.

The following are a number of reasons why this text should be adopted for use.

Comprehensive Coverage of Therapeutic Modalities Used in a Clinical Setting

The purpose of this text is to provide a theoretically based but practically oriented guide to the use of therapeutic modalities for the student therapist. It is intended for use in courses where various clinically oriented techniques and methods are presented.

The chapters in this text are divided into six parts. Each chapter discusses (1) the physiologic basis for use, (2) clinical applications, (3) specific techniques of application through the use of related laboratory activities, and (4) relevant individual case studies for each therapeutic modality.

Part I—Foundations of Therapeutic Modalities begins with a chapter that discusses the scientific basis for using therapeutic modalities and classifies the modalities in a logical order in relation to the electromagnetic and acoustic spectra. Guidelines for selecting the most appropriate modalities for use in different phases of the healing process are presented. A new chapter that deals specifically with the role of therapeutic modalities in wound healing has been added to this edition. Pain is discussed, in terms of neurophysiologic mechanisms of pain and the role of therapeutic modalities in pain management.

Part II—Electrical Modalities includes detailed discussions of the principles of electricity, electrical stimulating currents, iontophoresis, and biofeedback. Based on reviewer comments and the needs of the majority of physical therapy curriculums, a chapter that deals with the principles of electrophysiologic evaluation and testing has been added in this third edition. Although this is not a therapeutic modality per se, electrophysiologic testing is commonly taught in classes that cover electrical modalities and thus the decision was made to include this topic in this text.

Part III—Thermal Modalities discusses those modalities which produce a change in tissue temperatures including the shortwave and microwave diathermies, infrared modalities, and ultrasound.

Part IV—Light Therapy includes chapters on both low-level laser and ultraviolet therapy.

Part V—Mechanical Modalities includes chapters on traction and intermittent compression.

Part VI—Other Modalities includes a chapter on therapeutic massage. A new chapter has been added in this section which discusses a new modality that is beginning to be used by physical therapists called extracorporal shockwave therapy.

Part VII—Summary, Chapter 19 is intended to clearly and succinctly summarize the effects of the therapeutic modalities discussed throughout this text on the various physiologic systems of the body.

Based on Scientific Theory

This text discusses various concepts, principles, and theories that are supported by scientific research, factual evidence, and previous experience of the authors in dealing with various conditions. The material presented in this text has been carefully researched by the contributing authors to provide up-to-date information on the theoretical basis for employing a particular modality in a specific injury situation. Additionally, the manuscript for this text has been carefully reviewed by therapists, who are considered experts in their field to ensure that the material reflects factual and current concepts for modality use.

Timely and Practical

Certainly, therapeutic modalities used in a clinical setting are important tools for the therapist. This text provides the student with a comprehensive resource which should be used in student instruction on the theoretical basis and practical application of the various modalities. It should serve as a needed guide for the student therapist who is interested in knowing not only how to use a modality but also why that particular modality is most effective in a given situation.

The authors who have contributed to this text have a great deal of clinical experience. Each of these individuals has also at one time or another been involved with the formal classroom education of the student therapist. Thus this text has been directed at the student therapist who will be asked to apply the theoretical basis of modality use to the clinical setting.

Several other texts are available that discuss the use of selected physical modalities in various patient populations. This is the most comprehensive text on therapeutic modalities available in any specific discipline.

Pedagogic Aids

The aids this text uses to facilitate its use by students and instructors include:

Objectives   These goals are listed at the beginning of each chapter to introduce students to the points that will be emphasized.

Figures and Tables   Essential points on each chapter are illustrated with clear visual materials.

Summary   Each chapter has a summary that outlines the major points covered.

Review Questions   Designed to help the student review the material presented in each chapter by answering a series of thought-provoking questions.

Glossary of Key Terms   Each chapter contains a glossary of terms for quick reference.

References   A list of up-to-date references is provided at the end of each chapter for the student who wishes to read further on the subject being discussed.

Case Studies   A series of clinically based case studies are presented to enhance student understanding of how these modalities may be applied to a specific patient.

Lab Activities   Lab activities are included to guide the student through the setup and application of the various modalities.

Appendices A chart of trigger points and a comprehensive list of manufacturers of therapeutic modality equipment is provided.

How to Use the Laboratory Activities

There are a wide variety of laboratory activities found throughout this book.

Theory, biophysical principles, and range of potential clinical medicine applications for the various physical agent modalities will be found in this text. The activities are intended to provide the student or interested reader with a systematic and sequential method of completing a therapeutic modality application. The initial performance of a therapeutic procedure should proceed in a logical stepwise fashion. They are structured to allow both the instructor or supervisor and the student the ability to assess competency in a partial or complete fashion culminating in the independent ability to safely and effectively provide a therapeutic modality treatment.

Each therapeutic modality application has a separate sequential check list. Similarities will be noted in certain aspects of treatment application and completion. Space is provided for up to three separate instructors/supervisors to "sign off" (initial and date) the successful completion and demonstration of each element of the complete application. A Master Competency Check List is provided to document the successful completion of the individual therapeutic modality checklist and when the student is deemed competent to independently provide that treatment. This system documents the acquisition of skills necessary for effective physical agent modality application and ensures accountability by the student and instructor/supervisor to patients and other concerned parties.

Competency in the skillful application of therapeutic modalities is gained through diligent and frequent practice. Use of these activities in the manner described will guide the user in productive practice and successful acquisition of essential skills. Students are encouraged to practice each of the procedures on themselves first; thereby gaining an appreciation of the sensations associated with that particular modality. Further practice with a variety of lab partners will result in the development of the desired competence and confidence with any manufacturer's equipment.

ACKNOWLEDGMENTS

I would like to thank Michael Brown for his assistance in this project from the very beginning. His advice and direction have certainly helped in its completion.

I would also like to thank my wife, Tena, and our two boys, Brian and Zachary, for putting up with me when I get going with a project like this. Sometimes it's not easy.

MASTER COMPETENCY CHECK LIST

THERAPEUTIC MODALITY	EXAMINER		
	1	2	3
Positioning			
Electrical stimulation			
Analgesia			
Muscle reeducation			
Muscle strengthening			
Iontophoresis			
Biofeedback			
Shortwave diathermy			
Infrared physical agents			
Thermotherapy			
Hydrocollator pack			
Paraffin bath			
Infrared lamp			
Cryotherapy			
Ice massage			
Ice pack			
Gel cold pack			
Vapocoolant spray			
Cryo/Cuff			
Hydrotherapy			
Warm whirlpool			
Cold whirlpool			
Contrast bath			
Fluidotherapy			
Ultraviolet			
Low-power laser			
Ultraviolet			
Direct contact			
Bladder coupling			
Underwater coupling			
Phonophoresis			
Mechanical traction			
Cervical			
Lumbar			
Intermittent compression			
Massage			

THERAPEUTIC MODALITIES

in

Rehabilitation

PART ONE

FOUNDATIONS OF THERAPEUTIC MODALITIES

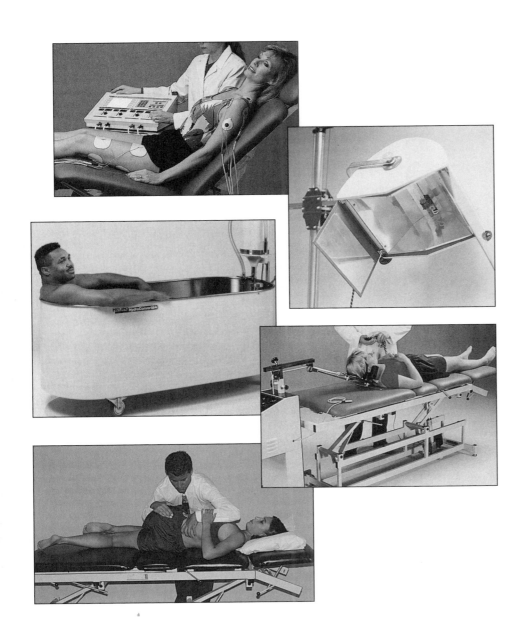

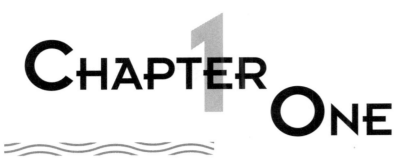

CHAPTER ONE

THE SCIENCE OF THERAPEUTIC MODALITIES

WILLIAM E. PRENTICE

OBJECTIVES

Following completion of this chapter, the student therapist will be able to:

✓ Define what radiant energy is, explain its physical properties, and indicate how it is produced.

✓ Analyze the relationship between wavelength and frequency.

✓ Apply the laws governing the effects of electromagnetic radiations to the various therapeutic modalities.

✓ Argue how the therapist might best make use of electromagnetic radiations to produce a specific physiologic response in the various biologic tissues of the body.

✓ Compare the physiologic effects produced by each therapeutic modality.

✓ Differentiate between the electromagnetic and acoustic spectra.

There is considerable confusion among even the most experienced therapists regarding the relationship of the various therapeutic modalities to the **electromagnetic** and **acoustic spectra**. Electrical stimulating currents, shortwave and microwave diathermy, the infrared modalities, ultraviolet therapy, and low-power lasers are all therapeutic agents that emit a type of energy with wavelengths and frequencies that can be classified as electromagnetic radiations.[6] **Ultrasound** and extracorporeal shock wave therapy are forms of radiation whose wavelengths and frequencies of vibration are best classified in the acoustic rather than the electromagnetic spectrum. Each of the modalities that make use of these varying types of energy will be discussed in the following chapters.

acoustic spectrum The range of frequencies and wavelengths of sound waves.

electromagnetic spectrum The range of frequencies and wavelengths associated with radiant energy.

RADIANT ENERGY

Radiation is a process by which energy in various forms travels through space.[1,15] Most of us are familiar with the effects of radiation from the sun. Sunlight is a type of radiant energy, and we know that it not only makes objects visible but also produces heat. The sun emits radiant energy as a result of high-intensity chemical reactions. This radiant energy in the form of sunlight travels through space at about 300 million meters per second and eventually reaches earth, where its effects may be felt or seen. However, the sun is not the only object capable of producing this radiant energy.

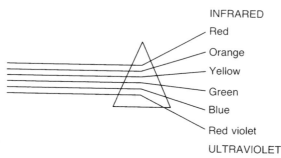

•**Figure 1-1** When a beam of light is shone through a prism, the various electromagnetic radiations in visible light are refracted and appear as a distinct band of color called a spectrum.

infrared The portion of the electromagnetic spectrum associated with thermal changes located adjacent to the red portion of the visible light spectrum.

ultraviolet The portion of the electromagnetic spectrum associated with chemical changes located adjacent to the violet portion of the visible light spectrum.

All matter produces energy that radiates in the form of heat. The sun produces radiation through chemical reactions. However, when a sufficiently intense chemical or electrical force is applied to any object, radiant energy in various forms can be produced by movement of electrons. Many of the therapeutic modalities to be discussed in this text produce radiant energy (i.e., the infrared modalities, the diathermies, ultraviolet, lasers, and the electrical stimulating modalities).[4,12]

If a ray of sunlight is passed through a prism, it will be broken down into various regions of colors (Fig. 1-1). Each of these colors represents a different form of radiant energy. They appear because the various forms of radiant energy are **refracted** or change direction as a result of differences in wavelength and frequency of each color, thus resulting in distinct bands of color called a spectrum. These color variations that we can detect with our eyes are referred to as visible light or luminous radiations. It becomes apparent when looking at this colorful display that there is a region of red at one end of the spectrum and a region of violet at the other end. When passed through a prism, the type of radiant energy refracted the least appears as the color red, whereas that refracted the most is violet.[12]

This beam of sunlight passing through the prism is also propagating forms of radiant energy that are not visible to our eyes.[13] If a thermometer is placed close to the red end of the spectrum, heat will be detected. Likewise, a photographic plate placed close to the violet end of the spectrum will indicate chemical changes. The form of radiant energy that produces heat and is located in the spectrum beyond the visible red portion is referred to as the **infrared** radiation region. The form of radiant energy that produces chemical changes and is located beyond the violet end of the visible spectrum is called the **ultraviolet** radiation region (Fig. 1-2). Ultraviolet, infrared, and visible light rays are produced by heat. As the temperature increases in a particular substance, the vibration of molecules tends to increase the activity of the electrons. The movement of electrons produces electromagnetic waves. The higher the temperature, the greater the frequency of electromagnetic waves produced. These electromagnetic waves produced by heat are usually absorbed by many objects and have little penetration.[7,11]

It is known that other forms of radiation beyond the infrared and ultraviolet portions of the spectrum may be produced when an electrical force is applied.[12] Beyond the infrared portion of the spectrum lie several large regions of radiations known as the **diathermies**; these include radio, television, and nerve and muscle stimulating currents. Beyond the ultraviolet end of the spectrum lies the high-frequency ionizing and penetration radiation region (i.e., x-rays, alpha, beta, and gamma rays).[13]

diathermy The application of high-frequency electrical energy that is used to generate heat in body tissue as a result of the resistance of the tissue to the passage of energy.

ELECTROMAGNETIC RADIATIONS

All of these various classifications of radiations collectively constitute the electromagnetic spectrum (Fig. 1-2). All the electromagnetic radiations lying within this spectrum have several theoretical characteristics in common[2]:

Region	Clinically Used Wavelength	Clinically Used Frequency*	Estimated Effective Depth of Penetration	Physiologic Effects
Electrical stimulating currents	3×10^8 to 75,000 km	1–4000 Hz	Effects may occur anywhere between electrodes	Pain modulation, muscle contraction, relaxation, ion movement
Commercial radio and television**				
Shortwave diathermy	22 m 11 m	13.56 MHz 27.12 MHz	3 cm	Deep tissue temperature increase, vasodilation, increased blood flow
Microwave diathermy	69 cm 33 cm 12 cm	433.9 MHz 915 MHz 2450 MHz	5 cm	Deep tissue temperature increase, vasodilation, increased blood flow
Infrared				
Cold packs (8°F)	111,000 A	2.70×10^{12} Hz		Superficial temperature decrease
Cold whirlpool (63°F)	99,514 A	3.01×10^{12} Hz		Vasoconstriction— decreased blood flow
Hot whirlpool (99°F)	93,097 A	3.22×10^{12} Hz	1 cm	Vasoconstriction— decreased blood flow
Paraffin bath (117°F)	90,187 A	3.32×10^{12} Hz		Analgesia
Hydrocollar (170°F)	82,457 A	3.63×10^{12} Hz		Superficial temperature increase
Luminous IR (1341°F)	28,860 A	1.04×10^{13} Hz		Vasodilation— increased blood flow
Nonluminous IR (3140°F)	14,430 A	2.08×10^{13} Hz		
Red	**Laser**			
Visible light	GaAs 9100 A	3.30×10^{13} Hz	5 cm	Pain modulation and wound healing
	HeNe 6328 A	4.74×10^{13} Hz	10–15 mm	
Violet				
Ultraviolet				Superficial chemical changes
UV-A	3200–4000 A	9.38×10^{13}–7.50×10^{13} Hz		Tanning effects
UV-B	2900–3200 A	1.03×10^{14}–9.38×10^{13} Hz	2 mm	Bactericidal
UV-C	2000–2900 A	1.50×10^{14}–1.03×10^{14} Hz		
Ionizing radiation (x-rays, gamma rays, cosmic rays)**				

* Calculated using $C = \lambda \times F$, C = velocity (3×10^8 m/sec), λ = wavelength, F = frequency.
** Although these fall under the classification of electromagnetic energy, they have nothing to do with therapeutic modalities and thus current no further discussion in this text.

•**Figure 1-2** Electromagnetic spectrum.

1. They may be produced when sufficiently intense electrical or chemical forces are applied to any material.
2. They all travel readily through space at an equal velocity.
3. Their direction of travel is always in a straight line.
4. They may be reflected, refracted, absorbed, or transmitted, depending on the specific medium that they strike.

The luminous, infrared, and ultraviolet rays in sunlight travel in waves through a vacuum or space at a velocity of about 300 million meters per second and all reach the earth at about the same time. These rays are emitted from chemical reactions taking place on the sun, and each type of radiation possesses its own individual physical characteristics. The basis of differentiation between the different regions of the electromagnetic spectrum is defined by analyzing the wavelengths and frequencies of the radiations within this spectrum.

The electromagnetic radiations produced by the different modalities all share the same physical characteristics as any other type of electromagnetic radiation. However, when these radiations come in contact with various biologic tissues, the velocity and direction of travel will be altered within the various types of tissues.[2]

WAVELENGTH AND FREQUENCY

Wavelength is defined as the distance between the peak of one wave and the peak of either the preceding or succeeding wave. **Frequency** is defined as the number of wave oscillations or vibrations occurring in 1 second and is expressed in hertz (Hz) units.

Each of the various types of radiation in the electromagnetic spectrum has a specific wavelength and frequency of vibrations. Since it is accepted theoretically that all forms of electromagnetic radiation are produced simultaneously, travel at a constant velocity through space, and reach earth at the same time, it follows that longer wavelengths must have shorter frequencies and shorter wavelengths must have higher frequencies.

$$\text{Velocity} = \text{wavelength} \times \text{frequency}$$
$$C = \lambda \times F$$

Thus an inverse or reciprocal relationship exists between wavelength and frequency. Velocity is a constant 3×10^8 m/sec.[14] Therefore, if we know the wavelength, frequency can be calculated.

LAWS GOVERNING THE EFFECTS OF ELECTROMAGNETIC RADIATIONS

When electromagnetic radiations strike or come in contact with various objects, several things may happen.[2] Some rays may be **reflected**, whereas others are **transmitted** through the tissues, where they may be refracted. Still others penetrate to deeper layers where they may be **absorbed** (Fig. 1-3). Generally, those radiations that have the longest wavelengths tend to have the greatest depths of penetration regardless of their frequency. It must be added, however, that a number of other factors, which are discussed later, can also contribute to the depth of penetration.

ARNDT-SCHULTZ PRINCIPLE

The purpose of using therapeutic modalities is to stimulate a specific body tissue to perform its normal function. This stimulation will only occur if energy produced by the electrotherapeutic device is absorbed by the tissue.[2] The **Arndt-Schultz principle** states that no reactions or changes can occur in the body tissues if the amount of energy absorbed is insufficient to stimulate the absorbing tissues. The goal of the therapist

Arndt-Schultz principle No reactions or changes can occur in the body tissues if the amount of energy absorbed is insufficient to stimulate the absorbing tissues.

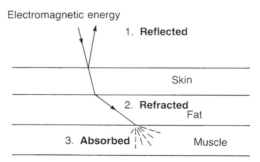

•**Figure 1-3** When electromagnetic radiations contact human tissues, they may be refracted, reflected, or absorbed. Energy that is transmitted through the tissues must be absorbed before any physiologic changes can take place.

should be to deliver sufficient energy in one form or another to stimulate the tissues to perform their normal function, while realizing that too much energy absorbed in a given period of time may seriously impair normal function and, if severe enough, may cause irreparable damage.[5] An example would be using an electrical stimulating current to create a muscle contraction. To achieve the depolarization of a motor nerve, the intensity of the current must be increased until enough energy is made available and is absorbed by that nerve to facilitate a depolarization.

LAW OF GROTTHUS-DRAPER

The inverse relationship that exists between energy absorption by a tissue and energy penetration to deeper layers is described by the **Law of Grotthus-Draper**. When electromagnetic energy strikes the surface of the skin, several things can happen to it. A portion of the energy may be *reflected* (bounce off) from the surface producing no physiologic response. That portion of the electromagnetic energy that is not reflected will penetrate into the tissues (skin layers), and some of it will be absorbed superficially. Again, if the amount of energy absorbed is sufficient to stimulate the target tissue, some physiologic response will occur (e.g., vasodilation of a blood vessel).[2]

> **Law of Grotthus-Draper** If the energy is not absorbed by the superficial tissues it will penetrate to deeper tissues.

The energy that is not absorbed superficially will continue to penetrate through the deeper layers of tissue (fat and muscle). At tissue interfaces (where skin meets fat or where fat meets muscle), the differences in density of the two tissues can cause that penetrating electromagnetic energy to be *refracted*, to alter its direction of transmission. If the target tissue is a motor nerve and your treatment goal is to provide enough energy to cause a depolarization of that motor nerve, then once again, enough energy must be absorbed by that nerve to cause a depolarization. An example showing application of the Law of Grotthus-Draper could be when using an ultrasound treatment to increase tissue temperature in the gluteus maximus muscle. Using ultrasound at a frequency of 1 MHz would be more effective than at 3 MHz, since less would be absorbed superficially at 1 MHz, and thus more energy would penetrate to the deeper muscle tissue.

COSINE LAW

Radiant energy is more easily transmitted to deeper tissues if the source of radiation is at a right angle to the area being radiated. Thus the smaller the angle between the propagating ray and the right angle, the less radiation reflected and the greater the absorption. This principle, known as the **cosine law**, is extremely important in the chapters dealing with the diathermies, ultraviolet light, and infrared heating, since the effectiveness of these modalities is based to a large extent on how they are positioned with regard to the patient (Fig. 1-4). An example showing the application of the cosine law could be when doing an ultrasound treatment, the surface of the applicator should be kept as flat on the skin surface as possible. This allows the acoustic energy coming from

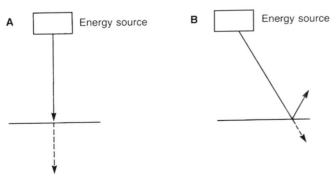

•**Figure 1-4** The cosine law states that the smaller the angle between the propagating ray and the right angle, the less radiation reflected and the greater absorbed. Thus the energy absorbed in **A.** would be greater than in **B.**

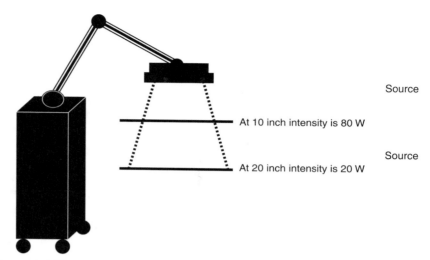

Source

At 10 inch intensity is 80 W

Source

At 20 inch intensity is 20 W

•**Figure 1-5** The inverse square law states that the intensity of the radiation striking a particular surface varies inversely with the square of the distance from the source.

the applicator to strike the surface as close to 90 degrees as possible, thus minimizing the amount of energy reflected.

INVERSE SQUARE LAW

The intensity of the radiation striking a particular surface is known to vary inversely with the square of the distance from the source.[3] For example, when using an infrared heating lamp to heat the low back region, the intensity of heat energy at the skin surface with the lamp positioned at a distance of 10 inches will be four times greater than if the lamp is placed at a 20-inch distance. This principle, known as the **inverse square law**, obviously is of great consequence when setting up a specific modality to achieve a desired physiologic effect (Fig. 1-5). Regardless of the path this transmitted energy takes, the physiologic effects are apparent only when the energy is absorbed by a specific tissue. All physical modalities emitting electromagnetic radiations are subject to the relationship between **absorption** and **transmission** of energy. The modalities that emit radiations with relatively longer wavelengths have the ability to transmit energy through the superficial tissue layers, thus penetrating to the deeper tissues where it is absorbed.

THE APPLICATION OF THE ELECTROMAGNETIC SPECTRUM TO THERAPEUTIC MODALITIES

Electromagnetic Modalities
- Electrical stimulating currents
- Biofeedback
- Iontophoresis
- Shortwave diathermy
- Microwave diathermy
- Infrared modalities
- Ultraviolet therapy
- Low-power laser

The therapeutic modalities discussed in detail in later chapters (with the exception of ultrasound, massage, traction, intermittent compression, and extracorporeal shock wave therapy) all emit radiations with physical characteristics that may be classified as electromagnetic.

Figure 1-2 represents the electromagnetic spectrum and places all of the modalities in order based on wavelengths and corresponding frequencies. It is apparent, for example, that the electrical stimulating currents have the longest wavelength and the lowest frequency and, all other factors being equal, therefore should have the greatest depth of penetration. As we move down the chart, the wavelengths in each region become progressively shorter and the frequencies progressively higher. Shortwave and microwave diathermy, the various sources of infrared heating, and the ultraviolet regions have progressively less depth of penetration.[10]

It should be mentioned that the regions labeled as radio and television frequencies, visible light, and high-frequency ionizing and penetrating radiations certainly fall under the classification of electromagnetic radiations. However, they do not have application as therapeutic modalities and, although extremely important to our everyday way of life, warrant no further consideration in the context of this discussion.

Electrical Stimulating Currents

The electrical stimulating currents that affect nerve and muscle tissue have the longest wavelengths and the lowest frequencies of any of the modalities. The wavelengths of electrical stimulating units are extremely long, ranging somewhere around 15,000 km. Clinically used frequencies range from 1 to 4000 Hz. Most stimulators have the flexibility to alter the frequency output of the device to elicit a desired physiologic response. The nerve and muscle stimulating currents are capable of (1) pain modulation either through stimulation of cutaneous sensory nerves at high frequencies (TENS [transculaneous electrical nerve stimulators]) or through production of β-endorphin at lower frequencies (electroaccutherapy); (2) producing muscle contraction and relaxation or tetany, depending on the type of current (alternating or direct) and frequency (Russian currents); (3) facilitating soft-tissue and bone healing through the use of subsensory microcurrents low intensity stimulator (LIS); and (4) producing a net movement of ions through the use of continuous direct current and thus eliciting a chemical change in the tissues (iontophoresis; see Chapter 7).[14] The electrical stimulating currents and their various physiologic effects are discussed in detail in Chapter 6.

Electromyographic Biofeedback

Electromyographic biofeedback is a therapeutic procedure that uses electronic or electromechanical instruments to accurately measure, process, and feed back reinforcing information via auditory or visual signals. Clinically, it is used to help the patient develop greater voluntary control in terms of either neuromuscular relaxation or muscle reeducation following injury. Biofeedback is discussed in Chapter 8.

Shortwave and Microwave Diathermy

The diathermies are considered to be high-frequency currents because they have more than 1 million cycles per second. When impulses of such a short duration come in contact with human tissue, there is not sufficient time for ion movement to take place. Consequently, there is no stimulation of either motor or sensory nerves. The energy of this rapidly vibrating electrical current produces heat as it passes through tissue cells, resulting in a temperature increase. Shortwave diathermy may be either continuous or pulsed. Both continuous shortwave as well as microwave diathermy are used primarily for their thermal effects, whereas pulsed shortwave is used for its nonthermal effects.

The electrotherapeutic shortwave and microwave devices have preset frequencies and wavelengths that cannot be altered. Shortwave diathermy units are set at either (1) 13.56 MHz (1 MHz = 10 million Hz) with a corresponding wavelength of 22 m; or (2) 27.12 MHz with a wavelength of 11 m.[5]

Microwave units have shorter wavelengths than do shortwave diathermy units and are set at wavelengths of 33 or 12 cm with respective frequencies of 915 or 2450 MHz. The depth of penetration with microwave is a bit deeper than with shortwave because the amount of energy when using microwave is concentrated in one spot rather than spread out over a large area.[5] This is discussed in more detail in Chapter 10.

Infrared Modalities

Perhaps the greatest confusion over the relationship between electromagnetic radiations and therapeutic modalities is associated with the infrared region. We tend to think of the infrared modalities as being the luminous and nonluminous infrared bakers or lamps only, when in fact the largest number of modalities used by therapists actually emit radiations with wavelengths and frequencies that clearly fall within this infrared region. Cold packs, hydrocollator packs, whirlpools, paraffin baths, and contrast baths are all infrared modalities.[7]

Earlier it was stated that any object heated (or cooled) to a temperature different than the surrounding environment will dissipate heat through radiation to the other

Treatment Tip
When treating low back pain, the therapist may choose to use infrared heating modalities, shortwave or microwave diathermy, or ultrasound, all of which have the ability to produce heat in the tissues. Ultrasound has a greater depth of penetration than any of the electromagnetic modalities since acoustic energy is more effectively transmitted through dense tissue than is electromagnetic energy.

materials with which it comes in contact. The infrared modalities are used to produce a local and occasionally a generalized heating or cooling of the superficial tissues. It is generally accepted that the infrared modalities have a maximum depth of penetration of 1 cm or less. The infrared modalities can elicit either increases or decreases in circulation depending on whether heat or cold is used. They are also known to have analgesic effects as a result of stimulation of sensory cutaneous nerve endings.

The infrared region of the spectrum is located adjacent to the red end of the visible light region. The wavelengths of the infrared modalities are obviously much shorter than are those of the electrical stimulating currents and the diathermies and are expressed in angstrom (Å) units; 1 Å is equal to 10^{-10} m.

Both the infrared and ultraviolet wavelengths are temperature dependent. Those modalities with the lower temperature have the longer wavelength. This means that an ice pack has a longer wavelength and thus a greater depth of penetration than does a hydrocollator pack. Temperatures used with the infrared modalities range from 0°C with ice to more than 3000°C with the infrared lamps. The wavelengths in this temperature range fall between 10,000 and 105,000 Å with corresponding frequencies ranging between 2×10^{12} and 4×10^{13} Hz.

It should be pointed out that an angstrom unit is an extremely small unit of measure and thus the differences in depth of penetration are not great between any of the infrared modalities. The critical factor is the superficial increase or decrease in tissue temperature that elicits the same physiologic response regardless of wavelength.

LASER

Of the modalities discussed in this book, the low-power **laser** is certainly the newest used by the therapist. The word laser is an acronym for *light amplification by stimulated emission of radiation*. Laser is a form of electromagnetic radiation that is classified within both the infrared and visible light portions of the spectrum.

Lasers are either high power or low power. High-power lasers are used in surgery for purposes of incision, coagulation of vessels, and thermolysis, owing to their thermal effects. The low-power or cold laser produces little or no thermal effects but seems to have some significant clinical effect on soft-tissue and fracture healing as well as pain management through stimulation of acupuncture and trigger points.

Two types of low-power lasers are used by therapists: the helium-neon laser (HeNe) and the gallium-arsenide laser (GaAs). The HeNe laser has a wavelength of 632.8 nm and a direct depth of penetration to 0.8 mm, although there may be some indirect effects up to 10–15 mm. The GaAs laser has a wavelength of 910 nm and can penetrate indirectly as much as 5 cm. The laser as a therapeutic tool is discussed in Chapter 13.

ULTRAVIOLET LIGHT

The ultraviolet portion of the electromagnetic spectrum is adjacent to the violet end of the visible light region. As stated previously, the radiations in the ultraviolet region are undetectable by the human eye. However, if a photographic plate is placed at the ultraviolet end, chemical changes will be apparent. Although an extremely hot source (7000–9000°C) is required to produce ultraviolet wavelengths, the physiologic effects of ultraviolet are mainly chemical in nature and occur entirely in the cutaneous layers of skin. The maximum depth of penetration with ultraviolet is about 1 mm. The wavelengths with ultraviolet range between 2000 and 4000 Å. The ultraviolet region is subdivided into three different areas: near ultraviolet or UV-A (3200–4000 Å); middle ultraviolet or UV-B (2900–3200 Å); and far ultraviolet or UV-C (2000–2900 Å). Clinically used frequencies with ultraviolet range between 7×10^{13} and 7×10^{14} Hz.[5,9,14] Although rarely used by the therapist, the application of ultraviolet therapy is discussed in Chapter 14.

Treatment Tip

When setting up a patient for treatment using either microwave diathermy or ultraviolet therapy, it is critical that the therapist consider the angle at which the electromagnetic energy is striking the body surface to ensure that most of the energy will be absorbed and not reflected. It is also essential to know the distance that these modalities should be placed from the surface to achieve the desired amount of energy in the target tissues.

Treatment Tip

The therapist may use ultraviolet light to treat skin lesions. Since the wavelength of ultraviolet energy is short, the depth of penetration is minimal, and thus the therapeutic effects are primarily superficial. Also, the ultraviolet region of the electromagnetic spectrum is known to produce chemical effects in biologic tissue, which may be helpful in facilitating healing.

THE ACOUSTIC SPECTRUM AND ULTRASOUND

One additional therapeutic modality frequently used by therapists is ultrasound. Ultrasound devices produce a type of energy that must be classified as acoustic rather than electromagnetic energy. Ultrasound is frequently classified along with shortwave and microwave diathermy as a deep-heating, "conversion"-type modality, and it is certainly true that all of these are capable of producing a temperature increase in human tissue to a considerable depth. However, ultrasound is a mechanical vibration, a sound wave, produced and transformed from high-frequency electrical energy.[5] Ultrasound must be considered a type of acoustic vibration rather than a type of electromagnetic radiation.

Acoustic and electromagnetic radiations have very different physical characteristics. When acoustic vibrations are produced, they travel at a velocity that is significantly lower than electromagnetic radiations. Electromagnetic waves travel at approximately 300 million meters per second, whereas sound waves travel at speeds from hundreds to several thousand meters per second.

The relationship between velocity, wavelength, and frequency is a bit different with acoustic energy than with electromagnetic energy, even though the inverse relationship between wavelength and frequency still exists. The distinction lies in the fact that the velocity of travel is much greater for electromagnetic energy than for acoustic energy. Therefore, wavelengths are considerably shorter in acoustic vibrations than in electromagnetic radiations at any given frequency.[5] For example, ultrasound traveling in the atmosphere has a wavelength of approximately 0.3 mm, whereas electromagnetic radiations have wavelengths of 297 m at a similar frequency.

We stated that electromagnetic radiations were capable of traveling through space or a vacuum. As the density of the transmitting medium is increased, the velocity of travel significantly decreases as a result of **refraction**, **reflection**, or absorption by the molecules in the medium. Acoustic vibrations will not be transmitted at all through a vacuum since they depend on conduction through molecular collisions. The more dense the transmitting medium, the greater the velocity of travel. In human tissue ultrasound has a much greater velocity of transmission in bone tissue (3500 m/sec), for example, than in fat tissue (1500 m/sec).

Frequencies of ultrasound wave production are between 700,000 and 1 million cycles per second. Frequencies up to around 20,000 Hz are detectable by the human ear. Thus the ultrasound portion of the acoustic spectrum is inaudible. Ultrasound generators are generally set at a standard frequency of 1–3 MHz (1000 kHz). The depth of penetration with ultrasound is much greater than with any of the electromagnetic radiations. At a frequency of 1 MHz, 50 percent of the energy produced will penetrate to a depth of about 5 cm. The reason for this great depth of penetration is that ultrasound travels very well through homogeneous tissue (e.g., fat tissue), whereas electromagnetic radiations are almost entirely absorbed. Thus when therapeutic penetration to deeper tissues is desired, ultrasound is the modality of choice.[8,11]

Therapeutic ultrasound traditionally has been used to produce a tissue temperature increase through thermal physiologic effects. However, it is also capable of enhancing healing at the cellular level as a result of its nonthermal physiologic effects. The clinical usefulness of therapeutic ultrasound is discussed in greater detail in Chapter 12.

EXTRACORPOREAL SHOCK WAVE THERAPY (ESWT)

Extracorporeal shock wave therapy (ESWT) is a relatively new noninvasive modality used in the treatment of both soft-tissue and bone injuries. ESWT was first used in the early 1980s in lithotripsy units used to fragment kidney and ureteral stones. The *shock waves*, in contrast to the connotation of being an electrical shock, are actually pulsed high-pressure, short-duration (<1 m/sec) sound waves. This acoustic energy is concentrated in a small focal area (2–8 mm in diameter) and is trasmitted through a coupling medium to a target region with little attenuation. Treatment uses a sequence of 1000–4000 shock wave pulses at 1–4 pps and lasts for 15–30 minutes.

acoustic energy Produced by ultrasound devices.

Over the last several years, a number of investigators, primarily in Europe and North America, have used this modality successfully in treating plantar fasciitis, medial/lateral epicondylitis, and nonunion fractures. It appears that although all the mechanisms by which shock waves affect bone are not yet understood, it is generally accepted that ESWT does have a stimulatory effect on osseous tissue. ESWT is discussed in detail in Chapter 18.

SUMMARY

1. Radiant energy may be produced when a sufficiently intense chemical or electrical force is applied to any object.
2. Electrical stimulating currents, shortwave and microwave diathermy, the infrared modalities, and ultraviolet therapy are all classified as portions of the electromagnetic spectrum according to corresponding wavelengths and frequencies associated with each region.
3. All electromagnetic radiations travel at the same velocity; thus wavelength and frequency are inversely related.
4. Radiations may be reflected, refracted, absorbed, or transmitted in the various tissues.
5. Those radiations with the longer wavelengths tend to have the greatest depth of penetration.
6. The purpose of using any therapeutic modality is to stimulate a specific tissue to perform its normal function.
7. Ultrasound and extracorporeal shock wave therapy are both forms of acoustic energy and are best propagated through dense tissue (e.g., biologic); thus they are extremely effective in reaching deep tissues.

REVIEW QUESTIONS

1. What is radiant energy and how it is produced?
2. What is the relationship between wavelength and frequency?
3. What are the characteristics of electromagnetic energy?
4. Which of the therapeutic modalities produce electromagnetic energy?
5. What is the purpose of using a therapeutic modality?
6. According to the Law of Grotthus-Draper, what happens to electromagnetic energy when it comes in contact with and/or penetrates human biologic tissue?
7. Explain the cosine and inverse square laws relative to tissue penetration of electromagnetic energy.
8. Which of the therapeutic modalities produces acoustic energy?
9. What are the differences between electromagnetic energy and acoustic energy?

REFERENCES

1. Fosbinder, R.A.: Electromagnetic radiation, Semin. Radiol. Technol. 10(3):84–88, 2002.
2. Gasos, J., Stavroulakis, P.: Biological effects of electromagnetic radiation, New York, 2003, Springer-Verlag.
3. Goats, G.C.: Appropriate use of the inverse square law, Physiotherapy 74(1):8, 1988.
4. Goldman, L.: Introduction to modern phototherapy, Springfield, IL, 1978, Charles C Thomas.
5. Griffin, J., Karselis, T.: Physical agents for physical therapists, Springfield, IL., 1978, Charles C Thomas.
6. Hitchcock, R.T., Patterson, R.M.: Radio-frequency and ELF electromagnetic energies: a handbook for healthcare professionals, New York, 1995, Van Nostrand Reinhold.
7. Lehmann, J.F., Guy, A.W.: Ultrasound therapy. Proc Workshop on Interaction of Ultrasound and Biological Tissues. Washington, DC, HEW Pub. (FDA 73:8008), Sept., 1972.

8. Lehmann, J., editor: Therapeutic heat and cold, ed. 2, New Haven, CT, 1982, Elizabeth Licht.

9. Licht, S.: Therapeutic electricity and ultraviolet radiation, New Haven, CT, 1959, Elizabeth Licht.

10. Nadler, S.F.: Complications from therapeutic modalities: results of a national survey of athletic trainers, Arch. Phys. Med. Rehabil. 84(6):849–853, 2003.

11. Schriber, W.: A manual of electrotherapy, Philadelphia, PA 1975, Lea & Febiger.

12. Sears, F., Zemansky, M., and Young, H.: University physics, Reading, MA, 1976, Addison-Wesley.

13. Smith, G.: Introduction to classical electromagnetic radiation, Boston, MA, 1997, Cambridge University Press.

14. Stillwell, K.: Therapeutic electricity and ultraviolet radiation, Baltimore, MD, 1983, Williams & Wilkins.

15. Venes, D., Thomas, C.L.: Taber's Cyclopedic Medical Dictionary, Philadelphia, PA, 2001, F.A. Davis.

SUGGESTED READINGS

Goodgold, J., Eberstein, A.: Electrodiagnosis of neuromuscular diseases, Baltimore, MD, 1972, Williams & Wilkins.

Jehle, H.: Charge fluctuation forces in biological systems, Ann. NY Acad. Sci. 158:240–255, 1969.

Koracs, R.: Light therapy, Springfield, IL, 1950, Charles C Thomas.

Licht, S., editor: Electrodiagnosis and electromyography, ed. 3, New Haven, CT, 1971, Elizabeth Licht.

Scott, P., Cooksey, F.: Clayton's electrotherapy and actinotherapy, London, 1962, Bailliere, Tindall and Cox.

GLOSSARY

absorption Energy that stimulates a particular tissue to perform its normal function.

acoustic spectrum The range of frequencies and wavelengths of sound waves.

Arndt-Schultz principle No reactions or changes can occur in the body if the amount of energy absorbed is not sufficient to stimulate the absorbing tissues.

cosine law Optimal radiation occurs when the source of radiation is at right angles to the center of the area being radiated.

diathermy The application of high-frequency electrical energy used to generate heat in body tissue as a result of the resistance of the tissue to the passage of energy.

electromagnetic spectrum The range of frequencies and wavelengths associated with radiant energy.

frequency The number of cycles or pulses per second.

infrared The portion of the electromagnetic spectrum associated with thermal changes located adjacent to the red portion of the visible light spectrum.

inverse square law The intensity of radiation striking a particular surface varies inversely with the square of the distance from the radiating source.

Law of Grotthus-Draper Energy not absorbed by the tissues must be transmitted.

radiation (1) The process of emitting energy from some source in the form of waves. (2) A method of heat transfer through which heat can be either gained or lost.

reflection The bending back of light or sound waves from a surface that they strike.

refraction The change in direction of a sound wave or radiation wave when it passes from one medium or type of tissue to another.

transmission The propagation of energy through a particular biologic tissue into deeper tissues.

ultrasound A portion of the acoustic spectrum located above audible sound.

ultraviolet The portion of the electromagnetic spectrum associated with chemical changes located adjacent to the violet portion of the visible light spectrum.

wavelength The distance from one point in a propagating wave to the same point in the next wave.

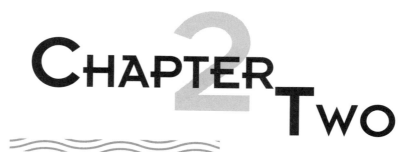

CHAPTER TWO

THE HEALING PROCESS AND GUIDELINES FOR USING THERAPEUTIC MODALITIES

WILLIAM E. PRENTICE

OBJECTIVES

Following completion of this chapter, the student therapist will be able to:

- ✓ Define inflammation and its associated signs and symptoms.
- ✓ Clarify how therapeutic modalities should be used in rehabilitation of various conditions.
- ✓ Compare the physiologic events associated with the three phases of the healing process.
- ✓ Formulate a plan for how specific modalities can be used effectively during each phase of healing and provide a rationale for their use.
- ✓ Categorize the indications and contraindications for using the various modalities discussed throughout this book.

Therapeutic modalities, when used appropriately, can be extremely useful tools in the rehabilitation of the injured patient. Like any other tool, their effectiveness is limited by the knowledge, skill, and experience of the person using them. For the therapist, decisions regarding how and when a modality may be best employed should be based on a combination of theoretical knowledge and practical experience. Modalities should not be used at random, nor should their use be based on what has always been done before. Instead, consideration must be given to what should work best in a specific clinical situation.

In any program of rehabilitation, modalities should be used primarily as adjuncts to therapeutic exercise and not at the exclusion of range-of-motion and strengthening exercises. Rehabilitation protocols and progressions must be based primarily on the physiologic responses of the tissues to injury and on an understanding of how various tissues heal. Thus the therapist must understand the healing process to be effective in incorporating therapeutic modalities into the rehabilitative process.

There are many different approaches and ideas regarding the use of modalities in injury rehabilitation. Therefore, no "cookbook" exists for modality use. Instead, therapists should make their own decisions from the available options in a given clinical situation about which modality will be most effective.

UNDERSTANDING THE HEALING PROCESS

Clinical decisions on how and when therapeutic modalities may best be used should be based on recognition of signs and symptoms as well as some awareness of the time frames associated with the various phases of the healing process.[12–14] The therapist must have a sound understanding of that process in terms of the sequence of the various phases of healing that take place.

Basically, the healing process consists of the inflammatory response phase, the fibroblastic-repair phase, and the maturation-remodeling phase. It must be stressed that although the phases of healing are presented as three separate entities, the healing process is a continuum.[23] Phases of the healing process overlap one another and have no definitive beginning or end points.[5]

INFLAMMATORY-RESPONSE PHASE

Once a tissue is injured, the process of healing begins immediately (Fig. 2-1).[1,7] The destruction of tissue produces direct injury to the cells of the various soft tissues. Cellular injury results in altered metabolism and the liberation of materials that initiate the inflammatory response. Cellular injury is characterized symptomatically by redness, swelling, tenderness, and increased temperature.[2,11]

Cellular Response

Inflammation is a process by means of which **leukocytes** and other **phagocytic cells** and exudate are delivered to the injured tissue. This cellular reaction generally is protective, tending to localize or dispose of injury by-products (e.g., blood, damaged cells) through phagocytosis, thus setting the stage for repair. Locally, vascular effects, disturbances of fluid exchange, and migration of leukocytes from the blood to the tissues occur.[18]

Signs of Inflammation
- Redness
- Swelling
- Tenderness to touch
- Increased temperature

Vascular Reaction

The vascular reaction involves vascular spasm, formation of a platelet plug, blood coagulation, and growth of fibrous tissue.[17] The immediate response to damage is a vasoconstriction of the vascular walls that lasts for approximately 5–10 minutes. This spasm presses the opposing endothelial linings together to produce a local anemia that is rapidly replaced by hyperemia of the area owing to dilation. This increase in blood flow is transitory and gives way to slowing of the flow in the dilated vessels, which then progresses to stagnation and stasis. The initial effusion of blood and plasma lasts for 24–36 hours.

Chemical Mediators

Three chemical mediators, *histamine*, *leucotaxin*, and *necrosin*, are important in limiting the amount of exudate and swelling following injury. Histamine released from the injured mast cells causes vasodilation and increased cell permeability, owing to swelling of endothelial cells, and then separation between the cells. Leucotaxin is responsible for margination in which leukocytes line up along the cell walls. It also increases cell permeability locally, thus affecting passage of the fluid and white blood cells through cell walls by diapedesis to form exudate. Therefore, vasodilation and active hyperemia are important in exudate (plasma) formation and supplying leukocytes to the injured area. Necrosin is responsible for phagocytic activity. The amount of swelling that occurs is directly related to the extent of vessel damage.

Function of Platelets

Platelets do not normally adhere to the vascular wall. However, injury to a vessel disrupts the endothelium and exposes the collagen fibers. Platelets adhere to the collagen

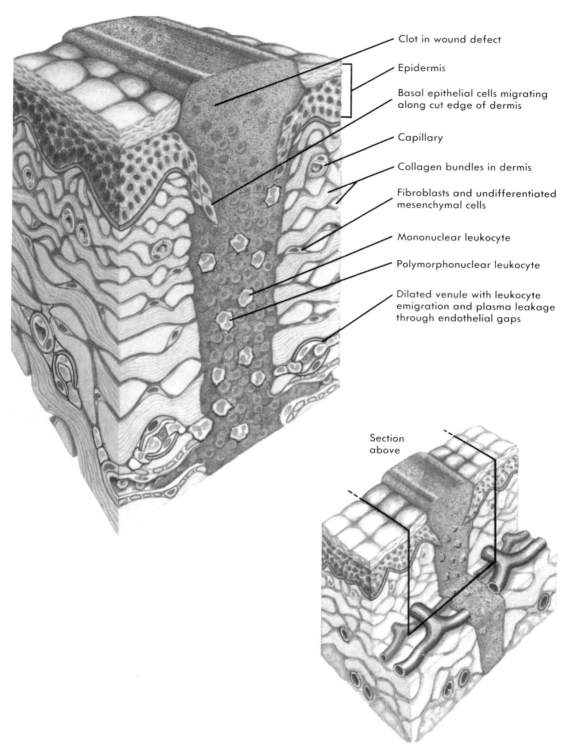

•**Figure 2-1** The inflammatory response phase.

fibers to create a sticky matrix on the vascular wall, to which additional platelets and leukocytes adhere and eventually form a plug. These plugs obstruct local lymphatic fluid drainage and thus localize the injury response.

Clot Formation

The initial event that precipitates clot formation is the conversion of *fibrinogen* to *fibrin*. This transformation occurs because of a cascading effect beginning with the release of a protein molecule called *thromboplastin* from the damaged cell. Thromboplastin causes *prothrombin* to be changed into *thrombin*, which in turn causes the conversion of fibrinogen into a very sticky fibrin clot that shuts off the blood supply to the injured area. Clot formation begins around 12 hours following injury and is completed by 48 hours.

As a result of a combination of these factors, the injured area becomes walled off during the inflammatory stage of healing. The leukocytes phagocytize most of the foreign debris toward the end of the inflammatory phase, setting the stage for the fibroblastic phase. This initial inflammatory response lasts for approximately 2–4 days following initial injury.

Chronic Inflammation

A distinction must be made between the acute inflammatory response as described in the preceding section and chronic inflammation. Chronic inflammation occurs when the acute inflammatory response does not eliminate the injuring agent and fails to restore tissue to its normal physiologic state. Chronic inflammation involves the replacement of leukocytes with *macrophages*, *lymphocytes*, and *plasma cells*. These cells accumulate in a highly vascularized and innervated loose connective tissue matrix in the area of injury.[9]

The specific mechanisms that convert an acute to a chronic inflammatory response currently are unknown; however, they seem to be associated with situations that involve overuse or overload with cumulative microtrauma to a particular structure.[4,9] Likewise, there is no specific time frame in which the classification of acute is changed to chronic inflammation.

In Chronic Inflammation Leukocytes Are Replaced with
- Macrophages
- Lymphocytes
- Plasma cells

FIBROBLASTIC-REPAIR PHASE

During the fibroblastic phase of healing, proliferative and regenerative activity leading to scar formation and repair of the injured tissue follows the vascular and exudative phenomena of inflammation (Fig. 2-2).[8] The period of scar formation referred to as **fibroplasia** begins within the first few hours following injury and may last for as long as 4–6 weeks. During this period many of the signs and symptoms associated with the inflammatory response subside. The patient may still indicate some tenderness to touch and will usually complain of pain when particular movements stress the injured structure. As scar formation progresses, complaints of tenderness or pain gradually disappear.[15]

During this phase, growth of endothelial capillary buds into the wound is stimulated by a lack of oxygen. Thus, the wound is now capable of healing aerobically. Along with increased oxygen delivery comes an increase in blood flow that delivers nutrients essential for tissue regeneration in the area.[3]

The formation of a delicate connective tissue called *granulation* tissue occurs with the breakdown of the fibrin clot. Granulation tissue consists of fibroblasts, collagen, and capillaries. It appears as a reddish granular mass of connective tissue that fills in the gaps during the healing process.

As the capillaries continue to grow into the area, fibroblasts accumulate at the wound site, arranging themselves parallel to the capillaries. Fibroblastic cells begin to synthesize an *extracellular matrix* that contains protein fibers of *collagen* and *elastin*, a *ground substance* that consists of nonfibrous proteins called *proteoglycans*, *glycosaminoglycans*, and fluid. On about day 6 or 7, fibroblasts also begin producing collagen fibers that are deposited in a random fashion throughout the forming scar. As the collagen continues to proliferate, the tensile strength of the wound rapidly increases in proportion to the rate of collagen synthesis.[20] As the tensile strength increases, the number of fibroblasts diminishes to signal the beginning of the maturation phase.

This normal sequence of events in the repair phase leads to the formation of minimal scar tissue. Occasionally, a persistent inflammatory response and continued release of inflammatory products can promote extended fibroplasia and excessive fibrogenesis that can lead to irreversible tissue damage.[19] Fibrosis can occur in synovial structures, as is the case with adhesive capsulitis in the shoulder; in extraarticular articular tissues including tendons and ligaments; in bursa; or in muscle.

Granulation Tissue Consists of
- Capillaries
- Collagen
- Fibroblasts

The Extracellular Matrix Contains
- Collagen
- Elastin
- Ground substance

fibroplasia The period of scar formation that occurs during the fibroblastic-repair phase.

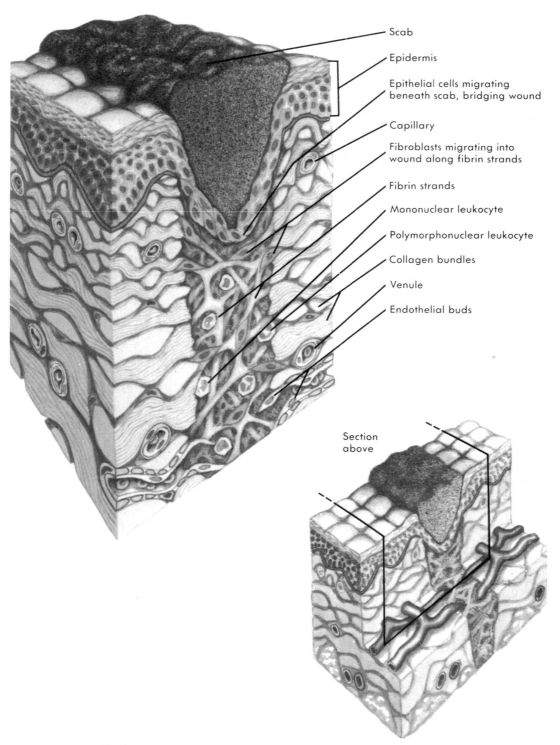

Scab

Epidermis

Epithelial cells migrating beneath scab, bridging wound

Capillary

Fibroblasts migrating into wound along fibrin strands

Fibrin strands

Mononuclear leukocyte

Polymorphonuclear leukocyte

Collagen bundles

Venule

Endothelial buds

Section above

•**Figure 2-2** The fibroblastic-repair phase.

MATURATION-REMODELING PHASE

The maturation-remodeling phase of healing is a long-term process (Fig. 2-3). This phase features a realignment or remodeling of the collagen fibers that make up the scar tissue according to the tensile forces to which that scar is subjected. Ongoing breakdown and synthesis of collagen occur with a steady increase in the tensile strength of the scar matrix. With increased stress and strain, the collagen fibers realign in a position

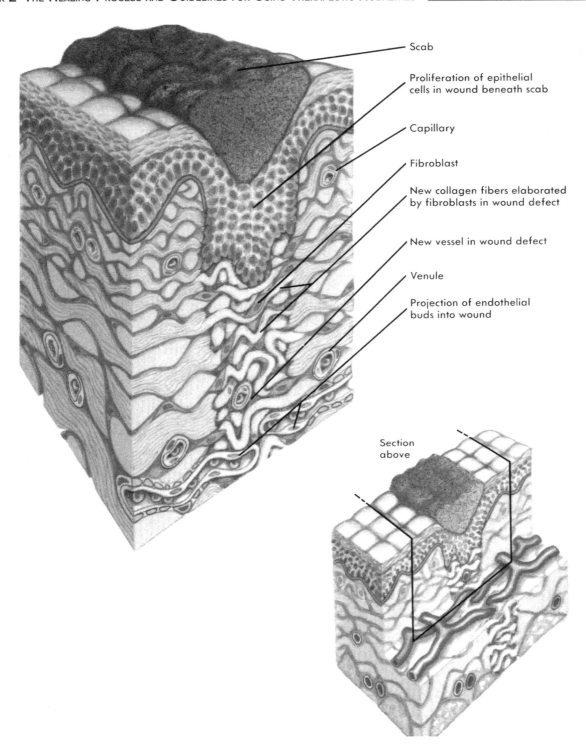

- Scab
- Proliferation of epithelial cells in wound beneath scab
- Capillary
- Fibroblast
- New collagen fibers elaborated by fibroblasts in wound defect
- New vessel in wound defect
- Venule
- Projection of endothelial buds into wound

Section above

•**Figure 2-3** The maturation-remodeling phase.

of maximum efficiency parallel to the lines of tension. The tissue gradually assumes normal appearance and function, although a scar is rarely as strong as the normal injured tissue. Usually by the end of approximately 3 weeks, a firm, strong, contracted, nonvascular scar exists. The maturation phase of healing may require several years to be totally complete.

Factors That Impede Healing
- Extent of injury
- Edema
- Hemorrhage
- Poor vascular supply
- Separation of tissue
- Muscle spasm
- Atrophy
- Corticosteroids
- Keloids and hypertrophic scars
- Infection
- Humidity, climate, and oxygen tension
- Health, age, and nutrition

FACTORS THAT IMPEDE HEALING

Extent of Injury

The extent of the inflammatory response is determined by the extent of the tissue injury. **Microtears** of soft tissue involve only minor damage and most often are associated with overuse. **Macrotears** involve significantly greater destruction of soft tissue and result in clinical symptoms and functional alterations. Macrotears generally are caused by acute trauma.

Edema

The increased pressure caused by swelling retards the healing process, causes separation of tissues, inhibits neuromuscular control, produces reflexive neurologic changes, and impedes nutrition in the injured part. Edema is best controlled and managed during the initial first aid management period.[22]

Hemorrhage

Bleeding occurs with even the smallest amount of damage to the capillaries. Bleeding produces the same negative effects on healing as does the accumulation of edema, and its presence produces additional tissue damage and thus exacerbation of the injury.

Poor Vascular Supply

Injuries to tissues with a poor vascular supply heal poorly and slowly. This is likely related to a failure in the delivery of phagocytic cells initially and also of fibroblasts necessary for formation of scar.

Separation of Tissue

Mechanical separation of tissue can significantly impact the course of healing. A wound that has smooth edges that are in good apposition will tend to heal by primary intention with minimal scarring. Conversely, a wound that has jagged separated edges must heal by second intention with granulation tissue filling the defect and excessive scarring.[16]

Muscle Spasm

Muscle spasm causes traction on the torn tissue, separates the two ends, and prevents approximation. Both local and generalized ischemia may result from spasm.

Atrophy

Wasting away of muscle tissue begins immediately with injury. Strengthening and early mobilization of the injured structure retards atrophy.

Corticosteroids

Use of corticosteroids in the treatment of inflammation is controversial. Steroid use in the early stages of healing has been demonstrated to inhibit fibroplasia, capillary proliferation, and collagen synthesis, and increases in tensile strength of the healing scar. Steroid use is debatable in the later stages of healing and with chronic inflammation.

Keloids and Hypertrophic Scars

Keloids occur when the rate of collagen production exceeds the rate of collagen breakdown during the maturation phase of healing. This process leads to hypertrophy of scar tissue, particularly around the periphery of the wound.

Infection

The presence of bacteria in the wound can delay healing and may cause excessive granulation tissue and large deformed scars.

Humidity, Climate, and Oxygen Tension

Humidity significantly influences the process of epithelization. Occlusive dressings stimulate the epithelium to migrate twice as fast without crust or scab formation. The formation of a scab occurs with dehydration of the wound and traps wound drainage, which promotes infection. Keeping the wound moist provides an advantage for the necrotic debris to go to the surface and be shed.

Oxygen tension relates to the neovascularization of the wound, which translates into optimal saturation and maximal tensile strength development. Circulation to the wound can be affected by ischemia, venous stasis, hematomas, and vessel trauma.

Health, Age, and Nutrition

The elastic qualities of the skin decrease with aging. Degenerative diseases such as diabetes and arteriosclerosis also become a concern of the older patient and may affect wound healing. Nutrition is important for wound healing. In particular, vitamins C (scurvy), K (clotting), and A and E (collagen synthesis); zinc for the enzyme systems; and amino acids play critical roles in the healing process.

INJURY MANAGEMENT USING MODALITIES

Traditionally in a clinical setting, injuries have been classified as being either **acute injuries** that result from trauma or **chronic injuries** that result primarily from overuse. This operational definition is not necessarily correct. If active inflammation is present that includes the classic symptoms of tenderness, swelling, redness, and so on, the injury should be considered acute and must be treated accordingly, using rest, ice, compression, and elevation.[7] Even if active inflammation persists for months following initial injury it should still be considered acute. Classification of an injury should be made according to the existing signs and symptoms that indicate the various stages of the healing process, and not according to time frames or mechanisms of injury. Once the signs of acute inflammation are no longer present, the injury may be considered to be chronic. Inflammation may be considered chronic when the normal cellular response in the inflammatory process is altered, replacing leukocytes with macrophages and plasma cells, along with degeneration of the injured structure.

Based on this definition of acute and chronic injury, the rehabilitation progression following injury may be determined by the four phases of healing. These phases overlap, and the estimated time frames for each phase show extreme variability between patients. Table 2-1 summarizes the various modalities that may be used in each of the four phases.

INITIAL ACUTE INJURY PHASE

Modality use in the initial treatment phase should be directed toward limiting the amount of swelling and reducing pain that occurs acutely. The acute phase is marked by swelling, pain to touch or with pressure, and pain on both active and passive motion. In general, the less initial swelling, the less the time required for rehabilitation. Traditionally, the modality of choice has been and still is ice.

Cryotherapy is known to produce vasoconstriction, at least superficially and perhaps indirectly in the deeper tissues, and thus limits the bleeding that always occurs with injury. Ice bags, cold packs, and ice massage may all be used effectively. Cold baths should be avoided because the extremities must be placed in a gravity-dependent position. Cold whirlpools also place the extremities in the gravity-dependent position and produce a massaging action that is likely to retard clotting. The importance of applying ice immediately following injury for limiting acute swelling through vasoconstriction has probably been overemphasized. The initial use of ice is more important for producing analgesia, which occurs through stimulation of sensory cutaneous nerves that blocks or reduces pain by way of the gating mechanism.

Treatment Tip
Immediately following injury the therapist should use cryotherapy, some type of compression device, along with elevation to control swelling initially. Additionally, electrical stimulating currents may be used to help provide analgesia, and ultrasound can be used to facilitate healing.

TABLE 2-1   **Clinical Decision Making on the Use of Various Therapeutic Modalities in Treatment of Acute Injury**

Phase	Approximate Time Frame	Clinical Picture	Possible Modalities Used	Rationale for Use
Initial acute	Injury—day 3	Swelling, pain to touch, pain on motion	CRYO ESC IC LPL ULTRA Rest	↓ Swelling, ↓ pain ↓ Pain ↓ Swelling ↓ Pain Nonthermal effects to ↑ healing
Inflammatory response	Days 2—6	Swelling subsides, warm to touch, discoloration, pain to touch, pain on motion	CRYO ESC IC LPL ULTRA Range of motion	↓ Swelling, ↓ pain ↓ Pain ↓ Swelling ↓ Pain Nonthermal effects to ↑ healing
Fibroblastic-repair	Days 4—10	Pain to touch, pain on motion, swollen	THERMO ESC LPL IC ULTRA Range of motion Strengthening	Mildly ↑ circulation ↓ Pain—muscle pumping ↓ Pain Facilitate lymphatic flow Nonthermal effects to ↑ healing
Maturation-remodeling	Day 7—recovery	Swollen, no more pain to touch, decreasing pain on motion	ULTRA ESC LPL SWD MWD Range of motion Strengthening Functional activities	Deep heating to ↑ circulation ↑ Range of motion, ↑ strength ↓ Pain ↓ Pain Deep heating to ↑ circulation Deep heating to ↑ circulation

CRYO, cryotherapy; *ESC*, electrical stimulating currents; *IC*, intermittent compression; *LPL*, low-power laser; *MWD*, microwave diathermy; *SWD*, shortwave diathermy; *THERMO*, thermotherapy; *ULTRA*, ultrasound; ↓, decrease; ↑, increase.

Immediate compression has been demonstrated to be an effective technique for limiting swelling. An intermittent compression device may be used to provide even pressure around an injured extremity. The pressurized sleeve mechanically reduces the amount of space available for swelling to accumulate. Units that combine both compression and cold have been shown to be more effective in reducing swelling than using compression alone. Regardless of the specific techniques selected, cold and compression should always be combined with elevation to avoid any additional pooling of blood in the injured area owing to the effects of gravity.

Electrical stimulating currents may also be used in the initial phase for pain reduction. Parameters should be adjusted to maximally stimulate sensory cutaneous nerve fibers, again to take advantage of the gate control mechanism of pain modulation. Intensities that produce muscle contractions should be avoided because they may increase clotting time.

Ultrasound has been demonstrated to be effective in facilitating the healing process when used immediately following injury and certainly within the first 48 hours. Low spatial-averaged intensities below 0.2 W/cm^2 produce nonthermal physiologic effects that alter the permeability of cell membranes to sodium and calcium ions important in healing.

The low-power laser has also been shown to be effective in pain modulation through the stimulation of trigger points and may be used acutely.

The injured part should be rested and protected for at least the first 48–72 hours to allow the inflammatory phase of the healing process to proceed naturally.

INFLAMMATORY-RESPONSE PHASE

The inflammatory response phase begins as early as day 1 and may last as long as day 6 following injury. Clinically, swelling begins to subside and eventually stops altogether. The injured area may feel warm to the touch, and some discoloration usually is apparent. The injury is still painful to the touch, and pain is elicited on movement of the injured part.

As in the initial injury stage, modalities should be used to control pain and reduce swelling. Cryotherapy should still be used during the inflammatory stage. Ice bags, cold packs, or ice massages provide analgesic effects. The use of cold also reduces the likelihood of swelling, which may continue during this stage. Swelling subsides completely by the end of this phase.

It must be emphasized that heating an injury too soon is a bigger mistake than prolonged use of ice. Many therapists elect to stay with cryotherapy for weeks following injury; in fact, some never switch to the superficial heating techniques. This procedure is simply a matter of personal preference that should be dictated by experience. Once swelling has stopped, the therapist may elect to begin contrast baths with a longer cold-to-hot ratio.

An intermittent compression device may be used to decrease swelling by facilitating resorption of the by-products of the inflammatory process by the lymphatic system. Electrical stimulating currents and low-power laser can be used to help reduce pain.

After the initial stage, the patient should begin to work on active and passive range of motion. Decisions regarding how rapidly to progress with exercise should be determined by the response of the injury to that exercise. If exercise produces additional swelling and markedly exacerbates pain, then the level or intensity of the exercise is too great and should be reduced. Therapists should be aggressive in their approach to rehabilitation, but the approach will always be limited by the healing process.

FIBROBLASTIC-REPAIR PHASE

Once the inflammatory response has subsided, the fibroblastic-repair phase begins. During this phase of the healing process, fibroblastic cells are laying down a matrix of collagen fibers and forming scar tissue. This stage may begin as early as 4 days after the injury and may last for several weeks. At this point, swelling has stopped completely. The injury is still tender to the touch but is not as painful as during the last stage. Pain is also less on active and passive motion.

Treatments may change during this stage from cold to heat, once again using increased swelling as a precautionary indicator. Thermotherapy techniques including hydrocollator packs, paraffin, or eventually warm whirlpool may be safely employed. The purpose of thermotherapy is to increase circulation to the injured area to promote healing. These modalities can also produce some degree of analgesia.

Intermittent compression can be used once again to facilitate removal of injury by-products from the area. Electrical stimulating currents can be used to assist this process by eliciting a muscle contraction and thus inducing a muscle pumping action. This aids in facilitating lymphatic flow. Electrical currents can once again be used for modulation of pain, as can stimulation of trigger points with the low-powered laser.

The therapist must continue to stress the importance of range-of-motion and strengthening exercises and progress them appropriately during this phase.

MATURATION-REMODELING PHASE

The maturation-remodeling phase is the longest of the four phases and may last for several years, depending on the severity of the injury. The ultimate goal during this maturation stage of the healing process is return to activity. The injury is no longer painful to the touch, although some progressively decreasing pain may still be felt on motion. The collagen fibers must be realigned according to tensile stresses and strains placed on them. Virtually all modalities may be used safely during this stage; thus, decisions should be based on what works most effectively in a given situation.

At this point some type of heating modality is beneficial to the healing process. The deep-heating modalities of ultrasound or shortwave and microwave diathermy should be used to increase circulation to the deeper tissues. Ultrasound is particularly useful during this period since collagen absorbs a high percentage of the available acoustic energy. Increased blood flow delivers the essential nutrients to the injured area to promote healing, and increased lymphatic flow assists in breakdown and removal of waste products. The superficial heating modalities are certainly less effective at this point.

Electrical stimulating currents can be used for a number of purposes. As before, they may be used in pain modulation. They also may be used to stimulate muscle contractions for the purpose of increasing both range of motion and muscular strength.

Low-power laser can also assist in modulating pain. If pain is reduced, therapeutic exercises may be progressed more quickly.

The Role of Progressive Controlled Mobility in the Maturation Phase

Wolff's Law states that both bone and soft tissue will respond to the physical demands placed on them, causing them to remodel or realign along lines of tensile force.[21] Therefore, it is critical that injured structures be exposed to progressively increasing loads, particularly during the remodeling phase. Controlled mobilization has been shown to be superior to immobilization for scar formation, revascularization, muscle regeneration, and reorientation of muscle fibers and tensile properties in animal models.[19] However, immobilization of the injured tissue during the inflammatory response phase will likely facilitate the process of healing by controlling inflammation, thus reducing clinical symptoms. As healing progresses to the repair phase, controlled activity directed toward return to normal flexibility and strength should be combined with protective support or bracing. Generally, clinical signs and symptoms disappear at the end of this phase.

As the remodeling phase begins, aggressive active range-of-motion and strengthening exercises should be incorporated to facilitate tissue remodeling and realignment. To a great extent, pain will dictate rate of progression. With initial injury, pain is intense and tends to decrease and eventually subside altogether as healing progresses. Any exacerbation of pain, swelling, or other clinical symptoms during or following a particular exercise or activity indicates that the load is too great for the level of tissue repair or remodeling. The therapist must be aware of the timelines required for the process of healing and realize that being overly aggressive can interfere with that process.

OTHER CONSIDERATIONS IN TREATING INJURY

During the rehabilitation period following injury, patients must alter their daily routines to allow the injury to heal sufficiently. Consideration must be given to maintaining levels of strength, flexibility, neuromuscular control, and cardiorespiratory endurance.

Modality use should be combined with anti-inflammatory medication, particularly during the initial acute and acute inflammatory phases of rehabilitation.

Treatment Tip
Therapeutic exercises should begin on day one following injury. The point is that modalities should be used to facilitate the patient's effort to actively exercise the injured part and not in place of the active exercise.

INDICATIONS AND CONTRAINDICATIONS

Table 2-2 presents a summary list of indications for using the various modalities. This list should aid the therapist in making decisions regarding the appropriate use of a therapeutic modality in a given clinical situation.

TABLE 2-2   Indications for Therapeutic Modalities

Therapeutic Modality	Physiologic Resources (Indications for Use)
Electrical stimulating currents—high voltage	Pain modulation Muscle reeducation Muscle pumping contractions Retard atrophy Muscle strengthening Increase range of motion Fracture healing Acute injury
Electrical stimulating currents—low voltage	Wound healing Fracture healing Iontophoresis
Electrical stimulating currents—interferential	Pain modulation Muscle reeducation Muscle pumping contractions Fracture healing Increase range of motion
Electrical stimulating currents—Russian	Muscle strengthening
Electrical stimulating currents— MENS	Fracture healing Wound healing
Shortwave and microwave diathermy	Increase deep circulation Increase metabolic activity Reduce muscle guarding/spasm Reduce inflammation Facilitate wound healing Analgesia Increase tissue temperatures over a large area
Cryotherapy—cold packs, ice massage	Acute injury Vasoconstriction—decreased blood flow Analgesia Reduce inflammation Reduce muscle guarding/spasm
Thermotherapy—hot whirlpool, paraffin, hydrocollator, infrared lamps	Vasodilation—increased blood flow Analgesia Reduce muscle guarding/spasm Reduce inflammation Increase metabolic activity Facilitate tissue healing
Low-power laser	Pain modulation (trigger points) Facilitate wound healing

SUMMARY

1. The three phases of the healing process are the inflammatory-response phase, fibroblastic-repair phase, and maturation-remodeling phase, which occur in sequence but overlap one another in a continuum.

2. Factors that may impede the healing process include edema, hemorrhage, lack of vascular supply, separation of tissue, muscle spasm, atrophy, corticosteroids, hypertrophic scars, infection, climate and humidity, age, health, and nutrition.

3. During the initial first-aid management of injury, all efforts should be directed at minimizing swelling and controlling pain.

4. In the inflammatory-response phase, the modalities used should attempt to minimize the inflammatory response but should not interfere with the process.

5. During the fibroblastic-repair phase, the modalities selected should function to increase blood and lymphatic flow to remove by-products of inflammation.

6. The modalities used during the maturation-remodeling phase should be integrated with therapeutic exercise to help facilitate realignment of collagen and to increase the tensile strength of the scar.

REVIEW QUESTIONS

1. How should the therapist incorporate therapeutic modalities into a rehabilitation program for various musculoskeletal injuries?

2. What are the physiologic events associated with the inflammatory response phase of the healing process?

3. How can you differentiate between acute and chronic inflammation?

4. How is collagen laid down in the area of injury during the fibroblastic repair phase of healing?

5. Explain Wolff's law and the importance of controlled mobility during the maturation-remodeling phase of healing.

6. What are some of the factors that can have a negative impact on the healing process?

7. Why is the immediate care provided following acute injury so important to the healing process and the course of rehabilitation?

8. What specific modalities may be incorporated into treatment during the inflammatory-response phase?

9. What specific modalities may be incorporated into treatment during the fibroblastic-repair phase?

10. What are the specific indications and contraindications for using the various modalities?

REFERENCES

1. Bryant, M.: Wound healing, CIBA Clin. Symp. 29(3):2–36, 1977.

2. Carrico, T., Mehrhof, A., and Cohen, I.: Biology and wound healing, Surg. Clin. North Am. 64(4):721–734, 1984.

3. Cheng, N.: The effects of electrocurrents on A.T.P. generation, protein synthesis and membrane transport, J. Orthop. Rel. Res. 171:264–272, 1982.

4. Fantone, J.: Basic concepts in inflammation. In Leadbetter, W., Buckwalter, J., and Gordon, S., editors. Sports-induced inflammation, Park Ridge, IL, 1990, American Academy of Orthopaedic Surgeons.

5. Fernandez, A., Finlew, J.: Wound healing: helping a natural process, Postgrad. Med. 74(4):311–318, 1983.

6. Fleischli J.G., Laughlin, T.J.: Electrical stimulation in wound healing. J. Foot Ankle Surg. 36:457, 1997.

7. Hart, J.: Inflammation 1: its role in the healing of acute wounds, J. Wound Care 11(6):205–209, 2002.

8. Hettinga, D.: Inflammatory response of synovial joint structures. In Gould J., Davies, G., editors. Orthopaedic and sports physical therapy, St. Louis, MO, 1990, C.V. Mosby.

9. Houghton, P.E.: Effects of therapeutic modalities on wound healing: a conservative approach to the management of chronic wounds, Phys. Ther. Rev. 4(3):167–182, 1999.

10. Leadbetter, W.: Introduction to sports-induced soft-tissue inflammation. In Leadbetter, W., Buckwalter, J., and Gordon, S., editors. Sports-induced inflammation, Park Ridge, IL, 1990, American Academy of Orthopaedic Surgeons.

11. Leadbetter, W., Buckwalter, J., and Gordon, S.: Sports-induced inflammation, Park Ridge, IL, 1990, American Academy of Orthopaedic Surgeons.

12. Marchesi, V.: Inflammation and healing. In Kissane J., editor. Anderson's pathology, ed. 8, St. Louis, MO, 1985, C.V. Mosby.

13. Montbriand, D.: Rehab products: equipment focus. Making progress: modalities can jumpstart the healing process, Advanced Magazine for Directors of Rehabilitation 11(7):69–70, 72, 80, 2002.

14. Prentice, W.: Arnheim's principles of athletic training, ed. 11, St. Louis, MA, 2003, McGraw-Hill.

15. Riley, W.: Wound healing, Am. Fam. Phys. 24:5, 1981.

16. Robbins, S., Cotran, R., and Kumar, V.: Pathologic basis of disease, ed. 3, Philadelphia, PA, 1984, W.B. Saunders.

17. Rywlin, A.: Hemopoietic system. In Kissane J.M., editor. Anderson's pathology, ed. 8, St. Louis, MO, 1985, C.V. Mosby.

18. Udermann, B.E.: Inflammation: the body's response to injury, Int. Sports J. 3(2)19–24, 1999.

19. Wahl, S., Renstrom, P.: Fibrosis in soft-tissue injuries. In Leadbetter, W., Buckwalter, J., and Gordon, S., editors. Sports-induced inflammation, Park Ridge, IL, 1990, American Academy of Orthopaedic Surgeons.

20. Weintraub, W.: Tendon and ligament healing: a new approach to sports and overuse injury, St. Paul, MN, 2003, Paradigm Publications.

21. Wolff, J.: Gesetz der transformation der knochen, Berlin, 1892, Aug. Hirschwald.

22. Woo, S.L-Y., Buckwalter, J., editors. Injury and repair of musculoskeletal soft tissues, Park Ridge, IL, 1988, American Academy of Orthopaedic Surgeons.

23. Young, T.: The healing process, Pract. Nurs. 22(10):38, 40, 43, 2001.

24. Zachezewski, J.: Flexibility for sports. In Sanders, B., editor. Sports physical therapy, Norwalk, CT, 1990, Appleton & Lange.

GLOSSARY

acute injury An injury in which active inflammation is present that includes the classic symptoms of tenderness, swelling, redness, and so on.

chronic injury An injury in which the normal cellular response in the inflammatory process is altered, replacing leukocytes with macrophages and plasma cells, along with degeneration of the injured structure.

fibroplasia The period of scar formation that occurs during the fibroblastic-repair phase.

macrotears Significant damage to soft tissues caused by acute trauma, which result in clinical symptoms and functional alterations.

microtears Minor damage to soft tissue most often associated with overuse.

CHAPTER THREE

THE ROLE OF THERAPEUTIC MODALITIES IN WOUND HEALING

PAMELA E. HOUGHTON

OBJECTIVES

Following completion of this chapter, the student therapist will be able to:

- ✓ Explain cellular and physiologic actions of commonly used modalities on wound healing.
- ✓ Review of clinical research evidence of effectiveness of modalities for delayed or non-healing wounds.
- ✓ Describe application techniques, stimulus parameters, and treatment schedules commonly used when treating chronic wounds with these modalities.
- ✓ Review indications, contraindications, and potential risks of each of the modalities.
- ✓ Use informaiton provided in the chapter to select the best modality for a particular type of chronic wound.

To determine the best modality for the treatment of a particular chronic wound, it is imperative that the physical therapist have an awareness of the experimental research evidence available that provides information about the cellular and systemic effects of these modalities on the biologic systems in general and on the processes of wound healing specifically. Therapies that halt the destructive chronic inflammatory process and help restore the normal balance of tissue promoters and inhibitors may accelerate closure of chronic wounds. Understanding how and where these modalities work within the healing processes allows the clinician to make a better choice of modality to facilitate the healing of wounds.

SUPERFICIAL HOT AND COLD

Both superficial hot and cold therapies are commonly used to treat musculoskeletal conditions following injuries. When cold is applied to the skin, vasoconstriction of cutaneous arterioles is stimulated immediately. Reduction in blood vessel lumen diameter causes a significant restriction of local blood flow to the subcutaneous tissue. Local vasoconstriction induced by hypothermia reduces fluid filtration into the interstitium and thus reduces the potential for edema to develop. In addition, the slower metabolism that occurs when tissue temperatures are lowered results in the release of fewer inflammatory mediators and reduced edema formation following tissue injury. Lower rates of metabolism also reduce oxygen demand of tissues and minimize the chances of further injury of tissues with limited blood perfusion due to ischemia. Both human[154] and animal[100] studies have shown that mild tissue cooling is effective in reducing acute inflammation and tissue swelling.

While cold application may be beneficial to control excess inflammation during the early phases of tissue repair, it has been shown to increase the incidence of wound infection[88] and interfere with the blood coagulation cascade.[130] In addition, continued hypothermia throughout the healing process can interfere with the development of optimal tissue strength[45] and limit recovery postoperatively.[138] Persistent inhibition of the inflammatory process deprives the healing process of key chemical mediators responsible for stimulating new tissue formation. In addition, vasoconstriction produced by cryotherapy reduces local blood flow at the site of injury and interferes with the delivery of oxygen to fuel tissue healing.

Elevation of local tissue temperature at the site of tissue in the later stages of the healing process has been purported to accelerate tissue repair. A key mechanism of action by which a thermal agent accelerates the healing process is via heat-induced vasodilation which provides increased blood supply and improved tissue oxygenation. Other beneficial effects of therapeutic heat include alteration of enzymatic activity of chronic wound fluid, stimulation of fibroblast proliferation and metabolism, and improved phagocytic activity of inflammatory cells.[125]

Modalities capable of producing local increases in tissue temperature include continuous shortwave diathermy, infrared lamps, continuous ultrasound, hydrocollator packs, and immersion in warm whirlpools. Recently, improved healing of chronic wounds has been demonstrated by the application of heat using a specially designed noncontact dressing that creates a moist wound environment and delivers sufficient thermal energy so as to maintain normal tissue temperature.[124]

HYDROTHERAPY

One method of delivering superficial heat or cold to healing tissues is by immersing the affected body part or limb in hydrotherapy tanks filled with either warm, tepid, or cool water. Wound cleansing using hydrotherapy removes necrotic and devitalized tissue, cleanses the wound surface of loosely adherent yellow fibrinous or gelatinous exudate, and takes away any foreign contaminants, or harmful residues of topical agents. Niederhuber et al.[110] and Bohannon[11] reported whirlpool with agitation removed surface bacteria especially when whirlpool treatment is followed by spraying of the skin surface. Hydrotherapy treatments have also been shown to increase the rate of granulation tissue formation.[12]

The removal of foreign matter and nonviable tissue using this nonspecific type of mechanical debridement will aid wound healing indirectly and help reduce bacterial burden within the wound. Additional benefits of hydrotherapy treatments of wounds covered with thick eschar are that the immersion will help soften the eschar and help facilitate subsequent debridement, provided it is carried out soon after hydrotherapy. Based on this mechanism of action of hydrotherapy, this therapeutic modality is indicated for nonhealing wounds that have substantial amounts of necrotic tissue. According to the Agency for Health Care Policy and Research (AHCPR) guidelines for the treatment of pressure ulcers, whirlpool treatments should be discontinued when debriding objectives have been met (i.e., the wound bed is clean).[9]

Elevating water temperature of the whirlpool can have additional therapeutic benefits including increasing changes in local circulation and reducing patients' perception of pain. Hydrotherapy treatments in whirlpools have been shown to improve comfort of surgical wounds postoperatively.[101] Some suggest hydrotherapy treatments may be useful for persons with mild arterial compromise. However, increased cellular activity produced by immersion in warm water could produce relative tissue ischemia if arterial disease is pronounced and local vascular supply cannot meet increased demands for nutrients and oxygen. In addition, heat-induced vasodilation and release of vasoactive substances can also be detrimental if treating persons with concurrent venous disease. McCulloch and Boyd reported that prolonged hydrotherapy treatment (greater than 5 min) of chronic venous leg ulcers when the unbandaged lower extremity is immersed in the dependent position can result in increased venous hypertension and vascular congestion leading to limb edema.[96] Ogiwara demonstrated recently that ankle dorsiflexion/plantarflexion exercises performed while the limb was immersed in the whirlpool tank were unable to offset edema formation due to limb dependency during hydrotherapy.[114]

Nonimmersion hydrotherapy techniques have become more popular recently. Pulsed lavage involves the delivery of an irrigating solution under pressure produced by an electronically powered device combined with suction to remove effluent. Some reports suggest that hydrotherapy delivered using this nonimmersion pulsed lavage technique has greater improvements in granulation tissue formation and removes surface contaminants more completely than traditional hydrotherapy treatments using only limb immersion. Pulsed lavage has been suggested to cleanse deep wounds with undermining. This form of nonimmersion hydrotherapy treatment may be useful with persons who have physical limitations or medical conditions that prevent water immersion.[64]

Most published protocols for the use of whirlpool on chronic wounds suggest that the limb should be immersed in water of a neutral temperature (92–96°F) for 10–20 minutes. Treatment times should be reduced if tissue maceration is produced. Water temperature is often selected based on arterial blood supply and venous return of the patient's limb. Warm water can be used to help improve blood supply and help with patient discomfort, whereas water temperatures should be employed with individuals at risk of developing venous congestion. However, whirlpools using water temperatures above or below body surface temperature should only be used on healthy individuals in whom local circulation is not compromised and cardiovascular status is normal. Hydrotherapy treatments should be discontinued once the wound bed is clean and devoid of necrotic tissue. Rinsing the limb after the limb is removed from the hydrotherapy tank is recommended to further aid the removal of bacteria and contaminants on the skin and wound surface.

Care must be taken to ensure that agitation produced by the turbines within the hydrotherapy tank does not result in excessive pressures that can cause mechanical damage to fragile new tissue deposited in the wound bed. Pressures produced by whirlpool turbines have not been documented and may vary greatly between manufactured models. There are reports in the literature of increased wound infection such as *Pseudomonas aeruginosa* for individuals using whirlpool.[142] This may occur because prolonged water immersion causes superhydration of the skin and can interfere with the normal skin defenses to bacteria. Appropriate protocols outlined by the Centers for Disease Control are employed for cleaning, disinfecting, sterilizing, and culturing of the hydrotherapy units should be carried out to reduce the occurrence of these water-borne infections. Other safety considerations when using this modality include the use of appropriate grounding of turbine units and the use of ground fault circuit breakers, and caution when transferring patients to and from the tank.

ELECTRICAL STIMULATION

Endogenous bioelectrical potentials have been measured across the skin of many animals including humans.[49] This potential formed by the separation of charged ions across the epidermis, is believed to be responsible for the formation of a current of injury that occurs whenever the insulative skin layer is disrupted by injury allowing charged particles to move down their concentration gradient. The presence of this small but measurable current of injury within a wound is strongly correlated with successful healing outcomes.[99]

In vitro studies have demonstrated that electrical stimulation can promote several activities of the inflammatory cells involved in the initial phases of tissue repair. It can induce cell migration to the site of injury through galvanotaxis,[116] stimulate inflammatory cell degranulation,[128] and release important chemical mediators such as growth factors and chemoattractants.[164] Electrical stimulation can also induce inflammatory cell proliferation so that a greater number of these cells are able to respond to the tissue injury.[14] These cellular actions of electrical currents on the inflammatory cells can speed the resolution of the inflammatory phase of tissue repair so that new tissue formation may begin sooner following injury.

Electrically induced activity of inflammatory cells may also underlie reduced edema formation observed following injury in animal models treated with electrical stimulation.[28,147] Reed documented that the application of electrical current reduced microvessel leakage and limited posttraumatic edema formation.[127] Whether electrical stimulation can produce similar effects on postraumatic edema in a clinical situation with human subjects has not been investigated sufficiently. In one clinical study that examined swelling postacute injury in humans, treatment using high-voltage pulsed galvanic current (HVPC) was found to be as effective as compression therapy at reducing posttraumatic swelling.[59]

Experimental research performed using various animal models has revealed that local application of electrical current to wounded skin,[5,6,18,24,102] or surgically incised ligaments[2,50,89] and tendons[108,118] results in improved collagen deposition,[5,6,50,108] accelerated collagen maturation and organization,[2] and greater tensile strength.[18,89,118,141] Stimulation of new tissue formation may in part, be due to direct action of electrical currents on fibroblasts. Application of electrical current to cultured fibroblasts has been shown to enhance collagen synthesis and secretion,[14,22] stimulate fibroblast proliferation,[14] increase the number of receptor sites for certain growth factors,[47] and direct fibroblast migration.[36,44]

Possible intracellular mechanisms that underlie these fibroblastic responses to electrical currents include activation of transcription and translation of mRNA to make available important protein precursors,[163] increased ATP production to supply necessary energy demands,[22] membrane permeability which would allow increased intracellular stores of calcium,[162] and production of membrane receptors for important cytokines such as epidermal growth factor.[47]

Epithelial cell activity during repair also seems to be affected by electrical current. In particular, in vitro studies have shown that epithelial cell proliferation[164] and differentiation[66] can be activated in epidermal cells by electrical stimulation. In addition, keratinocyte migration can be influenced by the application of an electrical field,[29,163] and the synthesis and secretion of growth factors by epithelial cells can be stimulated to a greater extent by the application of an electrical current.[164] Correspondingly, several authors have reported that exogenous application of electrical currents to various animal models can accelerate wound reepithelialization.[24,102]

In addition to accelerated activities of fibroblasts and epithelial cells during the proliferative stage of healing, electrical current has also been shown to augment angiogenesis. Clinical studies have detected a greater density of capillaries within newly formed granulation tissue analyzed in tissue biopsies taken from individuals with chronic venous leg wounds when they were pretreated with electrical current.[74]

Results from studies in which electrical currents have been applied to cultures of bacteria commonly found in chronic wounds suggest that electrical current may have bactericidal properties. Kincaid, Lavoie, Szuminsky and colleagues showed HVPC applied using negative electrode can directly affect bacterial growth and replication.[78,146] These in vitro reports need to be supported by clinical studies where the effects of electrical current on the amount and type of bacteria present in chronic wounds is investigated using physiologic levels of electrical currents applied using standard application techniques.

Increased local vasodilation and improved tissue oxygenation have been reported to occur in individuals with peripheral vascular disease following treatment with electrical current.[34] Gilcreast et al.[56] and Faghri et al.[46] have demonstrated that electrical stimulation can enhance perfusion of ischemic limbs. In addition, Im et al.[71] showed enhanced survival rates of skin flaps pretreated with electrical stimulation which was attributed to improved blood perfusion observed in skin flaps under the negatively charged cathode.

Treatment with HVPC with negative polarity produced greater increases in local blood flow of rats than did positive polarity stimulation.[147] Some reports suggest elevations in blood flow can be enhanced by stimulating the muscle pump with the use of relatively high intensity stimulation that is sufficient to produce intermittent neuromuscular contraction.[46] However, there are also reports that suggest only low intensity stimulation without muscle contraction can also produce significant blood flow changes.[105] Restoration of impaired local circulation by application of electrical currents would promote tissue healing by supplying required nutrients including oxygen and help to wash out of accumulated waste products produced by the injured tissue. Improved local circulation would also help remove inflammatory mediators that may contribute to local edema and pain.

In addition to the benefits of electrical stimulation on the tissue healing process, transcutaneous electrical nerve stimulation (TENS) has long been recognized to have analgesic properties. There are several published clinical reports that have shown electrical currents which are similar to those used to treat delayed healing can reduce an individual's perception of pain (refer to Chapter 6). Reducing pain caused by injuries or nonhealing wounds can indirectly aid the healing process by offsetting many of the adverse effects of stress on the healing process and ultimately improving the patient's quality of life.

The most common application technique for electrical stimulation of chronic wounds involves using a monopolar setup in which the active electrode placed directly into the wound bed using specialized electrodes composed of sterile conductive material with a larger dispersive electrode is placed on intact skin proximal to the wound (Fig. 3-1). This direct application technique involves preparing the wound bed with electroconductive material. This is usually done by packing the wound loosely with gauze soaked with hydrogel and/or saline (Fig. 3-2). Careful removal of wound dressings and judicious use of universal precautions and equipment decontamination procedures are also required so as to avoid excessive wound manipulation, cross contamination of equipment and infection of the therapist.

Several different stimulus parameters have been shown to be effective in accelerating wound closure. Stimulus intensity and frequency are adjusted so as to produce a strong tingling sensation or in the case of desensate skin, the stimulus intensity is adjusted to a submotor level. Recommendations regarding the polarity that should be used for the active electrode, which is placed into the wound bed, vary greatly. A recent review by Kloth and McCulloch suggested that the polarity of the active electrode should be varied at different times during the wound healing process depending on the stage of wound repair and the type of cell you wish to attract into the wound area.[81]

Initially, low intensity direct current (LIDC) was the electrical waveform utilized predominantly in several earlier studies, whereas pulsed currents have since been employed more recently due to greater comfort and less risk of causing tissue pH changes. HVPC is a common type of pulsed current employed in the treatment of chronic wounds. HVPC is a specialized form of pulsed current that has a twin-peaked monophasic waveform composed of two pulses of very short duration and relatively high pulse amplitude (Fig. 3-3). The unidirectional flow of ions produced by this form of monophasic pulsed current produces a small net charge under the active electrode that is thought to be important in producing physiologic responses such as edema reduction, circulatory changes, bactericidal effects, and directing cell motility by galvanotaxis. While the optimal stimulus parameters and treatment schedules for the use of

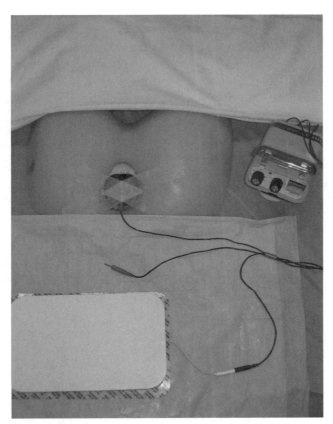

•**Figure 3-1** Application technique for electrical stimulation (HVPC) where the active electrode is applied directly to the wound bed while a large dispersive electrode is placed on intact skin distant from the wound site.

electrical stimulation on chronic wounds have not yet been agreed on, it appears that beneficial results can be obtained regardless of stimulus parameters used provided 300–500 uC/sec of electrical charge is delivered.[83]

Treatment schedules reported in the literature vary from as little as 1-hour treatments given three times weekly for 4 weeks to as much as 8 hours daily. It should be noted that in order to achieve optimal results with this modality, wound desiccation and the use of pertrolatum-based products in the wound bed must be avoided. In addition, it may be best to optimize the wound environment by coordinating electrotherapy treatments with the timing of wound dressing changes.

Application of electrical currents using asymmetrical biphasic waveforms applied through electrodes on the periulcer skin and distance acupuncture points. More recently HVPC applied for extended periods of time using garments made of specialized conductive material have also been shown to accelerate healing of a variety of types of chronic wounds (Fig. 3-4). Both these indirect application techniques shown in Figs. 3-4 and 3-5 have obvious practical advantage, however, the treatment protocols require much longer or more frequent application times (4.5–8 h/day). Studies in comparison of healing times produced by direct and indirect application techniques of electrical current have not yet been performed.

Adverse effects associated with electrical stimulation of chronic wounds include only minor discomforts associated with tingling sensations that are produced. The risk of electrical shock is minimal, especially considering that most portable electrical stimulation devices are battery powered. Chemical burns induced by pulsed electrical current are very unlikely since tissue pH changes have been shown to be minimal during application of HVPC.[109]

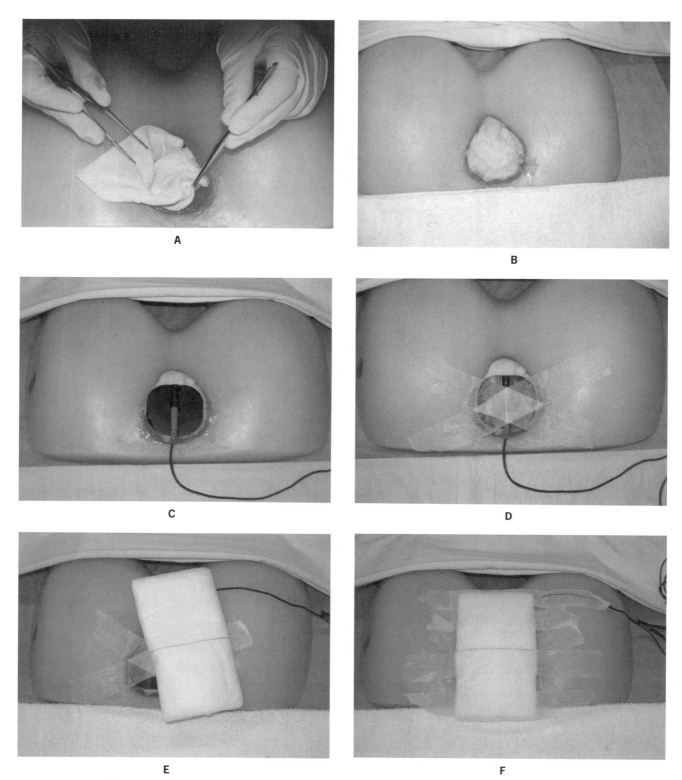

•**Figure 3-2** Preparation of the wound bed with electroconductive material and placement of the active electrode in the wound bed. **A and B.** Gauze soaked in hydrogel is loosely packed into the wound bed. **C and D.** A clean electrode is placed over the wound packing and secured in place with tape. **E and F.** The active electrode is further held in place by covering with a large cotton dressing.

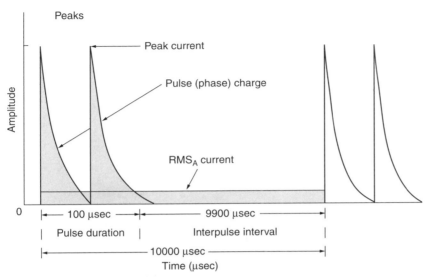

•Figure 3-3 Waveform of high-voltage pulsed galvanic current (HVPC).

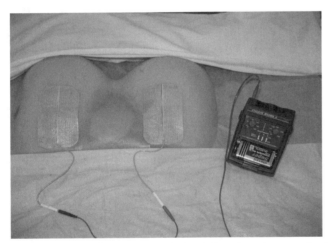

•Figure 3-4 Application technique for electrical stimulation where two equally sized electrodes are placed on either side of the wound and connected to a stimulator that delivers asymmetrical biphasic current.

ULTRASOUND

Cell culture studies have provided convincing evidence that ultrasound can alter the activity of cells known to be important in the inflammatory phase of healing. Stimulation of phagocytic activity of inflammatory cells such as macrophages and neutrophils has been reported.[30] This debridement action of ultrasound would be important in the initial stages of recovery from injury to clear the area of dead or devitalized material. Ultrasound has been shown to stimulate degranulation of inflammatory cells like macrophages[160] and mast cells.[37] This results in the release of numerous chemical mediators that in turn have been shown to activate other key cells in the healing process such as fibroblasts.[159] Thus, the effects of ultrasound during inflammation appear to help to reactivate the healing process by stimulating the natural debridement process and by causing the release of the body's endogenous source of growth factors and other cytokines at the local site of injury.

Examination of the temporal pattern of changes in the histologic composition of tissues obtained from animal models following injury treated with ultrasound are in the

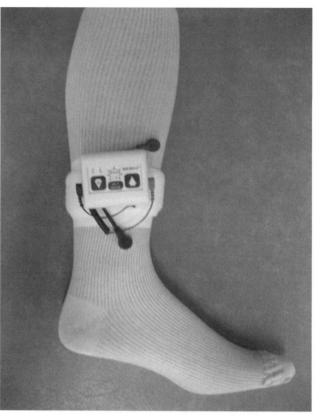

•**Figure 3-5** Silver-based conductive garments are used to deliver low levels of HVPC using a stimulator programmed to turn off and on over an extended treatment period. (Photo provided courtesy of Prizm Medical, Duluth, Georgia).

inflammatory phase of repair for a much shorter period of time following injury.[159] Although some researchers have referred to the effects of ultrasound on this phase of repair as "anti-inflammatory",[63] it is probably more likely the "proinflammatory" effects of ultrasound that are responsible for stimulating progression through the inflammatory phase of healing, which would allow more rapid deposition of new tissue to occur at the site of injury and completion of the repair process to occur sooner. Fyfe and Chahl reported that application of a similar treatment regime to edema produced experimentally in rat ankle joints caused an initial augmentation of swelling at 30 minutes posttreatment and this was followed by a greater reduction in swelling in ultrasound-treated ankles compared to control animals at 48 hours posttreatment.[51] This temporal pattern of changes to ankle joint swelling following ultrasound treatment is consistent with the theory that ultrasound initially stimulates the inflammatory phase of repair, which in turn results in a more rapid resolution of the edema and progression to subsequent phases of tissue repair.

Ultrasound has been found to effect several processes within the fibroblast—a key cell responsible for controlling production and degradation of extracellular matrix postinjury. Cell culture studies have shown that ultrasound can stimulate fibroblasts to synthesize and secrete collagen.[62] Ultrasound can also stimulate fibroblasts to proliferate resulting in a greater number of fibroblasts available to produce more collagen.[32] Further study of the mechanisms underlying ultrasound-induced fibroblastic activity has revealed that ultrasound can act directly to alter fibroblast function by producing calcium influx[3] and changing plasma membrane permeability.[33] Ultrasound treatment of experimentally placed skin lesions in animals has been shown in many studies to be associated with elevated levels of markers of collagen production such as procollagen mRNA expression and hydroxyl-proline concentrations.[38]

Studies examining the effects of ultrasound on healing tendons has revealed that collagen laid down under the direction of ultrasound is better organized and of greater tensile strength.[52,72,143] Producing scar tissue of greater breaking strength is an important functional advantage when referring to the healing of soft tissues such as ligaments and tendons. However, care needs to be taken when extrapolating to the clinical situation results obtained using experimentally produced injuries of ligaments and tendons of animals.

While many sources describe changes in local circulation as one of the physical effects of ultrasound, an examination of research studies performed to assess changes in skeletal blood flow in response to ultrasound treatments has produced inconclusive results.[132] Some reports suggest that ultrasound induces vascular changes such as production of blood stasis,[39] hemolysis,[155] increased vascular permeability, transient vasoconstriction,[132] and production of oxygen-free radicals.[94] All of these effects on blood vessels could interfere with local tissue perfusion. However, most of these potentially deleterious effects of ultrasound were associated with the application of quite high intensities of ultrasonic energy ($2–3$ W/cm^2).[39,155]

In summary, ultrasound has been shown to alter scar tissue formation through its actions on cellular processes in all phases of tissue repair but during the inflammatory phase of repair in particular. Ultrasound promotes the release of chemical mediators from inflammatory cells that in turn attract and activate fibroblasts to the site of injury and by directly stimulating collagen production during the proliferative stage of repair. Some research that is available suggests improved healing is more often associated with ultrasound treatments administered early in the healing process.[152] Jackson et al.[72] demonstrated that ultrasound administered soon after tissue injury during the inflammatory phase of repair produced improved tendon breaking strength, and that continued ultrasound treatments throughout the healing phase did not produce any further improvements in tensile strength of repaired tendons. Gan et al.[52] demonstrated that improvements obtained when ultrasound was administered within 7 days of injury were not observed if the commencement of ultrasound treatments was delayed. Therefore, it is possible that the proinflammatory effect of ultrasound occurring early in the healing process, which causes the body to produce its own mediators of tissue repair, is the critical action of this modality and is sufficient to kick start scar tissue formation and optimize collagen production, organization, and ultimately functional strength.

Sound waves have been administered to chronic wounds using both direct and indirect application techniques. With either application method the same ultrasound equipment used for other musculoskeletal disorders can be employed to treat chronic wounds. With the direct application technique, the wound bed is filled with sterile hydrogel and covered with a specialized dressing (Fig. 3-6) used as a conducting medium to deliver mechanical energy produced by ultrasound directly to the base of the wound bed. Ultrasound can also produce beneficial effects by application of low levels of ultrasound (Spatial Average Temporal Peak Intensity [SATP] = 1.0 W/cm^2; duty cycle = 20%; 3 MHz) to the periulcer skin for 5 min/5 cm^2 (Fig. 3-7). This indirect application method of pulsed ultrasound to the periulcer skin has tremendous practical advantages since it prevents the risk of wound contamination and the tissue dehydration and cooling that can occur when wound dressings are removed. Applying ultrasound to the periulcer skin employs similar equipment and application techniques as used by therapists to treat other musculoskeletal disorders. Therefore, minimal specialized training is required to use therapeutic ultrasound in wound care. Accelerated wound closure also has to be achieved by delivering low-frequency sound waves (30 kHz) from a large stationary sound head immersed in a water bath.

Although high doses of ultrasound have the potential to cause tissue cavitation, use of relatively low doses of ultrasound in wound treatment protocols have not yielded any reports of ultrasound-induced adverse effects. The risks of burns produced by this modality are minimal since it is used in a pulsed or interrupted mode that minimizes the accumulation of heat within the tissue.

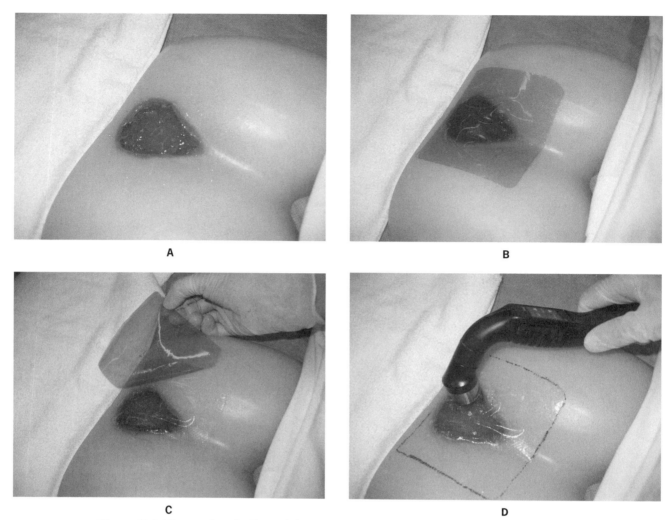

•**Figure 3-6** Ultrasound application technique used to deliver sound waves directly to the wound bed. **A.** Wound bed is filled with sterile hydrogel. **B and C.** Covered with transparent hydrogel sheet dressing. **D.** Ultrasound gel is applied over dressing and the sound head is applied to the gel to deliver sound waves directly to the wound bed.

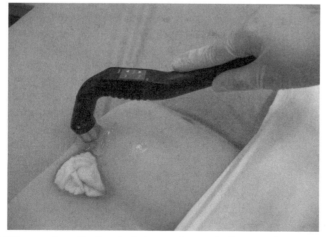

•**Figure 3-7** Ultrasound application technique using an indirect method where ultrasound is applied through gel to the periulcer skin. Wound packing is left in the wound during treatment to keep unwanted gel from the wound bed.

LASER

There are several in vitro studies performed using cultures of various types of cells known to be important in facilitating the healing process including macrophages,[12] neutrophils, mast cell[13] and lymphocytes,[115] as well as fibroblasts,[111,122,140] endothelial cells,[12] and epithelial cells.[161]

Biologic processes observed to be altered by administration of laser to cell cultures include protein synthesis,[140] cell growth and differentiation,[122] cell proliferation,[115] cell motility,[111] phagocytosis,[76] and cell degranulation.[12,161] Intracellular mechanisms of action to produce these cellular changes have also been investigated and proposed. They include activation of DNA synthesis to facilitate cell proliferation,[115,140] increase in transcription and translation of mRNA to make available important protein precursors,[161] and change in membrane permeability to stimulate physiologic changes such as nerve depolarization and stimulation of the influx of extracellular stores of calcium.[42] Calcium influx is, in turn, known to be an important intracellular signal for numerous cell processes including cell movement and phagocytosis, secretion of cytoplasmic granules containing potent chemical mediators, alteration in receptor binding affinity to facilitate intercellular communication, and activation of mitochondrial production of ATP via oxidative metabolism to make available energy to fuel increased needs of the photoactivated cell.

These direct actions of laser observed in these in vitro studies are believed to underlie several cell processes known to be important during the inflammatory phase of tissue repair. Several reports have documented the ability of laser to stimulate cell degranulation causing the release of potent inflammatory mediators as prostaglandins, growth factors,[158] and histamine[41] from various different types of leukocytes involved in the inflammatory phase of tissue repair. Laser irradiation of rat skin stimulated mast cell accumulation at the site of irradiation and a greater percentage of those mast cells present were found to be degranulated in previously traumatized skin.[41] Laser applied to macrophages in culture stimulates the release of chemical mediators into the cell culture supernatant that in turn was shown to be capable of activating fibroblast cell function.[12] Similarly, cell cultures of T lymphocytes exposed to laser were found to release an angiogenic factor that stimulated endothelial cell proliferation.[1]

Other effects of laser on white blood cells include the ability of laser to activate the phagocytic abilities, stimulate leukocyte proliferation, and promote migration of white blood cells toward the site of injury.[76] This laser-induced activation of many processes within the inflammatory phase of repair would promote the natural debridement action of leukocytes and help to clean foreign or dead and devitalized tissues within the injury site. Some reports suggest that laser effects are anti-inflammatory. Laser was found to produce a small but significant decrease in experimentally induced inflammation and edema produced by the inflammatory irritant carrageenin.[67]

Laser treatment of animals with injured tissues has resulted in increased collagen deposition[10] and that this augmentation of collagen production was associated with a concomitant improvement in the tensile strength of surgically incised skin[15,86] and tendons.[126] There also exist several other studies that have reported no benefit of laser on wound healing and breaking strength.[4,16,60,144] These negative findings tend to occur more commonly in studies where laser treatment regimes result in the administration of relatively low amounts of light energy to the wound bed (less than 1 J/cm^2)[70,136] or where the sham control group to which the effects of laser treatments are compared has been located within the same animal.[15,60,95]

Some reports suggest that laser can alter growth and replication of bacteria commonly found in chronic wounds.[156] However, recent reports have shown that the effects of laser applied to cultures of bacteria are dependent on the amount of laser energy delivered and wavelength of the light source with certain treatment protocols, actually causing a stimulation of bacterial growth.[113] Until factors that control the response of bacteria to laser are more completely understood, the use of laser on wounds contaminated with bacteria should be done cautiously.

Although there are numerous research studies that suggest laser therapy can have profound physiologic effects on tissue healing, there are a number of factors that can impact the tissue response to laser irradiation. Some stimulus parameters believed to influence the effects of laser therapy include laser wavelength, energy density, power density, pulse frequency, and treatment schedule. In addition to the laser parameters provided by the equipment, the biologic response to laser is also affected by changes within the host tissue such as tissue type and hydration, skin pigmentation, local blood flow, and basal level of tissue activity. More research is required to fully appreciate the influence that these and other factors have on the ability of laser therapy to produce the desired response.

A similar laser application technique used for the treatment of other musculoskeletal disorders has been described for the treatment of chronic wounds. Laser sources are often applied in contact to points equally distributed around the periulcer skin (Fig. 3-8). A transparent film barrier is often employed in conjunction with a contact point application technique to prevent cross contamination of the laser equipment. As with all light therapies, it is important to keep the angle and distance from the light source consistent when applying laser treatments. A noncontact, sweeping technique can also be used to deliver laser energy to the wound base. However, this would result in significantly less light energy delivered to the wound tissue and therefore laser treatment doses used with this noncontact application technique need to be increased accordingly. A multitude of different laser sources, wavelengths of light, dosimetry, treatment techniques, and treatment schedules have been reported in the literature. As a result, recommendations for treatment parameters to be used with laser treatments of chronic wounds cannot be provided at this time.

While scarcity of evidence from good, clinical research to support the use of laser in the treatment of chronic wounds is a disadvantage, an advantage of using this modality is the relatively minor safety precautions and risk. In addition, there are few medical conditions for which laser therapy is contraindicated for use. Nausea and dizziness have been reported to occur in 2 percent of patients following laser treatments.[57] Light therapies used in wound care do not produce tissue temperature elevations, therefore the risk of causing skin burns is minimal. However, exposure to eyes can cause severe retinal damage, and therefore both the therapist and patient must wear appropriate eye protection during treatment.

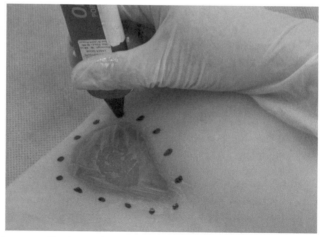

•**Figure 3-8** Laser application technique where laser tip is applied perpendicularly in contact to periulcer skin covered with transparent film. This procedure is carried for a specified period of time depending on the desired light energy delivered to the wound and is repeated to points evenly distributed around the wound.

Regardless of the treatment protocol selected to treat with laser therapy, careful documentation of treatment setup and parameters is critical. This documentation will help provide consistent delivery of laser energy and limit the number of variables that may be inadvertently changed during laser treatments. In this way, the therapist can systematically change laser treatment parameters while monitoring improvement in wound status in order to optimize a protocol for that patient who has a particular set of host factors.

ULTRAVIOLET LIGHT

The type of ultraviolet light is important in determining the tissue response. Light of shorter wavelength (180–250 nm) named ultraviolet light-C (UVC) is the type of ultraviolet light most commonly used in the treatment of chronic wounds. Effects of ultraviolet light that would be beneficial to the wound healing cascade include stimulation of epithelial migration and proliferation; release of chemical mediators, which in turn produce stimulated local cutaneous blood flow or erythema;[131,133] and bactericidal effects.[61] Bactericidal effects are greatest for shorter wavelengths of light (UVC) due to direct effects of UVC on nuclear material of the bacterium.[61] UVC exposure inhibits growth of in vitro cultures of bacteria commonly found to colonize chronic wounds.[65] Furthermore, a dose-dependent inhibition of UVC treatment on bacteria colonization of chronic pressure ulcers has been reported.[17] Recently, UVC has been shown to inhibit the in vitro growth of antibiotic-resistant bacteria (methicillin-resistant *Staphylococcus aureus* [MRSA] and vancomycin-resistant *Enterococcus faecalis* [VRE]).[26] Thai et al.[149] have demonstrated that a single exposure of UVC applied to superficial chronic wounds colonized with multiple bacteria including MRSA resulted in a significant reduction in the amount of bacteria detected using semiquantitative swabs. In addition, it has been demonstrated that successive treatments of UVC lasting 180 seconds each could eliminate MRSA detected using surface swabs in chronic infected wounds.[150] This result is extremely exciting given the fact that one of the most pressing problems today in both the acute-care-hospital and extended-care settings is the morbidity or mortality occurring in debilitated patients as a result of MRSA and VRE infections. This antibacterial effect of UVC that peaks at a wavelength of 254 nm is believed to speed healing via removal of a bioburden to the natural debridement system and thereby allowing more rapid progress through the inflammatory phase of wound healing.

Small, portable, relatively cost-effective lamps, which deliver ultraviolet light at specific wavelengths, are available commercially (254 nm). By using specific wavelength of UVC, potentially carcinogenic effects of UVA and UVB wavelengths can be reduced, and the risks of skin burns can be virtually eliminated. Since even thin transparent dressings have been shown to block the transmission of shorter wavelengths of light such as UVC, wound dressings must be removed and the wound must be properly cleansed prior to the UVC treatment. The amount of light energy delivered is known to be dependent on the duration of the treatment, the distance, and the angle of the light source.

Application methods for UVC in wounds are simplified by maintaining the UVC lamp at a consistent angle (perpendicular to the body surface) and distance (approximately 2.5 cm or 1 in) from the wound (refer to Fig. 3-9). In this way the desired response can be obtained by altering only the treatment time. In vitro studies have shown that bacteria kill rates of 100 percent can be obtained after 90 seconds of exposure to UVC.[26] Clinical case studies suggest that repeated treatments of longer durations (180 sec) are required to reduce bacteria counts from chronic wounds.[150] The same exposure time can be used daily throughout the treatment period until the clinical signs of wound infection are no longer observed. Cotton drapes and/or a thick petroleum jelly covering are often used on the periulcer skin to ensure that UVC is only

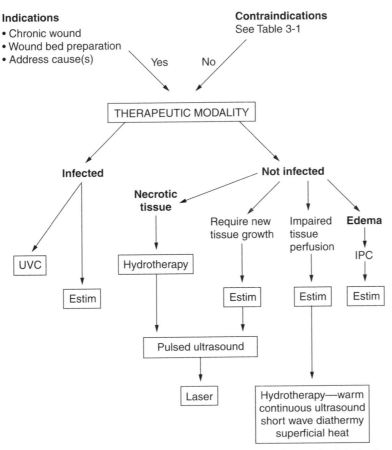

Figure 3-14 Algorithm to help clinicians choose the best modality to stimulate healing of non-healing wounds (for contraindications, see Table 3–1).

superficial heat, pulsed ultrasound, or laser. Several reports suggest that local application of electrical currents will induce vasodilation and improve tissue oxygenation. There is some evidence that suggests thermal modalities such as warm whirlpool and other superficial heating agents can improve local blood flow. These modalities as well as deeper heating agents such as continuous ultrasound or short-wave diathermy should only be considered with caution for use on chronic wounds with mild circulatory compromise when the potential for inducing tissue ischemia has been ruled out and the presence of intact sensation has been confirmed. Clinical research evidence to show laser and pulsed ultrasounds can increase local blood flow is limited.

Noninfected wounds that are clear of most necrotic tissue and require new tissue formation to help fill in and close over the wound defect should be treated with modalities capable of stimulating granulation tissue production such as electrical stimulation, ultrasound, or laser. Based on strong laboratory and clinical research electrical stimulation should be considered first, in particular for chronic pressure ulcers. There is also good experimental and clinical research evidence to support the use of pulsed ultrasound on chronic venous ulcers. Administration of pulsed ultrasound to the periulcer skin would be particularly appropriate if access to the wound bed is not possible or if metal is present in the wound bed. Given the relative paucity of clinical research evidence to support the use of laser and the lack of appreciation of how various biologic and technical factors influence results produced by this modality, laser therapy for

CASE STUDY 3-1
ELECTRICAL STIMULATION: WOUND CARE

Background: A 57-year-old woman sustained a complete spinal cord injury at the T3 level in a motor vehicle accident 15 years ago. She has developed a stage III pressure ulcer over the right greater trochanter, and has been referred for wound care. The ulcer is circular, 8 cm in diameter, and 3 cm deep at the deepest point. There is a moderate amount of yellow and green exudate with a mild odor. The wound bed is yellow, the wound margins are intact, and there is no undermining detected. The patient notes that the wound is not painful.

Impression: Stage III pressure ulcer.

Treatment Plan: The source of the ulcer appears to be an improperly fitted wheelchair, resulting from a gradual weight gain over the past 10 years. Therefore, the initial treatment is to obtain a wheelchair of the correct width to relieve pressure on the ulcer. Wound care was initiated on a daily schedule, consisting of pulsed lavage to debride the necrotic tissue. Following each session, the wound was dressed with gauze, which was removed at the next session using the lavage (wet-to wet-dressings).

Response: After seven treatment sessions, there was no exudate and the wound bed was red. Pulsed lavage was then discontinued, and a hydrogel dressing was applied, with changes as needed. After 6 weeks, the wound size and appearance were unchanged. Therefore, treatment with pulsatile monophasic (high volt) electrical stimulation was initiated on a 5-day per week schedule. Treatment parameters were negative polarity (cathode) for the treatment electrode, 100 pps (continuous mode), 200 V amplitude, and 60-minute duration. The treatment electrode was formed by packing the wound with sterile gauze moistened with sterile saline. The dispersive electrode (anode) was a moistened pad with a surface area of 75 cm^2 (three times the active electrode size) placed over the anterior thigh. The wound was dressed with sterile gauze following each treatment, with a hydrogel dressing

used for weekend periods. After 20 sessions (4 weeks), the wound had decreased to 1.6 cm in diameter (an 80% reduction), and was 0.5 cm deep. Electrical stimulation was discontinued, and a foam sheet dressing was used. The wound was completely closed 6 weeks later, and the patient was discharged.

Discussion Questions

- What tissues were injured/affected?
- What symptoms were present?
- What phase of the injury-healing continuum did the patient present for care in? What are the physical agent modality's biophysical effects? (direct/indirect/ depth/tissue affinity)
- What are the physical agent modality's indications/contraindications?
- What are the parameters of the physical agent modality's application/dosage/duration/frequency in this case study?
- What other physical agent modalities could be utilized to treat this injury or condition? Why? How?
- Why was electrical stimulation not used from the beginning of the episode of care? Why was sharp debridement not used to remove the necrotic tissue?
- What is the role of nutrition in the treatment of this patient?
- What other wound care products (dressings) would have been appropriate?
- Why was the wheelchair issue addressed first in the care of this patient?

The rehabilitation professional employs physical agent modalities to create an optimum environment for tissue healing while minimizing the symptoms associated with the trauma or condition.

patients with chronic wounds should be considered if electrical stimulation or ultrasound is contraindicated or impractical.

In all cases when using therapeutic modalities to accelerate the healing of chronic wounds, changes in wound status should be monitored at least weekly using valid and reliable outcome measures. Lack of progression of chronic wounds may also be a missed causative agent, and therefore another assessment of the patient to review underlying causes and current wound care therapy is warranted. If wound improvements are not detected after a few weeks of treatment with the chosen modality, then alteration in stimulus parameters should be initiated. If it continues then another treatment modality should be offered to the client.

SUMMARY

1. Before applying therapeutic modality to individuals with chronic wounds, review the wound management program and ensure that the wound environment is optimized and the primary etiology of the wound has been sufficiently addressed.
2. The list of contraindications for various modalities varies greatly across resources. Consult the literature provided with specific equipment in use.
3. Before selecting a modality to accelerate a chronic wound, the clinician should understand the primary action of the modality on the healing process.
4. Hydrotherapy is indicated to help cleanse necrotic tissue and surface contaminants from chronic wounds and should be discontinued when the wound is clean.
5. Administration of pulsed ultrasound during the inflammatory phase of repair can accelerate natural debridement and release chemical mediators that can stimulate subsequent steps involved in tissue repair.
6. Comparatively, electrical stimulation therapy presently has the greatest number of well-designed, randomized, controlled clinical trials documenting its ability to accelerate healing and promote closure of chronic wounds.
7. Many best practice recommendations and guidelines produced in North America suggest that electrotherapy should be considered to treat individuals with chronic pressure ulcers.
8. Pneumatic compression therapy combined with stockings and bandages can reduce chronic edema associated with chronic venous ulcers.
9. UVC can kill bacteria and may be helpful in the treatment of wounds contaminated with bacteria that are resistant to other antimicrobial therapy.

REVIEW QUESTIONS

Select answers for questions 1–6 from the choice of modalities listed below.

    A. Pneumatic compression therapy   D. Electrical stimulation therapy
    B. UVC therapy   E. Pulsed ultrasound
    C. Laser therapy   F. Hydrotherapy

1. What modalities require direct application of the emitted energy to the wound bed and therefore require prior removal of all wound dressings?
2. What modalities need to be applied perpendicular to the tissue surface in order to optimize energy delivery to the target structure?
3. What modalities could be used on patients with wounds in which the wound and surrounding skin are very painful to touch?
4. What modalities would be best to treat
   a. chronic wounds that are delayed in healing because of an excessive bacterial load?
   b. wounds filled with necrotic tissue?
   c. deep wounds requiring new tissue formation to fill in wound defect?
   d. diabetic foot wounds in individuals with concurrent mild peripheral vascular disease?

5. What modalities act on the wound healing process to
   a. activate the inflammatory process?
   b. improve local blood flow?
   c. stimulate new tissue formation?
   d. improve wound strength?
   e. reduce tissue edema?
6. For what modality is the best clinical research evidence available to support their use on
   a. chronic pressure ulcers?
   b. chronic venous ulcers?
7. Describe a clinical scenario in which a client would most likely benefit from the use of therapeutic modalities to accelerate wound closure.
8. What factors can alter the biologic response to laser therapy and should be monitored, controlled, and documented with each treatment?

REFERENCES

1. Agaiby, A.D., Ghali, L.R., Wilson, R., and Dyson, M.: Laser modulation of angiogenic factor production by T-lymphocytes, Lasers Surg. Med. 26:357–363, 2000.
2. Akai, M., Oda, H., Shirasaki, Y., and Tateishi, T.: Electrical stimulation of ligament healing, Clin. Orthop. 235:296–301, 1988.
3. Al-Karmi, A.M., Dinno, M.A., Stoltz, D.A., Crum, L.A., and Matthews, J.C.: Calcium and the effects of ultrasound on frog skin, Ultrasound Med. Bio. 20:73–81, 1994.
4. Allendorf, J.D.F., Bessler, M., Huang, J., Kayton, M.L., Laird, D., Nowygrod, R., et al.: Helium-neon laser irradiation at fluences of 1, 2 and 4 J/cm² failed to accelerated wound healing as assessed by both wound contracture rate and tensile strength, Lasers Surg. Med. 20:340–345, 1997.
5. Alvarez, O., Mertz, P., Smerbeck, R., and Eaglstein, W.: The healing of superficial skin wounds is stimulated by external electrical current, J. Invest. Dermatol. 81:144–148, 1983.
6. Bach, S., Bilgrav, K., Gottrup, F., and Jorgensen, T.E.: The effect of electrical current on healing skin incision, Eur. J. Surg. 157:171–174, 1991.
7. Baker, L., Chambers, R., DeMuth, S., and Villar, F.: Effects of electrical stimulation on wound healing in patients with diabetic ulcers, Diabetes Care 20:405–412, 1997.
8. Baker, L., Rubayi, S., Villar, F., and DeMuth, S.: Effect of electrical stimulation waveform on healing of ulcers in human beings with spinal cord injury, Wound Repair Regen. 4:21–28, 1996.
9. Bergstrom, N., Bennett, M.A., Carlson, C.E., et al.: Clinical practice guideline number 15 : treatment of pressure ulcers, Rockville, MD, US Department of Health and Human Services, Public Health Services, Agency for Health Care Policy and Research: AHCPR Publication 95-065, 1995.
10. Bischt, D., Gupta, S.C., Misra, V., Mital, V.P., and Sharma, P.: Effect of low intensity laser radiation on healing of open skin wounds in rats, Indian J. Med. Res. 100:43–46, 1994.
11. Bohannon, R.W.: Whirlpool versus whirlpool rinse for removal of bacteria from a venous stasis ulcer, Phys. Ther. 62:304–308, 1982.
12. Bolton, P.A., Young, S., and Dyson, M.: Macrophage responsiveness to light therapy—a dose response study, LLLT 101–106, 1991.
13. Bouma, M.G., Buurman, W.A., and van den Wildenberg, F.A.J.M.: Low energy laser irradiation fails to modulate the inflammatory function of human monocytes and endothelial cells, Lasers Surg. Med. 19:207–221, 1996.
14. Bourguignon, G.J., Bourguignon, L.Y.W.: Electric stimulation of protein and DNA synthesis in human fibroblasts, FASEB J. 1:398–402, 1987.
15. Braverman, B., McCarthy, R.J., Ivankovich, A.D., Forde, D.E., Overfield, M., and Bapna, M.S.: Effect of helium-neon and infrared laser irradiation of wound healing in rabbits, Lasers Surg. Med. 9:50–58, 1989.
16. Broadley, C., Broadley, K.N., Disimone, G., Reinisch, L., and Davidson, J.M.: Low-energy helium-neon laser irradiation and the tensile strength of incisional wounds in the rat, Wound Repair Regen. 3:512–517, 1995.
17. Burger, A., Jordaan, A.J., and Schoombee, G.E.: The bactericidal effect of ultraviolet light on infected pressure sores, S. Afr. J. Physiother. 41(2):55–57, 1985.
18. Burgess, E., Hollinger, J., Bennett, S., Schmitt, J., Buck, D., Shannon, R., et al.: Charged beads enhance cutaneous wound healing in Rhesus non-human primates, Plast. Reconstr. Surg. 102:2395–2403, 1998.
19. Callam, M.J., Dale, J.J., Harper, D.R., and Ruckley, C.V.: A controlled trial of weekly ultrasound therapy in chronic leg ulceration, Lancet 2(8552):204–206, 1987.
20. Cameron, M.H.: Physical agents in rehabilitation: from research to practice, ed. 2, W.B. Saunder's, Toronto, 2003.
21. Carley, P.J., and Wainapel, S.F.: Electrotherapy for acceleration of wound healing: low intensity direct current, Arch. Phys. Med. Rehabil. 66:443–446, 1985.

22. Cheng, N., Hoof, H.V., Bockx, E., Hoogmartens, M.J., et al.: The effects of electric currents on ATP generation, protein synthesis, and membrane transport in rat skin, Clin. Orthop. 171:264–272, 1982.

23. Cherry, G.W., Wilson, J.: The treatment of ambulatory venous ulcer patients with warming therapy, Ostomy Wound Manage. 45:65–70, 1999.

24. Chu, C.S., McManus, A.T., Manson, A.D., Okerberg, C.V., and Pruitt, B.A.: Multiple graft harvestings from deep partial-thickness scald wounds healed under the influence of weak direct current, J. Trauma 30:1044–1050, 1990.

25. Coleridge-Smith, P., Sarin, S., Hasty, J., and Scurr, J.H.: Sequential gradient pneumatic compression enhances venous ulcer healing: a randomized trial, Surgery 108:871–875, 1990.

26. Conner Kerr, T.A., Sullivan, P.K., Gaillard, J., Franklin, M.E., and Jones, R.M.: The effects of ultraviolet radiation on antibiotic resistant bacteria in vitro, Ostomy Wound Manage. 44(10):50–56, 1990.

27. Consortium of Spinal Cord Medicine: Pressure Ulcer Prevention and Treatment Following Spinal Cord Injury: A Clinical Practice Guideline for Health Care Professionals, Sponsored by Paralyzed Veterans of America, pp. 43–45, 2000.

28. Cook, H.A., Morales, M., La Rosa, E.M., Dean, J., Donnelly, M.K., McHugh, P., et al.: Effects of electrical stimulation on lymphatic flow and limb volume in the rat, Phys. Ther. 74:1040–1046, 1994.

29. Cooper, M.S., Schilwa, M.: Electrical and ionic controls of tissue cell locomotion in DC electric field, J. Neurosci. Res. 13:223–244, 1985.

30. Crowell, J.A., Kusserow, B.K., and Nyborg, W.L.: Functional changes in white blood cells after microsonation, Ultrasound Med. Biol. 3:185, 1997.

31. Cullum, N., Nelson, E.A., Fletcher, A.W., and Sheldon, T.A.: Compression for venous leg ulcers, The Cochrane Library Issue 4, 2003.

32. De Deyne, P., Kirsch-Volders, M.: In Vitro effects of therapeutic ultrasound on the nucleus of human fibroblasts, Phys. Ther. 75:629–634, 1995.

33. Dinno, M.A., Dyson, M., Young, S.R., Mortimer, A.J., Hart, J., and Crum, L.A.: The significance of membrane changes in the safe and effective use of therapeutic and diagnostic ultrasound, Phys. Med. Biol. 34:1543–1552, 1989.

34. Dodgen, P.W., Johnson, B.W., Baker, L.L., and Chambers, R.B.: The effects of electrical stimulation on cutaneous oxygen supply in diabetic older adults, Phys. Ther. 67:793–793, 1987.

35. Dolynchuk, K., Keast, D., Campbell, K., Houghton, P.E., Orsted, H., and Sibbald, G.: Best practice guidelines for the treatment pressure ulcers, Ostomy Wound Manage. 46(11):38–53, 2000.

36. Dunn, M.G., Doillon, C.J., Berg, R.A., Olson, R.M., and Silver, F.H.: Wound healing using a collagen matrix: effect of DC electrical stimulation, J. Biomed. Mater. Res. App. Biomater. 22:191–206, 1988.

37. Dyson, M., Luke, D.A.: Induction of mast cell degranulation in skin by ultrasound, IEEE Trans. UFFC 133:194–201, 1986.

38. Dyson, M., Pond, J.B., Joseph, J., and Warwick, R.: The stimulation of tissue regeneration by means of ultrasound, Clin. Sci. 35:273–285, 1968.

39. Dyson, M., Woodward, B., and Pond, J.B.: Flow of red blood cells stopped by ultrasound, Nature 232:572–573, 1971.

40. Dyson, M., Suckling, J.: Stimulation of tissue repair by ultrasound: a survey of the mechanisms involved, Physiotherapy 64:105–108, 1978.

41. El Sayed, S.O., Dyson, M.: Effect of laser pulse repetition rate and pulse duration on mast cell number and degranulation, Lasers Surg. Med. 19:433–437, 1996.

42. Enwemeka, C.S.: Laser biostimulation of healing wounds: specific effects and mechanisms of action, JOPST 9(10):333–338, 1988.

43. Erickson, C.A., Nuccitelli R.: Embryonic fibroblast motility and orientation can be influenced by physiological electric fields, J. Cell Biol. 98:296–307, 1984.

44. Eriksson, S.V., Lundenberg, T., and Malm, M.: A placebo controlled trial of ultrasound therapy in chronic leg ulceration, Scand. J. Rehabil. Med. 23:211–213, 1991.

45. Esclamado, R.M., Damiano, G.A., and Cummings, C.W.: Effect of local hypothermia on early wound repair, Arch. Otolaryngol. Head Neck Surg. 116:803–808, 1990.

46. Faghri, P., Votto, J., and Hovorka, C.: Venous hemodynamics of the lower extremities in response to electrical stimulation, Arch. Phys. Med. Rehabil. 79:842–848, 1998.

47. Falanga, V., Bourguignon, G.J., and Bourguignon, L.Y.W.: Electrical stimulation increases the expression of fibroblast receptors for transforming growth factor-beta, Abstr. Wound Repair Regen. 88:488, 1987.

48. Feedar, J., Kloth, L., and Gentzkow, G.: Chronic dermal ulcer healing enhanced with monophasic pulsed electrical stimulation, Phys. Ther. 71:639–649, 1991.

49. Foulds, I.S., Barker, A.T.: Human skin battery potentials and their possible role in wound healing, Br. J. Dermatol. 109:515–522, 1983.

50. Fujita, M., Hukuda, S., and Doida, Y.: The effect of constant direct electrical current on intrinsic healing in the flexor tendon in vitro, J. Hand Surg.—Br. 17:94–98, 1992.

51. Fyfe, M.C., Chahl, L.A.: The effect of single or repeated applications of "therapeutic" ultrasound on plasma extravasation during silver nitrate induced inflammation of the rat hindpaw ankle joint in vivo, Ultrasound Med. Biol. 11:273–283, 1985.

52. Gan, B.S., Huys, S., Sherebrin, M.H., and Scilley, C.G.: The effects of ultrasound treatment on flexor tendon healing in the chicken limb, J. Hand Surg. 20B:809–814, 1995.

53. Gardner, S.E., Frantz, R.A., and Schmidt, F.L.: Effect of electrical stimulation on chronic wound healing: a meta-analysis, Wound Repair Regen. 7:495–503, 1999.

54. Gault, W., Gatens, P.: Use of low intensity direct current in management of ischemic skin ulcers, Phys. Ther. 56:265–269, 1976.

55. Gentzkow, G.D., Alon, G., Taler, G.A., Eltorai, I.M., and Montroy, R.E.: Healing of refractory stage III and IV pressure ulcers by a new electrical stimulation device, Wounds 5:160–172, 1993.

56. Gilcreast, D., Stotts, N.A., Froelicher, E., Baker, L., and Moss, K.: Effect of electrical stimulation on foot skin perfusion in persons with or at risk for diabetic foot ulcers, Wound Repair Regen. 6:434–441, 1998.

57. Gogia, P.P.: Low-energy laser in wound management. In Gogia, P.P., editor. Clinical wound management, Thorofare, NJ, Slack, pp. 165–172, 1995.

58. Griffin, J., Tooms, R., Mendius, R., Clifft, J., Vander Zwaag, R., and El-Zeky, F.: Efficacy of high voltage pulsed current for healing of pressure ulcers in patients with spinal cord injury, Phys. Ther. 71:433–444, 1991.

59. Griffin, J.W., Newsome, L.S., Stralka, S.W., and Wright, P.E.: Reduction of chronic posttraumatic hand edema: a comparison of high voltage pulsed current intermittent pneumatic compression, and placebo treatments, Phys. Ther. 170:279–286, 1990.

60. Hall, G., Anneroth, G., Schennings, T., Zetterqvist, L., and Ryden, H.: Effect of low level energy laser irradiation on wound healing. An experimental study in rats, Swed. Dent. J. 18:29–34, 1994.

61. Hall, J.D., Mount, D.W.: Mechanism of DNA replication and mutagenesis in ultraviolet-irradiated bacteria and mammalian cells, Prog. Nucleic Acid Res. Mol. Biol. 25:53–126, 1981.

62. Harvey, W., Dyson, M., Pond, J., and Grahame, R.: The 'in vitro' stimulation of protein synthesis in human fibroblasts by therapeutic levels of ultrasound, Rheumatol. Rehabil. 14: 237–240, 1975.

63. Hashish, I., Harvey, W., and Harris, M.: Anti-inflammatory effects of ultrasound therapy: evidence for a major placebo effect, Br. J. Rheumatol. 25:77–81, 1986.

64. Haynes, L.J., Brown, M.H., Handley, B.C., et al.: Comparison of Pulsavac and sterile whirlpool regarding the promotion of tissue granulation (abstract), Phys. Ther. 74(Suppl.):54, 1994.

65. High, A.S., High, J.P.: Treatment of infected skin wounds using ultra-violet radiation an in vitro study, Physiotherapy 89:359–360, 1983.

66. Hinsenkamp, M., Jercinovic, A., de Graef, C., Wilaert, F., and Heenen, M.: Effects of low frequency pulsed electrical current on Keratinocytes in vitro, Bioelectromagnetics 18:250–254, 1997.

67. Honmura, A., Yanase, M., Obata, J., and Haruki, E.: Therapeutic effect of ga-al-as diode laser irradiation on experimentally induced inflammation in rats, Lasers Surg. Med. 12:441–449, 1992.

68. Horwitz, L.R., Burke, T.J., and Carnegie, D.: Augmentation of wound healing using monochromatic infrared energy, Adv. Wound Care 12:35–40, 1999.

69. Houghton, P.E., Kincaid, C.B., Lovell, M., Campbell, K.E., Keast, D.H., Woodbury, M.G., and Harris, K.A.: Effect of electrical stimulation on chronic leg ulcer size and appearance, Phys. Ther. 83(1):17–28, 2003.

70. Hunter, J., Leonard, L., Wilson, R., Snider, G., and Dixon, J.: Effects of low energy laser on wound healing in a porcine model, Lasers Surg. Med. 3:285–290, 1984.

71. Im, M.J., Lee, W.P.A., and Hoopes, J.E.: Effect of electrical stimulation on survival of skin flaps in pigs, Phys. Ther. 70:37–40, 1990.

72. Jackson, B.A., Schwane, J.A., and Starcher, B.C.: Effect of ultrasound therapy on the repair of Achilles tendon injuries in rats, Med. Sci. Sports Exerc. 23:171–176, 1991.

73. Johannsen, F., Nyholm, A., and Karlsmark, T.: Ultrasound therapy in chronic leg ulceration: a meta-analysis, Wound Repair Regen. 6:121–126, 1998.

74. Junger, M., Zuder, D., Steins, A., Hahn, M., and Klyscz, T.: Treatment of venous ulcers with low frequency pulsed current (Dermapulse): effects on cutaneous microcirculation, Hautartz 18:897–903, 1997.

75. Kaada, B.: Promoted healing of chronic ulceration by transcutaneous nerve stimulation (TNS), VASA 12:262–269, 1983.

76. Karu, Ti., Ryabykh, T.P., Fedoseyeva, G.E., and Puchkova, N.I.: Helium-neon laser induced respiratory burst of phagocytic cells, Lasers Surg. Med. 9:585–588, 1989.

77. Katelaris, P.M., Fletcher, J.P., Little, J.M., McEntyre, R.J., and Jeffcoate, KW.: Electrical stimulation in the treatment of chronic venous ulceration, Aust. N.Z. J. Surg. 57:605–607, 1987.

78. Kincaid, C.B., Lavoie, K.H.: Inhibition of bacterial growth in vitro following stimulation with high voltage, monophasic, pulsed current, Phys. Ther. 69:651–655, 1989.

79. Kitchen, S.: Electrotherapy: evidence-based practice, ed. 11, Toronto, 2002, Churchill Livingstone.

80. Kloth, L., Feedar, J.: Acceleration of wound healing with high voltage, monophasic, pulsed current, Phys. Ther. 68:503–508, 1988.

81. Kloth, L.C., McCulloch, J.M.: Wound healing alternatives management, ed. 3, Philadelphia, PA, 2002, F.A. Davis.

82. Kloth, L.C., et al.: Effects of normothermic dressing on pressure ulcer healing, Adv. Skin Wound Care 13:69–74, 2000.

83. Kloth, L.C.: Proceedings of Symposium on Advanced Wound Care. Proceedings of the 13th Annual meeting of the American Association of Wound Care (AAWC) and Medical Research Forum, Dallas, TX, April 1–6, 2000.

84. Kloth, L.C., McCulloch, J.M.: Promotion of wound healing with electrical stimulation, Adv. Wound Care 9:42–45, 1996.

85. Kolari, P.I., Pekanmaki, K.: Intermittent pneumatic compression in healing of venous ulcers, Lancet 2:1108, 1986.

86. Kovacs, I., Mester, E., and Gorog, P.: Laser-induced stimulation of the vascularization of the healing wound. An ear chamber experiment, Experientia 15:341–343, 1974.

87. Kunimoto, B., Gulliver, W., Cooling, M., Houghton, P., Orsted, and Sibbald, R.G.: Recommendations for practice: prevention and treatment of venous leg ulcers, Ostomy Wound Manage. 47(2):34–50, 2001.

88. Kurz, A., Sessler, K.I., and Lenhardt, R.: Perioperative normothermia to reduce the incidence of surgical-wound infection and shorten hospitalization, N. Engl. J. Med. 334:1209–1215, 1996.

89. Litke, D.S., Dahners, L.E.: Effects of different levels of direct current on early ligament healing in a rat model, J. Orthop. Res. 12:683–688, 1994.

90. Lundeberg, T., Nordstrom, F., Brodda-Jansen, G., Eriksson, S.V., Kjartansson, J., and Samuelson, U.E.: Pulsed ultrasound does not improve healing of venous ulcers, Scand. J. Rehabil. Med. 22:195–197, 1990.

91. Lundeberg, T.C.M., Eriksson, S.V., and Malm, M.: Electrical nerve stimulation improves healing of diabetic ulcers, Ann. Plast. Surg. 29:328–330, 1992.

92. Mackie, R.M., Elwood, J.M., and Hawk, J.L.M.: Links between exposure to ultraviolet radiation and skin cancer, J.R. Coll. Physicians Lond. 21:91–96, 1987.

93. Malm, M., Lundeberg, T.: Effect of low power gallium arsenide laser on healing of venous ulcers, Scand. J. Plast. Reconstr. Hand Surg. 25:249–251, 1991.

94. Maxwell, L.: Therapeutic ultrasound: its effects on the cellular and molecular mechanisms of inflammation and repair, Physiotherapy 78:421–426, 1992.

95. McCaughan, J., Bethel, B., Johnston, T., and Janssen, W.: Effect of low-dose argon irradiation on rate of wound closure, Lasers Surg. Med. 5:607–614, 1985.

96. McCulloch, J.M., Boyd, V.B.: The effects of whirlpool and the dependent position on lower extremity volume, J. Orthop. Sports Phys. Ther. 16(4):169–173, 1992.

97. McCulloch, J.M., Marler, K.C., Neal, M.B., et al.: Intermittent pneumatic compression improves venous ulcer healing, Adv. Wound Care 7:22–26, 1994.

98. McDiarmid, T., Burns, P.N., Lewith, G.T., and Machin, D.: Ultrasound and the treatment of pressure sores, Physiotherapy 71:66–70, 1985.

99. McGinnis, M.E., Vanable, J.W.: Wound epithelium controls stump currents, Develop. Biol. 116:174–18, 1986.

100. McMaster, W.C., Liddle, S.: Cryotherapy influence on post-traumatic limb edema, Clin. Orthop. 150:283–287, 1980.

101. Meeker, B.J.: Description of the effects of whirlpool therapy on postoperative pain and surgical wound healing, Louisiana State University Medical CTR in New Orleans School of Nursing, D.N.S. 109, 1994.

102. Mertz, P.M., Davis, S.C., Cazzaniga, A.L., Cheng, K., Reich, J.D., and Eaglstein, W.H.: Electrical stimulation: acceleration of soft tissue repair by varying the polarity, Wounds 5:153–15, 1993.

103. Mester, A.F., Mester, A.: Wound healing, Low Level Laser Therapy (LLLT), 7–15, 1989.

104. Michlovitz, S.L.: Thermal agents in rehabilitation, ed. 3, Philadelphhia, PA, 1996, F.A. Davis.

105. Mohr, T., Akers, T.K., and Wessman, H.C.: Effect of high voltage stimulation on blood flow in the rat hind limb, Phys. Ther. 67:526–533, 1987.

106. Mulder, G., Robinson, J., and Seeley, J.: Study of sequential compression treatment of non healing chronic venous ulcers, Wounds 3:111–115, 1990.

107. Mulder, G.D.: Treatment of open-skin wounds with electric stimulation, Arch. Phys. Med. Rehabil. 72:375–377, 1991.

108. Nessler, J.P., Mass, D.P.: Direct-current electrical stimulation of tendon healing in vitro, Clin. Orthop. 217:303–312, April 1987.

109. Newton, R., Karselis, T.: Skin pH following high voltage pulsed galvanic stimulation, Phys. Ther. 63:1593–1596, 1983.

110. Niederhuber, S., Stribley, R.F., and Koepke, G.H.: Reduction of skin bacterial load with use of therapeutic whirlpool, Phys. Ther. 55(5):482–486, 1975.

111. Noble, P.B., Shields, E.D., Blecher, P.D.M., and Bentley, K.C.: Locomotory characteristics of fibroblasts within a three-dimensional collagen lattice: modulation by a helium/neon soft laser, Lasers Surg. Med. 12:669–674, 1992.

112. Nussbaum, E.L., Biemann, I., and Mustard, B.: Comparison of ultrasound/ultraviolet-C and laser for treatment of pressure ulcers in patients with spinal cord injury, Phys. Ther. 74:812–825, 1994.

113. Nussbaum, E.L., Lilge, L., and Mazzulli, T.: Effects of 630,660,810, and 905 nm Laser irradiation delivering radiant exposure of 1–50 J/cm^2 on three species of bacteria in vitro, J. Clin. Laser Med. Surg. 20(6):325–333, 2002.

114. Ogiwara, S.: Calf muscle pumping and rest positions during and/or after whirlpool therapy, J. Phys. Ther. Sci. 13(2):99–105, 2001.

115. Ohta, A., Abergel, R.P., and Uitto, J.: Laser modulation of human immune system: inhibition of lymphocyte proliferation by a gallium-arsenide laser at low energy, Lasers Surg. Med. 7:199–201, 1987.

116. Orida, N., Feldman, J.D.: Directional protrusive pseudopodial activity and motility in macrophages induced by extracellular electric fields, Cell Motil. 2:243–255, 1982.

117. Ovington, L.G.: Dressings and adjunctive therapies: AHCPR guidelines revisited, Ostomy Wound Manage. 45(1A):94S–106S, 1999.

118. Owoeye, I., Spielholz, NI., and Nelson, A.J.: Low-intensity pulsed galvanic current and the healing of tenotomized rat achilles tendons: preliminary report using load-to-break measurements, Arch. Phys. Med. Rehabil. 68:415–418, 1987.

119. Pekanmaki, K., Kolari, P.J., and Kiistala, U.: Intermittent pneumatic compression treatment for post-thrombotic leg ulcers, Clin. Exp. Dermatol. 12:350–353, 1987.

120. Peschen, M., Weichenthal, M., Schopf, E., and Vanscheidt, W.: Low frequency ultrasound treatment of chronic venous leg ulcers in an outpatient therapy, Acta Derm. Venereol. (Stockh.) 77:311–314, 1997.

121. Peters, E.J., Armstrong, D.G., Wunderlich, R.P., Bosma, J., Stacpoole-Shea, S., and Lavery, L.A.: The benefit of electrical stimulation to enhance perfusion in persons with diabetes mellitus, J. Foot Ankle Surg. 37(5):396–400, 1998.

122. Pourreau-Schneider, N., Ahmed, A., Soudry, M., Jacquemier, J., Kopp, F., Franquin, J.C., et al.: Helium-neon laser treatment transforms fibroblasts into myofibroblasts, Am. J. Pathol. 137: 171–178, 1990.

123. Prentice, W.E.: Therapeutic modalities for physical therapists, ed. 2, McGraw-Hill Medical Publishing Division, 1999, New York.

124. Price, P., Bale, S., Crook, H., and Harding, K.G.: The effect of a radiant heat dressing on pressure ulcers, J. Wound Care 9:201–205, 2000.

125. Rabkin, J.M., Hunt, T.K.: Local heat increases blood flow and oxygen tension in wounds, Arch. Surg. 122:221–225, 1987.

126. Reddy, G.K., Stehno-Bittel, L., and Enwemeka, C.S.: Laser photostimulation of collagen production in healing rabbit Achilles tendons, Lasers Surg. Med. 22:281–287, 1998.

127. Reed, B.V.: Effect of high voltage pulsed electrical stimulation on microvascular permeability to plasma proteins, Phys. Ther. 4:491–495, 1988.

128. Reich, J.D., Cazzaniga, A.L., Mertz, P.M., Kerdel, F.A., and Eaglstein, W.H.: The effect of electrical stimulation on the

number of mast cells in healing wounds, J. Am. Acad. Dermatol. 25:40–46, 1991.

129. Roche, C., West, J.: A controlled trial investigating the effect of ultrasound on venous ulcers referred from general practitioners, Physiotherapy 12:475–477, 1984.

130. Rohrer, M.J., Natale, A.M.: Effect of hypothermia on the coagulation cascade, Crit. Care Med. 10:1402–1405, 1992.

131. Rosario, R., Mark, G.J., Parrish, J.A., and Mihm, M.C.: Histological changes produced in skin by equally erythemogenic doses of UV-A, UV-B, UV-C and UV-A with psoralens, Br. J. Dermatol. 101:299–308, 1979.

132. Rubin, M.J., Etchison, M.R., Condra, K.A., Franklin, T.D., and Snoddy, A.M.: Acute effects of ultrasound on skeletal muscle oxygen tension, blood flow and capillary density, J. Med. Biol. 16:271–277, 1990.

133. Sachsenmaier, C., Radler-Pohlm, A., Zinck, R., et. al.: Involvement of growth factor receptors in the mammalian UVC response, Cell 78:963–972, 1994.

134. Santilli, S.M., Valusek, P.A., and Robinson, C.: Use of a noncontact radiant heat bandage for the treatment of chronic venous stasis ulcers, Adv. Wound Care 12:89–93, 1999.

135. Santoianni, P., Monfrecola, G., Martellotta, D., and Ayala, F.: Inadequate effect of helium-neon laser on venous leg ulcers, Photodermatology 1:245–249, 1984.

136. Saperia, D., Glassberg, E., Lyons, R.F., Abergel, P., Baneux, P., Castel, J.C., et. al.: Demonstration of elevated type I and type III procollagen mRNA levels in cutaneous wounds treated with helium-neon laser, Biochem. Biophys. Res. Commun. 138: 1123–1128, 1986.

137. Schindl, A., Schindl, M., and Schindl, L.: Successful treatment of a persistent radiation ulcer by low power laser therapy, J. Am. Acad. Dermatol. 37:646–649, 1997.

138. Scott, E.M., Leaper, D.J., Clark, M., and Kelly, P.J.: Effects of warming therapy on pressure ulcers—a randomised trial, AORN J. 73(5):921–938, 2001.

139. Shuttleworth, E., Banfield, K.: Light relief, Wound Care 70–78, 1996.

140. Skinner, S., Gage, J., Wilce, P., and Shaw, R.: A preliminary study of the effects of laser radiation on collagen metabolism in cell culture, Aust. Dent. J. 41:188–192, 1996.

141. Smith, J., Romansky, N., Vomero, J., and Davis, R.: The effect of electrical stimulation on wound healing in diabetic mice, J. Am. Podiatry Assoc. 74:71–75, 1984.

142. Solomon, S.L.: Host factors in whirlpool-associated pseudomonas Aeruginosa skin disease, Infect. Control 16:402–406, 1985.

143. Stevenson, J.H., Pang, C.Y., Lindsay, W.K., and Zuker, Rm.: Functional, mechanical and biochemical assessment of ultrasound therapy on tendon healing in the chicken toe, Plast. Reconstr. Surg. 77:965–970, 1986.

144. Surinchak, J.S., Alago, M.L., Bellamy, R.F., Stuck, B.E., and Belkin, M.: Effects of low-level energy lasers on the healing of full-thickness skin defects, Lasers Surg. Med. 2:267–274, 1983.

145. Sussman, C.: Wound care: a collaborative practice manual for phys. therapic and nurses. Gaithersburg, MD, 1998, Aspen Publications.

146. Szuminsky, N.J., Albers, A.C., Unger, P., and Eddy, J.G.: Effect of narrow, pulsed high voltages on bacterial viability, Phys. Ther. 74:660–667, 1994.

147. Taylor, K., Fish, D.R., Mendel, F.C., and Burton, H.W.: Effect of a single 30-minute treatment of high voltage pulsed current on edema formation in frog hind limbs, Phys. Ther. 72:63–68, 1992.

148. ter Riet, G., Kessels, A.G.H., and Knipschild, P.: A randomized clinical trial of ultrasound in the treatment of pressure ulcers, Phys. Ther. 76(12):1301–1311, 1996.

149. Thai, T.P., Houghton, P.E., Campbell, K.E., Keast, D.H., and Woodbury. M.G.: Effects of ultraviolet light C (UVC) on bacterial colonization of chronic wounds, Ostomy Wound Manage. 2004 (in press).

150. Thai, T.P., Houghton, P.E., Campbell, K.E., Keast., D.H., and Woodbury, M.G.: The role of ultraviolet light C (UVC) in the treatment of chronic wounds with MRSA, Ostomy Wound Manage. 48(11):52–60, 2002.

151. Trengove, N.J., Stacey, M.C., MacAuley, S., Bennett, N., Gibson, J., Burslem, F., Murphy, G., and Schultz, G.: Analysis of acute and chronic wound environments: the role of proteases and their inhibitors, Wound Repair Regen. 7(6):442–452, 1999.

152. Turner, S.M., Powell, E.S., and Ng, C.S.S.: The effect of ultrasound on the healing of repaired cockerel tendon: is collagen cross-linkage a factor? J. Hand Surg. 14B:428–433, 1989.

153. Weichenthal, M., Mohr, P., Stegmann, W., and Brejtbart, E.W.: Low frequency ultrasound treatment of chronic venous ulcers, Wound Repair Regen. 5:18–22, 1997.

154. Weston, M., Taber, C., Casagranda, L., and Cornwall, M.: Changes in local blood volume during gel pack application to traumatized ankles, J. Orthop. Sports Phys. Ther. 19:197–199, 1994.

155. Williams, A.R., Miller, D.L., and Gross, D.R.: Haemolysis in vivo by therapeutic intensities of ultrasound, Ultrasound Med. Biol. 12:501–509, 1986.

156. Wilson, M., Yianni, C.: Killing of methicillin-resistant staphylococcus aureus by low power laser light, J. Med. Microbiol. 42:62–66, 1997.

157. Wood, J.M., Evans, P.E., Schallreuter, K.U., Jacobson, W.E., Swift, R., Newman, J., White, C., and Jacobson, M.: A multicenter study on the use of pulsed low-intensity direct current for healing chronic stage II and stage III decubitus ulcers, Arch. Dermatol. 129:999–1009, 1993.

158. Young, S., Bolton, P., Dyson, M., Harvey, W., and Diamantopoulos, C.: Macrophage responsiveness to light therapy, Lasers Surg. Med. 9:497–505, 1989.

159. Young, S.R., Dyson, M.: Effect of therapeutic ultrasound on the healing of full-thickness excised skin lesions, Ultrasonics 28:175–179, 1990.

160. Young, S.R., Dyson, M.: Macrophage responsiveness to therapeutic ultrasound, Ultrasound Med. Biol. 16:809–816 1990.

161. Yu, H-S., Chang, K-L., Yu, C-L., Chen, J-W., and Chen, G-S.: Low-energy helium-neon laser irradiation stimulates interleukin-1 alpha and interleukin-8 release from cultured human keratinocytes, J. Invest. Dermatol. 107:593–596, 1996.

162. Zhao, M., Dick, A., Forrester, J.V., and McCaig, C.D.: Electric field-directed cell motility involves up-regulated expression and asymmetric redistribution of the epidermal growth factor receptors and is enhanced by fibronectin and laminin, Mol. Biol. Cell 10:1259–1276, 1999.

163. Zhao. M., McCaig., C.D., Fernandez, A.A., Forrester, J.V., and Araki-Sasaki, K.: Human corneal epithelial cells reorient and migrate cathodally in a small applied electric field, Curr. Eye Res. 16:973–984, 1997.

164. Zhuang, H., Wang, W., Seldes, R.M., Tahernia, A.D., Fan, H., and Brighton, C.T.: Electrical stimulation induces the level of TGF-β1 mRNA in osteoblastic cells by a mechanism involving calcium/calmodulin pathway, Biochem. Biophys. Res. Commun. 237:225–229, 1997.

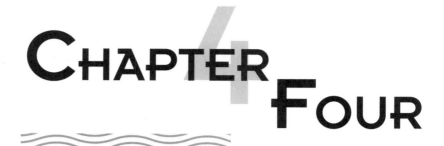

CHAPTER FOUR

MANAGING PAIN WITH THERAPEUTIC MODALITIES

CRAIG R. DENEGAR and
PHILLIP B. DONLEY

OBJECTIVES

Following completion of this chapter, the student therapist will be able to:

- ✔ Compare the various types of pain, and appraise their positive and negative effects.
- ✔ Choose a technique for assessing pain.
- ✔ Analyze the characteristics of sensory receptors.
- ✔ Examine how the nervous system relays information about painful stimuli.
- ✔ Distinguish the different neurophysiologic mechanisms for pain control for the therapeutic modalities used by therapists.
- ✔ Predict how pain perception can be modified by cognitive factors.

UNDERSTANDING PAIN

The International Association for the Study of Pain (IASP) defines **pain** as "an unpleasant sensory and emotional experience associated with actual or potential tissue damage, or described in terms of such damage."[24] Pain is a subjective sensation with more than one dimension and an abundance of descriptors of its qualities and characteristics. In spite of its universality, pain is composed of a variety of human discomforts, rather than being a single entity.[22] The perception of pain can be subjectively modified by past experiences and expectations. Much of what we do to treat patients' pain is to change their perceptions of pain.[4]

Pain does itself have a purpose. It warns us that there is something wrong and can provoke a withdrawal response to avoid further injury. It also results in muscle spasm and guarding or protection of the injured part. However, pain can persist after it is no longer useful. It can become a means of enhancing disability and inhibiting efforts to rehabilitate the patient. Prolonged spasm, which leads to circulatory deficiency, muscle atrophy, disuse habits, and conscious or unconscious guarding, may lead to a severe loss of function.[18] Chronic pain may become a disease state in itself. As defined by the IASP, chronic pain is "a persistent pain that is not amendable, as a rule, to treatments based on specific remedies, or through the routine methods of pain control such as nonnarcotic analgesics."[25] Often lacking an identifiable cause, chronic pain can totally disable a patient.

Research in recent years has led to a better understanding of pain and pain relief. This research also has raised new questions, although leaving many unanswered. We now have better explanations for the analgesic properties of the physical agents we use, as well as a better understanding of the psychology of pain. Newer physical agents, such as laser, and recent improvements to older agents, such as diathermy and transcutaneous electrical nerve simulators, offer new approaches to the treatment of musculoskeletal injury and pain. The evolution of the treatment of pain is, however, incomplete. Not even the mechanisms for the analgesic response to the simplest therapeutic modalities, heat and cold, have been fully described.[35]

The control of pain is an essential aspect of caring for the injured patient. The therapist has several therapeutic agents with analgesic properties from which to choose. The selection of a therapeutic agent should be based on a sound understanding of its physical properties and physiologic effects. This chapter does not provide a complete explanation of neurophysiology, pain, and pain relief. Several physiology textbooks provide extensive discussions of human neurophysiology and neurobiology to supplement this chapter. Instead, this chapter presents an overview of some theories of pain control, intended to provide a stimulus for the therapist to develop his or her own rationale for using modalities in the plan of care for patients treated. Ideally, it will also facilitate growth in the body of evidence from which improved responses to the therapeutic agents used in the treatment of pain can be derived.

Many of the modalities discussed in later chapters have analgesic properties. Often, they are employed to reduce pain and permit the patient to perform therapeutic exercises. Some understanding of what pain is, how it affects us, and how it is perceived is essential for the therapist who uses these modalities.

TYPES OF PAIN

Traditionally, pain has been categorized as either **acute** or **chronic**. Acute pain is experienced when tissue damage is impending and after injury has occurred. Pain lasting for more than 6 months is generally classified as chronic.[6] More recently, the term **persistent pain** has been used to differentiate chronic pain that defies intervention from conditions where continuing (persistent) pain is a symptom of a treatable condition.[14,30] There is more research devoted to chronic pain and its treatment, but acute and persistent confront the therapist most often.

The patient's pain experience provides the physical therapist with the foundation of the examination and diagnostic process. The site or pattern of pain, however, is not necessarily the site of the tissue lesion. **Referred pain**, which also may be either acute or chronic, is pain that is perceived to be in an area that seems to have little relation to the existing pathology. For example, injury to the spleen often results in pain in the left shoulder. This pattern, known as Kehr's sign, is useful for identifying this serious injury and arranging prompt emergency care. Referred pain can outlast the causative events because of altered reflex patterns, continuing mechanical stress on muscles, learned habits of guarding, or the development of hypersensitive areas, called **trigger points**.

Irritation of nerves and nerve roots can cause radiating pain. Pressure on the lumbar nerve roots associated with a herniated disc or a contusion of the sciatic nerve can result in pain radiating down the lower extremity to the foot.

Deep somatic pain is a type that seems to be sclerotomic (associated with a **sclerotome**, a segment of bone innervated by a spinal segment). There is often a discrepancy between the site of the disorder and the site of the pain.

PAIN ASSESSMENT

The patient's perception of pain can differ markedly from person to person, as can the terminology used to describe the type of pain experienced. The therapist commonly asks the patient to describe what the pain feels like during an injury evaluation.

Terms like "sharp," "dull," "aching," "throbbing," "burning," "piercing," "localized," and "generalized" are often used by the patient. It is sometimes difficult for the therapist to infer what exactly is causing a particular type of pain. For example, "burning" pain is often associated with some injury to a nerve, but certainly there are other injuries that may produce what the patient is perceiving as "burning" pain. Thus verbal descriptions of the type of pain should be applied with caution.

Pain is a complex phenomenon that is difficult to evaluate and quantify because it is subjective and is influenced by attitudes and beliefs of the therapist and patient. Quantification is hindered by the fact that pain is a very difficult concept to put into words.[1]

Although obtaining an accurate and standardized assessment of pain is problematic, several tools have been developed to assist the clinician in evaluating patients and monitoring changes in their condition over time. These pain profiles identify the type of pain, quantify the intensity of pain, evaluate the effect of the pain experience on the patient's level of function, and assess the psychosocial impact of pain.

The pain profiles are useful. They compel the patient to verbalize the pain and thereby provide an outlet for the patient and provide the therapist a better understanding of the pain experience. They assess the psychosocial response to pain and injury. The pain profile can assist with the evaluation process by improving communication and directing the therapist toward appropriate diagnostic tests. These assessments also assist the therapist in identifying which therapeutic agents may be effective and when they should be applied. Finally, these profiles provide a standard measure to monitor treatment progress.[12]

PAIN ASSESSMENT SCALES

The following profiles are used in the evaluation of acute and chronic pain associated with illnesses and injuries.

Visual Analog Scales

Pain Assessment Techniques
- Visual analog scales
- Pain charts
- McGill Pain Questionnaire
- Activity Pattern Indicators Profile
- Numeric pain scales

Visual analog scales are quick and simple tests completed by the patient (Fig. 4-1). These scales consist of a line, usually 10 cm in length, the extremes of which are taken to represent the limits of the pain experience. One end is defined as "NO PAIN" and the other as "SEVERE PAIN." The patient is asked to mark the line at a point corresponding to the severity of the pain. The distance between "NO PAIN" and the mark represents pain severity. A similar scale can be used to assess treatment effectiveness by placing "NO PAIN RELIEF" at one end of the scale and "COMPLETE PAIN RELIEF" at the other. These scales can be completed daily or more often as pre- and posttreatment assessments.[16]

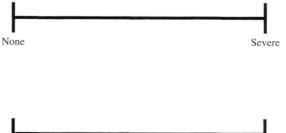

•**Figure 4-1** Visual analog scales.

Pain Charts

Pain charts can be used to establish spatial properties of pain. These two-dimensional graphic portrayals are completed by the patient to assess the location of pain and a number of subjective components. Simple line drawings of the body in several postural positions are presented to the patient (Fig. 4-2). The patient draws or colors the pictures in areas that correspond to the pain experience. Different colors are used for different sensations. For example, blue for aching pain, yellow for numbness or tingling, red for burning pain, and green for cramping pain. Descriptions can be added to the form to enhance the communication value. The form could be completed daily.[19]

McGill Pain Questionnaire

The McGill Pain Questionnaire (MPQ) is a tool with 78 words that describe pain (Fig. 4-3). These words are grouped into 20 sets that are divided into four categories, representing dimensions of the pain experience. Completion of the MPQ may take 20 minutes and is often frustrating for patients who do not speak English well. It is commonly administered to patients with low back pain. When administered every 2–4 weeks it has demonstrated changes in status very clearly.[22]

Activity Pain Indicators Profile

The Activity Pattern Indicators Pain Profile measures patient activity. It is a 64-question, self-report tool that may be used to assess functional impairment associated with pain. The instrument measures the frequency of certain behaviors such as housework, recreation, and social activities.[14]

Numeric Pain Scales

The most common acute pain profile used in outpatient clinics today is a numeric pain scale. The patient is asked to rate his or her pain on a scale from 1 to 10, with 10 representing the worst pain experienced or imaginable. The question is asked before and after treatment. When treatments provide pain relief, patients are asked about the extent and duration of the relief. In addition, the patient may be asked to estimate the portion of the day in which he or she experiences pain and about specific activities that

Treatment Tip
There are a number of pain evaluation tools, including visual analog scales, pain charts, the McGill Pain Questionnaire, the Activity Pattern Indicators Profile, and numeric pain scales. Numeric pain scales, in which patients are asked to rate their pain on a scale from 1 to 10, are perhaps the most widely used in the clinical setting.

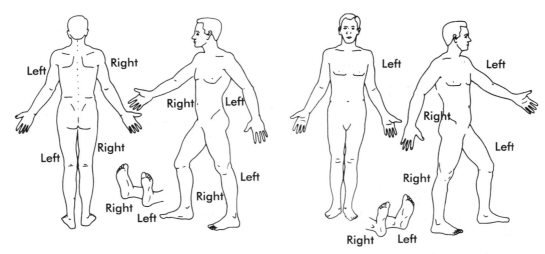

•**Figure 4-2** The pain chart. Use the following instructions: "Please use all of the figures to show me exactly where all your pains are and where they radiate to. Shade or draw with blue marker. Only the patient is to fill out this sheet. Please be as precise and detailed as possible. Use yellow marker for numbness and tingling. Use red marker for burning or hot areas and green marker for cramping. Please remember: blue = pain; yellow = numbness and tingling; red = burning or hot areas; green = cramping." (Used with permission from Melzack, R.: Pain measurement and assessment, New York, 1983, Raven Press.)

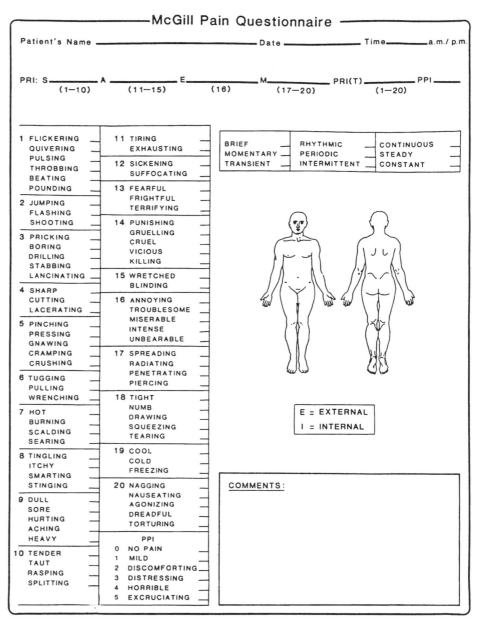

•Figure 4-3 McGill Pain Questionnaire. The descriptors fall into four major groups: Sensory, 1–10; affective, 11–15; evaluative, 16; and miscellaneous, 17–20. The rank value for each descriptor is based on its position in the word set. The sum of the rank values is the pain rating index (PRI). The present pain intensity (PPI) is based on a scale of 0–5. (Used with permission from Melzack, R.: Pain measurement and assessment, New York, 1983, Raven Press.)

increase or decrease pain. When pain affects sleep, the patient may be asked to estimate the amount of sleep gotten in the previous 24 hours. In addition, the amount of medication required for pain can be noted. This information helps the therapist assess changes in pain, select appropriate treatments, and communicate more clearly with the patient about the course of recovery from injury or surgery.

All of these scales help the patient communicate the severity and duration of his or her pain and appreciate changes that occur. Often in a long recovery, patients lose sight of how much progress has been made in terms of the pain experience and return to functional activities. A review of these pain scales often can serve to reassure the patient, foster a brighter, more positive outlook, and reinforce the commitment to the plan of treatment.

Documentation

The efficacy of many of the treatments used by therapists has not been fully substantiated. These scales are one source of data that can help therapists identify the most effective approaches to managing common injuries. These assessment tools can also be useful when reviewing a patient's progress with physicians and third-party payers.

TISSUE SENSITIVITY

The four structures most sensitive to damaging (noxious) stimuli are (1) the **periosteum** and **joint capsule**; (2) subchondral bone, tendons, and ligament; (3) muscle and cortical bone; and (4) the synovium and articular cartilage. A variety of "silent" fractures produce little or no pain. Different anatomic tissues exhibit varying degrees of sensitivity to pain. **Avulsion fractures** tend to be quite painful, because they tear away the periosteum. Musculoskeletal pain usually is spread over a large area unless it is close to the surface. For example, a hamstring strain usually results in pain over the posterior thigh, whereas an acromioclavicular sprain usually localizes over the joint.

periosteum A highly vascularized and innervated membrane lining the surface of bone.

GOALS IN MANAGING PAIN

Regardless of the cause of pain, its reduction is an essential part of treatment. Pain signals the patient to seek assistance and often is useful in establishing a diagnosis. Once the injury or illness is diagnosed, pain serves little purpose. Medical or surgical treatment or immobilization is necessary to treat some conditions, but physical therapy and an early return to activity are appropriate following many injuries. The physical therapist's objectives are to encourage the body to heal through exercise designed to progressively increase functional capacity and to return the patient to work and recreational and other activities as swiftly and safely as possible. Pain will inhibit therapeutic exercise. The challenge for the physical therapist is to control acute pain and protect the patient from further injury while encouraging progressive exercise in a supervised environment.

PAIN PERCEPTION AND NEURAL TRANSMISSION

SENSORY RECEPTORS

There are several types of sensory receptors in the body, and the physical therapist should be aware of their existence and the types of stimuli that activate them (Table 4-1). Activation of some of these sense organs with therapeutic agents will decrease the patient's perception of pain.

Six different types of receptor nerve endings are commonly described.

1. Meissner's corpuscles are activated by light touch.
2. Pacinian corpuscles respond to deep pressure.
3. Merkel's corpuscles respond to deep pressure, but more slowly than pacinian corpuscles, and also are activated by hair follicle deflection.
4. Ruffini corpuscles in the skin are sensitive to touch, tension, and possibly heat; those in the joint capsules and ligaments are sensitive to change in position.
5. Krause's end bulbs are thermoreceptors that react to a decrease in temperature and touch.[30]
6. Pain receptors, called **nociceptors** or **free nerve endings**, are sensitive to extreme mechanical, thermal, or chemical energy.[3] They respond to noxious stimuli, namely, to impending or actual tissue damage (e.g., cuts, burns, sprains). The term **nociceptive** is from the Latin *nocere*, to damage, and is used to imply pain information. These organs respond to superficial forms of heat and cold, analgesic balms, and massage.

TABLE 4-1   **Some Characteristics of Selected Sensory Receptors**

Type of Sensory Receptors	Stimulus		Receptor	
	General Term	Specific Nature	Term	Location
Mechanoreceptors	Pressure	Movement of hair in a hair follicle	Afferent nerve fiber	Base of hair follicles
		Light pressure	Meissner's corpuscle	Skin
		Deep pressure	Pacinian corpuscle	Skin
		Touch	Merkel's touch corpuscle	Skin
Nociceptors	Pain	Distension (stretch)	Free nerve endings	Wall of gastrointestinal tract, pharynx, skin
Proprioceptors	Tension	Distension	Corpuscles of Ruffini	Skin and capsules in joints and ligaments
		Length changes	Muscle spindles	Skeletal muscle
		Tension changes	Golgi tendon organs	Between muscles and tendons
Thermoreceptors	Temperature change	Cold	Krause's end bulbs	Skin
		Heat	Corpuscles of Ruffini	Skin and capsules in joints and ligaments

From Previte J.J. *Human physiology*, New York, 1983, McGraw-Hill.

Proprioceptors found in muscles, joint capsules, ligaments, and tendons provide information regarding joint position and muscle tone. The muscle spindles react to changes in length and tension when the muscle is stretched or contracted. The Golgi tendon organs also react to changes in length and tension within the muscle. See Table 4-1 for a more complete listing.

Some sensory receptors respond to phasic activity and produce an impulse when the stimulus is increasing or decreasing, but not during a sustained stimulus. They adapt to a constant stimulus. Meissner's corpuscles and pacinian corpuscles are examples of such receptors.

Tonic receptors produce impulses as long as the stimulus is present. Examples of tonic receptors are muscle spindles, free nerve endings, and Krause's end bulbs. The initial impulse is at a higher frequency than later impulses, which occur during sustained stimulation.

Accommodation is the decline in generator potential and the reduction of frequency that occurs with a prolonged stimulus or with frequently repeated stimuli. If some physical agents are used too often or for too long the receptors may adapt to or accommodate the stimulus and reduce their impulses. The accommodation phenomenon can be observed with the use of superficial hot and cold agents, such as ice packs and hydrocollator packs.

As a stimulus becomes stronger, the number of receptors excited increases and the frequency of the impulses increases. This provides more electrical activity at the spinal cord level, which may facilitate the effects of some physical agents.

NEURAL TRANSMISSION

afferent Conduction of a nerve impulse toward an organ.

Afferent nerve fibers transmit impulses from the sensory receptors toward the brain, whereas **efferent** fibers, such as motor neurons, transmit impulses from the brain toward the periphery.[35] First-order or primary afferents transmit the impulses from the sensory receptor to the dorsal horn of the spinal cord (Fig. 4-4). There are four

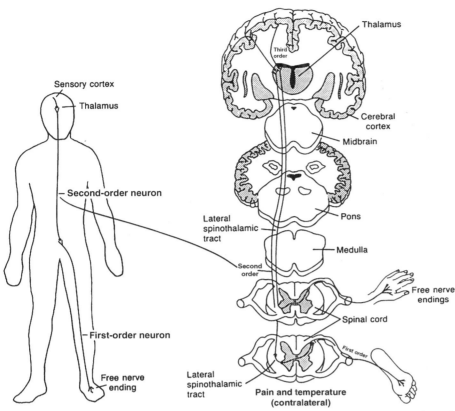

•**Figure 4-4** The lateral spinothalamic tract carries impulses of pain and temperature from the sensory receptors to the cortex.

different types of first-order neurons (Table 4-2). Note that A-alpha and A-beta fibers are characterized as being large-diameter afferents and A-delta and C fibers as small-diameter afferents.

Second-order afferent fibers carry sensory messages from the dorsal horn to the brain. Second-order afferent fibers are categorized as wide dynamic range or nociceptive specific. The wide dynamic range second-order afferents receive input from A-beta, A-delta, and C fibers. These second-order afferents serve relatively large, overlapping receptor fields. The nociceptive-specific second-order afferents respond exclusively to noxious stimulation. They receive input only from A-delta and C fibers. These afferents serve smaller receptor fields that do not overlap. All of these neurons synapse with third-order neurons that carry information to various brain centers where the input is integrated, interpreted, and acted on.

FACILITATORS AND INHIBITORS OF SYNAPTIC TRANSMISSION

For information to pass between neurons, a transmitter substance must be released from one neuron terminal (presynaptic membrane), enter the synaptic cleft, and attach to a receptor site on the next neuron (postsynaptic membrane). In the past, all the activity within the synapse was attributed to **neurotransmitters**, such as acetylcholine. The neurotransmitters, when released in sufficient quantities, are known to cause depolarization of the postsynaptic neuron. In the absence of the neurotransmitter, no depolarization occurs.

It is now apparent that several compounds that are not true neurotransmitters can facilitate or inhibit synaptic activity. These compounds are classified as biogenic amine transmitters or neuroactive peptides. **Serotonin** and **norepinephrine** are examples of biogenic amine transmitters. About two dozen neuroactive peptides have been identified, including **substance P, glutamate, neurokinen, enkephalins**, and **β-endorphin**.[3]

neurotransmitter Substance that passes information between neurons. It is released from one neuron terminal (presynaptic membrane), enters the synaptic cleft, and attaches (binds) to a receptor on the next neuron (postsynaptic membrane). Substance P, enkephalins, serotonin, methionine, acetylcholine, and leucine enkephalin are neurotransmitters.

TABLE 4-2   **Classification of Afferent Neurons**

Size	Type	Group	Subgroup	Diameter (Micrometers)	Conduction Velocity m/sec	Receptor	Stimulus
Large	A α	I	1a	12–20 (22)	70–120	Proprioceptive mechanoreceptor	Muscle velocity and length change, muscle shortening of rapid speed
	A α	I	1b				
	A β	II	Muscle	6–12	36–72	Proprioceptive mechanoreceptor	Muscle length information from touch and pacinian corpuscles
	A β	II	Skin			Cutaneous receptors	Touch, vibration, hair receptors
	A δ	III	Muscle	1–5 (6)	6(12)–36(80)	75% mechanoreceptors and thermoreceptors	Temperature change
Small	A δ	III	Skin			25% nociceptors, mechanoreceptors, and thermoreceptors (hot and cold)	Noxious, mechanical, and temperature (>45°C, <10°C)
	C	IV	Muscle	0.3–1.0	0.4–1.0	50% mechanoreceptors and thermoreceptors	Touch and temperature
	C	IV	Skin			50% nociceptors, 20% mechanoreceptors, and 30% thermoreceptors (hot and cold)	Noxious, mechanical, and temperature (>45°C, <10°C)

β-Endorphin serotonin, and enkephalin are important in the body's (endogenous) pain control mechanisms.[2]

Enkephalin is an **endogenous** (made by the body) **opioid** that inhibits the depolarization of second-order nociceptive nerve fibers. It is released from **interneurons**, enkephalin neurons with short axons. The enkephalins are stored in nerve-ending vesicles found in the **substantia gelatinosa** and several areas of the brain. When released, enkephalin may bind to presynaptic or postsynaptic membranes.[3]

Norepinephrine is a biogenic amine transmitter that is released by the depolarization of some neurons and that binds to the postsynaptic membranes. Norepinephrine is found in several areas of the nervous system, including a tract that descends from the pons that inhibits synaptic transmission between first-order and second-order nociceptive fibers, thus decreasing pain sensation.[17]

Other endogenous opioids may be active analgesic agents. These neuroactive peptides are released into the central nervous system and have an action similar to that of morphine, an opiate analgesic. There are specific receptors located at strategic sites, called binding sites, to receive these compounds. β-Endorphin, a 31-amino acid peptide, and **dynorphin** have potent analgesic effects. These are released within the central nervous system by mechanisms that are not fully understood at this time.

NOCICEPTION

A nociceptive neuron is a neuron that transmits pain signals. Its cell body is in the dorsal root ganglion near the spinal cord. Approximately 25 percent of the myelinated A-delta and 50 percent of the unmyelinated C fibers contact nociceptors and are considered nociceptive, afferent neurons (see Table 4-2). Pain is initiated by a chemical stimulus. Injury to a cell due to trauma triggers the formation and release of **prostaglandin** and **bradykinin,** which sensitize the nociceptors in and around the area of injury by lowering the depolarization threshold. This is referred to as **primary hyperalgesia**, in which the nerve's threshold to noxious stimuli is lowered, thus enhancing the pain response. Over a period of several hours **secondary hyperalgesia** occurs, as chemicals spread throughout the surrounding tissues, increasing the size of the painful area and creating hypersensitivity. Once a nociceptor is stimulated, it releases a neuropeptide (substance P) that initiates the electrical impulses along the afferent fiber toward the spinal cord. Substance P also serves as a transmitter substance between the first- and second-order afferent fibers at the dorsal horn of the spinal column (Fig. 4-4).

The A-delta and C fibers that transmit sensations of pain and temperature have different diameters (A-delta are larger) and different conduction velocities (A-delta are faster). The C fibers also are connected to more of the nociceptive-specific second-order afferents. These differences result in two qualitatively different types of pain, termed fast and slow.[3] Fast pain is brief, well-localized, and well-matched to the stimulus— for example, the initial pain of an unexpected pinprick. Slow pain is an aching, throbbing, or burning sensation that is poorly localized and less specifically related to the stimulus. There is a delay in the perception of slow pain following injury, but the pain will continue long after the noxious stimulus is removed. Fast pain is transmitted over the larger, faster-conducting A-delta afferent neurons and originates from receptors located in the skin. Slow pain is transmitted by the C afferent neurons and originates from both superficial tissue (skin) and deeper tissue (ligaments and muscles).[3]

The various types of afferent fibers follow different courses as they ascend toward the brain. Some A-delta and most C afferent neurons enter the spinal cord through the dorsolateral tract of Lissauer and synapse in marginal zone (lamina 1) or the substantia gelatinosa (lamina 2) with a second-order neuron.[17] Most nociceptive second-order neurons ascend to higher centers along one of three tracts—(1) the lateral spinothalamic tract; (2) spinoreticular tract; or (3) spinoencephalic tract—with the remainder ascending along the spinocervical tract or as projections to the cuneate and gracile nuclei of the medulla.[17] Approximately 90 percent of the wide dynamic range second-order afferents terminate in the thalamus.[17] Third-order neurons project to the sensory cortex and numerous other centers in the central nervous system. These projections allow us to

serotonin A neurotransmitter found in neurons descending in the dorsolateral tract.

enkephalin Neurotransmitter proteins that block the passage of noxious stimuli from first- to second-order afferents. They inhibit the release of substance P and are produced by enkephalinergic neurons.

endogenous opioids Opiate-like neuroactive peptide substances made by the body.

nociceptive Pain information or signals or pain stimuli.

CASE STUDY 4-1
MANAGING ACUTE PAIN

Background: Stacey is a 21-year-old college basketball player referred for physical therapy the day after athroscopic surgery to remove loose bodies and a tear in the medial meniscus of her left knee.

Impression: She is typical of patients presenting the day following acute injury and surgery. She is experiencing considerable discomfort and demonstrates inhibition of the quadriceps muscles and an unwillingness to flex and extend the knee.

Treatment: Stacey was treated with an ice bag around the knee for 20 minutes, being careful to protect the common peroneal nerve on the posterior lateral aspect of the knee. Following cold application she was encouraged to perform quadriceps setting and heel slides.

Response: Her volitional control of the quadriceps improved and she left the clinic able to perform a straight leg raise without a lag. She was also able to move the knee from extension to 50 degrees of flexion. She was sent home with instructions to use cold three to four times daily followed by the previously described exercises. Stacey demonstrated active range of motion from terminal extension to 115 degrees of flexion and good control of the quadriceps on return to the clinic 5 days later. Her rehabilitation progressed well and she returned to playing basketball within 3 weeks in preparation for the upcoming season.

Surgery results in acute pain and the associated guarding, splinting, and neuromuscular inhibition. When active muscle contractions and range of motion exercises can be performed safely, the use of therapeutic modalities can assist the patient regain function. In this case, cold was selected because of the acute presentation and the ease of use at home. TENS also would have been appropriate, either alone or in combination with cold. It is also important to appreciate the effects of pain-free movement on the recovery process. Movement lessens the sensation of stiffness postoperatively and provides large-diameter afferent input into the dorsal horn, which may relieve pain through a gating mechanism or the stimulation of enkephalin interneurons.

The rehabilitation professional employs physical agent modalities to create an optimum environment for tissue healing while minimizing the symptoms associated with the trauma or condition.

Discussion Questions

- What tissues were injured/affected?
- What symptoms were present?
- What phase of the injury-healing continuum did the patient present for care in?
- What are the physical agent modality's biophysical effects (direct/indirect/depth/tissue affinity)?
- What are the physical agent modality's indications/contraindications?
- What are the parameters of the physical agent modality's application/dosage/duration/frequency in this case study?
- What other physical agent modalities could be utilized to treat this injury or condition? Why? How?

perceive pain. They also permit the integration of past experiences and emotions that form our response to the pain experience. These connections are also believed to be parts of complex circuits that the therapist may stimulate to manage pain. Most analgesic physical agents are believed to slow or block the impulses ascending along the A-delta and C afferent neuron pathways through direct input into the dorsal horn or through descending mechanisms. These pathways are discussed in more detail in the following section.

NEUROPHYSIOLOGIC EXPLANATIONS OF PAIN CONTROL

The neurophysiologic mechanisms of pain control through stimulation of cutaneous receptors have not been fully explained. Much of what is known and current theory are the result of work involving electroacupuncture and transcutaneous electrical nerve stimulation.[34] However, this information often provides an explanation for the analgesic response to other modalities, such as massage, analgesic balms, and moist heat.

The concepts of the analgesic response to cutaneous receptor stimulation presented here were first proposed by Melzack and Wall and Castel.[7,23] These models essentially present three analgesic mechanisms:

Mechanisms of Pain Control
- Blocking ascending pathways
- Blocking descending pathways
- Release of β-endorphin

1. Stimulation from ascending A-beta afferents results in the blocking of impulses (pain messages) carried along A-delta and C afferent fibers.
2. Stimulation of descending pathways in the dorsolateral tract of the spinal cord by A-delta and C fiber afferent input results in a blocking of the impulses carried along the A-delta and C afferent fibers.
3. The stimulation of A-delta and C afferent fibers causes the release of endogenous opioids (β-endorphin), resulting in a prolonged activation of descending analgesic pathways.

These theories or models are not necessarily mutually exclusive. Recent evidence suggests that pain relief may result from combinations of dorsal horn and central nervous system activity.[2,9]

A decrease in input along nociceptive afferents also results in pain relief. Cooling afferent fibers decreases the rate at which they conduct impulses. Thus, a 20-minute application of cold is effective in relieving pain because of the decrease in activity, rather than an increase in activity along afferent pathways.

BLOCKING PAIN IMPULSES WITH ASCENDING A-BETA INPUT

Pain modulation caused by sensory stimulation and the resultant increase in the impulses in the large-diameter (A-beta) afferent fibers was proposed by the gate control theory of pain (Fig. 4-5).[23] Impulses ascending on these fibers stimulate the substantia

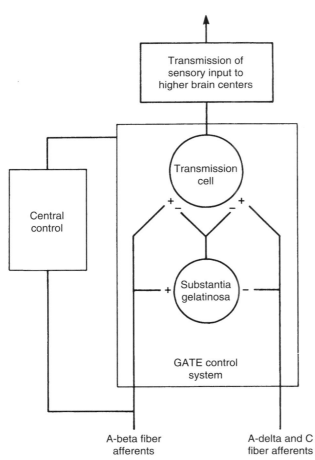

•**Figure 4-5** The gate control system. Increases A-beta input and stimulates the substantia gelatinosa that inhibits the flow of afferent input to sensory centers.

substantia gelatinosa (SG) Melzack and Wall proposed that the SG is responsible for closing the gate to painful stimuli.

efferent Conduction of a nerve impulse away from an organ.

periaqueductal gray A midbrain structure that plays an important role in descending tracts that inhibit synaptic transmission of noxious input in the dorsal horn.

gelatinosa as they enter the dorsal horn of the spinal cord. Stimulation of the substantia gelatinosa inhibits synaptic transmission in the large and small (A-delta and C) fiber afferent pathways. The "pain message" carried along the smaller-diameter fibers is not transmitted to the second-order neurons and never reaches sensory centers. The balance between the input from the small- and large-diameter afferents determines how much of the pain message is blocked or gated.

The concept of sensory stimulation for pain relief, as proposed by the gate control theory, has empirical support. Rubbing a contusion, applying moist heat, or massaging sore muscles decreases the perception of pain. The analgesic response to these treatments is attributed to the increased stimulation of large-diameter afferent fibers.

The gate control theory also proposes that A-delta and C fiber impulses inhibit the substantia gelatinosa, facilitating the perception of pain. The sensation of pain does not diminish rapidly, because free nerve endings do not accommodate and the afferent impulses from them "open the gate" to further pain message transmission.

The discovery and isolation of endogenous opioids in the 1970s led to new theories of pain relief. Castel introduced an endogenous opioid analog to the gate control theory (Fig. 4-6).[7] This theory proposes that increased neural activity in A-alpha and A-beta primary afferent pathways triggers a release of enkephalin from **enkephalin interneurons** found in the dorsal horn. These neuroactive amines inhibit synaptic transmission in the A-delta and C fiber afferent pathways. The end result, as in the gate control theory, is that the pain message is blocked before it reaches sensory levels.

DESCENDING PAIN CONTROL MECHANISMS

The gate control theory proposed a second analgesic mechanism that involves descending efferent fibers.[23] The central control, originating in higher centers of the central nervous system, could affect the dorsal horn gating process. Impulses from the thalamus and brain stem (**central biasing**) are carried into the dorsal horn on efferent fibers in the dorsal or dorsal lateral paths (or tracts). Impulses from the higher centers act to close the gate and block transmission of the pain message at the dorsal horn synapse. Through this system, it was theorized, previous experiences, emotional influences, sensory perceptions, and other factors could influence the transmission of the pain message and the perception of pain.

Castel offers an endogenous opioid model of descending influence over dorsal horn synapse activity (Fig. 4-7).[7] Stimulation of the **periaqueductal gray** region of the midbrain and the **raphe nucleus** in the pons and medulla by ascending neural input, especially from A-delta and C fiber afferents, and possibly central biasing, activates the descending mechanism. The periaqueductal gray stimulates the raphe nucleus. The raphe nucleus in turn sends impulses along serotonergic efferent fibers in the dorsal lateral tract, which synapse with enkephalin interneurons. The interneurons release

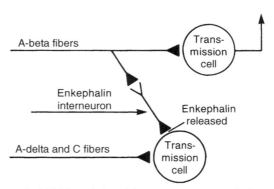

•**Figure 4-6** Presynaptic inhibition of dorsal horn synapse transmission owing to A-beta fiber stimulation at enkephalin interneurons.

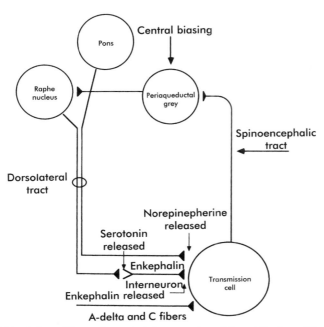

•Figure 3-7 Stimulation of the periaqueductal gray region of the midbrain and the raphe nucleus in the pons and medulla by ascending neural input, especially from A-delta and C fiber afferents, and possibly central biasing, activates the descending mechanism.

enkephalin into the dorsal horn, inhibiting the synaptic transmission of impulses to the second-order afferent neurons.

A second descending, norandrenergic pathway projecting from the pons to the dorsal horn has also been identified.[17] The significance of these parallel pathways is not fully understood. It is also not known if these norandrenergic fibers directly inhibit dorsal horn synapses or stimulate the enkephalin interneurons.

This model provides a physiologic explanation for the analgesic response to brief, intense stimulation. The analgesia following accupressure and the use of some transcutaneous electrical nerve simulators (TENS), such as point simulators, is attributed to this descending pain control mechanism.

BETA-ENDORPHIN AND DYNORPHIN

There is evidence that stimulation of the small-diameter afferents (A-delta and C) can stimulate the release of other endogenous opioids.[8,10,20,28,29,31,32] Beta-endorphin (BEP) and dynorphin are neuroactive peptides with potent analgesic effects. The term **endorphin** refers to an opiatelike substance produced by the body. The mechanisms regulating the release of BEP and dynorphin have not been fully elucidated. However, it is apparent that these large endogenous substances play a role in the analgesic response to some forms of stimuli used in the treatment of patients in pain.

In the anterior pituitary gland, it shares the prohormone propiomelanocortin (POMC) with adrenocorticotropin (ACTH). BEP does not readily cross the blood-brain barrier[3] and the anterior pituitary gland is not the sole source of BEP.[11] The neurons in the hypothalamus that send projections to the PAG and noradrenergic nuclei in the brain stem contain BEP. Prolonged (20–40 minutes) small diameter afferent fiber stimulation via electroacupuncture has been thought to trigger the release of BEP.[32] It is possible that BEP released from these neurons by stimulation of the hypothalamus is responsible for the analgesic response to the treatments[6] (Fig. 4-8). Once again, further

enkephalinergic interneurons Neurons with short axons that release enkephalin. They are widespread in the central nervous system and are found in the substantia gelatinosa, nucleus raphae magnus, and periaqueductual gray matter.

β-endorphin A neurohormone derived from proopiomelanocortin (POMC).

ACTH Adrenocorticotrophic hormone. This hormone stimulates the release of glucocorticoids (cortisol) from the adrenal glands.

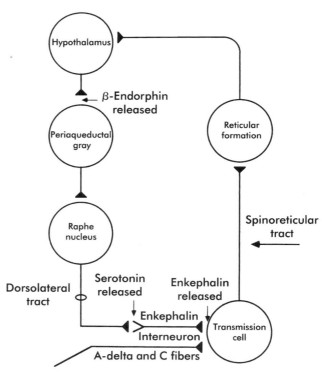

•**Figure 4-8** The neurons in the hypothalamus that send projections to the periaqueductal gray and noradrenergic nuclei in the brain stem contain β-endorphin. It is possible that β-endorphin released from these neurons by stimulation of the hypothalamus is responsible for the analgesic response to the treatments.

research is needed to clarify where and how these substances are released and how the release of BEP affects neural acitivity and pain perception.

Dynorphin, a more recently isolated endogenous opioid, is found in the PAG, ros-troventral medulla, and the dorsal horn.[17] It has been demonstrated that dynorphin is released during electroacupuncture.[15] Dynorphin may be responsible for suppressing the response to noxious mechanical stimulation.[17]

SUMMARY OF PAIN CONTROL MECHANISMS

The body's pain control mechanisms are probably not mutually exclusive. Rather, analgesia is the result of overlapping processes. It is also important to realize that the theories presented are only models. They are useful in conceptualizing the perception of pain and pain relief. These models will help the therapist understand the effects of therapeutic modalities and form a sound rationale for modality application. As more research is conducted and as the mysteries of pain and neurophysiology are solved, new models will emerge. The physical therapist should adapt these models to fit new developments.

COGNITIVE INFLUENCES

Pain perception and the response to a painful experience is not solely a sensory phenom-enon. The pain experience may be heightened by anxiety and in those suffering from depression. Past pain experiences as well as cultural influences may serve to heighten or suppress the responses to the perception of pain. The process of cognitive appraisal, where the patient is assisted in evaluating the pain experience can substantially alter the response to the painful stimulus. Take for example, patients seeking care for shoulder pain. They present convinced that they have suffered a torn rotator cuff, that surgery is necessary, and the recovery will be a long and painful process. Through the examination process, the clinician reaches a diagnosis of glenohumeral impingement syndrome with a low probability of substantial rotator cuff pathology. While the clinician carefully explains why the diagnosis of impingement syndrome is far more plausible and what should be done to treat the shoulder, patients are appraising this new information. If patients leave convinced that their shoulder pain is due to impingement and that the plan of care is reasonable, they also likely leave less anxious about their condition. Thus, through cognitive appraisal the pain experience has been altered. The clinician must also be mindful that pain can occur in the absence of local pathologic processes. In addition, pain memory, which is associated with old injuries, may result in pain perception and pain response that are out of proportion to a new, often minor, injury. The treatment of psychologic dysfunction is beyond the scope of practice of the physical therapist. Recognition that an individual patient's complaints are likely not due to musculoskeletal origins, be it referred from a diseased organ or due to somatization, should prompt the physical therapist to refer the patient for evaluation and treatment by an appropriated qualified provider.

PAIN MANAGEMENT

How should the physical therapist approach pain? First, the source of the pain must be identified. Unidentified pain may hide a serious disorder, and treatment of such pain may delay the appropriate treatment of the disorder. Once a diagnosis has been made, many physical agents can provide pain relief. The physical therapist should match the therapeutic agent to each patient's situation; and it must be understood that the pain system differs between patients and thus it cannot be assumed that every patient is similar in sensitivities or responses to external stimuli. Casts and braces may prevent the application of ice or moist heat. However, TENS electrodes often can be positioned under a cast or brace for pain relief. Following acute injuries, ice may be the therapeutic agent of choice because of the effect of cold on the inflammatory process. There is not one "best" therapeutic agent for pain control. The physical therapist must select the therapeutic agent that is most appropriate for each patient based on the knowledge of the modalities and professional judgment. In no situation should the physical therapist apply a therapeutic agent without first developing a clear rationale for the treatment.

In general, physical agents can be used to accomplish the following:

1. Stimulate large-diameter afferent fibers. This can be done with TENS, massage, and analgesic balms.
2. Decrease pain fiber transmission velocity with cold or ultrasound.
3. Stimulate small-diameter afferent fibers and descending pain control mechanisms with acupressure, deep massage, or TENS over acupuncture points or trigger points.[31]
4. Stimulate a release of BEP or other endogenous opioids through prolonged small-diameter fiber stimulation with TENS.[33]

Other useful pain control strategies include the following.

1. Encourage central biasing through cognitive processes, such as motivation, tension diversion, focusing, relaxation techniques, positive thinking, thought stopping, and self-control.
2. Minimize the tissue damage through the application of proper first aid and immobilization.
3. Maintain a line of communication with the patient. Let the patient know what to expect following an injury. Pain, swelling, dysfunction, and atrophy will occur following injury. The patient's anxiety over these events will increase his or her perception of pain. Often, a patient who has been told what to expect by someone he or she trusts will be less anxious and suffer less pain.

CASE STUDY 4-2
MANAGING CHRONIC PAIN

Background: Linda is a 31-year-old resident in oral surgery. She was referred for physical therapy for complaints of upper back and neck pain with frequent headaches. She states that she has been experiencing the symptoms off and on for about 2 years. Her symptoms are worse at the end of the work day, especially on days she is in the operating room. There is no history of trauma to the affected region.

Physical exam reveals a forward head, rounded shoulder posture, spasm of the cervical paraspinal and trapezius muscles, and very sensitive trigger points throughout the region.

Impression: Her symptoms were consistent with pain of myofascial origin secondary to posture, job-related stress, and fatigue of the postural muscles.

Treatment: She was treated with TENS over the trigger points using a Neuroprobe, soft tissue mobilization, and instructed in a routine of postural exercises. She was encouraged to perform postural exercises and relaxation activities during breaks in her schedule. Linda returned to the clinic indicating she had experienced near complete relief following her first visit for about 6 hours. The stimulation of trigger points was repeated and Linda was instructed in the use of a TENS unit with conventional parameters over her most sensitive trigger point. She had access to the TENS unit through the surgical clinic where she worked.

Response: Linda was seen for two additional visits. She indicated her compliance with the exercise program, which was subsequently expanded into a general conditioning program with an emphasis on upper body endurance. She also indicated that her symptoms were becoming much less severe and less frequent and that the home TENS unit gave her a means of controlling her pain before it became severe enough to affect her activities. Over the subsequent several months, Linda completed her residency without additional care for her neck and upper back.

Myofascial pain or pain of soft tissue origin has several causes, many of which may contribute to a single individual's symptoms. Poor posture, stress, repetitive microtrauma, and acute injuries can combine to cause a pain pattern that is often difficult to understand. The keys to management are to identify the causative factors and help the patient address them. In this case Linda had to recondition postural muscles to restore balance between antagonistic groups. Her long hours of standing over operating tables had contributed to her postural deficits. She also became more aware of how she responded to stressors and began using relaxation techniques with which she was familiar.

Her four visits to physical therapy enabled us to identify the causes of Linda's pain, break the pain spasm cycle, desensitize her trigger points, and initiate a program of progressive, pain-free exercises. Pain control is essential in the management of myofascial pain. Exercise that is painful further sensitizes trigger points and promotes the use of inefficient, antalgic movement patterns.

The rehabilitation professional employs physical agent modalities to create an optimum environment for tissue healing while minimizing the symptoms associated with the trauma or condition.

Discussion Questions
- What tissues were injured/affected?
- What symptoms were present?
- What phase of the injury-healing continuum did the patient present for care in?
- What are the physical agent modality's biophysical effects (direct/indirect/depth/tissue affinity)?
- What are the physical agent modality's indications/contraindications?
- What are the parameters of the physical agent modality's application/dosage/duration/frequency in this case study?
- What other physical agent modalities could be utilized to treat this injury or condition? Why? How?

4. Recognize that all pain, even psychosomatic pain, is very real to the patient.
5. Encourage supervised exercise to encourage blood flow, promote nutrition, increase metabolic activity, and reduce stiffness and guarding if the activity will not cause further harm to the patient.

The physician may choose to prescribe oral or injectable medications in the treatment of the patient. The most commonly used medications are classified as analgesics, anti-inflammatory agents, or both. The therapist should become familiar with these drugs and note if the patient is taking any medications. It is also important to work with the referring physician to assure that the patient takes the medications appropriately.

The physical therapist's approach to the patient has a great impact on the success of the treatment. The patient will not be convinced of the efficacy and importance of the treatment unless the therapist appears confident about it. The physical therapist must make the patient a participant rather than a passive spectator in the treatment and rehabilitation process.

The goal of most treatment programs is to encourage early pain-free exercise. The physical agents used to control pain do little to promote tissue healing. They should be used to relieve acute pain following injury or surgery or to control pain and other symptoms, such as swelling, to promote progressive exercise. The physical therapist should not lose sight of the effects of the physical agents or the importance of progressive exercise in restoring the patient's functional ability.

Reducing the perception of pain is as much an art as a science. Selection of the proper physical agent, proper application, and marketing are all important and will continue to be so even as we increase our understanding of the neurophysiology of pain. There is still the need for a good empirical rationale for the use of a physical agent. The therapist is encouraged to keep abreast of the neurophysiology of pain and the physiology of tissue healing to maintain a current scientific basis for selecting modalities and managing the pain experienced by his or her patients.

SUMMARY

1. Pain is a response to a noxious stimulus that is subjectively modified by past experiences and expectations.
2. Pain is classified as either acute or chronic and can exhibit many different patterns.
3. Early reduction of pain in a treatment program will facilitate therapeutic exercise.
4. Stimulation of sensory receptors via the therapeutic modalities can modify the patient's perception of pain.
5. Four mechanisms of pain control may explain the analgesic effects of physical agents:
   a. Decreased transmission of input along nociceptive pathways.
   b. Dorsal horn modulation owing to the input from large-diameter afferents through a gate control system, the release of enkephalins, or both.
   c. Descending efferent fiber activation owing to the effects of small fiber afferent input on higher centers, including the thalamus, raphe nucleus, and periaqueductal gray region.
   d. The central release of endogenous opioids including β-endorphin through prolonged small-diameter afferent stimulation.
6. Pain perception may be influenced by a variety of cognitive processes mediated by the higher brain centers.
7. The selection of a therapeutic modality for controlling pain should be based on current knowledge of neurophysiology and the psychology of pain.
8. The application of physical agents for the control of pain should not occur until the diagnosis of the injury has been established.
9. The selection of a therapeutic modality for managing pain should be based on establishing the primary cause of pain.

REVIEW QUESTIONS

1. What is a basic definition of pain?
2. What are the different types of pain?

3. What are the different assessment scales available to help the therapist determine the extent of pain perception?
4. What are the characteristics of the various sensory receptors?
5. How does the nervous system relay information about painful stimuli?
6. Describe how the gate control mechanism of pain modulation may be used to modulate pain.
7. How do the descending pain control mechanisms function to modulate pain?
8. What are the opiate-like substances, and how do they act to modulate pain?
9. How can pain perception can be modified by cognitive factors?
10. How can the therapist help modulate pain during a rehabilitation program?

REFERENCES

1. Addison, R.: Chronic pain syndrome, Am. J. Med. 77:54, 1985.
2. Anderson, S., Ericson, T., and Holmgren, E.: Electroacupuncture affects pain threshold measured with electrical stimulation of teeth, Brain 63:393–396, 1973.
3. Berne, R., Levy, M.: Physiology, St. Louis, MO, 1988, C.V. Mosby.
4. Bishop, B.: Pain: its physiology and rationale for management, Phys. Ther. 60:13–37, 1980.
5. Bonica, J.: The management of pain, Philadelphia, PA, 1990, Lea & Febiger.
6. Bowsher, D.: Central pain mechanisms. In Wells, P., Frampton, V., and Bowsher, D., editors. Pain management in physical therapy. Norwalk, CT, 1988, Appleton & Lange.
7. Castel, J.: Pain management: acupuncture and transcutaneous electrical nerve stimulation techniques, Lake Bluff, IL, 1979, Pain Control Services.
8. Chapman, C., Benedetti, C.: Analgesia following electrical stimulation: partial reversal by a narcotic antagonist, Life Sci. 26:44–48, 1979.
9. Cheng, R., Pomeranz, B.: Electroacupuncture analgesia could be mediated by at least two pain relieving mechanisms: endorphin and non-endorphin systems, Life Sci. 25:1957–1962, 1979.
10. Clement-Jones, V., McLaughlin, L., and Tomlin, S.: Increased beta-endorphin but not met-enkephalin levels in human cerebrospinal fluid after electroacupuncture for recurrent pain, Lancet 2:946–948, 1980.
11. Denegar, G., Perrin, D., and Rogol, A.: Influence of transcutaneous electrical nerve stimulation on pain, range of motion and serum cortisol concentration in females with induced delayed onset muscle soreness, JOSPT 11:101–103, 1989.
12. Dickerman, J.: The use of pain profiles in clinical practice, Fam. Pract. Recert. 14(3):35–44, 1992.
13. Fedorczyk, J.: The role of physical agents in modulating pain. J. Hand Ther. 10:110–121, 1997.
14. Gatchel, R.: Million behavioral health inventory: its utility in predicting physical functioning patients with low back pain. Arch. Phys. Med. Rehabil. 67:878, 1986.
15. Ho, W., Wen, H.: Opioid-like activity in the cerebrospinal fluid of pain patients treated by electroacupuncture. Neuropharmacology 28:961–966, 1989.
16. Huskisson, E.: Visual analogue scales. Pain measurement and assessment. In Melzack, R., editor. Pain measurement and assessment, New York, 1983, Raven Press.
17. Jessell, T., Kelly, D.: Pain and analgesia. In Kandel, E., Schwartz, J., and Jessell T., editors. Principles of neural science, Norwalk, CT, 1991, Appleton & Lange.
18. Kuland, D.N.: The injured athletes' pain, Curr. Concepts Pain 1:3–10, 1983.
19. Margoles, M.: The pain chart: spatial properties of pain. In Melzack, R., editor. Pain measurement and assessment, New York, 1983, Raven Press.
20. Mattacola, C., Perrin, D., Gansneder, B.: A comparison of visual analog and graphic rating scales for assessing pain following delayed onset muscle soreness. J. Sport Rehabil. 6:38–46, 1997.
21. Mayer, D., Price, D., and Rafii, A.: Antagonism of acupuncture analgesia in man by the narcotic antagonist naloxone, Brain Res. 121:368–372, 1977.
22. Melzack, R.: Concepts of pain measurement. In Melzack, R., editor. Pain measurement and assessment, New York, 1983, Raven Press.
23. Melzack, R., Wall, P.: Pain mechanisms: a new theory, Science 150:971–979, 1965.
24. Merskey, H., Albe Fessard, D., and Bonica, J.: Pain terms: a list with definitions and notes on usage, Pain 6:249–252, 1979.
25. Merskey, H., Bogduk, N.: Classification of chronic pain. Definitions of chronic pain syndromes and definition of pain terms, ed. 2, Seattle, 1994, International Association for the Study of Pain.
26. Millan, M.J.: Descending control of pain. Prog. Neurobiol. 66:355–474, 2002.
27. Pomeranz, B., Chiu, D.: Naloxone blockade of acupuncture analgesia: enkephalin implicated, Life Sci. 19:1757–1762, 1976.
28. Pomeranz, B., Paley, D.: Electro-acupuncture hypoalgesia is mediated by afferent impulses: an electrophysiological study in mice, Exp. Neurol. 66:398–402, 1979.

29. Pomeranz, B., Paley, D.: Brain opiates at work in acupuncture, New Scientist 73:12–13, 1975.

30. Previte, J.: Human physiology, New York, 1983, McGraw-Hill.

31. Salar, G., Job, I., and Mingringo, S.: Effects of transcutaneous electrotherapy on CSF beta-endorphin content in patients without pain problems, Pain 10:169–172, 1981.

32. Sjoland, B., Eriksson, M.: Increased cerebrospinal fluid levels of endorphins after electro-acupuncture, Acta Physiol. Scand. 100:382–384, 1977.

33. Sjolund, B., Eriksson, M.: Electroacupuncture and endogenous morphines, Lancet 2:1085, 1976.

34. Wen, H., Ho, W., and Ling, N.: The influence of electroacupuncture on naloxone induces morphine withdrawal: elevation of immunoassayable beta-endorphin activity in the brain but not in the blood, Am. J. Clin. Med. 7:237–240, 1979.

35. Willis, W., Grossman, R.: Medical Neurobiology, ed. 3, St. Louis, MO, 1981, C.V. Mosby.

36. Wolf, S.: Neurophysiologic mechanisms in pain modulation: relevance to TENS. In Manheimer, J., Lampe, G. editors. Clinical applications of TENS, Philadelphia, PA, 1984, F.A. Davis.

GLOSSARY

accommodation Adaptation by the sensory receptors to various stimuli over an extended period of time.

ACTH Adrenocorticotropic hormone. This hormone stimulates the release of glucocorticoids (cortisol) from the adrenal glands.

afferent Conduction of a nerve impulse away from an organ.

avulsion fracture A fracture in which a small piece of bone is torn away by an attached tendon or ligament.

beta-endorphin A neurohormone derived from proopiomelanocortin (POMC). It is similar in structure and properties to morphine. Beta-endorphin has a half-life of 4 hours.

bradykinin A chemical formed in injured tissue as part of the inflammatory process that vasodilates small arterioles.

central biasing A theory of pain modulation where higher centers such as the cerebral cortex influence the perception of and response to pain.

dynorphin An endogenous opioid derived from the prohormone prodynorphin.

efferent Conduction of a nerve impulse toward an organ.

endogenous opioids Opiatelike substances made by the body.

endorphins Endogenous opioids whose actions have analgesic properties (i.e., β-endorphin).

enkephalin Neurotransmitter proteins that block the passage of noxious stimuli from first- to second-order afferents. They inhibit the release of substance P and are produced by enkephalinergic neurons.

enkephalinergic interneurons Neurons with short axons that release enkephalin. They are widespread in the central nervous system and are found in the substantia gelatinosa, nucleus raphae magnus, and periaqueductal gray matter.

focusing Narrowing attention to the appropriate stimuli in the environment.

interneurons Neurons contained entirely in the central nervous system. They have no projections outside the spinal cord. Their function is to serve as relay stations within the central nervous system.

joint capsule Ligamentous structure that surrounds and encapsulates a joint.

neurotransmitter Substance that passes information between neurons. It is released from one neuron terminal (presynaptic membrane), enters the synaptic cleft, and attaches (binds) to a receptor on the next neuron (postsynaptic membrane). Substance P, enkephalins, serotonin, methionine, and leucine enkephalin are neurotransmitters.

nociceptive Pain information or signals of pain stimuli.

norepinephrine A neurotransmitter.

opiate receptors Neurons that have receptors that bind to opiate substances.

periaqueductal gray A midbrain structure that plays an important role in descending tracts that inhibit synaptic transmission of noxious input in the dorsal horn.

periosteum A highly vascularized and innervated membrane lining the surface of bone.

polymodal nociceptors Small unmyelinated afferent fibers that have high threshold axons and respond only to cutaneous stimulation (pain, deep pressure, and temperature). C fibers are examples of these.

prostaglandins Irritants that are synthesized locally during injury in tissue from a fatty acid precursor (arachidonic acid). They act with bradykinin to amplify pain by sensitizing afferent neurons to chemical and mechanical stimulation. Aspirin is thought to be capable of interrupting the process. Prostaglandins are powerful vasodilators. They induce erythema, increase leakage of plasma from vessels, and attract leukocytes to an injured area.

raphe nucleus Part of the brain that is known to inhibit pain impulses being transmitted through the ascending system.

referred pain (referred myofascial pain) When nociceptive impulses reach the dorsal gray matter, they converge and their summation can depolarize internuncial neurons over several spinal segments, causing the individual to feel pain in distal areas innervated by these segments.

reticular formation A network of neurons that extends through the length of the spinal column, brain stem, and into the basal regions of the diencephalon and telencephalon. The cell bodies lie in diffuse groups within the brain stem. The reticular formation receives input from and/or sends output to most central nervous system structures.

sclerotome A segment of bone innervated by a spinal segment.

sensitization Prolonged depolarization of nociceptive neurons that results in continuous stimulation. Most sensory receptors are rendered less sensitive after prolonged stimulation. This is not the case with nociceptive neurons.

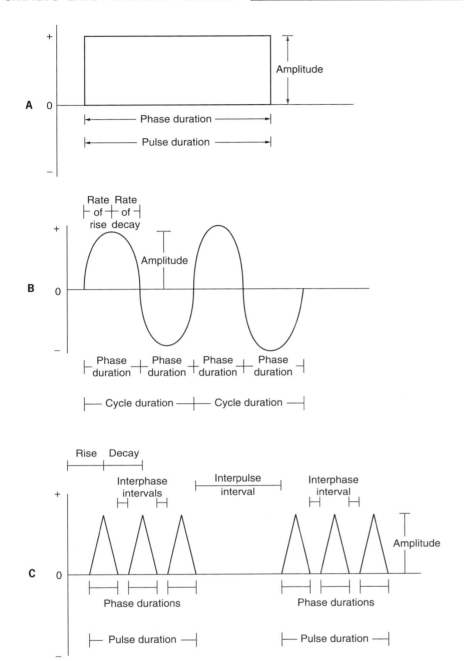

•**Figure 5-4** Characteristics of **A.** DC current, **B.** AC current, and **C.** PC current.

interphase interval. With pulsatile currents there is always a short period of time when current is not flowing between the two phases called the **interpulse interval** (Fig. 5-4C).

PULSE AMPLITUDE

The amplitude of each pulse reflects the intensity of the current, the maximum amplitude being the tip or highest point of each phase (see Fig. 5-4). Amplitude is measured in amperes, microamps (μA), or milliamps (mA). The term amplitude is synonymous with the terms voltage and current intensity. Voltage is measured in volts, microvolts (μV), or millivolts (mV). The higher the amplitude, the greater the peak voltage or intensity. However, the peak amplitude should not be confused with the total amount of current being delivered to the tissues.

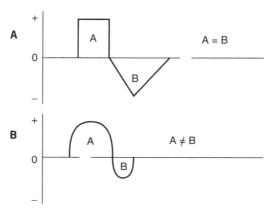

•**Figure 5-5** Asymmetric waveforms. **A.** Balanced asymmetrical current. **B.** Unbalanced asymmetrical current.

On electrical generators that produce short-duration pulses, the total current produced (c/sec) is low compared to peak current amplitudes owing to long interpulse intervals that have current amplitudes of zero. Thus, the **total current** (average), or the amount of current flowing per unit of time, is relatively low, ranging from as low as 2 to as high as 100 mA on some interferential generators. Total current can be increased by either increasing pulse duration or increasing pulse frequency or by some combination of the two (Fig. 5-6).

PULSE CHARGE

pulse charge The total amount of electricity being delivered to the patient during each pulse.

The term **pulse charge** refers to the total amount of electricity being delivered to the patient during each pulse (measured in columbs or microcolumbs). With monophasic current, the phase charge and the pulse charge are the same and always greater than zero. With biphasic current, the pulse charge is equal to the sum of the phase charges. If the pulse is symmetric, the net pulse charge is zero. In asymmetric pulses the net pulse charge is greater than zero, which is a DC current by definition.[1]

PULSE RATE OF RISE AND DECAY TIMES

Amplitude = voltage = current intensity

The **rate of rise** in amplitude, or the rise time, refers to how quickly the pulse reaches its maximum amplitude in each phase. Conversely, **decay time** refers to the time in which a pulse goes from peak amplitude to 0 V. The rate of rise is important physiologically because of the **accommodation** phenomenon, in which a fiber that has been subjected to a constant level of depolarization will become unexcitable at that same intensity or

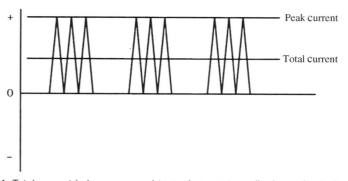

•**Figure 5-6** Total current is low compared to peak current amplitudes owing to long interpulse intervals.

amplitude. Rate of rise and decay times are generally short, ranging from nanoseconds (billionths of a second) to milliseconds (thousandths of a second) (see Fig. 5-3).

By observing the different waveforms, it is apparent that the sine wave has a gradual increase and decrease in amplitude for alternating, direct, and pulsatile currents (see Fig. 5-3A–C). The rectangular wave has an almost instantaneous increase in amplitude, which plateaus for a period of time and then abruptly falls off (see Fig. 5-3D–F). The spiked wave has a rapid increase and decrease in amplitude (see Fig. 5-3G–I). The shape of these waveforms as they reach their maximum amplitude or intensity is directly related to the excitability of nervous tissue. The more rapid the increase in amplitude or the rate of rise, the greater the current's ability to excite nervous tissue.

Many DC generators make use of a twin peak spiked pulse of very short duration (170 μsec) and peak amplitudes as high as 500 V (Fig. 5-7). Combining a high peak intensity with a short phase duration produces a very comfortable type of current as well as an effective means of stimulating sensory, motor, and pain fibers.[28]

The effects of the various waveforms on biologic tissue are discussed in Chapter 6.

rate of rise How quickly a waveform reaches its maximum amplitude.

PULSE DURATION

The **duration** of each pulse indicates the length of time current is flowing in one cycle. With monophasic current, the phase duration is the same as the pulse duration and is the time from initiation of the phase to its end. With **biphasic current**, the pulse duration is determined by the combined phase durations. In some electrotherapeutic devices the duration is preset by the manufacturer. Other devices have the capability of changing duration. The phase duration may be as short as a few microseconds or may be a long-duration direct current that flows for several minutes.

With pulsatile currents, and in some instances with alternating and direct currents, the current flow is off for a period of time. The combined time of the pulse duration and the interpulse interval is referred to as the **pulse period** (see Fig. 5-4).

biphasic current Another name for alternating current, in which the direction of current flow reverses direction.

PULSE FREQUENCY

Pulse **frequency** indicates the number of pulses or cycles per second. Each individual pulse represents a rise and fall in amplitude. As the frequency of any waveform is increased, the amplitude tends to increase and decrease more rapidly. The muscular and nervous system responses depend on the length of time between pulses and on how the pulses or waveforms are modulated.[20] Muscle responds with individual twitch contractions to pulse rates of less than 50 pps. At 50 pps or greater a tetanic contraction will result, regardless of whether the current is biphasic, monophasic, or polyphasic.

frequency The number of cycles or pulses per second.

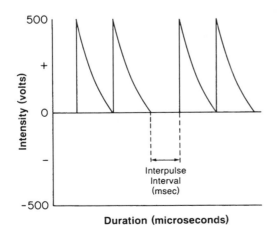

•**Figure 5-7** Most DC generators produce a twin peak spiked pulse of short duration and high amplitude.

Stimulators have been clinically labeled as either low-, medium-, or high-frequency generators, and a great deal of misunderstanding exists over how these frequency ranges are classified.[1] Generally, all stimulating units are low-frequency electrical generators that deliver between one and several hundred pulses per second. Recently, a number of so-called medium-frequency generators have been developed that have frequencies of 2500 to as high as 10,000 pps. However, these high-frequency pulses are in reality groups of pulses combined as **bursts** that range in frequency from 1 to 200 pps These modulated bursts are capable of producing a physiologically effective frequency of stimulation only in this 1 to 200 pps range owing to the limitations of the absolute refractory period of nerve cell membranes. Therefore, many of the claims of equipment manufacturers relative to medium-frequency generators are inaccurate.[1]

CURRENT MODULATION

The physiologic responses to the various waveforms depend to a large extent on current modulation. **Modulation** refers to any alteration in the amplitude, duration, or frequency of the current during a series of pulses or cycles.

CONTINUOUS CURRENT

With continuous current the amplitude of current flow remains the same for several seconds or perhaps minutes. Continuous current is usually associated with long pulse duration monophasic current (Fig. 5-8A). With monophasic current, flow is always in a uniform direction. In the discussion of physiologic responses to electrical currents, it was indicated that positive and negative ions are attracted toward poles or, in this case, electrodes of opposite polarity. This accumulation of charged ions over a period of time creates either an acidic or alkaline environment that may be of therapeutic value. This therapeutic technique has been referred to as **medical galvanism**. The technique of **iontophoresis** also uses continuous monophasic current to transport ions into the tissues (see Chapter 7). If the amplitude is great enough to produce a muscle contraction, the contraction will occur only when the current flow is turned on or off. Thus, with direct continuous current, there will be a muscle contraction both when the current is turned on and when it is turned off.

Burst Modulation

Burst modulation occurs when pulsatile or alternating current flows for a short duration (milliseconds) and then is turned off for a short time (milliseconds) in a repetitive cycle (Fig. 5-8B and C). With pulsatile currents, sets of pulses are combined. These combined pulses are most commonly referred to in the literature as **bursts**, but they have also been called *packets*, *envelopes*, or *pulse trains*.[17] The interruptions between individual bursts are called interburst intervals. The interburst interval is much too short to have any effect on a muscle contraction. Thus, the physiologic effects of a burst of pulses will be the same as with a single pulse.[1] Some machines allow the therapist to change the burst duration and/or the interburst interval.

Beat Modulation

A beat modulation will be produced when two interfering alternating current waveforms with differing frequencies are delivered to two separate pairs of electrodes through separate channels within the same generator (see Fig. 6-27). The two pairs of electrodes are set up in a crisscrossed or cloverleaf-like pattern so that the circuits interfere with one another (see Fig. 6-28). This interference pattern produces a beat frequency equal to the difference in frequency between the two alternataing current frequencies. As an example, one circuit may have a fixed frequency of 4000 Hz, while the other is set at a frequency of 4100 Hz, thus creating a beat frequency of 100 beats per second. This type of beat-modulated alternating current is referred to as interferential current and will be discussed further in Chapter 6.

Current Modulation
- Continuous
- Burst
- Beat
- Ramping

bursts A combined set of three or more pulses; also referred to as packets or envelopes.

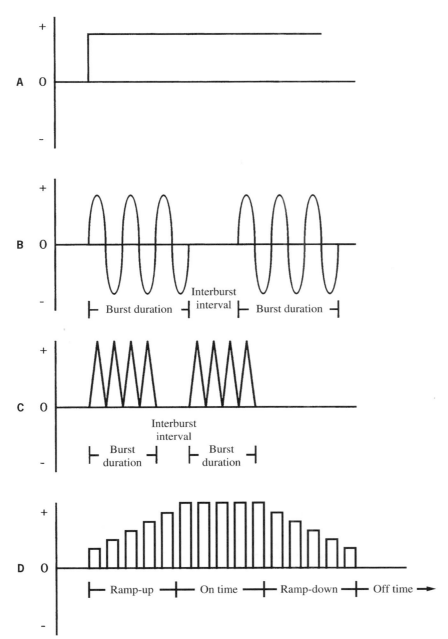

•**Figure 5-8** Current may be modulated using **A.** continuous current, **B.** burst modulated alternating current, **C.** burst modulated pulsatile current, and **D.** ramp-up and ramp-down modulation.

Ramping Modulation

In **ramping** modulation, also called surging modulation, current amplitude will increase or ramp-up gradually to some preset maximum and may also decrease or ramp-down in intensity (Fig. 5-8D). Ramp-up time is usually preset at about one-third of the on time. The ramp-down option is not available on all machines. Most modern stimulators allow the therapist to set the on and off times between 1 and 10 seconds. Ramping modulation is used clinically to elicit muscle contraction and is generally considered to be a very comfortable type of current since it allows for a gradual increase in the intensity of a muscle contraction.

ramping Another name for surging modulation, in which the current builds gradually to some maximum amplitude.

ELECTRICAL CIRCUITS

The path of current from a generating power source through various components back to the generating source is called an electrical **circuit**.[4] A closed circuit is one in which electrons are flowing, and in an open circuit the current flow ceases. Electronic circuits are not ordinarily composed of single elements; they often encompass several branches or components with different resistances. The current in each branch may be easily calculated if the individual resistances are known and if the amount of voltage applied to the circuit is also known.[6]

With the development of the microelectronics industry, we all know that electrical circuits can be extremely complex. However, all electrical circuits have several basic components. There is a power source, which is capable of producing voltage. There is some type of conducting medium or pathway that current travels along and that carries the flowing electrons. Finally, there is some component or group of components that are driven by this flowing current. These driven elements provide resistance to electrical flow.[6]

SERIES AND PARALLEL CIRCUITS

The components that provide resistance to current flow may be connected to one another in one of two different patterns, a **series circuit** or a **parallel circuit**. The main difference between these two is that in a series circuit there is only one path for current to get from one terminal to another. In a parallel circuit, two or more routes exist for current to pass between the two terminals.

series circuit A circuit in which there is only one path for current to get from one terminal to another.

In a series circuit the components are placed end-to-end (Fig. 5-9). The number of amperes of an electrical current flowing through a series circuit is exactly the same at any point in that circuit. The resistance to current flow in this total circuit is equal to the resistance of all the components in the circuit added together.

$$R_T = R_1 + R_2 + R_3$$

Electrical energy is required to force the current through the resistor, and this energy is dissipated in the form of heat. Consequently, there is a decrease in voltage at each component such that the total voltage at the beginning of the circuit is equal to the sum of the voltage decreases at each component.

$$V_T = VD_1 + VD_2 + VD_3$$

parallel circuit A circuit in which two or more routes exist for current to pass between the two terminals.

In a parallel circuit, the component resistors are placed side by side and the ends are connected (Fig. 5-10). Each of the resistors in a parallel circuit receives the same voltage.

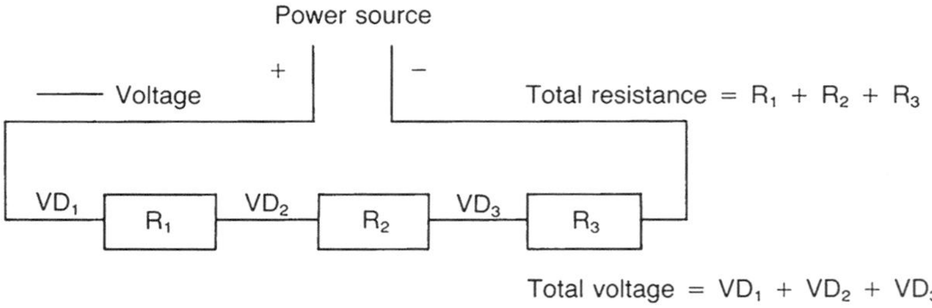

•**Figure 5-9** In a series circuit, the component resistors are placed end to end. The total resistance to current flow is equal to the resistance of all the components added together. There is a voltage decrease at each component such that the sum of the voltage decreases is equal to the total voltage.

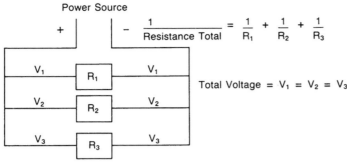

Power Source

$$\frac{1}{\text{Resistance Total}} = \frac{1}{R_1} + \frac{1}{R_2} + \frac{1}{R_3}$$

Total Voltage $= V_1 = V_2 = V_3$

•**Figure 5-10** In a parallel circuit the component resistors are placed side by side and the ends are connected. The current flow in each of the pathways is inversely proportional to the resistance of the pathway. The total voltage is the sum of the voltages at each component.

The current passing through each component depends on its resistance. Therefore, the total voltage will be exactly the same as the voltage at each component.

$$V_T = V_1 = V_2 = V_3$$

Each additional resistance added to a parallel circuit in effect decreases the total resistance. Adding an alternative pathway, regardless of its resistance to current flow, improves the ability of the current to get from one point to another. The current will, in general, choose the pathway that offers the least resistance. The formula for determining total resistance in a parallel circuit according to Ohm's law is:

$$\frac{1}{R_T} = \frac{1}{R_1} + \frac{1}{R_2} + \frac{1}{R_3}$$

Thus, component resistors connected in a series circuit have a higher resistance and lower current flow, and resistors in a parallel circuit have a lower resistance and a higher current flow.

The electrical modalities, in general, make use of some combination of both series and parallel circuits.[11] For example, to elicit a muscle contraction, the electrodes from an electrical stimulating unit are placed on the skin (Fig. 5-11). The current from those electrodes must pass directly through the skin and fat. The total resistance to current flow seen by the electrical stimulating unit is equal to the combined resistances at each electrode. This passage of current through the skin is basically a series circuit.

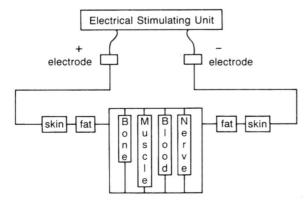

•**Figure 5-11** The electrical circuit that exists when electrons flow through human tissue is in reality a combination of a series and parallel circuit.

After the current passes through the skin and fat, it comes in contact with a number of different types of biologic tissues (bone, connective tissue, blood, muscle). The current has several different pathways through which it may reach the muscle to be stimulated. The total current traveling through these tissues is the sum of the currents in each different type of tissue, and because there are additional tissues through which current may travel, the total resistance is effectively reduced. Thus, in this typical application of a therapeutic modality, both parallel and series circuits are used to produce the desired physiologic effect.

CURRENT FLOW THROUGH BIOLOGIC TISSUES

As stated previously, electrical current tends to choose the path that offers the least resistance to flow or, stated differently, the material that is the best conductor.[28] The conductivity of the different types of tissue in the body is variable. Typically, tissue that is highest in water content and consequently highest in ion content is the best conductor of electricity.

The skin has different layers that vary in water content, but generally the skin offers the primary resistance to current flow and is considered an insulator. Skin preparation for the purpose of reducing electrical impedance is of primary concern with electrodiagnostic apparatus, but it is also important with electrotherapeutic devices (see Chapter 8). The greater the impedance of the skin, the higher the voltage of the electrical current must be to stimulate underlying nerve and muscle. Chemical changes in the skin can make it more resistant to certain types of current. Thus, skin impedance is generally higher with direct current than with alternating current.[14]

Blood is a biologic tissue that is composed largely of water and ions and is consequently the best electrical conductor of all tissues. Muscle is composed of about 75 percent water and depends on the movement of ions for contraction. Muscle tends to propagate an electrical impulse much more effectively in a longitudinal direction than transversely. Muscle tendons are considerably more dense than muscle, contain relatively little water, and are considered poor conductors. Fat contains only about 14 percent water and is thought to be a poor conductor. Peripheral nerve conductivity is approximately six times that of muscle. However, the nerve generally is surrounded by fat and a fibrous sheath, both of which are considered to be poor conductors. Bone is extremely dense, contains only about 5 percent water, and is considered to be the poorest biologic conductor of electrical current. It is essential for the therapist to understand that many biologic tissues will be stimulated by an electrical current. Selecting the appropriate treatment parameters is critical if the desired tissue response is to be attained.[13]

PHYSIOLOGIC RESPONSES TO ELECTRICAL CURRENT

The effects of electrical current passing through the various tissues of the body may be thermal, chemical, or physiologic.[24]

All electrical currents cause a rise in temperature in a conducting tissue.[20] The tissues of the body possess varying degrees of resistance, and those of higher resistance should heat up more when electrical current passes through. As indicated in previous chapters, the diathermies generate a continuous high-frequency electrical current that is designed to produce a tissue temperature increase. The electrical currents used for stimulation of nerve and muscle have a relatively low average current flow that produces minimal thermal effects.

Basically, electrical currents are used to produce either muscle contractions or modification of pain impulses through effects on the motor and sensory nerves. This function is dependent to a great extent on selecting the appropriate treatment parameters based on the principles identified in this chapter.[20]

tetany Muscle condition that is caused by hyperexcitation and results in cramps and spasms.

Treatment Tip
To produce a tetanic muscle contraction, current intensity should be increased sufficiently to produce a muscle contraction and then the frequency adjusted to approximately 50 pps. This will produce a tetanic contraction regardless of whether AC, DC, or pulsed current is being used.

Treatment Tip
Only a long-duration continuous DC current is capable of producing ion movement. Continuous DC current can also elicit a muscle contraction when the current is turned on and off.

Electrical currents are also used to produce chemical effects. Most biologic tissue contains negatively and positively charged ions. A direct current flow will cause migration of these charged particles toward the pole of opposite polarity. At the positive pole the negatively charged particles cause an acid reaction in which there is coagulation of protein and hardening of the tissues. At the negative pole the positively charged particles produce an alkaline reaction, liquefying protein, and causing softening of the tissues.

SAFETY IN THE USE OF ELECTRICAL EQUIPMENT

Electrical safety in the clinical setting should be of maximal concern to the professional therapist. Too often there are reports of patients being electrocuted as a result of faulty electrical circuits in whirlpools. This type of accident can be avoided by taking some basic precautions and acquiring an understanding of the power distribution system and electrical grounds.[10]

The typical electrical circuit consists of a source producing electrical power, a conductor that carries the power to a resistor or series of driven elements, and a conductor that carries the power back to the power source.

Electrical power is carried from generating plants through high-tension power lines carrying 2200 V. The power is decreased by a transformer and is supplied in the wall outlet at 220 or 120 V with a frequency of 60 Hz. The voltage at the outlet is alternating current, which means that one of the poles, the "hot" or "live" wire, is either positive or negative with respect to other neutral lines. Theoretically, the voltage of the neutral pole should be zero. Actually, the voltage of the neutral line is about 10 V. Thus, both hot and neutral lines carry some voltage with respect to the earth, which has zero voltage. The voltage from either of these two leads may be sufficient to cause physiologic damage.

The two-pronged plug has only two leads, both of which carry some voltage. Consequently, the electrical device has no true **ground**. The term true ground literally means the electrical circuit is connected to the earth or the ground, which has the ability to accept large electrical charges without becoming charged itself. The ground will continually accept these charges until the electrical potential has been neutralized. Therefore, any electrical charge that may be potentially hazardous (i.e., any electricity escaping from the circuit) is almost immediately neutralized by the ground. If an individual were to come in contact with a short-circuited instrument that was not grounded, the electrical current would flow through that individual to reach the ground.

Electrical devices that have two-pronged plugs generally rely on the chassis or casing of the power source to act as a ground. The danger with the two-pronged plug devices is that there is no true ground. Therefore, if an individual were to touch the casing of the instrument while in contact with some object or instrument that has a true ground, an electrical shock may result. With three-pronged plugs, the third prong is grounded directly to the earth and all excess electrical energy theoretically should be neutralized through this.

By far the most common mechanism of injury from therapeutic devices results when there is some damage, breakdown, or short circuit to the power cord. When this happens, the casing of the machine becomes electrically charged. In other words, there is a voltage leak, and in a device that is not properly grounded electrical shock may occur (Fig. 5-12).

The magnitude of the electrical shock is a critical factor in terms of potential health danger (Table 5-2). Shock from electrical currents flowing at 1 or less mA will not be felt and is referred to as **microshock**. Shock from a current flow greater than 1 mA is called **macroshock**. Currents that range between 1 and 15 mA produce a tingling sensation or perhaps some muscle contraction. Currents flowing at 15–100 mA cause a painful electrical shock. Currents between 100 and 200 mA may result in

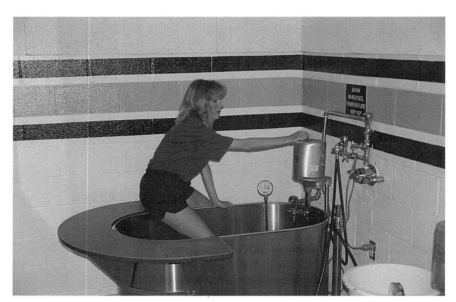

•Figure 5-12 There is danger of electrical shock when a therapeutic device is not properly grounded. This is a major problem in a whirlpool.

fibrillation of cardiac muscle or respiratory arrest. When current flow is above 200 mA, there is rapid burning and destruction of tissue.[18]

Most electrotherapeutic devices (e.g., muscle stimulators, ultrasound, and the diathermies) are generally used in dry environments. All new electrotherapeutic equipment being produced has three-pronged plugs and is thus grounded to the earth. However, in a wet or damp area the three-pronged plug may not provide sufficient protection from electrical shock.

We know that the body will readily conduct electricity because of its high water content. If the body is wet or if an individual is standing in water, the resistance to electrical flow is reduced even more. Thus if a short should occur, the shock could be as much as five times greater in this damp or wet environment. The potential danger that exists with whirlpools or tubs is obvious. The ground on the whirlpool will supposedly conduct all current leakage from a faulty motor or power cord to the earth. However, an individual in a whirlpool is actually a part of that circuit and is subject to the same current levels as any other component of the circuit. Small amounts of current therefore can be potentially harmful, no matter how well the apparatus is grounded. For this reason in 1981 the National Electrical Code required that all health care facilities using whirlpools and tubs install **ground-fault interruptors (GFI)** (Fig. 5-13). These devices constantly compare the amount of electricity flowing from the wall outlet to the whirlpool turbine with the amount returning to the outlet. If there is any leakage in current flow detected, the ground-fault circuit breaker will automatically interrupt current flow in as little as one-fortieth of a second, thus shutting off current flow and

Treatment Tip
The National Electrical Code requires that all whirlpools have ground-fault interruptors installed to automatically shut off current flow. In addition the therapist should not allow the patient to turn the whirlpool on or off. This is especially important when the patient is already in contact with the water. Extension cords or multiple adaptors should never be used in the hydrotherapy area.

TABLE 5-2	Physiologic Effects of Electrical Shock at Varying Magnitudes	
Intensity (mA)	**Physiologic Effects**	
0–1	Imperceptible	
1–15	Tingling sensation and muscle contraction	
15–100	Painful electrical shock	
100–200	Cardiac or respiratory arrest	
>200	Instant tissue burning and destruction	

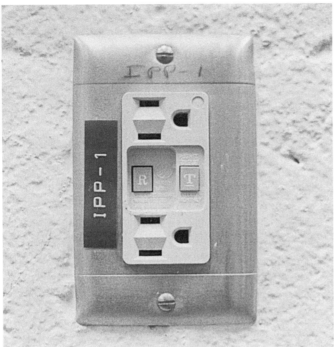

•**Figure 5-13** A typical ground-fault interruptor.

ground-fault interruptors (GFI) A safety device that automatically shuts off current flow and reducing the chances of electrical shock.

reducing the chances of electrical shock.[21] These devices may be installed either in the electrical outlet or in the circuit-breaker box.

Regardless of the type of electrotherapeutic device being used and the type of environment, the following safety practices should be considered.

1. The entire electrical system of the building or training room should be designed or evaluated by a qualified electrician. Problems with the electrical system may exist in older buildings or in situations where rooms have been modified to accommodate therapeutic devices (e.g., putting a whirlpool in a locker room where the concrete floor is always wet or damp).

2. It should not be assumed that all three-pronged wall outlets are automatically grounded to the earth. The ground must be checked.

3. The therapist should become very familiar with the equipment being used and any potential problems that may exist or develop. Any defective equipment should be removed from the clinic immediately.

4. The plug should not be jerked out of the wall by pulling on the cable.

5. Extension cords or multiple adaptors should never be used.

6. Equipment should be reevaluated on a yearly basis and should conform to National Electrical Code guidelines. If a clinic or training room is not in compliance with this code, then there is no legal protection in a lawsuit.

7. Common sense should always be exercised when using electrotherapeutic devices. A situation that appears to be potentially dangerous may in fact result in injury or death.

SUMMARY

1. Electrons move along a conducting medium as an electrical current.

2. A volt is the electromotive force that produces a movement of electrons; an ampere is a unit of measurement that indicates the rate at which electrical current is flowing.

3. Ohm's law expresses the relationship between current flow voltage and resistance. The current flow is directly proportional to the voltage and inversely proportional to the resistance.

4. Electrotherapeutic devices generate three different types of current, alternating (AC) or biphasic, direct (DC) or monophasic, or pulsatile (PC) or polyphasic, which are capable of producing specific physiologic changes when introduced into biologic tissue.

5. Confusion exists relative to the terminology used to describe electrotherapeutic currents, but all therapeutic electrical generators are transcutaneous electrical stimulators, regardless of whether they deliver biphasic, monophasic, or polyphasic currents through electrodes attached to the skin.

6. The term pulse is synonymous with waveform, which indicates a graphic representation of the shape, direction, amplitude, duration, and pulse frequency of the electrical current being produced by the electrotherapeutic device, as displayed by an instrument called an oscilloscope.

7. Modulation refers to any alteration in the magnitude or any variation in duration of a pulse (or pulses) and may be continuous, interrupted, burst, or ramped.

8. The main difference between a series and a parallel circuit is that in a series circuit there is a single pathway for current to get from one terminal to another, and in a parallel circuit two or more routes exist for current to pass.

9. The electrical circuit that exists when electron flow is through human tissue is in reality a combination of both a series and a parallel circuit.

10. The effects of electrical current moving through biologic tissue may be chemical, thermal, or physiologic.

11. Electrical safety is critical when using electrotherapeutic devices. It is the responsibility of the therapist to make sure that all electrical modalities conform to the National Electrical Code.

REVIEW QUESTIONS

1. How are the following electrical terms defined: potential difference, ampere, volt, ohm, and watt?

2. What is the mathematical expression of Ohm's law and what does it represent?

3. What are the three different types of electrical current?

4. What is a transcutaneous electrical stimulator and how is it related to a TENS unit?

5. What are the different types of waveforms that may be produced by electrical stimulating generators?

6. What are the various pulse characteristics of the different waveforms?

7. How can electrical currents be modulated?

8. What are the differences between series and parallel circuits?

9. How does electrical current travel through various types of biologic tissue?

10. What steps can the therapist take to ensure safety of the athlete when using electrical modalities?

REFERENCES

1. Alon, G.: Principles of electrical stimulation. In Nelson, R., Currier, D., editors. Clinical electrotherapy, Norwalk, CT, 1999, Appleton & Lange.
2. American Physical Therapy Association: Electrotherapeutic terminology in physical therapy: APTA section on clinical electrophysiology, Alexandria, VA, 2000, American Physical Therapy Association.
3. Bergueld, P.: Electromedical instrumentation: a guide for medical personnel, Cambridge, 1980, Cambridge University Press.

4. Carlos, J.: Clinical electrotherapy part I: physiology and basic concepts. PT—Magazine Phys. Ther. 6(4):44, 1998.
5. Chamishion, R.: Basic medical electronics, Boston, MA, 1964, Little, Brown.
6. Cohen, H., Brunilik, J.: Manual of electroneuromyography, ed. 2, New York, Harper & Row.
7. Cook, T., Barr, J.: Instrumentation. In Nelson, R., Currier, D., editors. Clinical electrotherapy, Norwalk, CT, 1991, Appleton & Lange.
8. Cromwell, L., Arditti, M., and Weibell, F.: Medical instrumentation for health care, Englewood Cliffs, NJ, 1976, Prentice-Hall.
9. DeDomenico, G.: Basic guidelines for interferential therapy, Sydney, Australia, 1981, Theramed.
10. Gersch, M.R.: Electrotherapy in rehabilitation, Philadelphia, PA, 2000, F.A. Davis.
11. Griffin, J., Karselis, T.: Physical agents for physical therapists, Springfield, IL, 1988, Charles C Thomas.
12. Holcomb, W.R.: A practical guide to electrical therapy. J. Sport Rehabile. 6(3):272–282, 1997.
13. Kahn, I.: Principles and practice of electrotherapy, Philadelphia, PA, 2000, Elsevier Health Sciences.
14. Kitchen, S., Bazin, S.: Electrotherapy: evidence-based practice, Wernersville, PA, 2001, Harcourt Health Sciences.
15. Kloth, L., Cummings, J.: Electrotherapeutic terminology in physical therapy, Alexandria, VA, 1990, Section on Clinical Electrophysiology and the American Physical Therapy Association.
16. Licht, S.: Therapeutic electricity and ultraviolet radiation, vol. IV, ed. 2, Baltimore, MD, 1969, Waverly.
17. McLoda, T.A., Carmack, J.A.: Optimal burst duration during a facilitated quadriceps femoris contraction. J. Athl. Train. 35(2):145–150, 2000.
18. Myklebust, B., Kloth, L.: Electrodiagnostic and electrotherapeutic instrumentation: characteristics of recording and stimulation systems and principles of safety. In Gersh, M.R.: Electrotherapy in rehabilitation, Philadelphia, PA, 2001, F.A. Davis.
19. Myklebust, B., Robinson, A.: Instrumentation. In Snyder-Mackler, L., Robinson, A. editors. Clinical electrophysiology, electrotherapy and electrotherapy and electrophysiologic testing, Baltimore, MD, 1995, Williams & Wilkins.
20. Nalty, T., Sabbahi, M.: Electrotherapy clinical procedures manual, New York, 2001, McGraw-Hill.
21. Porter, M., Porter, J.: Electrical safety in the training room, Athl. Train. 16(4):263–264, 1981.
22. Reed, A., Low, J.: Electrotherapy explained: principles and practices, Burlington, MA, 2000, Elsevier Science and Technology.
23. Robinson, A.: Basic concepts and terminology in electricity. In Snyder-Mackler, L., Robinson, A. editors. Clinical electrophysiology, electrotherapy and electrotherapy and electrophysiologic testing, Baltimore, MD, 1995, Williams & Wilkins.
24. Shriber, W.: A manual of electrotherapy, ed. 4, Philadelphia, PA, 1975, Lea & Febiger.
25. Stillwell, G.: Therapeutic electricity and ultraviolet radiation, ed. 3, Baltimore, MD, 1983, Williams & Wilkins.
26. Valkenberg, V.: Basic electricity, Clifton Park, NY, 1995, Delmar Learning.
27. Watkins, A.: A manual of electrotherapy, ed. 3, Philadelphia, PA, 1968, Lea & Febiger.
28. Wolf, S.: Electrotherapy: clinics in physical therapy, vol. 2, New York, 1981, Churchill Livingstone.
29. Zbar, P., Rockmaker, G., Bates, D.: Basic electricity: a text-lab manual, New York, 2000, McGraw-Hill.

SUGGESTED READINGS

Alon, G.: Electrical stimulators, Chattanooga, TN, 1985, Chattanooga Corporation. (Video presentation).
Alon, G.: High voltage stimulation: a monograph, Chattanooga, TN, 1984, Chattanooga Corporation.
Alon, G., Allin, J., and Inbar, G.: Optimization of pulse duration and pulse charge during TENS, Aust. J. Physiother. 29:195, 1983.
Baker, L., McNeal, D., and Benton, L.: Neuromuscular electrical stimulation: a practical guide, Downey, CA, 1993, Rancho Los Amigos Hospital.
Benton, L., Baker, L., and Bowman, B.: Functional electrical stimulation: a practical clinical guide, Downey, CA, 1980, Rancho Los Amigos Hospital.
Binder, S.: In Wolf, S., editor. Electrotherapy, New York, 1981, Churchill Livingstone.
Bowman, B., Baker, L.: Effects of waveform parameters on comfort during transcutaneous neuromuscular electrical stimulation, Ann. Biomed. Eng. 13:59–74, 1985.
Brown, I.: Fundamentals of electrotherapy, course guide, Madison, WI, 1963, University of Wisconsin Press.
Campbell, J.: A critical appraisal of the electrical output characteristics of ten TENS units, Clin. Phys. Physiol. Meas. 3:141, 1982.
Geddes, L.: A short history of electrical stimulation of excitable tissue, Physiologist 27:1, 1984.
Geddes, L., Baler, L.: Applied biomedical instrumentation, New York, 1975, Wiley.
Kottke, F.: Handbook of physical medicine and rehabilitation, ed. 3, Philadelphia, PA, 1982, W.B. Saunders.
Lane, J.: Electrical impedances of superficial limb tissues, epidermis, dermis, and muscle sheath, Ann. N.Y. Acad. Sci. 238:812, 1974.
Licht, S.: Electrodiagnosis and electromyography, vol. 1, ed. 3, Baltimore, MD, 1971, Waverly.
Mannheimer, J., Lampe, G.: Clinical transcutaneous electrical nerve stimulation, Philadelphia, PA, 1984, F.A. Davis.
Nelson, R., Currier, D.: Clinical electrotherapy, Norwalk, CT, 1999, Appleton & Lange.
Newton, R.: Electrotherapeutic treatment: selecting appropriate wave form characteristics. Clinton, NJ, 1984, Preston.

Newton, R.: Electrotherapy: selecting wave form parameters, paper presented at the American Physical Therapy Association Conference, Washington, DC, 1981.

Reismann, M.: A comparison of electrical stimulators eliciting muscle contraction, Phys. Ther. 64:751, 1984.

Scott, P: Clayton's electrotherapy and actinotherapy, eds. 5 and 7, Baltimore, MD, 1965 and 1975, Williams & Wilkins.

Sunderland, S.: Nerves and nerve injuries, Baltimore, MD, 1968, Williams & Wilkins.

Wadsworth, H., Chanmugan, A.: Electrophysical agents in physical therapy, Marickville, Australia, 1983, Science Press.

Ward, A.: Electricity waves and fields in therapy, Marickville, Australia, 1980, Science Press.

Glossary

accommodation Adaptation by the sensory receptors to various stimuli over an extended period of time.

alternating current Current that periodically changes its polarity or direction of flow.

ampere Unit of measure that indicates the rate at which electrical current is flowing.

amplitude The intensity of current flow as indicated by the height of the waveform from baseline.

average current The amount of current flowing per unit of time.

biphasic current Another name for alternating current, in which the direction of current flow reverses direction.

bursts A combined set of three or more pulses; also referred to as packets or envelopes.

circuit The path of current from a generating source through the various components back to the generating source.

conductance The ease with which a current flows along a conducting medium.

conductors Materials that permit the free movement of electrons.

coulomb Indicates the number of electrons flowing in a current.

current The flow of electrons.

decay time The time required for a waveform to go from peak amplitude to 0 V.

direct current Galvanic current that always flows in the same direction and may flow in either a positive or negative direction.

duration Sometimes also referred to as pulse width. Indicates the length of time the current is flowing.

electrical current The net movement of electrons along a conducting medium.

electrical impedance The opposition to electron flow in a conducting material.

electrical potential The difference between charged particles at a higher and lower potential.

electron Fundamental particles of matter possessing a negative electrical charge and very small mass.

faradic current An asymmetric biphasic waveform seldom used on modern electrical generators.

filter Changes pulsating DC current to smooth DC.

frequency The number of cycles or pulses per second.

ground A wire that makes an electrical connection with the earth.

ground-fault interruptors (GFI) A safety device that automatically shuts off current flow and reduces the chances of electrical shock.

high-voltage current Current in which the waveform has an amplitude of greater than 150 V with a relatively short pulse duration.

insulators Materials that resist current flow.

interpulse interval The interruptions between individual pulses or groups of pulses.

intrapulse interval The period of time between individual pulses.

ion A positively or negatively charged particle.

iontophoresis Uses continuous direct current to drive ions into the tissues.

low-voltage current Current in which the waveform has an amplitude of less than 150 V.

macroshock An electrical shock that can be felt and has a leakage of electrical current of greater than 1 mA.

medical galvanism Creates either an acidic or alkaline environment that may be of therapeutic value.

microcurrent electrical nerve stimulator (MENS) Used primarily in tissue healing. The current intensities are too small to excite peripheral nerves.

microshock An electrical shock that is imperceptible because of a leakage of current of less than 1 mA.

modulation Refers to any alteration in the magnitude or any variation in the duration of an electrical current.

monophasic current Another name for direct current, in which the direction of current flow remains the same.

neuromuscular electrical stimulator (NMES) Also called an electrical muscle stimulator (EMS), it is used to stimulate muscle directly, as would be the case with denervated muscle where peripheral nerves are not functioning.

ohm A unit of measure that indicates resistance to current flow.

Ohm's law The current in an electrical circuit is directly proportional to the voltage and inversely proportional to the resistance.

oscillator Used to produce and output a specific waveform, which may be different from that used to power or drive the stimulating unit.

output amplifier Used to magnify or increase the amplitude of the voltage output of the generator and control it at a specific level.

parallel circuit A circuit in which two or more routes exist for current to pass between the two terminals.

phases That portion of the pulse that rises above or below the baseline for some period of time.

polyphasic current (PC) Current that contains three or more grouped phases in a single pulse and that is used in interferential and "Russian" currents.

pulsatile currents Contain 3 or more pulses grouped togather and can be unidirectional or bidirectional.

pulse An individual waveform.

pulse charge The total amount of electricity being delivered to the patient during each pulse.

pulse period The combined time of the pulse duration and the interpulse interval.

ramping Another name for surging modulation, in which the current builds gradually to some maximum amplitude.

rate of rise How quickly a waveform reaches its maximum amplitude.

rectifier Converts AC current to pulsating DC current.

regulator Produces a specific controlled voltage output.

resistance The opposition to electron flow in a conducting material.

series circuit A circuit in which there is only one path for current to get from one terminal to another.

tetany Muscle condition that is caused by hyperexcitation and results in cramps and spasms.

transcutaneous electrical nerve stimulator (TENS) A transcutaneous electrical stimulator used to stimulate peripheral nerves.

transcutaneous electrical stimulator All therapeutic electrical generators regardless of whether they deliver AC, DC, or pulsed currents through electrodes attached to the skin.

transformer Reduces the amount of voltage from the power supply.

volt The electromotive force that must be applied to produce a movement of electrons. A measure of electrical power.

voltage The force resulting from an accumulation of electrons at one point in an electrical circuit, usually corresponding to a deficit of electrons at another point in the circuit.

watt A measure of electrical power (watt = volt × ampere).

waveform The shape of an electrical current as displayed on an oscilloscope.

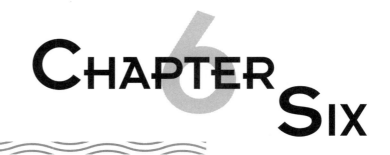

CHAPTER SIX

ELECTRICAL STIMULATING CURRENTS

DANIEL N. HOOKER

OBJECTIVES

Following completion of this chapter, the student therapist will be able to:

- ✓ Explain muscle and nerve responses to electrical stimulation.
- ✓ Describe nonexcitatory cell and tissue responses to electrical stimulation.
- ✓ Articulate the uses of electrically stimulated muscle contractions.
- ✓ Establish the various treatment parameters that must be considered with electrical stimulating currents.
- ✓ Determine the effect of noncontractable stimulation on edema.
- ✓ Compare techniques for modulating pain through the use of electrical stimulating currents.
- ✓ Differentiate between specialized electrical current generators in relation to physiologic changes and benefits.
- ✓ Identify problems that might respond to electrical stimulation.

Often the physical therapist uses electrical currents for treatment in an effort to create a quick cure for the physical problems suffered by his or her patients. Although electrical treatments can provide dramatic results at times, this is the exception rather than the rule. The use of electricity in treating an injury can be beneficial, but the therapist must base this use on facts about the effects of electricity on biologic tissues. The treatment program must be tailored toward influencing the problems identified in the evaluation. Electrical therapy should not be used in a "shotgun" approach if we are to maximize the effectiveness of this modality.

The clinical use of electrotherapy has changed as the changing technology has enabled equipment manufacturers to design and promote their latest product lines. Modern electronics have opened the doors to electronic equipment that could conceivably generate any electrical output desired. Wave shapes, amplitudes, and frequencies can be manipulated so that any combination is possible.

Research is lagging behind commercial development, as usual. Experts will continue to disagree with or challenge the interpretations of the results of the research that has been and will be conducted. Researchers in the biologic responses find it difficult to isolate one variable for experimentation and maintain control of all the other variables that could affect their results. Deciding whether the results of a study are significant for cause and effect, are merely a chance happening, or are significant but not directly caused by the manipulation of the experimental variable, becomes very difficult for the clinician. There are more questions than answers in this field of research.

Electrotherapy of the future is moving toward attempts at controlling cellular and tissue function with externally generated electrical currents. The therapist will need the concepts of **bioelectromagnetics**, the study of biologic tissues' electrical and magnetic properties, to apply and understand the therapeutic outcomes of the next generation of electrical modalities. Knowledge of the electric properties of cells, intercellular and intracellular communication, bioelectric potentials, tissue currents, strain-generated electric potentials, and the biologic effects of other nonionizing energy will be essential for the expert clinician to use present and future electrical modalities for maximum therapeutic benefit.[24,25]

PHYSIOLOGIC RESPONSE TO ELECTRICAL CURRENTS

Electricity has an effect on each cell and tissue that it passes through.[24,121] The type and extent of the response are dependent on the type of tissue and its response characteristics (e.g., how it normally functions and how it grows or changes under normal stress) and the nature of the current applied (i.e., direct or alternating, intensity, duration, voltage, and density). The tissue should respond to electrical energy in a manner similar to that in which it normally functions or grows. These statements are true within a certain range of current parameters, but current density above critical levels can cause coagulation and tissue destruction.[4] Clinically, therapists use electrical currents for the following reasons.

Physiologic Responses
- Excitatory
- Nonexcitatory

1. To create muscle contraction through nerve or muscle stimulations.
2. To stimulate sensory nerves to help in treating pain.
3. To create an electrical field in biologic tissues to stimulate or alter the healing process.
4. To create an electrical field on the skin surface to drive ions beneficial to the healing process into or through the skin.

As electricity moves through the body's conductive medium, changes in physiologic functioning can occur at various levels of the total system. Four levels can be readily identified from the functional standpoint.

1. Cellular
2. Tissue
3. Segmental
4. Systematic

Therapeutic Uses of Electricity
- Muscle contraction
- Sensory stimulation
- Ion movement

As in all classification systems, there is some overlap and assignment to one level may be arbitrary. The effects can be defined as follows.

1. Cellular level: This can be broken down into five major effects.
   a. Excitation of nerve cells
   b. Changes in cell membrane permeability
   c. Protein synthesis
   d. Stimulation of fibroblast, osteoblast
   e. Modification of microcirculation
2. Tissue level: This requires multiple cellular events.
   a. Skeletal muscle contraction
   b. Smooth muscle contraction
   c. Tissue regeneration

CASE STUDY 6-1
Electrical Stimulating Currents: Strengthening of Innervated Muscle

Background: A 22-year-old woman sustained a severe grade II medial collateral ligament sprain of the left knee 3 days ago in an auto accident, and is being treated with plaster immobilization for 3 weeks. She is not able to generate a maximal isometric quadriceps contraction voluntarily. The cast has been modified to accommodate electrodes over the femoral nerve and the motor point of the vastus medialis muscle. There are no restrictions on the amount of force she is allowed to produce during a knee extension effort.

Impression: Grade II medial collateral ligament (MCL) sprain of the left knee, with inability to generate maximal isometric force of the knee extensors.

Treatment Plan: A 5-day per week schedule of electrical stimulation was initiated. A polyphasic waveform was selected, with a 2500 Hz carrier wave, with an effective frequency of 50 Hz (10 msec on, 10 msec off). The stimulator was set to ramp the current up for 6 seconds, then maintain the current at a specific amplitude for 10 seconds, then drop to zero with no ramp; rest time was 50 seconds, giving an effective duty cycle of 1:5 (10 sec on, 50 sec off). Each treatment session began with 10 repetitions at a comfortable stimulus amplitude, followed by three sets of 10 repetitions each with the maximal amount of current tolerable. A 2-minute rest separated the sets. During the 10 seconds on time, the current amplitude was adjusted to the maximal amount the patient was able to tolerate. The patient was encouraged to contract the quadriceps femoris muscle group as the current was delivered.

Response: The patient's tolerance for the electrical stimulation gradually increased during the first week, then reached a plateau; this plateau was maintained for the next 2 weeks. Upon removal of the cast, there was no measurable or visible atrophy of the left thigh. A rehabilitation program of active range of motion, strengthening exercise, and functional activities was initiated, and the patient returned to full, pain-free activity 3 weeks following cast removal.

Discussion Questions:
- What tissues were injured or affected?
- What symptoms were present?
- What phase of the injury-healing continuum did the patient present for care in?
- What are the physical agent modality's biophysical effects (direct, indirect, depth, and tissue affinity)?
- What are the physical agent modality's indications and contraindications?
- What are the parameters of the physical agent modality's application, dosage, duration, and frequency in this case study?
- What other physical agent modalities could be used to treat this injury or condition? Why? How?

The rehabilitation professional employs physical agent modalities to create an optimum environment for tissue healing while minimizing the symptoms associated with the trauma or condition.

---

ionic channels in the wall that allow passive ion movement along the electrochemical gradients (Fig. 6-8C).

The only difference between excitable and nonexcitable cell membranes is the presence of voltage-gated sodium ion channels. In the excitatory cells, these ion channels generate the action potentials once a depolarizing stimulus causes the membrane to become more permeable to the outside Na^+. The Na^+ channels are triggered to open, and Na^+ ions move into the cell causing a brief reversal of charge. The charge reversal causes these ion channels to close, and the normal membrane potential returns.

The cell membrane is not only an outside covering but also is intimately involved with internal cell structures as an intercellular membrane, surrounds organelles, and supports the internal structure of the cell. This intercellular membrane can then exercise control of the movement of substances out from the cytoplasm or into the cytoplasm from the organelles. This movement is controlled by the same type electrochemical gradients and selective ion channels as that used in maintaining the cell wall (Fig. 6-8).[24,25]

CASE STUDY 6-2
ELECTRICAL STIMULATING CURRENTS: REEDUCATION OF INNERVATED MUSCLE (2)

Background: A 16-year-old male underwent arthroscopic partial medial meniscectomy on the right knee yesterday. He is to begin ambulation with crutches, weight bearing as tolerated, today. Clinic policy states that patients must be able to produce an active quadriceps femoris contraction prior to crutch-walking instruction. However, the patient is unable to produce an active contraction of the quadriceps femoris muscle. There is minimal pain and swelling, but after working with the patient for 15 minutes, he remains unable to contract the quadriceps femoris.

Impression: Status postarthroscopic surgery on the right knee with inhibition of quadriceps femoris control.

Treatment Plan: Using a pulsatile monophasic waveform generator, a course of electrical stimulation was initiated. The cathode (active, negative polarity) was placed over the motor point of the vastus mediails, and the anode (inactive, positive polarity) was placed on the posterior thigh. The frequency was set at 40 pps. Using an uninterrupted (1:0) duty cycle, the amplitude was set to a level that produced a visible contraction, but was below the pain threshold. After establishing the stimulus amplitude, the duty cycle was then adjusted to deliver 15 seconds of stimulus followed by 15 seconds of rest; the current was not ramped, so the effective duty cycle was 1:1. The patient was encouraged to contract the quadriceps femoris during the stimulation for the first five stimulations, then was asked to contract the quadriceps femoris before the stimulus was delivered.

Response: After 20 repetitions of the stimulus, the patient was able to initiate a contraction of the quadriceps femoris before the current was delivered. The electrical stimulation was discontinued, and the patient was able to continue to contract the quadriceps femoris voluntarily. He was then instructed in crutch walking, and routine postoperative rehabilitation was initiated.

Discussion Questions

- What tissues were injured/affected?
- What symptoms were present?
- What phase of the injury-healing continuum did the patient present for care in?
- What are the physical agent modality's biophysical effects (direct/indirect/depth/tissue affinity)?
- What are the physical agent modality's indications/contraindications?
- What are the parameters of the physical agent modality's application/dosage/duration/frequency in this case study?
- What other physical agent modalities could be utilized to treat this injury or condition? Why? How?
- Why was the patient unable to contract the quadriceps femoris following surgery?
- Why was the ability to contract the quadriceps femoris a prerequisite to crutch ambulation?
- What is the difference (pathway and physiology) between the voluntary muscle contraction and the induced (stimulated) contraction?
- How did the electrical stimulation assist the patient in regaining the ability to voluntarily contract the muscle?
- What is a viable alternative approach to assisting this patient?
- What would you suspect if there were no responses to the electrical stimulation?
- Why was the amplitude of stimulus set below the pain threshold?

The rehabilitation professional employs physical agent modalities to create an optimum environment for tissue healing while minimizing the symptoms associated with the trauma or condition.

Intercellular Structures

The internal cell structure is also made up of a dense network of hollow microtubules. These microtubules can be built and dismantled by the cell relatively rapidly and are **dipoles** with the negatively charged end directed centrally and the positive end directed peripherally. The microtubes are very active in cell function, moving materials such as neurotransmitters along the surface of the cell, making cilia move, moving organelles around within the cell, acting as sensors of the extracellular environment. The microtubes also form the mitotic spindle in the cell division process (Fig. 6-8). Because of its ability to change rapidly and help in cell movement and intracellular movement, the microtubes are probably significant actors in the organization of the cells during wound healing and regeneration.

CASE STUDY 6-3
ELECTRICAL STIMULATING CURRENTS: REEDUCATION OF INNERVATED MUSCLE

Background: A 23-year-old man experienced a Sunderland Grade V lesion of the left radial nerve as a result of an open fracture of the humerus sustained in a motorcycle accident. The injury occurred 2 years ago. There was an unsuccessful primary repair of the nerve injury; because there was no evidence of reinnervation, a sural nerve graft was completed 1 year ago. Again, there was no evidence of reinnervation, so the distal attachment of the flexor carpi radialis (FCR) was transferred to the posterior aspect of the base of the third metacarpal to provide wrist extension. The tendon transfer was completed 3 weeks ago. The wrist and forearm have been immobilized until yesterday, and the patient has been referred for rehabilitation. The surgeon has cleared the patient for gentle FCR contraction.

Impression: Posttendon transfer with lack of voluntary control.

Treatment Plan: Using a pulsatile biphasic waveform generator, a course of therapeutic electrical stimulation was initiated. A bipolar electrode arrangement was used, with one electrode over the motor point of the FCR and the other electrode approximately 4 cm distal, over the FCR. The pulse rate was set at 40 pps, and the effective duty cycle was set at 5:5 (5 sec on, 5 sec off), with a 2-second ramp-up and a 2-second ramp-down (so the total time the current was delivered was 7 sec, with 7 sec between stimulations). The current amplitude was adjusted to achieve a palpable contraction of the FCR, but no wrist motion, and the treatment time was set to 12 minutes, so as to achieve approximately 50 contractions.

Response: Treatment was conducted daily for 3 weeks, with gradual increases in the current amplitude and number of repetitions. At this time, the patient was able to initiate wrist extension independent of the electrical stimulation, and was discharged to a home program.

Discussion Questions:

- What tissues were injured or affected?
- What symptoms were present?
- What phase of the injury-healing continuum did the patient present for care in?
- What are the physical agent modality's biophysical effects (direct, indirect, depth, and tissue affinity)?
- What are the physical agent modality's indications and contraindications?
- What are the parameters of the physical agent modality's application, dosage, duration, and frequency in this case study?
- What other physical agent modalities could be used to treat this injury or condition? Why? How?
- What structures are involved with a Sunderland Grade V peripheral nerve injury?
- What is involved in a sural nerve graft? What was the surgeon trying to achieve?
- What factors led to the failure of the primary radial nerve repair and the sural graft?
- Why did the surgeon wait nearly a year after the primary repair to do the sural graft and nearly a year after the sural graft to perform the tendon transfer?
- Will wrist extension in the absence of extensor digitorum communis function really increase the patient's function? Why or why not?

The rehabilitation professional employs physical agent modalities to create an optimum environment for tissue healing while minimizing the symptoms associated with the trauma or condition.

Normal cells are signaled and respond to changes when messages contact the outer projections of the cell wall. Likewise, messages from within the cell can be sent outside the cell. The message can be chemical, such as hormones, or possibly be an electromagnetic energy coded message. Once the message is received, the signal is conveyed across the membrane to the cell's interior. The message is then transferred to another message system or switchboard that activates the cell's response to the message. The message may speed the cell up, make it move, stimulate production of extracellular proteins, or increase the secretions of that cell (Fig. 6-8A and B).[25]

Electrical Circuits in Tissue

Many cells are physically united with neighboring cells of like structure and collectively perform as one tissue. The cell membranes are bound together by junctions between the outer projections of each cell membrane. These specialized junctions allow direct

CASE STUDY 6-4
ELECTRICAL STIMULATING CURRENTS: STRENGTHENING OF INNERVATED MUSCLE (2)

Background: A 33-year-old woman sustained an isolated rupture of the left anterior cruciate ligament (ACL) 2 weeks ago while skiing. Three days ago, she underwent an arthroscopically assisted intraarticular reconstruction of the ACL using an autologous patellar-ligament graft. She is now weight-bearing as tolerated with axillary crutches, is using a removable splint, and has been cleared for accelerated rehabilitation.

Impression: Postoperative ACL reconstruction.

Treatment Plan: In addition to the standard active strengthening and range of motion exercise and physical agent modalities to control postoperative pain and swelling, a course of electrical stimulation for strengthening was initiated. The split was removed, and the patient was seated on an isokinetic testing and training device, with the left knee in 65 degrees of flexion and the device set at a speed of 0 degrees per second (isometric). A pulsatile polyphasic electrical stimulator was used, with electrodes placed over the motor points of the vastus medialis and vastus lateralis muscles. The stimulator produced a 2500-Hz carrier wave, with an effective frequency of 50 Hz (10 msec on, 10 msec off). A 2-second ramp-up a 2-second ramp-down setting was selected, with a total duty cycle of 10:50 (so 14 sec on, 50 sec off), and the current amplitude was adjusted to maximal tolerance during every third stimulation. Fifteen cycles were administered, then the patient rested for 5 minutes; this was repeated twice, for a total of 45 contractions per treatment session. The patient was treated three times per week for a total of 5 weeks.

Response: A linear increase in force produced during electrical stimulation, as well as maximal isometric force

production, was recorded over the 5 weeks of treatment. The patient's gait and range of motion improved, and she was discharged to a home program at the end of treatment.

Discussion Questions:
- What tissues were injured or affected?
- What symptoms were present?
- What phase of the injury-healing continuum did the patient present for care in?
- What are the physical agent modality's biophysical effects (direct, indirect, depth, and tissue affinity)?
- What are the physical agent modality's indications and contraindications?
- What are the parameters of the physical agent modality's application, dosage, duration, and frequency in this case study?
- What other physical agent modalities could be used to treat this injury or condition? Why? How?
- What advantages are there to augmenting the ACL repair with the patellar tendon?
- Why was the training of the quadriceps femoris conducted at 65 degrees of flexion? What biomechanical factors favor training at this joint angle as opposed to full extension of the knee?
- What effect did the electrical stimulation have on the healing rate of the reconstruction? On the patient's return to function?

The rehabilitation professional employs physical agent modalities to create an optimum environment for tissue healing while minimizing the symptoms associated with the trauma or condition.

communication between adjacent cells. These specialized junction areas are called **gap junctions** and contain channels for ionic, electrical, and small molecule signaling. The cells connected by gap junctions can then act together when one cell receives an extracellular message, the tissue can be coordinated in its response by the gap junction's internal message system. Embryonic and regenerating tissues are particularly rich in gap junctions, and they probably play a significant role in tissue growth and differentiation (see Fig. 6-8B).

Cells are surrounded by a bonding medium of collagen, elastin, and hyaluronic acid gel. This extracellular matrix can also interact with the adjacent cell surface receptors to modify cell function, orientation and alignment, shape, movement, metabolic rate, and differentiation.[25]

Strain-Related Potentials

The previous discussion of cell structure points out that every cell surface carries a charge. Every support structure within the cell, membranes, or microtubes are dipoles. In effect, cell structures have similar properties to electrets (insulators carrying a permanent charge, similar to a permanent magnet). **Electrets** are capable of **piezoelectric activity**, in which mechanical deformation of the structure causes a change in the surface electrical charge of the structure. They are also capable of **electropiezo activity**, in which changing an electric surface charge would force the electret to change shape. This becomes important when considering the piezoelectric effect of bone and connective tissue and how this change in electrical surface activity may guide or stimulate growth and healing.

Most connective tissues also generate a tissue-based electrical potential in response to strain of the tissue. Tension on surfaces or distraction on the surface creates these **strain-related potentials (SRPs)**. Where there is compression, the strain-related potentials are negative. Where there is tension these SRPs are positive. Functionally, these strain-related potentials have helped provide an electromechanical explanation for Wolff's law governing bone's growth in response to mechanical stress. The controlling mechanism for these events is most likely some form of the intrinsic electrochemical responses discussed earlier in this chapter, as no specific hormonal or neurologic controls have been discovered. The stress-generated potential must signal the membranes of the osteoblast, osteocytes, and osteoclasts to add or take away bone in areas of compression or tension. The cells have the necessary mechanisms to receive and decode the strain information, and intrinsically the cells can respond appropriately to maintain the integrity of the tissue (Fig. 6-9).[9,20,25]

Cells are grouped together into tissues creating segmental units, and segmental units combine into a whole system. Each cell, considered an ionic battery when added together with other cells, can collectively summate the influence and generate potential differences across the surface of the body or between different areas of the same tissue. These endogenous currents with their polarity gradients seem to play a key role in guiding the development, growth, regeneration, and repair of the cells, tissues, and segments of our bodies.[24]

Normal Bioelectric Fields

Becker demonstrated a direct current bioelectric field that could be measured in salamanders and other animals. The spatial configuration of this field coincided with the arrangement of their central nervous systems, with the positive areas being located near the major nerve cell accumulations, that is, brain, brachial, and lumbar plexus areas. The negative areas were near the major peripheral nerve outflows from these areas.[10–12,24,25]

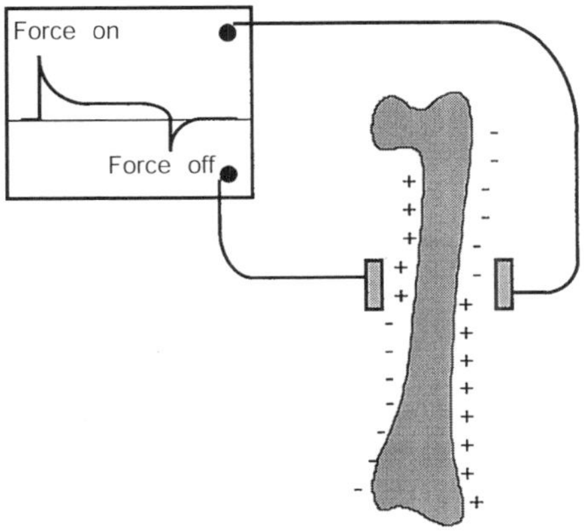

piezoelectric activity Changing electric surface charges of a structure forces the structure to change shape.

electrets Insulators carrying a permanent charge similar to a permanent magnet.

electropiezo activity Changing electric surface charges of a structure forces the structure to change shape.

strain related potentials Tissue-based electric potentials generated in response to strain for the tissue.

•**Figure 6-9** Electrical response of boney tissue to the momentary deforming stress of weight bearing.

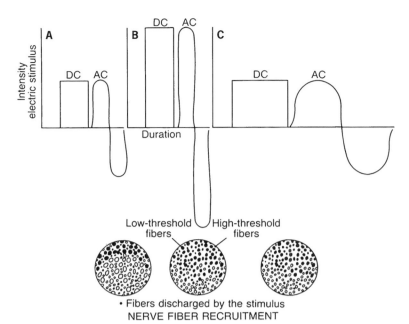

•**Figure 6-19** Recruitment of nerve fibers. **A.** A stimulus pulse at a duration-intensity just above threshold will excite the closest and largest fibers. Each electrical pulse of the same intensity at the same location will cause the same fibers to fire. **B.** Increasing the intensity will excite smaller fibers and fibers farther away. **C.** Increasing the duration will also excite smaller fibers and fibers farther away.

membranes (Fig. 6-19C). Greater numbers of nerve fibers then would react to the same intensity stimulus, because the current would be available for a longer period of time.[13,67,144] This method requires the use of a stimulator with an adjustable duration. The low-voltage stimulators usually are available with this parameter, whereas the high-voltage stimulators usually have a preset pulse duration.

POLARITY

During the use of any stimulator, an electrode that has a greater level of electrons is called the negative electrode or the cathode. The other electrode in this system has a lower level of electrons and is called the positive electrode or the anode. The negative electrode attracts positive ions and the positive electrode attracts negative ions and electrons. With AC waves, these electrodes change polarity with each current cycle.

With a direct current generator, the therapist can designate one electrode as the negative and one as the positive, and for the duration of the treatment the electrodes will provide that polar effect. The polar effect can be thought of in terms of three characteristics: (1) chemical effects, (2) ease of excitation, and (3) direction of current flow.[12,13,96,108,115,144]

Chemical Effects

Changes in pH under each electrode, a reflex vasodilation, and the ability to facilitate movement of oppositely charged ions through the skin into the tissue (iontophoresis) are all thought of as chemical effects. A tissue-stimulating effect is ascribed to the negative electrode. To create these effects, longer pulse durations (>1 min) are required.[12,52,110,115] The bacteriostatic effect was achieved at either the anode or cathode with intensities in the 5–10 mA range, although at 1 mA or below the greatest bacteriostatic effect was found at the cathode.[60] Another study using treatment times exceeding 30 minutes found some bacteriostatic effect of high-voltage pulsed currents.[78]

Chemical changes occur only with long duration continuous current.

Negative electrode = cathode
Positive electrode = anode

Muscle contraction = negative active electrode

Cathode = distal
Anode = proximal

Ease of Excitation of Excitable Tissue

The polarity of the active electrode usually should be negative when the desired result is a muscle contraction because of the greater facility for membrane depolarization at the negative pole. However, current density under the positive pole can be increased rapidly enough to create a depolarizing effect. Using the positive electrode as the active electrode is not as efficient, because it will require more current intensity to create an action potential. This may cause the patient to be less comfortable with the treatment. In treatment programs requiring muscle contraction or sensory nerve stimulation, patient comfort should dictate the choice of positive or negative polarity. Negative polarity usually is the most comfortable in this instance.[39,108,144]

Direction of Current Flow

In some treatment schemes, the direction of current flow also is considered important. Generally speaking, the negative electrode is positioned distally and the positive electrode proximally. This arrangement tries to replicate the naturally occurring pattern of electrical flow in the body.[12,99]

The direction of current flow could also influence shifting of the water content of the tissues and movement of colloids (fluid suspension of the intracellular fluid). Neither of these phenomena is well documented or understood, and further study is needed before clinical treatments are designed around these concepts.[105,117,144]

True polar effects can be substantiated when they occur close to the electrodes through which the current is entering the tissue. In laboratory situations in physics and physical therapy, polar effects occur in very close proximity to the electrode. To cause these effects, the current must flow through a medium. If the tissue to be treated is centrally located between the two electrodes, results cannot be assigned to polar effects.[12,65] Clinically, polar effects are an important consideration in iontophoresis, stimulating motor points or peripheral nerves, and in the biostimulative effect on nonexcitatory cells.

ELECTRODE PLACEMENT

When using any of the treatment protocols aimed at the electrical stimulation of sensory nerves for pain suppression, there are several guidelines that will help the therapist select the appropriate sites for electrode placement. Transcutaneous electrical nerve stimulation (TENS) uses similar-sized electrodes placed according to a pattern and moved in a trial-and-error pattern until pain is decreased. The following patterns may be used.

1. Electrodes may be placed on or around the painful area.
2. Electrodes may be placed over specific dermatomes, myotomes, or sclerotomes that correspond to the painful area.
3. Electrodes may be placed close to the spinal cord segment that innervates a painful area.
4. Peripheral nerves that innervate the painful area may be stimulated by placing electrodes over sites where the nerve becomes superficial and can be stimulated easily.
5. Vascular structures contain neural tissue as well as ionic fluids that would transmit electrical stimulating currents and may be most easily stimulated by electrode placement over superficial vascular structures.
6. Electrode placement over trigger point locations.[138]
7. Both acupuncture and trigger points have been conveniently mapped out and illustrated. A reference on acupuncture and trigger areas is included in Appendix A. The therapist should systematically attempt to stimulate the points listed as successful for certain areas and types of pain. If they are effective, the patient will have decreased pain. These points also can be identified using an ohm meter point locator to determine areas of decreased skin resistance.
8. Combinations of any of the preceding systems and bilateral electrode placement also can be successful.[83,84,96,148]
9. Crossing patterns, also referred to as an interferential technique, involve electrode application such that the electrical signals from each set of electrodes add together at some point in the body and the intensity accumulates. The electrodes are usually arranged in a crisscross pattern around the point to be stimulated (Fig. 6-20). If there is a specific superficial

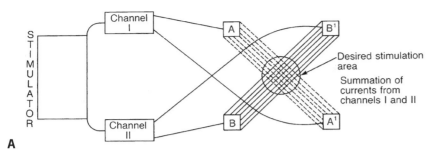

A

Treatment Tip
When using interferential current, the four electrodes should be set up in a square pattern with the target treatment area being in the center of the square so that the maximum interference will take place where the electric field lines cross at the center of the pattern.

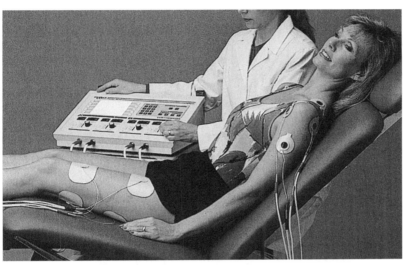

B

•**Figure 6-20 A.** Current flow would be from A to A′ and B to B′. As the currents cross the area of stimulation they summate in intensity. **B.** Application of electrodes in a crossing pattern for both the thigh and the shoulder.

area (e.g., medial collateral acromioclavicular joint) that you wish to stimulate, your electrodes should be relatively close together. They should be located so the area to be treated is central to the location of the electrodes. If there is poorly localized pain (general shoulder pain) that seems to be deeper in the joint or muscle area, spread your electrodes farther apart to give more penetration to the current.

The physical therapist should not be limited to any one system but should evaluate electrode placement for each patient. The effectiveness of sensory stimulation is closely tied in with proper electrode placement. As in all trial-and-error treatment approaches, a systematic, organized search is always better than a "shotgun," hit-or-miss approach. Numerous articles have identified some of the best locations for common pain problems, and these may be used as a starting point for the first approach.[83] If the treatment is not achieving the desired results, the electrode placement should be reconsidered.

THERAPEUTIC USES OF ELECTRICALLY INDUCED MUSCLE CONTRACTION

A variety of therapeutic gains can be made by electrically stimulating a muscle contraction:

1. Muscle reeducation
2. Muscle pump contractions
3. Retardation of atrophy
4. Muscle strengthening
5. Increasing range of motion

Any electrical stimulator—high-voltage, low-voltage, biphasic current, **hybrid current**, or TENS may be used to cause muscle contraction. The efficiency and effectiveness of treatment can be increased by following the protocols as closely as possible with the available equipment.

Muscle fatigue should be considered when deciding on treatment parameters. The variables that have an influence on muscle fatigue are the following.

1. Intensity: combination of the pulse stimulus' amplitude intensity and the pulse duration
2. The number of pulses or bursts per second
3. On time
4. Off time

Muscle force is varied by changing the intensity to recruit more or less motor units. Muscle force can also be varied to a certain degree by increasing the summating quality of the contraction with high burst or pulse rates. The greater the force, the greater the demands on the muscle, the greater the occlusion of muscle blood flow, the greater the fatigue. If high muscle forces are not required, the intensity and frequency can be adjusted to desired levels but fatigue can still be a factor. To minimize fatigue associated with forceful contractions, a combination of the lowest frequency and the higher intensity will keep the force constant.[15]

If high force levels are desired, then higher frequencies and intensities can be used. To keep the muscle fatigue as low as possible, the rest time between contractions should be at least 60 seconds for each 10 seconds of contraction time. A variable frequency train, in which a high-frequency then low-frequency stimulus are used, will also help minimize fatigue in repetitive functional electric stimulation.[15]

Neuromuscular-induced contraction at the higher torques are associated with patient perceptions of pain, either from the current used or the intensity of the contraction. This is often a limiting factor in the success of any of the following protocols. Each patient needs supervision and satisfactory therapist confidence for the most effective compliance with the treatment goals.[15,38,65]

When using electrical stimulation for muscle contraction, motor point stimulation can give the best individual muscle contraction. To find the motor point of a muscle, a probe electrode should be used to stimulate the muscle. Stimulation should be started in the approximate location of the desired motor point. (See Appendix A for motor point chart.) The intensity should be increased until contraction is visible, and the current intensity should be maintained at that level. The probe should be moved around until the best visible contraction for that current intensity is found; this is the motor point.[13,140] By choosing this location for stimulation, the current density can be increased in an area where numerous motor nerve fibers can be affected, maximizing the muscular response from the stimulation.

MUSCLE REEDUCATION

Muscular inhibition after surgery or injury is the primary indication for muscle reeducation. If the neuromuscular mechanisms of a muscle have not been damaged, then central nervous system inhibition of this muscle usually is a factor in loss of control. The atrophy of synaptic contacts that remain unused for long periods is theorized as a source of this sensorimotor alienation. The addition of electrical stimulation of the motor nerve provides an artificial use of the inactive synapses and helps restore a more normal balance to the system as the ascending sensory information will be reintegrated into the patient's movement control patterns. A muscle contraction usually can be forced by electrically stimulating the muscle. Forcing the muscle to contract causes an increase in the sensory input from that muscle. The patient feels the muscle contract, sees the muscle contract, and can attempt to duplicate this muscular response.[13,36,46,107] The object here is to reestablish control and not to create a strengthening contraction.

> **Treatment Tip**
> In a conventional TENS treatment, the goals is to provide as much sensory cutaneous input as possible. Thus, both the frequency and pulse duration should be set as high as the unit will allow. The intensity should be increased until a muscle contraction is elicited, then decreased slightly until the patient feels only a tingling sensation. If using a portable unit, the treatment may continue for several hours if necessary or until the pain subsides.

   Protocols for muscle reeducation do not list specific parameters to make this treatment more efficient, but the following criteria are essential for effective electrical stimulation.

1. Current intensity must be adequate for muscle contraction but comfortable for the patient.

2. Pulse per duration should be set as close as possible to chronaxie for motor neurons (300–600 μsec).

3. Pulses per second should be high enough to produce a tetanic contraction (35–55 pps) but adjusted so that muscle fatigue is minimized. Higher rates may be more fatigue producing than rates in the midrange of tetanic contraction.

4. On/off cycles should be based on the equipment parameters available and the therapist's preference in teaching the patient to regain control of the muscle. Currents that ramp up or down will require longer on-times so the effective current is on for 2–3 seconds. Off-times can either be a 1:1 contraction to recovery ratio or 1:4 or 5 depending on the therapist's preference or the patient's attention span and/or level of fatigue.

5. Interrupted or surged current must be used.

6. The patient should be instructed to allow just the electricity to make the muscle contract, allowing the patient to feel and see the response desired. Next, the patient should alternate voluntary muscle contractions with current-induced contractions.

7. Total treatment time should be about 15 minutes, but this can be repeated several times daily.

8. High-voltage pulsed or medium-frequency biphasic current may be most effective (see Fig. 6-20).[13,36,43]

MUSCLE PUMP CONTRACTIONS

Electrically induced muscle contraction can be used to duplicate the regular muscle contractions that help stimulate circulation by pumping fluid and blood through venous and lymphatic channels back into the heart.[33] A discussion of edema formation is included in Chapter 16. Using sensory level stimulation has also been found to decrease edema in sprain and contusion injuries in animals. That discussion is included elsewhere in this volume.

   Electrical stimulation of muscle contractions in the affected extremity can help in reestablishing the proper circulatory pattern while keeping the injured part protected.[44,45,66]

   The following criteria must be satisfied for the electrical treatment to be successful in helping to reduce swelling.

1. Current intensity must be high enough to provide a strong, comfortable muscle contraction.

2. Pulse duration is preset on most of the therapeutic generators. If adjustable, it should be set as close as possible to the duration needed for chronaxie (300–600 μsec) of the motor nerve to be stimulated.

3. Pulses per second should be in the beginnings of tetany range (35–50 pps).

4. Interrupted or surged current must be used.

5. On time should be 5–10 seconds.

6. Off time should be 5–10 seconds.

7. The part to be treated should be elevated.

8. The patient should be instructed to allow the electricity to make the muscles contract. Active range of motion may be encouraged at the same time if it is not contraindicated.

9. Total treatment time should be between 20 and 30 minutes; treatment should be repeated two to five times daily.

10. High-voltage pulsatile or medium-frequency biphasic current may be most effective (see Fig. 6-20).[36,46,111,114,128]

11. Use this protocol in addition to the normal ice for best effect.[49,105]

RETARDATION OF ATROPHY

Prevention or retardation of atrophy has traditionally been a reason for treating patients with electrically stimulated muscle contraction. The maintenance of muscle tissue, after an injury that prevents normal muscular exercise, can be accomplished by substituting

CASE STUDY 6-5
ELECTRICAL STIMULATING CURRENTS: PAIN MODULATION

Background: A 47-year-old man sustained a closed crush injury of the right foot in a construction accident 12 weeks ago. Radiographs revealed no bone injury, and the physical examination indicated that the neurovascular structures were intact. A pneumatic immobilization device was applied to the right leg in the emergency department, the patient was supplied with axillary crutches, and he was instructed to avoid weight bearing on the right foot until he was cleared by his family physician. The immobilization device was removed 6 weeks ago, and the patient was instructed to begin progressive weight bearing and to exercise the foot on his own. He has now been referred to you because of a progressive increase in burning pain in the foot and leg, with swelling and extreme sensitivity to touch. The patient refuses to bear weight on the foot and is not wearing a sock or shoe on the right foot.

Impression: Complex regional pain syndrome (CRPS) type I (aka Reflex Sympathetic Dystrophy).

Treatment Plan: A pulsatile biphasic current was delivered to the right leg, with electrodes over the anterior and posterior compartments. The frequency was 2 pps, and the amplitude was above the patient's pain threshold but below pain tolerance; a strong muscular twitch response was elicited. The current was delivered without interruption (duty cycle of 1:0) for 60 seconds. When the current was turned off, the patient's foot was brushed lightly with the therapist's hands. The process was repeated a total of 10 times in the initial treatment session, and the patient was instructed to attempt the brushing process at home.

Response: After the initial 60 seconds of current at the first treatment session, the patient was able to tolerate 5 seconds of light touch. After the tenth period of

stimulation, the patient was able to tolerate 45 seconds of moderate touch. Treatment was repeated 3 days per week for 2 weeks, at which time the patient was able to tolerate a sock and shoe, was partial weight-bearing, and continued the desensitization process on a home program.

Discussion Questions:

- What tissues were injured or affected?
- What symptoms were present?
- What phase of the injury-healing continuum did the patient present for care in?
- What are the physical agent modality's biophysical effects (direct, indirect, depth, and tissue affinity)?
- What are the physical agent modality's indications and contraindications?
- What are the parameters of the physical agent modality's application, dosage, duration, and frequency in this case study?
- What other physical agent modalities could be used to treat this injury or condition? Why? How?
- What is CRPS type I?
- What is the difference between CRPS type I and CRPS type II?
- Why was low-frequency TENS selected for this patient? Would other forms of TENS (e.g., conventional, hyperstimulation) have been effective? Why or why not?
- Is it likely that CRPS could have been prevented in this patient? How?

The rehabilitation professional employs physical agent modalities to create an optimum environment for tissue healing while minimizing the symptoms associated with the trauma or condition.

---

an electrically stimulated muscle contraction. The electrical stimulation reproduces the physical and chemical events associated with normal voluntary muscle contraction and helps to maintain normal muscle function.

Again, no specific protocols exist. In designing a program, the practitioner should try to duplicate muscle contractions associated with normal exercise routines. The following criteria can be used as guidelines in developing effective treatment protocols.

1. Current intensity should be as high as can be tolerated by the patient. This can be increased during the treatment as some sensory accommodation takes place. The contraction should be capable of moving the limb through the antigravity range or of achieving 25 percent or more of the normal **maximum voluntary isometric contraction (MVIC)** torque for the muscle. The higher torque readings seem to have the best results.

2. Pulse duration is preset on most of the therapeutic generators. If it is adjustable, it should be set as close as possible to the duration needed for chronaxie (300–600 μsec) of the motor nerve to be stimulated.

3. Pulses per second should be in the tetany range (50–85 pps).

4. Interrupted or surge-type current should be used.

5. On time should be between 6 and 15 seconds.

6. Off time should be at least 1 minute.

7. The muscle should be given some resistance, either gravity or external resistance provided by the addition of weights or by fixing the joint so that the contraction becomes isometric.

8. The patient can be instructed to work with the electrically induced contraction, but voluntary effort is not necessary for the success of this treatment.

9. Total treatment time should be 15–20 minutes, or enough time to allow a minimum of 10 contractions; some protocols have been successful with three sets of 10 contractions. The treatment can be repeated two times daily. Some protocols using battery-powered rather than line-powered units have advocated longer bouts with more repetitions probably because of low-contraction force.

10. A medium-frequency biphasic current stimulator is the machine of choice (see Fig. 6-20).[46,107,119,122,123]

MUSCLE STRENGTHENING

Muscle strengthening from electrical muscle stimulation has been used with some good results in patients with weakness or denervation of a muscle group.[86,90,141,142] The protocol is better established for this use, but more research is needed to clarify the procedures and allow us to generalize the results to other patient problems. The following summarizes the protocols used successfully.

1. Current intensity should be high enough to make the muscle develop 60 percent of the torque developed in a MVIC.

2. Pulse duration is preset on most therapeutic generators. If adjustable, it should be set as close as possible to the duration needed for chronaxie (300–600 μsec) of the motor nerve to be stimulated. In general longer pulse durations should include more nerves in response.

3. Pulses per second should be in the tetany range (70–85 pps).

4. Surged or interrupted current with a gradual ramp to peak intensity is most effective.

5. On time should be in the 10- to 15-second range.

6. Off time should be in the 50-second to 2-minute range.

7. Resistance usually is applied by immobilizing the limb. The muscle is then given an isometric contraction torque equal to or greater than 25 percent of the MVIC torque. The greater the percentage of torque produced, the better the results.

8. The patient can be instructed to work with the electrically induced contraction, but voluntary effort is not necessary for the success of the treatment.

9. Total treatment time should include a minimum of 10 contractions, but mimicking normal active resistive training protocols of three sets of 10 contractions can also be productive. Fatigue is a major factor in this setup. Electrical stimulation bouts should be scheduled at least three times weekly. Generally, strength gains will continue over the treatment course, but intensities may need to increase to keep pace with the most current maximum voluntary contraction torques.

10. A medium-frequency biphasic current stimulator is the machine of choice (see Fig. 6-20).[15,36–38,46,107,119,122,123]

INCREASING RANGE OF MOTION

Increasing the range of motion in contracted joints is also a possible and documented use of electrical muscle stimulation. Electrically stimulating a muscle contraction pulls the joint through the limited range. The continued contraction of this muscle group over an extended time appears to make the contracted joint and muscle tissue modify and lengthen. Reduction of contractures in patients with hemiplegia has been reported, although no studies have reported this type of use in contracted joints from athletic injuries or surgery. The protocol needed to affect joint contracture is the following.

1. Current intensity must be of sufficient intensity and duration to make a muscle contract strongly enough to move the body part through its antigravity range. Intensity should be increased gradually during treatment.

2. Pulse duration is preset on most of the therapeutic generators. If it is adjustable, it should be set as close as possible to the duration needed for chronaxie (300–600 μsec) of the motor nerve to be stimulated.

3. Pulses per second should be at the beginning of the tetany range (40–60 pps).

4. Interrupted or surged current should be used.

5. On time should be between 15 and 20 seconds.

6. Off time should be equal to or greater than on time, fatigue is a big consideration.

7. The stimulated muscle group should be antagonistic to the joint contracture, and the patient should be positioned so the joint will be moved to the limits of the available range.

8. The patient is passive in this treatment and does not work with the electrical contraction.

9. Total treatment time should be 90 minutes daily. This can be broken into three 30-minute treatments.

10. High-voltage pulsatile or medium-frequency biphasic current stimulators are the best choices (Fig. 6-21).

THE EFFECT OF NONCONTRACTILE STIMULATION ON EDEMA

Ion movement within biologic tissues is a basic theory in the electrotherapy literature. This is clearly seen in the action potential model of nerve cell depolarization. The effects of sensory-level stimulation on edema has been theorized to work on this principle. Research has not documented the effectiveness of this type of treatment, and therapists should continue to use other more proven mechanisms to decrease edema. See Chapter 14 for a discussion of edema formation.

Since 1987, numerous studies using rat and frog models have helped to more clearly define the effects of electrical stimulation on edema formation and reduction.[44,45,77,134,136] The muscle pumping theory discussed elsewhere in this volume has seemed the most viable way to effect this problem.[104] Most of the recent studies have focused on a sensory-level stimulation. Early theory supported the use of sensory-level direct current as a driving force to make the charged plasma protein ions in the interstitial spaces move in the direction of the oppositely charged electrode. Cook et al. demonstrated an increased lymphatic uptake of labeled albumin within rats treated with sensory level high-voltage stimulation.[33] However, there was no significant reduction in the limb volume. They hypothesized that the electric field introduced into the area of edema facilitated the movement of the charged proteins into the lymphatic channels. When the lymphatic channel volume increased, the contraction rate of the smooth muscle in the lymphatics increase. They also hypothesize that stimulation of sensory neurons may cause an indirect activation of the autonomic nervous system. This might cause release of adrenergic substances that would also increase the rate of lymph smooth muscle contraction and lymph circulation.

1. Extended treatment times, 1 hour.

2. Direct current stimulation with polarity arranged in correct fashion.

3. Electrodes arranged to pull or push plasma proteins into the lymphatic system and be moved back into the circulatory system via the thoracic duct.

Another proposed mechanism is that a microamp stimulation of the local neurovascular components in an injured area may cause a vasoconstriction and reduce the permeability of the capillary walls to limit the migration of plasma proteins into the interstitial spaces. This would retard the accumulation of plasma proteins and the associated fluid dynamics of the edema exudate. In a study on the histamine-stimulated leakage of plasma proteins, animals treated with small doses of electrical current produced

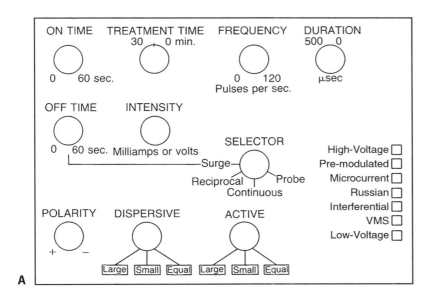

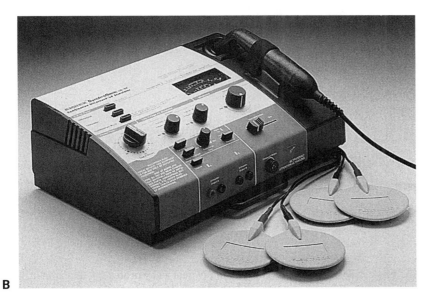

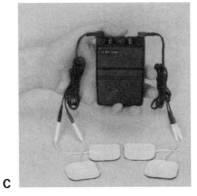

•Figure 6-21 A. Electrical stimulator control panel. B. High-volt unit. C. TENS.

less leakage. The underlying mechanisms were a reduced pore size in the capillary walls and reduced pooling of blood in the capillaries, which could have been initiated by hormonal, neural, mechanical, or electrochemical factors.

Theory on the exact mechanism of edema control from these methods remains cloudy and contradictory, but we do not have enough research findings to support trying an edema control electrical stimulation trial clinically.

The following is an edema control sensory stimulation protocol.

1. Current intensity of 30–50 V or 10 percent less than needed to produce a visible muscle contraction is most effective.
2. Preset short-duration currents on the high-voltage equipment are effective.
3. High-pulse frequencies (120 pps) are most effective.
4. Interrupted DC currents are most effective. Biphasic currents showed increases in volume.
5. The animals treated with a negative distal electrode had a significant treatment effect. The animals with a positive distal electrode showed no change.
6. Time of treatment after injury: The best results were reported when treatment began immediately after injury. Treatment started after 24 hours showed an effect on the accumulation of new edema volume but showed no effect on the existing edema volume.
7. A 30-minute treatment showed good control of volume for 4–5 hours.
8. The water immersion electrode technique was effective, but using surface electrodes was not effective.
9. High-voltage pulsed generators were effective, and low-voltage generators were not effective.[5,14,21,34,48,49,58,75,78,88,102,104,105,106,132,133]

STIMULATION OF DENERVATED MUSCLE

Electrical currents may be used to produce a muscle contraction in **denervated muscle**. A muscle that is denervated is one that has lost its peripheral nerve supply. The primary purpose for electrically stimulating denervated muscle is to help minimize the extent of atrophy during the period while the nerve is regenerating. Following denervation, the muscle fibers experience a number of progressive anatomic, biochemical, and physiologic changes that lead to a decrease in the size of the individual muscle fibers and in the diameter and weight of the muscle. Consequently, there will be a decrease in the amount of tension that can be generated by that muscle and an increase in the time required for the muscle to contract.[30,35] These degenerative changes progress until the muscle is reinnervated by axons regenerating across the site of the lesion. If reinnervation does not occur within 2 years, it is generally accepted that fibrous connective tissue will have replaced the contractile elements of the muscle and recovery of muscle function is not possible.[35]

A review of the literature indicates that the majority of studies support the use of electrical stimulation of denervated muscle. These studies generally indicate that muscle atrophy can be retarded, loss of both muscle mass and contractile strength can be minimized, and muscle fiber size can be maintained by the appropriate use of electrical stimulation.[31,61,64] Electrically stimulated contractions of denervated muscle may limit edema and venous stasis, thus delaying muscle fiber fibrosis and degeneration.[35] However, there also seems to be general agreement that electrical stimulation has little or no effect on the rate of nerve regeneration or muscle reinnervation.

A few studies have suggested that electrical stimulation of denervated muscle actually may interfere with reinnervation, thus delaying functional return.[91,120] These studies propose that the muscle contraction disrupts the regenerating neuromuscular junction retarding reinnervation, and that electrical stimulation may traumatize denervated muscle since it is more sensitive to trauma than normal muscle.[35,64,91]

TREATMENT PARAMETERS FOR STIMULATING DENERVATED MUSCLE

The following treatment parameters have been recommended for stimulating denervated muscle.

1. A current with an asymmetric, biphasic waveform with a pulse duration less than 1 msec may be used during the first 2 weeks.[79]

2. After 2 weeks, either an interrupted square wave direct current, a progressive exponential wave direct current, each with a long pulse duration of greater than 10 msec, or a sine wave alternating current with a frequency lower than 10 Hz will produce a twitch contraction.[35] The length of the pulse should be as short as possible but long enough to elicit a contraction.[135]

3. The current waveform should have a pulse duration equal to or greater than the chronaxie of the denervated muscle.

4. The amplitude of the current along with the pulse duration must be sufficient to stimulate a denervated muscle with a prolonged chronaxie while producing a moderately strong contraction of the muscle fibers.

5. The pause between stimuli should be 1:4 or 5 (15–40 mA) longer (about 3–6 sec) than the stimulus duration to minimize fatigue.[135]

6. Either a monopolar or bipolar electrode setup can be used with the small-diameter active electrode placed over the most electrically active point in the muscle. This may not be the motor point since the muscle is not normally innervated.

7. Stimulation should begin immediately following denervation using three stimulation treatments per day involving three sets of between 5 and 20 repetitions that can be varied according to fatigability of the muscle.[35]

8. The contraction needs to create muscle tension, so joints may need to be fixed, or isotonic contraction for end-range positions may be needed.

THERAPEUTIC USES OF ELECTRICAL STIMULATION OF SENSORY NERVES

Clinically, efforts are made to stimulate the sensory nerves to change the patient's perception of a painful stimulus coming from an injured area. To understand how to maximally affect the perception of pain through electrical stimulation, it is necessary to understand pain perception. The gate control theory, the descending or **central biasing** theory, and the opiate pain control theory are the theoretical basis for pain reduction phenomena. These theories are covered in depth in Chapter 4.

GATE CONTROL THEORY

Electrically stimulating the large sensory fibers when there is pain in a certain area will force the central nervous system to make the brain's recognition area aware of the electrical stimuli. As long as the stimuli are applied, the perception of pain is diminished. Electrical stimulation of sensory nerves will evoke the gate control mechanism and diminish awareness of painful stimuli. As long as the stimulation is causing firing of the sensory nerves, the gate to pain should be closed. If accommodation to the electrical stimulus occurs or if the stimulus stops, the gate is then open, and pain returns to perception.[16,20,83,84,87,98,99,102,118,119,123,144]

The physical dominance, enkephalin release model is used in treating pain from acute injuries, problems with the musculoskeletal system, or postoperative pain. The following criteria can be used as guidelines in developing effective treatment protocols.

1. Current intensity should be adjusted to tolerance but should not cause a muscular contraction, the higher the better.

2. Pulse duration (pulse width) should be 75–150 μsec or maximum possible on the machine.

3. Pulses per second should be 80–125, or as high as possible on the machine.

4. A transcutaneous electrical stimulator waveform should be used.

5. On time should be continuous mode.

6. Total treatment time should correspond to fluctuations in pain; the unit should be left on until pain is no longer perceived, turned off, then restarted when pain begins again.

7. If this treatment is successful, you will have some pain relief within the first 30 minutes of treatment.

8. If it is not successful, but you feel this is the best theoretical or most clinically applicable approach, change the electrode placements and try again. If this is not successful, then using a different theoretical approach may offer more help.

9. Any stimulator that can deliver this current is acceptable. Portable units are better for 24-hour pain control (see Fig. 6-20).[83,84,95]

DESCENDING PAIN CONTROL THEORY (CENTRAL BIASING THEORY)

Intense electrical stimulation of the smaller fibers (C fibers or pain fibers) at peripheral sites (trigger and acupoint) for short time periods causes stimulation of descending neurons, which then affect transmission of pain information by closing the gate at the spinal cord level (see Fig. 3-5).[23]

The central biasing setup is used on sharp chronic pain or severe pathologic pain. Changing the bias of the central nervous system and increasing the descending influences on the transmission of pain are best accomplished with the following protocols.

1. Current intensity should be very high, approaching a noxious level; muscular contraction is not desirable.

2. Pulse duration should be 10 msec.

3. Pulses per second should be 80.

4. On time should be 30 seconds to 1 minute.

5. Stimulation should be applied over trigger or acupuncture points.

6. Selection and number of points used varies according to the part treated.

7. A low-frequency, high-intensity generator is the stimulator of choice for central biasing (see Fig. 6-20).[23]

8. If this treatment is successful, pain will be relieved shortly after the treatment.

9. If this treatment is not successful, try different electrode setups by expanding the treatment points used.

OPIATE PAIN CONTROL THEORY

Electrical stimulation of sensory nerves may stimulate the release of enkephalin from local sites throughout the central nervous system and the release of β-endorphin from the pituitary gland into the cerebral spinal fluid. The mechanism that causes the release and then the binding of enkephalin and β-endorphin to some nerve cells is still unclear. It is certain that a diminution or elimination of pain perception is caused by applying an electrical current to areas close to the site of pain or to acupuncture or trigger points, both local and distant to the pain area.[23,29,92,98,101,119,125,149]

To use the influence of hyperstimulation analgesia and β-endorphin release, a point stimulation setup must be used.[93] A large dispersive pad and a small pad or hand-held probe point electrode are utilized in this approach. The point electrode is applied to the chosen site, and the intensity is increased until it is perceived by the patient. The probe is then moved around the area, and the patient is asked to report relative changes in perception of intensity. When a location of maximum-intensity perception is found, the current intensity is increased to maximum tolerable levels.[42] This is much the same as finding a motor point, as described earlier.[23,112]

Beta-endorphin stimulation may offer better relief for the deep aching or chronic pain similar to overuse injury's pain. Beta-endorphin production may be stimulated using the following protocols.

1. Current intensity should be high, approaching a noxious level: muscular contraction is acceptable.

CASE STUDY 6-6
ELECTRICAL STIMULATING: ANALGESIA

Background: A 52-year-old woman is 9 months post-hemilaminectomy and discectomy without fusion at L5-S1 due to a herniated disc with compromise of the S1 nerve root. The surgery resulted in relief of the peripheral pain, weakness, and sensory loss, but persistent pain in the lumbosacral spine and buttock prevents the patient from engaging in rehabilitation exercises effectively.

Impression: Status postspinal surgery with persistent postoperative pain; no neural deficit.

Treatment Plan: The patient was already being treated with a hot pack prior to exercise; conventional TENS was added to the treatment regimen. Electrodes were placed at the L3-4 interspace and over the greater trochanter. A pulsatile biphasic waveform was selected, with a rate of 60 pps, an amplitude between the sensory and motor thresholds, and a duty cycle of 1:0 (uninterrupted). The stimulation was delivered for the 10-minute heat application and remained in place during the therapeutic exercise, as well as for 30 minutes following the exercise.

Response: The patient experienced a 60 percent reduction in the symptoms during the exercise; this enabled the patient to perform the exercise through a greater range and with a greater effect. The effect of the TENS began to diminish after 8 weeks, but the pain had diminished to manageable levels such that the patient was able to continue the rehabilitation program without the TENS.

Discussion Questions

- What tissues were injured/affected?
- What symptoms were present?
- What phase of the injury-healing continuum did the patient present for care in?
- What are the physical agent modality's biophysical effects? (direct/indirect/depth/tissue affinity)
- What are the physical agent modality's indications/contraindications?
- What are the parameters of the physical agent modality's application/dosage/duration/frequency in this case study?
- What other physical agent modalities could be utilized to treat this injury or condition? Why? How?
- What factors led to the selection of conventional TENS?
- What would be the advantages and disadvantages of low TENS for this patient?
- What is the theoretical mechanism of action of conventional TENS?
- Why did the effect of the TENS diminish over time?
- Would you characterize the patient's pain as chronic or acute? Why? Are there different optimum forms of electrical stimulation for pain relief dependent on the nature of the pain?

The rehabilitation professional employs physical agent modalities to create an optimum environment for tissue healing while minimizing the symptoms associated with the trauma or condition.

2. Pulse duration should be 200 μsec to 10 msec.

3. Pulses per second should be between 1 and 5.

4. High-voltage pulsed current should be used.

5. On time should be 30–45 seconds.

6. Stimulation should be applied over trigger or acupuncture points.

7. Selection and number of points used varies according to the part and condition being treated.

8. A high-voltage pulsatile current or a low-frequency, high-intensity machine is best for this effect (see Fig. 6-20).[23,98,101]

9. If stimulation is successful, you should know at the completion of the treatment. The analgesic effect should last for several (6–7) hours.

10. If not successful, try expanding the number of stimulation sites. Add the same stimulation points on the opposite side of the body, add auricular (ear) acupuncture points, add more points on the same limb.

A combination of intense point stimulation and transcutaneous electrical nerve stimulation may be used. The transcutaneous electrical nerve stimulation applications should be used as much as needed to make the patient comfortable, and the intense point stimulation should be used on a periodic basis. Periodic use of intense point stimulation gives maximal pain relief for a period of time and allows some gains in overall pain suppression. Daily intense point stimulation may eventually bias the central nervous system and decrease the effectiveness of this type of stimulation.[67]

PLACEBO EFFECT OF ELECTRICAL STIMULATION

All three of these theories of sensory electrical stimulation produce their effects on the transmission lines of pain by interrupting or slowing the flow of pain information to the brain. The brain is the reception and interpretation center for these pain messages, and incorporating this area into your treatment can enhance the treatment's effects. This is crucial to a successful treatment because the therapist is trying to alter the patient's pain perception. This perceptual change is influenced by many factors at the cognitive and affective levels.

There is a major placebo effect in all that we do in providing any therapy to our patients. This placebo effect is a basic and extremely important tool to help us achieve the best results. Our attitude toward the patients and our presentation of the therapy to them are crucial. When the therapist demonstrates a sincere interest in the patient's problems, the patient uses that interest to add to his or her own conviction and motivation to get well.

When these factors are active, real physiologic changes occur that assist in the healing process. The therapist should not intentionally deceive the patient with a sham treatment but should use the treatment to have the best impact on the patient's perception of the problem and the treatment's effectiveness.

The treatment will work better if the patient has a profound belief in the treatment's ability to alleviate the problem. To gain the most from this effect, the patient needs to be intimately involved with the treatment. We must educate, encourage, and empower the patient to get better. Giving the patient the knowledge and ability to feel some control and to be self-determined in healing reduces the stress of injury and enhances the patient's recovery powers. In stressful situations any measure of control lessens the extent of the stress and results in the improvement of disease resistance or injury recovery factors that will improve treatment outcomes.[67]

CLINICAL USES OF LOW-VOLTAGE CONTINUOUS MONOPHASIC CURRENT

MEDICAL GALVANISM

The application of continuous low-voltage monophasic current causes several physiologic changes that can be used therapeutically. The therapeutic benefits are related to the polar and vasomotor effects and to the acid reaction around the positive pole and the alkaline reaction at the negative pole. The therapist must be concerned with the damaging effects of this variety of current. Acidic or alkaline changes can cause severe skin reactions.[144] These reactions occur only with low-voltage continuous direct current and are not likely with the high-voltage pulsed generators. The pulse duration of the high-voltage pulsatile generators is too short to cause these chemical changes.[110]

There is also a vasomotor effect on the skin, increasing blood flow between the electrodes. The benefits from this type of direct current are usually attributed to the increased blood flow through the treatment area.[144]

The following protocols for continuous low-voltage direct current can be used to give the greatest vasomotor effects.

1. Current intensity should be to the patient's tolerance; it should be increased as accommodation takes place. These intensities are in the mA range.
2. Continuous monophasic current should be used.

3. Pulses per second should be 0.

4. A low-voltage monophasic current stimulator is the machine of choice.

5. Treatment time should be between a 15-minute minimum and a 50-minute maximum.

6. Equal-sized electrodes are used over gauze that has been soaked in saline solution and lightly squeezed.

7. Skin should be unbroken (see Fig. 6-20).[74,108,112]

IONTOPHORESIS

Direct current has been used for many years to transport ions from the heavy metals into and through the skin for treatment of skin infections or for a counterirritating effect. Iontophoresis is discussed in detail in Chapter 7.

TREATMENT PRECAUTIONS WITH CONTINUOUS MONOPHASIC CURRENTS

Skin burns are the greatest hazard of any continuous monophasic current technique. These burns result from excessive electrical density in any area, usually from direct metal contact with skin or from setting the intensity too high for the size of the active electrode. Both these problems cause a very high density of current in the area of contact.[108,112]

FUNCTIONAL ELECTRICAL STIMULATION (FES)

Since the mid-1980s researchers have experimented with using computer-controlled electrical currents that stimulate the peripheral nervous system for the purpose of providing dynamic assistance in functional activities, such as walking or upper extremity function.[85] Used primarily in patients who have sustained spinal cord injury or suffered a stroke, **functional electrical stimulation (FES)** utilizes multiple-channel electrical stimulators controlled by a microprocessor to recruit muscles in a programmed synergistic sequence that will allow the patient to accomplish a specific functional movement pattern.[42,85] Even though this technique has been used effectively in short-term management of a variety of dysfunctions, there are many practical considerations for use that might impede or limit the long-term independent usefulness of FES by a patient.[9]

Currently, the majority of FES programs are limited to the use of surface electrodes that are difficult to adhere to the skin and to maintain positioning at the appropriate stimulation point.[63] For FES to be useful to the patient on a daily basis, the electrodes, and possibly the stimulator itself, will need to be implanted directly into the muscle or on a nerve.[1,53] Research is ongoing toward this end, but to date no acceptable system has been developed.

The existing computer control systems for FES also need to be refined if they are to be both useful and safe for the patient. The control systems must use either a preset activation sequence that will allow the patient to execute a specific task, or there must be some type of feedback from the stimulated neuromuscular systems so that the computer can make the appropriate movement corrections to ensure the safety of the patient. The development of a "closed-loop" feedback control system that would allow the computer to compensate for uneven terrain or to adjust the speed and frequency of movement presents a major challenge to researchers working in this area.[152]

functional electrical stimulation
Utilizes multiple channel electrical stimulators to recruit muscles in a programmed sequence that produces a functional movement pattern.

Although multichannel microprocessors may be preprogrammed to execute a variety of specific movement patterns, how those programs will be activated presents another obstacle for development of FES systems. Foot switches or crutch switches may potentially be used to trigger a desired response, although there are limitations to the number of switches that a spinal cord or stroke patient would actually be able to use.[42] Some of the upper extremity control devices have used movements of the contralateral shoulder to trigger a response. Verbal commands recognized by the computer also have been used to control stimulation of muscle in various functional tasks.[9]

Presently long-term independent use of FES is practical for only a few problems.[9] Certainly as new technologies continue to become available, ongoing clinical research will make FES increasingly practical for various patient populations. The future of FES holds many exciting possibilities for patients and therapists alike.

CLINICAL USES OF FES

FES has a number of clinical applications.[82] Initially, FES was used for stroke patients with a foot drop to assist dorsiflexion. Subsequently it was found to be more useful in treating patients with incomplete spinal cord injury who have good stance stability but are unable to achieve adequate flexion during the swing phase of gait.[9]

Functional electrical stimulation has been used with some success, enabling patients to stand, transfer, ambulate on level surfaces, and even ascend stairs on a limited basis using a walker or crutches in a closely supervised environment.[17,47,73,80,94,126] Spinal cord patients have used computer-controlled FES to allow them to exercise on bicycle ergometers to improve cardiorespiratory endurance and fitness.[8,19,139]

Control of muscles in the upper extremity using multiple-channel stimulation has allowed paraplegic patients to use the muscles of the hand and forearm of the paralyzed limb in functional grasp patterns. FES has also been used effectively in managing shoulder subluxation in the hemiplegic patient.[9]

SPECIALIZED ELECTRICAL CURRENTS

LOW-INTENSITY STIMULATORS (LIS)

LIS < 1 mA

Another type of low-voltage equipment is the low-intensity stimulator (LIS). The characteristic that distinguishes this type of generator is that the intensity of the stimulus is limited to 1000 μA or less in LIS, whereas the intensity of the standard low-voltage equipment can be increased into the mamp range.[3]

Generators that produce LIS were originally called microcurrent electrical neuromuscular stimulators (MENS). However, the stimulation pathway is not the usual neural pathway, and they are not designed to stimulate a muscle contraction. Consequently, this type of generator was subsequently referred to as a microcurrent electrical stimulator (MES). Low-intensity stimulator is the most recent and currently used term in an ongoing evolution of terminology relative to this type of stimulator.

Perhaps the most important point to emphasize is that currents generated by these devices are not substantially different from the currents discussed previously. These currents still have a direction, and both biphasic and monophasic waveforms are available. The currents also have amplitude (intensity), pulse duration, and frequency.

Low-intensity stimulator currents are defined as those of less than 1 mA or 1000 μA. The generators can generate a variety of waveforms from modified monophasic to biphasic square waves with frequencies from 0.3 to 50 Hz. The pulse durations are also variable and may be prolonged at the lower frequencies from 1 to 500 msec. This varies as the frequency changes or is preset when pulsatile currents are used. Many of these devices are made with an impedance-sensitive voltage that adapts the current to the impedance to keep the current constant as selected.[114]

If the current generator can be adjusted to allow increases of intensity above 1000 μA, the current becomes like those previously described in this text. If the current provokes an action potential in a sensory or motor nerve, the results on that tissue will be the same as previously described for other currents' sensation or muscle contraction.

Most of the literature on microcurrents and subsequently on low-intensity stimulators has been generated by researchers interested in stimulating the healing process in fractures and skin wounds. Subsequent research aimed at identifying why and how microcurrents work. The best researched areas of application of LIS-type currents is in the stimulation of bone formation in delayed union or nonunion of fractures of the long bones. Most of this research was done using implanted rather than surface electrodes, and most have used low-intensity direct current (LIDC) with the negative pole placed at the fracture site.[5,11,37] We are in danger of generalizing treatments for all problems based on success in this one area. These applications were intended to mimic the normal electrical field created during the injury and healing process.[4,48] At present these electrical changes are poorly understood, and the effects of adding additional electric current to the normal electrical activity created by the injury and healing process are still being investigated.

As can be seen in the previous sections on the bioelectric properties of cells and tissues, there are several possible theories that might explain the biostimulative effects of LIS currents and give the therapist some guidance in developing clinical protocols.

The current of injury, stress-generated potentials, cell metabolism stimulation, and bioelectric fields guiding growth are all natural events that low-intensity stimulation may augment, stimulate, or artificially replace.[24,25]

Low-intensity stimulation has been used for two major effects:

1. Analgesia of the painful area.
2. Biostimulation of the healing process, either for enhancing the process or for acceleration of its stages.[40]

Analgesic Effects of Low-Intensity Stimulation

The mechanism of analgesia created by LIS current does not fit into our present theoretical framework, as sensory nerve excitation is a necessary component of all three models of electroanalgesia stimulation. At best LIS can create or change the constant direct current flow of the neural tissues, which may have some way of biasing the transmission of the painful stimulus. Low-intensity stimulation may also make the nerve cell membrane more receptive to neurotransmitters that will block transmission. The exact mechanism has not yet been established. The research is not supportive of the effectiveness of LIS for pain reduction.[18,131] This lack of consensus and disagreement in the research gives the therapist limited security in devising an effective protocol. Most of the research uses delayed onset muscle soreness (DOMS) or cold-induced pain models, and results show no difference between LIS and placebo treatments.[2,7,21,42,55,62,71,72,81,100,116,118,137,145,147,153]

Promotion of Wound Healing

Low-intensity monophasic current has been used to treat skin ulcers that have poor blood flow. The treated ulcers show accelerated healing rates when compared with untreated skin ulcers.

The following protocol was used to promote wound healing.

1. Current intensity was 200–400 μA for normal skin and 400–800 μA for denervated skin.
2. Long pulse durations or continuous uninterrupted currents can be used.
3. Maximum pulse frequency.
4. Monophasic direct current is best but biphasic direct current is acceptable. Low-intensity stimulators can be used but other generators with intensities adjusted to subsensory levels also can be effective. A battery-powered portable unit is most convenient.
5. Treatment time was 2 hours followed by a 4-hour rest time.
6. Utilize two to three treatment bouts per day.
7. The negative electrode is positioned in the wound area for the first 3 days. The positive electrode should be positioned 25 cm proximal to the wound.
8. After 3 days the polarity is reversed and the positive electrode is positioned in the wound area.
9. If infection is present, the negative electrode should be left in the wound area until the signs of infection are not evident. The negative electrode remains in the wound for 3 days after the infection clears.
10. If the wound-size decreases plateau, then return the negative electrode to the wound area for 3 days.

Other protocols have been successful using the anode in the wound area for the entire time. High-voltage stimulation also has been used in a manner similar to the negative-positive model presented. The intensity was adjusted to give a microamp current.

LIS Effects
- Analgesia
- Fracture healing
- Wound healing
- Ligament and tendon healing

The mechanism by which LIS stimulates healing is elusive, but cells are stimulated to increase their normal proliferation, migration, motility, DNA synthesis, and collagen synthesis. Receptor levels for growth factor have also shown a significant increase when wound areas are stimulated.[22,26,27,52,54,57,69,89,107,140,146,151] The naturally occurring electrical potential gradients are enhanced following electrical stimulation.[55]

Promotion of Fracture Healing

The use of low-intensity direct current may be an adjunctive modality in the treatment of fractures, especially fractures prone to nonunion. Fracture healing may be accelerated by passing a monophasic current through the fracture site. Getting the current into the bony area without an invasive technique is difficult.[12,20,23,25,32,37,70,113,130]

Using a standard transcutaneous electrical nerve stimulation unit, Kahn reported favorable results in the electrical stimulation of callus formation in fractures that had nonunions after 6 months.[74] This information is based on a case study. Results of a more extensive population of nonunions have not been documented. Kahn used the following protocol.

1. Current intensity was just perceptible to the patient.
2. Pulse duration was the longest duration allowed on the unit (100–200 msec).
3. Pulses per second were set at the lowest frequency allowed on the unit (5–10 pps).
4. Standard monophasic or biphasic current in the transcutaneous electrical stimulating units were used.
5. Treatment time was from 30 minutes to 1 hour, three to four times daily.
6. A negative electrode was placed close to but distal to the fracture site. A positive electrode was placed proximal to the immobilizing device.
7. If four pads were used, the interferential placement described earlier was used.
8. Results were reassessed at monthly intervals (see Fig. 6-20).[74]

Promotion of Healing in Tendon and Ligament

There are only a few research studies on the biostimulative effect of electrical stimulation on tendon or ligament healing. Both tissues have been found to generate strain-generated electric potentials naturally in response to stress. These potentials help signal the tissue to grow in response to the stress according to Wolff's law.

In an experimental study on partial division of dog patellar tendons treated with 20 µA cathodal stimulation, the stimulated tendons showed 92 percent recovery of normal breaking strength at 8 weeks.[127]

Tendon stimulated in vitro in a culture medium showed increased fibroblastic cellular activity, tendon cellular proliferation, and collagen synthesis. The rate at which stimulated tendons demonstrated histologic repair at the injury site was also significantly accelerated over the control group.[109] Litke and Dahners studied rat medial collateral ligament (MCL) injuries treated with electrical simulation. The treated group showed statistical significance in the rupture force, stiffness, energy absorbed, and laxity.[91]

As can be seen by the previous sections, LIS current can be a valuable addition to the clinical armamentarium of the therapist, but it is untested clinically.

This is a case where more may not be better. For electricity to produce these effects (1) cells must be current-sensitive; (2) correct polarity orientation may be necessary; and (3) correct amounts of current will cause the cells to be more active in the healing process.

If results are not going correctly, then reduce the current and/or change polarity. Weak stimuli may increase physiologic activity, whereas very much stronger stimuli abolish or inhibit activity.

Most generators in use today are capable of low-intensity current. Simply turn the machine on but do not increase the intensity to threshold levels. This can also be a function of current density using electrode size and placement as well as intensity to keep current in the µamp range.

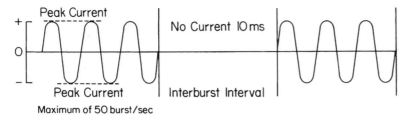

•**Figure 6-22** Russian current with pulsatile AC wave form and 10-msec interburst interval.

The therapist is certainly entitled to be very skeptical of the manufacturers' claims until more research is reported. Existing protocols for use are not well established, which leaves the therapist with an insecure feeling about this modality.

RUSSIAN CURRENTS (MEDIUM-FREQUENCY CURRENT GENERATORS)

This class of current generators was developed in Canada and the United States after the Russian scientist Yadou M. Kots presented a seminar on the use of electrical muscular stimulators to augment strength gain.[143] The stimulators developed after this presentation were termed "Russian current" generators. These stimulators have evolved and presently deliver a medium-frequency (2000–10,000 Hz) pulsatile biphasic waveform. The pulse can be varied from 50 to 250 μsec; the phase duration will be one-half of the pulse duration, or 25–125 μsec.[40] As the pulse frequency increases, the pulse duration decreases.[24,48,56] There are two basic waveforms: a sine wave and a square wave cycle with a fixed intrapulse interval.

The sine wave is produced in a burst mode that has a 50 percent duty cycle. According to strength-duration curve data, to obtain the same stimulation effect as the duration of the stimulus decreases, the intensity must be increased. The intensity associated with this duration of current could be considered painful.

To make this intensity of current tolerable, it is generated in 50-bursts-per-second envelopes with an interburst interval of 10 msec. This slightly reduces the total current but allows enough of a peak current intensity to stimulate muscle very well (Fig. 6-22). If the current continued without the burst effect, the total current delivered would equal the lightly shaded area in Fig. 6-23. When generated with the burst effect, the total current is decreased. Here the total current would equal the darkly shaded area in Fig. 6-24. This allows tolerance of greater current intensity by the patient. The other factor affecting patient comfort is the effect that frequency will have on the impedance of the tissue. Higher-frequency currents reduce the resistance to the current flow, again making this type of waveform comfortable enough that the patient may tolerate higher intensities. As the intensity increases, more motor nerves are stimulated, increasing the magnitude of the contraction. Because it is a fast-oscillating biphasic current, as soon as the nerve repolarizes it is stimulated again, producing a current that will maximally summate muscle contraction.[97]

Russian current A medium frequency (2000–10,000 Hz) polyphasic AC wave generated in 50-bursts-per-second envelopes.

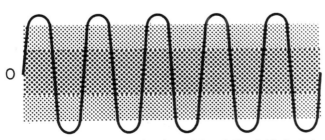

•**Figure 6-23** Russian current without an interburst interval. The light shaded area is equal to the total current.

CASE STUDY 6-7
ELECTRICAL STIMULATION: CONTROL OF SWELLING

Background: A 43-year-old woman recreational runner sustained a grade II ankle sprain (inversion stress) approximately 4 hours prior to presentation for treatment. She is ambulatory in a touch weight bearing mode with crutches and is not in acute distress. Positive signs are limited to the ankle, which demonstrates 3+/4 swelling, marked restriction in range of motion, and point tenderness over the anterior talo-fibular and calcaneal-fibular ligaments. There is no loss of ligamentous stability.

Impression: Grade II ankle sprain, with significant swelling.

Treatment Plan: In addition to therapeutic exercise, electrical stimulation was selected to assist in the reduction of the swelling. A monophasic pulsatile waveform generator was selected, and the cathode (negative polarity) was placed over the anterio-lateral aspect of the ankle, with the anode over the posterior leg. The pulse rate was set at 120 pps, with the amplitude between the sensory and motor thresholds. Stimulation was applied for 30 minutes daily.

Response: The swelling was reduced by approximately 30 percent after the initial treatment, but had returned the next day. Over the next 5 days, the swelling was markedly reduced following treatment, but regressed by about 50 percent by the next day. Electrical stimulation was discontinued after 7 days. A progressive rehabilitation program was initiated the first day, and the patient returned to full activity after 3 weeks.

Discussion Questions

- What tissues were injured/affected?
- What symptoms were present?
- What phase of the injury-healing continuum did the patient present for care in?
- What are the physical agent modality's biophysical effects (direct/indirect/depth/tissue affinity)?
- What are the physical agent modality's indications/contraindications?
- What are the parameters of the physical agent modality's application/dosage/duration/frequency in this case study?
- What other physical agent modalities could be utilized to treat this injury or condition? Why? How?
- Is electrical stimulation the most effective means to control the swelling in this patient's ankle? What approach might be more or equally effective?
- How will the swelling affect the healing of the injured tissues?
- How will the swelling affect the ability of the patient to perform therapeutic exercise?
- What are the physiological mechanisms for the swelling? For the resolution of the swelling?
- Why is the term "swelling" used in lieu of "edema" or "effusion"?

The rehabilitation professional employs physical agent modalities to create an optimum environment for tissue healing while minimizing the symptoms associated with the trauma or condition.

The frequency (pulses per second or, in this case, bursts per second) is also a variable that can be controlled. This would make the muscle respond with a twitch rather than a gradually increasing mechanical contraction. Gradually increasing the numbers of bursts interrupts the mechanical relaxation cycle of the muscle and causes more shortening to take place (see Fig. 6-18).[108]

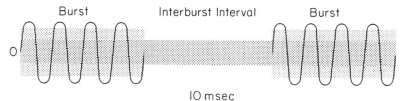

•**Figure 6-24** Russian current with an interburst interval. Dark shading represents total current, and light shading indicates total current without the interburst interval.

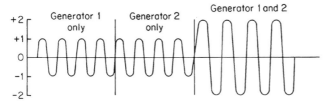

•**Figure 6-25** Sine wave from generator 1 and sine wave from generator 2 showing a constructive interference pattern.

INTERFERENTIAL CURRENTS

The research and use of interferential currents (IFC) has taken place primarily in Europe. An Austrian scientist, Ho Nemec, introduced the concept and suggested its therapeutic use. Nemec's concept resulted in the creation of a type of electrical generator that is difficult to understand, not because the theory is so complex, but because electrical engineers added so many options to the generator that the current can be modified substantially while still maintaining its basic waveform.

The theories and behavior of electrical waves are part of basic physics. This behavior is easiest to understand when continuous sine waves are used as an example.

With only one circuit, the current behaves as described earlier; if put on an oscilloscope, it looks like generator 1 in Fig. 6-25. If a second generator is brought into the same location, the currents may interfere with each other. This interference can be summative—that is, the amplitudes of the electric wave are combined and increase (Fig. 6-25). Both waves are exactly the same; if they are produced in phase or originate at the same time, they combine. This is called **constructive interference**.

If these waves are generated out of sync, generator 1 starts in a positive direction at the same time that generator 2 starts in a negative direction; the waves then will cancel each other out. This is called **destructive interference**; in the summation the waves end up with an amplitude of 0 (Fig. 6-26).

To make this more complex, assume that one generator has a slightly slower or faster frequency and that the generators begin producing current simultaneously. Initially, the electric waves will be constructively summated; however, because the frequencies of the two waves differ, they gradually will get out of phase and become destructively summated. When dealing with sound waves, we hear distinct beats as this phenomenon occurs. We borrow the term **beat** when describing this behavior. When any waveforms are out of phase but are combined in the same location, the waves will

constructive interference The combined amplitude of two distinct circuits increases the amplitude.

destructive interference Combined amplitude of two distinct circuits decreases the amplitude.

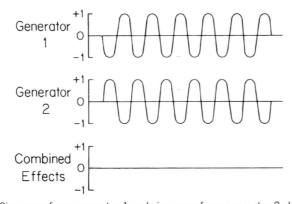

•**Figure 6-26** Sine wave from generator 1 and sine wave from generator 2 showing a destructive interference pattern.

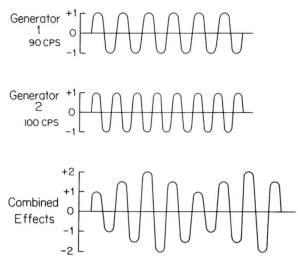

•**Figure 6-27** Sine wave from generator 1 at 90 cps and sine wave from generator 2 at 100 cps showing the heterodyne or beating pattern of interference.

cause a beat effect. The blending of the waves is caused by the constructive and destructive interference patterns of the waves and is called **heterodyne** (Fig. 6-27).[48,50]

The heterodyne effect is seen on an oscilloscope as a cyclic, rising and falling waveform.[129] The peaks or beat frequency in this heterodyne wave behavior occur regularly, according to the difference of each current; for example,

$$100 \, \text{pps} - 90 \, \text{pps} = 10 \, \text{pps beat frequency}$$

In electric currents, this beat frequency is, in effect, the stimulation frequency of the waveform, because the destructive interference negates the effects of the other part of the wave. The intensity (amplitude) will be set according to sensations created by this peak.[48] When using an interference current for therapy, the therapist should select the frequencies to create a beat frequency corresponding to his or her choices of frequency when using other stimulators; 20–50 pps for muscle contraction, 50–120 pps for pain management, and 1 pps for acustim pain relief.

When the electrodes are arranged in a square alignment and interferential currents are passed through a homogeneous medium, a predictable pattern of interference will occur. In this pattern, an electric field is created that resembles a four-petaled flower, with the center of the flower located where the two currents cross and the petals falling between the electric current force lines. The maximum interference effect takes place near the center, with the field gradually decreasing in strength as it moves toward the points of the petal (Fig. 6-28).[48]

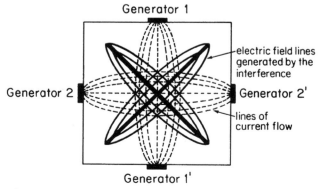

•**Figure 6-28** Square electrode alignment and interference pattern of current in a homogeneous medium.

Because the body is not a homogeneous medium, we cannot predict the exact location of this interference pattern; we must rely on the patient's perception. If the patient has a localized structure that is painful, locating the stimulation in the correct location is relatively easy. The therapist moves the electrode placement until the patient centers the feeling of the stimulus in the problem area.[48,50] When a patient has poorly localized pain, the task becomes more difficult. See the discussion in the electrode placement section for a general discussion on the effect of electrode movement. The engineers added features to the generators and created a scanning interferential current that moves the flower petals of force around while the treatment is taking place. This enlarges the effective treatment area. Additional technology and another set of electrodes create a three-dimensional flower effect when one looks at the electrical field. This is called a **stereodynamic interference current.**[48,50]

All these alterations and modifications are designed to spread the heterodyne effect throughout the tissue. Because it is controlled by a cyclic electrical pattern, however, we actually may be decreasing the current passed through the structures we are trying to treat. The machines seem complex but lack the versatility to do much more than the conventional TENS treatment.[108,124]

Nikolova[111] has used IFC for a variety of clinical problems and found them effective in dealing with pain problems (e.g., joint sprains with swelling, restricted mobility and pain, neuritis, retarded callus formation following fractures, pseudarthrosis).[101] These claims are supported by other researchers. Each of these researchers used slightly different protocols in treating the different clinical problems. To be successful in achieving the desired results with interferential currents, the therapist must thoroughly review existing protocols and acquire a good working knowledge of the application techniques.

stereodynamic interference current
Three distinct circuits blending and creating a distinct electrical wave pattern.

CONCLUSION

The world of electrical therapy is constantly changing, owing to the advances in research, engineering, and technology and because of the competitive pressures of the marketplace. Equipment manufacturers will develop a different machine and try to market it on the basis of a single feature of their product. The old adage "let the buyer beware" is certainly good advice. The more understanding of electrical currents the therapist has, the less likely he or she is to be "snowed" or confused by the sales spiel. Even more important, the greater the understanding, the easier it becomes to manipulate the treatment protocols to optimize results for each patient.[67]

SUMMARY

1. When an electrical system is applied to muscle or nerve tissue, the result will be tissue membrane depolarization, provided that the current has the appropriate intensity, duration, and waveform to reach the tissue's excitability threshold.

2. Nerve function and muscle contraction are the same regardless of the stimulation mechanism (i.e., natural or electrical).

3. Muscle and nerve tissue respond in an all-or-none fashion; there is no gradation of response.

4. Muscle contraction will change according to changes in current. As the frequency of the electrical stimulus increases, the muscle will develop more tension as a result of the summation of the contraction of the muscle fiber through progressive mechanical shortening. Increases in intensity spread the current over a larger area and increase the number of motor units activated by the current. Increases in the duration of the current also will cause more motor units to be activated.

Kostov, A., Andrews, B., and Popovic, D.: Machine learning in control of functional electrical stimulation systems for locomotion, IEEE Trans. Biomed. Eng. 42(6):541–551, 1995.

Kramer, J., Mendryk, S.: Electrical stimulation as a strength improvement technique: a review, J. Orthop. Sports Phys. Ther. 4:91, 1982.

Kues, J., Mayhew, T.: Concentric and eccentric force-velocity relationships during electrically induced submaximal contractions, Phys. Ther. 76(5):S17, 1996.

Lainey, C., Walmsley, R., and Andrew, G.: Effectiveness of exercise alone versus exercise plus electrical stimulation in strengthening the quadriceps muscle, Physiother. Can. 35:5, 1983.

Lampe, G.: Introduction to the use of transcutaneous electrical nerve stimulation devices, Phys. Ther. 58:1450, 1978.

Lane, J.: Electrical impedances of superficial limb tissue, epidermis, dermis and muscle sheath. Ann. N.Y. Acad. Sci. 238:812, 1974.

Latash, M., Yee, M., and Orpett, C.: Combining electrical muscle stimulation with voluntary contraction for studying muscle fatigue, Arch. Phys. Med. Rehabil. 75(1):29–35, 1994.

Laughman, R., Youdas, J., and Garrett, T.: Strength changes in the normal quadriceps femoris muscle as a result of electrical stimulation, Phys. Ther. 63:494, 1983.

LeDoux, J., Quinones, M.: An investigation of the use of percutaneous electrical stimulation in muscle reeducation, Phys. Ther. 61:678, 1981.

Leffman, D., Arnall, D., and Holmgren, P.: Effect of microamperage stimulation on the rate of wound healing in rats: a histological study, Phys. Ther. 74(3):195–200, 1994.

Levin, M., Hui-Chan, C.: Conventional and acupuncture-like transcutaneous electrical nerve stimulation excite similar afferent fibers, Arch. Phys. Med. Rehabil. 74(1):54–60, 1993.

Licht, S.: History of electrotherapy. In Stillwell, G.K., editor. Therapeutic electricity and ultraviolet radiation, ed. 3, Baltimore, 1983, Williams & Wilkins.

Litke, D., Dahners, L.: Effects of different levels of direct current on early ligament healing in a rat model, J. Orthop. Res. 12:683–688, 1992.

Livesley, E.: Effects of electrical neuromuscular stimulation on functional performance in patients with multiple sclerosis. Physiotherapy 78(12):914–917, 1992.

Loeser, J.: Nonpharmacologic approaches to pain relief. In Ng, L., Bonica, J., editors. Pain, discomfort and humanitarian care, New York, 1980, Elsevier.

Loesor, J., Black, R., and Christman, A.: A relief of pain by transcutaneous stimulation, J. Neurosurg. 42:308, 1975.

Long, D.: Cutaneous afferent stimulation for relief of chronic pain, Clin. Neurosurg. 21:257, 1974.

Macdonald, A., Coates, T.: The discovery of transcutaneous spinal electroanalgesia and its relief of chronic pain, Physiotherapy 81(11):653–661, 1995.

Mannneimer, C., Carlsson, C.: The analgesic effect of transcutaneous electrical nerve stimulation (TENS) in patients with rheumatoid arthritis. A comparative study of different pulse patterns, Pain 6:329, 1979.

Mannheimer, C., Lund, S., and Carlsson, C.: The effect of transcutaneous electrical nerve stimulation (TENS) on joint pain in patients with rheumatoid arthritis, Scand. J. Rheumatol. 7:13, 1978.

Mannheimer, J.: Electrode placements for transcutaneous electrical nerve stimulation, Phys. Ther. 58:1455, 1978.

Mao, W., Ghia, J., and Scott, D.: High versus low-intensity acupuncture analgesic for treatment of chronic pain: effects on platelet serotonin, Pain 8:331, 1980.

Markov, M.: Electric current and electromagnetic field effects on soft tissue: implications for wound healing, Wounds Compen. Clin. Res. Pract. 7(3):94–110, 1995.

Marvie, K.: A major advance in the control of post-operative knee pain, Orthopedics 2:129, 1979.

Massey, B., Nelson, R., and Sharkey, B.: Effects of high frequency electrical stimulation on the size and strength of skeletal muscle, J. Sports Med. Phys. Fit. 5:136, 1965.

Matsunaga, T., Shimada, Y., and Sato, K.: Muscle fatigue from intermittent stimulation with low and high frequency electrical pulses, Arch. Phys. Med. Rehabil. 80(1):48–53, 1999.

Mattison, J.: Transcutaneous electrical nerve stimulation in the management of painful muscle spasm in patients with multiple sclerosis, Clin. Rehabil. 7(1):45–48, 1993.

McMiken, D., Todd-Smith, M., and Thompson, C.: Strengthening of human quadriceps muscles by cutaneous electrical stimulation, Scand. J. Rehabil. Med. 15:25, 1983.

McQuain, M., Sinaki, M., and Shibley, L.: Effect of electrical stimulation on lumbar paraspinal muscles, Spine 18(13): 1787–1792, 1993.

Merrick, M.A.: Research digest. Unconventional modalities: microcurrent, Athl. Ther. Today 4(5):53–54, 1999.

Meyer, G., Fields, H.: Causalgia treated by selective large fibre stimulation of peripheral nerve, Brain 95:163, 1972.

Miller, B.F., Gruben, K.G., and Morgan, B.J.: Circulatory responses to voluntary and electrically induced muscle contractions in humans, Phys. Ther. 80(1):53–60, 2000.

Milner-Brown, H., Stein, R.: The relation between the surface electromyogram and muscular force, J. Physiol. 246:549, 1975.

Mohr, T., Carlson, B., and Sulentic, C.: Comparison of isometric exercise and high volt galvanic stimulation on quadriceps, femoris muscle strength, Phys. Ther. 65:606, 1985.

Mostowy, D.: An application of transcutaneous electrical nerve stimulation to control pain in the elderly, J. Gerontol. Nurs. 22(2):36–38, 1996.

Munsat, T., McNeal, D., and Waters, R.: Preliminary observations on prolonged stimulation of peripheral nerve in man, Arch. Neurol. 33:608, 1976.

Myklebust, J., editor. Neural stimulation, Boca Raton, FL, 1985, CRC Press.

Naess, K., Storm-Mathison, A.: Fatigue of sustained tetanic contractions. Acta Physiol. Scand. 34:351, 1955.

Owens, J., Malone, T.: Treatment parameters of high frequency electrical stimulation as established on the electrostim 180, J. Orthop. Sports Phys. Ther. 4:162, 1983.

Packman-Braun, R.: Misconceptions regarding functional electrical stimulation, Neurol. Rept. 19(3):17–21, 1995.

Pert, V.: TENS for pain in multiple sclerosis, Physiotherapy 77(3):227–228, 1991.

Petrofsky, J.: Functional electrical stimulation, a two-year study. J. Rehabil. 58(3):29–34, 1992.

Picaza, J., Cannon, B., and Hunter, S.: Pain suppression by peripheral stimulation, Part I. Observations with transcutaneous stimuli, Surg. Neurol. 4:105, 1975.

Pouran, D., Faghri, M., and Rodgers, M.: The effects of functional electrical stimulation on shoulder subluxation, arm function recovery, and shoulder pain in hemiplegic stroke patients, Arch. Phys. Med. Rehabil. 75(1):73–79, 1994.

Procacci, P., Zoppi, M., and Maresca, M.: Transcutaneous electrical stimulation in low back pain: a critical evaluation, Acupunct. Electrother. Res. 7:1, 1982.

Rabischong, E., Doutrelot, P., and Ohanna, F.: Compound motor action potentials and mechanical failure during sustained contractions by electrical stimulation in paraplegic, Paraplegia 33(12):707–714, 1995.

Rack, P., Westbury, D.: The effects of length and stimulus rate on tension in the isometric cat soleus muscle, J. Physiol. 204:443, 1969.

Ray, R., Samuelson, A.: Microcurrent versus a placebo for the control of pain and edema, J. Athl. Train. 31:S-48, 1996.

Reddana, P., Moortly, C., and Govidappa, S.: Pattern of skeletal muscle chemical composition during in vivo electrical stimulations, Ind. J. Physiol. Pharmacol. 25:33, 1981.

Rieb, L., Pomeranz, B.: Alterations in electrical pain thresholds by use of acupuncture-like transcutaneous electrical nerve stimulation in pain-free subjects, Phys. Ther. 72(9):658–667, 1992.

Rochester, L.: Influence of electrical stimulation of the tibialis anterior muscle in paraplegic subjects. 1. Contractile properties, Paraplegia 33(8):437–449, 1995.

Roeser, W., et al.: The use of transcutaneous nerve stimulation for pain control in athletic medicine. A preliminary report, Am. J. Sports Med. 4(5):210, 1976.

Romero, J., Sanford, T., and Schroeder, R.: The effects of electrical stimulation of normal quadriceps on strength and girth, Med. Sci. Sports Exerc. 14:194, 1982.

Rosenberg, M., Vutyid, L., and Bourbe, D.: Transcutaneous electrical nerve stimulation for the relief of post-operative pain, Pain 5:129, 1978.

Rowley, B., McKenna, J., and Chase, G.: The influence of electrical current on an infecting microorganism in wounds, Ann. N.Y. Acad. Sci. 238:543, 1974.

Schmitz, R., Martin, D., and Perrin, D.: The effects of interferential current of perceived pain and serum cortisol in a delayed onset muscle soreness model, J. Athl. Train. 29(2):171, 1994.

Seib, T., Price, R., and Reyes, M.: The quantitative measurement of spasticity: effect of cutaneous electrical stimulation, Arch. Phys. Med. Rehabil. 75(7):746–750, 1994.

Selkowitz, D.: Improvement in isometric strength of the quadricep femoris muscle after training with electrical stimulation, Phys. Ther. 65:186, 1985.

Shealey, C., Maurer, D.: Transcutaneous nerve stimulation for control of pain, Surg. Neurol. 2:45, 1974.

Simmonds, M., Wessel, J., and Scudds, R.: The effect of pain quality on the efficacy of conventional TENS, Physiotherapy (Can.) 44(3):35–40, 1992.

Sjolund, B., Eriksson, M.: The influence of naloxone on analgesia produced by peripheral conditioning stimulation, Brain Res. 173:295, 1979.

Sjolund, B., Terenius, L., and Eriksson, M.: Increased cerebrospinal fluid levels of endorphin after electroacupuncture, Acta Physiol. Scand. 100:382, 1977.

Smith, B., Betz, R., and Mulcahey, M.: Reliability of percutaneous intramuscular electrodes for upper extremity functional neuromuscular stimulation in adolescents with C5 injury, Arch. Phys. Med. Rehabil. 75(9):939–945, 1994.

Smith, B., Mulcahey, M., and Betz, R.: Quantitative comparison of grasp and release abilities with and without functional neuromuscular stimulation in adolescents with tetraplegia, Paraplegia 34(1):16–23, 1996.

Snyder-Mackler, L., Delitto, A., and Stralka, S.: Use of electrical stimulation to enhance recovery of quadriceps femoris muscle force production in patients following anterior cruciate ligament reconstruction, Phys. Ther. 74(10):901–907, 1994.

Standish, W., Valiant, G., and Bonen, and A.: The effects of immobilization and of electrical stimulation on muscle glycogen and myofibrillar ATPase, Can. J. Appl. Sports Sci. 7:267, 1982.

Stone, J.A.: Prevention and rehabilitation. Interferential electrical stimulation, Athl. Ther. Today 2(2):27, 1997.

Stone, J.A.: Prevention and rehabilitation. Microcurrent electrical stimulation, Athl. Ther. Today 2(6):15, 1997.

Stone, J.A.: Prevention and rehabilitation. "Russian" electrical stimulation, Athl. Ther. Today 2(3):27, 1997.

Szehi, E., David, E.: The stereodynamic interferential current—a new electrotherapeutic technique, Electromedica 48:13, 1980.

Szuminsky, N., Albers, A., and Unger, P.: Effect of narrow pulsed high voltages on bacterial viability, Phys. Ther. 74(7):660–667, 1994.

Taylor, M., Newton, R., and Personius, W.: The effects of interferential current stimulation for the treatment of subjects with recurrent jaw pain, abstract, Phys. Ther. 66:774, 1986.

Taylor, P., Hallet, M., and Flaherty, L.: Treatment of osteoarthritis of the knee with transcutaneous electrical nerve stimulation, Pain 11:233, 1981.

Terezhalmy, G., Ross, G., and Holmes-Johnson, E.: Transcutaneous electrical nerve stimulation treatment of TMJMPDS patients, Ear Nose Throat J. 61:664, 1982.

Thorsteinsson, G., Stonnington, H.: The placebo effect of transcutaneous electrical stimulation, Pain 5:31, 1978.

Walsh, D., Foster, N., and Baxter, G.: Transcutaneous electrical nerve stimulation parameters to neurophysiological and hypoalgesic effects, Phys. Ther. 76(5):552, 1996.

Weber, M., Servedio, F., and Woddall, W.: The effects of three modalities on delayed onset muscle soreness, J. Orthop. Sports Phys. Ther. 20(5): 236–242, 1994.

Wheeler, P., Wolcott, L., and Morris, J.: Neural considerations in the healing of ulcerated tissue by clinical electrotherapeutic application of weak direct current: findings and theory. In Reynolds, D., Sjoberg, A., editors. Neuroelectric research, Springfield, IL, 1971, Charles C Thomas, pp. 83–96.

Windsor, R., Lester, J.: Electrical stimulation in clinical practice. Phys. Sports Med. 21(2):85–86, 89–90, 91–92, 1993.

Wolf, S., Gersh, M., and Rao, V.: Examination of electrode placements and stimulating parameters in treating chronic pain with conventional transcutaneous nerve stimulation (TENS), Pain 11:37, 1981.

Wong, R., Jette, D.: Changes in sympathetic tone associated with different forms of transcutaneous electrical nerve stimulation in healthy subjects, Phys. Ther. 64:478, 1984.

Yarkony, G., Roth, E.: Neuromuscular stimulation in spinal cord injury: restoration of functional movement of the extremities. Part 1, Arch. Phys. Med. Rehabil. 73(1):78–86, 1992.

Yarkony, G., Roth, E., and Cybulski, J.: Neuromuscular stimulation in spinal cord injury II: prevention of secondary complications, Part 2, Arch. Phys. Med. Rehabil. 73(2):195–200, 1992.

Zecca, L., Ferrario, P., and Furia, G.: Effects of pulsed electromagnetic field on acute and chronic inflammation, Trans. Biol. Repair Growth Soc. 3:72, 1983.

GLOSSARY

absolute refractory period Brief time period (0.5 μsec) following membrane depolarization during which the membrane is incapable of depolarizing again.

action potential A recorded change in electrical potential between the inside and outside of a nerve cell, resulting in muscular contraction.

active electrode Electrode at which greatest current density occurs.

all-or-none response The depolarization of nerve or muscle membrane is the same once a depolarizing intensity threshold is reached; further increases in intensity do not increase the response. Stimuli at intensities less than threshold do not create a depolarizing effect.

anode Positively charged electrode in a direct current system.

beat Distinct wave pattern created by combining two distinct circuit electrical waves that blend into a gradual rising and falling wave.

bioelectromagnetics The study of biologic tissues' electrical and magnetic properties.

cathode Negatively charged electrode in a direct current system.

central biasing The use of hyperstimulation analgesia to bias the central nervous system against transmitting painful stimuli to the sensory recognition area. This occurs through hormonal influences created by brain stem stimulation.

chronaxie The duration of time necessary to cause observable tissue excitation, given a current intensity of two times rheobasic current.

constructive interference The combined amplitude of two distinct circuits increases the amplitude.

current density Amount of current flow per cubic area.

current of injury A bioelectric current produced by any type of cellular trauma that plays a key role in stimulating healing.

denervated muscle Muscle that has lost its peripheral nerve supply.

depolarization Process or act of neutralizing the cell membrane's resting potential.

destructive interference Combined amplitude of two distinct circuits decreases the amplitude.

dipoles Molecules whose ends carry opposite charge.

electrets Insulators carrying a permanent charge similar to a permanent magnet.

electropiezo activity Changing electric surface charges of a structure forces the structure to change shape.

frequency window selectivity Cellular responses may be triggered by a certain electrical frequency range.

functional electrical stimulation Utilizes multiple-channel electrical stimulators to recruit muscles in a programmed sequence that produces a functional movement pattern.

gap junctions Specialized junction areas connecting cells of like structure that contain channels for ionic, electrical, and small molecule signaling that pass messages from cell to cell.

heterodynes Cyclic rising and falling waveform of interferential current.

hybrid currents Currents that have waveforms containing parameters that are not classically alternating or direct.

impedance The resistance of the tissue to the passage of electrical current.

indifferent or dispersive electrode Large electrode used to spread out electrical charge and decrease current density at that electrode site.

maximum voluntary isometric contraction Peak torque produced by a muscular contraction.

piezoelectric activity Changing electric surface charges of a structure forces the structure to change shape.

resting potential The potential difference between the inside and outside of a membrane.

rheobase The intensity of current necessary to cause observable tissue excitation, given a long current duration.

Russian current A medium-frequency (2000 to 10,000 Hz) polyphasic AC wave generated in 50-bursts-per-second envelopes.

stereodynamic interference current Three distinct circuits blending and creating a distinct electrical wave pattern.

strain-related potentials Tissue-based electric potentials generated in response to strain for the tissue.

strength-duration curve A graphic illustration of the relationship between current intensity and current duration in causing depolarization of a nerve or muscle membrane.

summation of contractions Shortening of muscle myofilaments caused by increasing the frequency of muscle membrane depolarization.

tetanization This occurs when individual muscle twitch responses can no longer be distinguished and the responses force maximum shortening of the stimulated muscle fiber.

twitch muscle contraction A single muscle contraction caused by one depolarization phenomenon.

voltage-sensitive permeability The quality of some cell membranes that makes them permeable to different ions based on the electric charge of the ions. Nerve and muscle cell membranes allow negatively charged ions into the cell while actively transporting some positively charged ions outside the cell membrane.

LAB ACTIVITY

ELECTRICAL STIMULATION: ANALGESIA

DESCRIPTION:

Electroanalgesia is arguably the most common use of therapeutic electricity. The use of therapeutic electricity for analgesia is often referred to as transcutaneous electrical nerve stimulation or TENS; however, all forms of therapeutic electricity that do not use implanted or needle electrodes are "transcutaneous," and many forms stimulate nerves. Therefore, the term TENS should be discouraged. Although there are hundreds of different types of electrical stimulators available for use, there are essentially three levels in the body that may be affected.

The first level is the spinal gate. This level is activated by increasing the input to the spinal cord from large-diameter afferent neurons. The second level is referred to as the central bias mechanism, where intense small fiber afferent input activates a negative feedback loop through connections in the midbrain. Finally, some forms of electrical stimulation appear to stimulate the production of endogenous opiates, the endorphins.

Although stimulators have many different waveforms and modulations, there is no evidence that an "optimal" waveform exists. It is impossible to predict for an individual patient what type of current, what electrode configuration, what amplitude of stimulation, and so on, will provide relief of pain. Therefore, electroanalgesia is somewhat of a trial and error phenomenon. This does not mean the approach should be haphazard; a systematic approach, based on clinical experience, is best.

Generally, there are three types of stimulation for electroanalgesia; conventional, low-frequency, and hyperstimulation. Conventional generally has a pulse rate of 10–100 pps and is applied at an amplitude between sensory and motor thresholds. Low-frequency stimulation has a pulse rate of 1–5 pps, and an amplitude between motor and pain thresholds. Hyperstimulation generally uses a monophasic pulsatile current at a frequency of 1–128 pps and an amplitude to pain tolerance. Hyperstimulation is often referred to as point stimulation.

PHYSIOLOGIC EFFECTS:

Depolarization of peripheral nerves

THERAPEUTIC EFFECTS:

Inhibition of pain perception

INDICATIONS:

The obvious indication for electroanalgesia is pain. However, the cause of the pain should be identified prior to the use of electrical stimulation, and it must be remembered that the modulation of pain is not treating the cause of the pain.

CONTRAINDICATIONS:

- Pregnancy
- Implanted electrical pacing devices (e.g., cardiac pacemaker, bladder stimulator)
- Cardiac arrhythmia
- Over the carotid sinus area
- Hypersensitivity (i.e., the patient who has a strong aversion to electricity, or the patient with certain types of catheters or shunts)

ELECTRICAL STIMULATION: ANALGESIA

PROCEDURE	EVALUATION		
	1	2	3
1. Check supplies.			
a. Obtain towels or sheets for draping, conductant.			
b. Check stimulator, electrodes, and cables for charged battery, broken or frayed insulation, and so on.			
c. Ensure the amplitude controls are at zero.			
2. Question patient.			
a. Verify identity of patient (if not already verified).			
b. Verify the absence of contraindications.			
c. Ask about previous treatments for current condition, and check treatment notes.			
3. Position patient.			
a. Place patient in a well-supported, comfortable position.			
b. Expose body part to be treated.			
c. Drape patient to preserve patient's modesty, protect clothing, but allow access to body part.			
4. Inspect body part to be treated.			
a. Check light touch perception.			
b. Assess function of body part (e.g., ROM, irritability).			
5a. Apply conventional electrical stimulation.			
a. Place conductant on electrodes as indicated, secure electrodes to patient.			
b. Remind the patient to inform you when he or she feels something. Do not tell the patient what he or she will feel; for example, do not say, "Tell me when you feel a buzz or tingle."			
c. Adjust the pulse rate, pulse width, and mode of stimulation to desired settings if possible.			
d. Turn on the stimulator, and increase the amplitude slowly. Monitor the patient's response, not the stimulator.			
e. After the patient reports the onset of the stimulus, adjust the amplitude to a comfortable level, but make sure it is below motor threshold. If it is impossible to achieve suprasensory threshold stimulation without a motor response, turn the stimulator off and move the electrodes to another location.			
f. Set a timer for the appropriate treatment time and give the patient a signaling device. Make sure the patient understands how to use the signaling device.			
g. Recheck the patient after about 5 minutes. If the sensation has diminished, adjust the amplitude appropriately.			
5b. Apply low-frequency electrical stimulation.			
a. Place conductant on electrodes as indicated, secure electrodes to patient.			
b. Remind the patient to inform you when he or she feels something. Do not tell the patient what he or she will feel; for example, do not say, "Tell me when you feel a buzz or tingle."			

PROCEDURE	EVALUATION		
	1	2	3
c. Adjust the pulse rate, pulse width, and mode of stimulation to desired settings if possible.			
d. Turn on the stimulator, and increase the amplitude slowly. Monitor the patient's response, not the stimulator.			
e. After the patient reports the onset of the stimulus, adjust the amplitude to a comfortable level above motor threshold. The contraction should be just a twitch, not a strong contraction.			
f. Set a timer for the appropriate treatment time and give the patient a signaling device. Make sure the patient understands how to use the signaling device.			
g. Recheck the patient after about 5 minutes. If the sensation has diminished, adjust the amplitude appropriately.			
5c. Apply hyperstimulation electrical stimulation.			
a. Place conductant on "inactive" electrode, have the patient hold the electrode in his or her palm. Apply the conductant to points to be stimulated.			
b. If using electrical resistance to locate stimulation points, set sensitivity of ohm meter; set pulse rate, polarity, and length of stimulation to desired settings.			
c. Move the "active" electrode slowly in the area of the point to be stimulated until the area of minimal resistance is found; the pressure applied to the electrode must be constant.			
d. Tell the patient to report when the amplitude of stimulation is as high as he or she can tolerate. Activate the stimulation current, and increase the amplitude slowly. Monitor the patient's response, not the stimulator.			
e. After the patient reports that the stimulus is as much as he or she can tolerate, maintain constant pressure on the electrode. Stimulate the point two or three times, for 15–30 seconds each time.			
f. Repeat the process for each point to be stimulated.			
6. Complete treatment.			
a. When the treatment time is over, turn the intensity control to zero, and move the generator away from the patient; remove conductant with a towel.			
b. Remove material used for draping, assist the patient in dressing as needed.			
c. Have the patient perform appropriate therapeutic exercise as indicated.			
d. Clean the treatment area and equipment according to normal protocol.			
7. Assess treatment efficacy.			
a. Ask the patient how the treated area feels.			
b. Visually inspect the treated area for any adverse reactions.			
c. Perform functional tests as indicated.			

LAB ACTIVITY

ELECTRICAL STIMULATION: REEDUCATION

DESCRIPTION:

Electrical stimulation may be used to assist a patient in regaining the ability to voluntarily control a normally innervated muscle. Sometimes following surgery, a patient temporarily loses the ability to produce a muscle contraction. Probably the most common loss is of the quadriceps femoris following knee surgery. In addition, if a patient has undergone a tendon transfer, he or she may have difficulty recruiting the muscle to perform the new joint action.

The mechanism by which electrical stimulation aids in the recovery of volitional control of skeletal muscle is not clear, nor is the reason volitional control is lost following surgery. The probable method of action is via stimulation of joint, muscle, and skin proprioceptors when the muscle produces joint motion.

PHYSIOLOGIC EFFECTS:

Depolarization of peripheral nerves

THERAPEUTIC EFFECTS:

Recovery of volitional control of skeletal muscle

INDICATIONS:

The primary indication is loss of volitional control of a skeletal muscle following surgery or a tendon transfer.

CONTRAINDICATIONS:

- Pregnancy
- Implanted electrical pacing devices (e.g., cardiac pacemaker, bladder stimulator)
- Cardiac arrhythmia
- Over the carotid sinus area
- Hypersensitivity (i.e., the patient who has a strong aversion to electricity, or the patient with certain types of catheters or shunts)

ELECTRICAL STIMULATION: REEDUCATION

PROCEDURE	EVALUATION		
	1	2	3
1. Check supplies.			
a. Obtain towels or sheets for draping, conductant.			
b. Check stimulator, electrodes, and cables for charged battery, broken or frayed insulation, etc.			
c. Verify that the intensity control is at zero.			
2. Question patient.			
a. Verify identity of patient (if not already verified).			
b. Verify the absence of contraindications.			
c. Ask about previous exposure to electrotherapy, check treatment notes.			

PROCEDURE	EVALUATION		
	1	2	3
3. Position patient.			
a. Place patient in a well-supported, comfortable position.			
b. Expose body part to be treated.			
c. Drape patient to preserve patient's modesty, protect clothing, but allow access to body part.			
4. Inspect body part to be treated.			
a. Check light touch perception.			
b. Assess function of body part (e.g., ROM, irritability).			
5. Apply electrical stimulation for reeducation.			
a. Place conductant on electrodes as needed, secure electrodes to patient. Electrode location will vary depending on desired effect. Usually, the ideal location for the active electrode is over the motor point of the target muscle or the peripheral nerve trunk that supplies the target muscle.			
b. Remind the patient to inform you when he or she feels something. Do not tell the patient what he or she will feel; for example, do not say, "Tell me when you feel a buzz or tingle."			
c. Adjust the pulse rate, pulse width, and mode of stimulation to desired settings if possible.			
d. Turn on the stimulator, and increase the amplitude slowly. Monitor the patient's response, not the stimulator.			
e. After the patient reports the onset of the stimulus, adjust the amplitude to a comfortable level above motor threshold. Encourage the patient to try to volitionally contract the muscle before the stimulator does, and increase the force during the stimulation.			
f. Continue to monitor the patient during the duration of the treatment.			
6. Complete treatment.			
a. When the treatment time is over or the patient is able to control the muscle contraction, turn the intensity to zero, and move the generator away from the patient; remove conductant with a towel.			
b. Remove material used for draping, assist the patient in dressing as needed.			
c. Have the patient perform appropriate therapeutic exercise as indicated.			
d. Clean the treatment area and equipment according to normal protocol.			
7. Assess treatment efficacy.			
a. Ask the patient how the treated area feels.			
b. Visually inspect the treated area for any adverse reactions.			
c. Perform functional tests as indicated.			

LAB ACTIVITY

ELECTRICAL STIMULATION: STRENGTHENING

DESCRIPTION:

Electrical stimulation is often used for increasing skeletal muscle strength by itself or in conjunction with active exercise. However, there is no evidence the electrical stimulation by itself or in conjunction with active exercise is better than active exercise alone for muscle strengthening. Also, the increase in tension-developing capacity does not transfer to functional activities. Because of this, it is sometimes referred to as "electrical stimulation to increase isometric force development capacity."

PHYSIOLOGIC EFFECTS:

Depolarization of peripheral nerves

THERAPEUTIC EFFECTS:

Increase in isometric force development capacity

INDICATIONS:

The primary indication is muscle weakness. However, electrical stimulation is sometimes used in an attempt to prevent disuse atrophy during immobilization of a limb.

CONTRAINDICATIONS:

- Pregnancy
- Implanted electrical pacing devices (e.g., cardiac pacemaker, bladder stimulator)
- Cardiac arrhythmia
- Over the carotid sinus area
- Hypersensitivity (i.e., the patient who has a strong aversion to electricity, or the patient with certain types of catheters or shunts)

ELECTRICAL STIMULATION: STRENGTHENING

PROCEDURE	EVALUATION		
	1	2	3
1. Check supplies.			
a. Obtain towels or sheets for draping, conductant.			
b. Check stimulator, electrodes, and cables for charged battery, broken or frayed insulation, etc.			
c. Verify that the intensity control is at zero.			
2. Question patient.			
a. Verify identity of patient (if not already verified).			
b. Verify the absence of contraindications.			
c. Ask about previous exposure to electrotherapy, check treatment notes.			
3. Position patient.			
a. Place patient in a well-supported, comfortable position.			
b. Expose body part to be treated.			
c. Drape patient to preserve patient's modesty, protect clothing, but allow access to body part.			

PROCEDURE	EVALUATION		
	1	2	3
4. Inspect body part to be treated.			
a. Check light touch perception.			
b. Assess function of body part (e.g., ROM, irritability).			
5. Apply electrical stimulation for muscle strengthening.			
a. Place conductant on electrodes as indicated, secure electrodes to patient. Electrode location will vary depending on desired effect. Usually, the ideal location for the active electrode is over the motor point of the target muscle, or the peripheral nerve trunk that supplies the target muscle.			
b. Remind the patient to inform you when he or she feels something. Do not tell the patient what he or she will feel; for example, do not say, "Tell me when you feel a buzz or tingle."			
c. Adjust the pulse rate, pulse width, and mode of stimulation to desired settings if possible.			
d. Turn on the stimulator, and increase the amplitude slowly. Monitor the patient's response, not the stimulator.			
e. After the patient reports the onset of the stimulus, adjust the amplitude to as high a level as the patient can tolerate.			
f. Set a timer for the appropriate treatment time and give the patient a signaling device. Make sure the patient understands how to use the signaling device.			
g. Recheck the patient after about 5 minutes. If the sensation has diminished, adjust the amplitude appropriately.			
6. Complete treatment.			
a. When the treatment time is over, turn the intensity control to zero, move the generator away from the patient remove conductant with a towel.			
b. Remove material used for draping, assist the patient in dressing as needed.			
c. Have the patient perform appropriate therapeutic exercise as indicated.			
d. Clean the treatment area and equipment according to normal protocol.			
7. Assess treatment efficacy.			
a. Ask the patient how the treated area feels.			
b. Visually inspect the treated area for any adverse reactions.			
c. Perform functional tests as indicated.			

CHAPTER 7 SEVEN

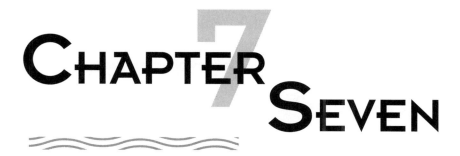

IONTOPHORESIS

WILLIAM E. PRENTICE

OBJECTIVES

Following completion of this chapter, the student therapist will be able to:

- ✓ Differentiate between iontophoresis and phonophoresis.
- ✓ Explain the basic mechanisms of ion transfer.
- ✓ Establish specific iontophoresis application procedures and techniques.
- ✓ Identify the different ions most commonly used in iontophoresis.
- ✓ Choose the appropriate clinical applications for using an iontophoresis technique.
- ✓ Establish precautions and concerns for using iontophoresis treatment.

Iontophoresis is a therapeutic technique that involves the introduction of ions into the body tissues by means of a direct electrical current.[15] Originally referred to as **ion transfer**, it was first described by LeDuc in 1903 as a technique of transporting chemicals across a membrane using an electrical current as a driving force.[54] Since that time there have been increases and decreases in the popularity and use of iontophoresis as a therapeutic technique. Recently new emphasis has been placed on iontophoresis, and it has become a commonly used technique in clinical settings. Iontophoresis has several advantages as a treatment technique in that it is a painless, sterile, noninvasive technique for introducing specific ions into the tissue that has been demonstrated to have a positive effect on the healing process.[21]

The therapist must be aware that most of the medications used in iontophoresis require a physician's prescription for use.

IONTOPHORESIS VERSUS PHONOPHORESIS

It is critical to point out the difference between iontophoresis and phonophoresis since the two techniques are often confused and occasionally the two terms are erroneously interchanged. It is true that both techniques are used to deliver chemicals to various biologic tissues. Phonophoresis, which is discussed in detail in Chapter 12, involves the use of acoustic energy in the form of ultrasound to drive whole molecules across the skin into the tissues, whereas iontophoresis uses an electrical current to transport ions into the tissues.

iontophoresis A therapeutic technique that involves the introduction of ions into the body tissues by means of a direct electrical current.

BASIC MECHANISMS OF ION TRANSFER

PHARMACOKINETICS OF IONTOPHORESIS

In an ideal drug delivery system, the goal is to maximize the therapeutic effects of a drug while minimizing adverse effects and simultaneously providing a high degree of patient compliance and acceptability.[80] Transdermal iontophoresis delivers medication at a constant rate so that the effective plasma concentration remains within a therapeutic window for an extended period of time. The therapeutic window refers to the plasma concentrations of a drug which should fall between a minimum concentration necessary for a therapeutic effect and the maximum effective concentration above which adverse effects may possibly occur.[80] Iontophoresis is able to facilitate the delivery of charged and high-molecular-weight compounds that cannot be effectively delivered by simply applying them to the skin. Iontophoresis is useful since it appears to overcome the resistive properties of the stratum corneum to charged ions.[80]

Iontophoresis decreases the absorption lag time, while it increases the delivery rate when compared with passive skin application. A primary advantage of iontophoresis is the ability to provide both a spiked and sustained release of a drug, thus reducing the possibility of developing a tolerance to the drug. The rate at which an ion may be delivered is determined by a number of factors including the concentration of the ion, the pH of the solution, molecular size of the solute, current density, and the duration of the treatment.

It appears that mechanisms of absorption of drugs administered by iontophoresis are similar to administration of drugs via other methods.[80] However, there are advantages of taking medication via transdermal iontophoresis relative to taking oral medications, because the medication is concentrated in a specific area and it does not have to be absorbed within the gastrointestinal tract. Additionally, transdermal administration is safer than administering a drug through injection.

MOVEMENT OF IONS IN SOLUTION

As defined in Chapter 5, **ions** are positively or negatively charged particles. Through the process of **ionization** soluble compounds such as acids, alkaloids, or salts dissociate or dissolve into ions, which are suspended in some type of solution.[16] The resulting solutions are called **electrolytes** in which ionic movement occurs. Ions will move or migrate within this solution according to the electrically charged currents acting on them. The term **electrophoresis** refers to the movement of ions in solution.

At any given instant, the electrode that has the greatest concentration of electrons is negatively charged and is referred to as the negative electrode or cathode. Conversely, the electrode with a lower concentration of electrons is called the positive electrode or anode. Negatively charged ions will be repelled from the negative electrode, and thus they move toward the positive electrode, creating an acidic reaction. Positively charged ions will tend to move toward the negative electrode and away from the positive electrode, resulting in an alkaline reaction.

The manner in which ions move in solution forms the basis for iontophoresis. Positively charged ions are carried into the tissues from the positive pole and negatively charged ions are introduced by the negative pole. Once they enter the tissues, the ions are picked up by the body's own charged ions, and electrolytes pick up the electrons and transport them, allowing flow of current between active and dispersive electrodes. Thus knowing the correct ion polarity and matching it with the appropriate electrode polarity is of critical importance in using iontophoresis.

MOVEMENT OF IONS THROUGH TISSUE

The force that acts to move ions through the tissues is determined by both the strength of the electrical field and the electrical impedance of tissues to current flow. The strength of the electrical field is determined by the current density. The difference in

ionization A process by which soluble compounds such as acids, alkaloids, or salts dissociate or dissolve into ions that are suspended in some type of solution.

acidic reaction The accumulation of negative ions under the positive pole that produces hydrochloric acid.

current density between the active and inactive or dispersive electrodes establishes a gradient of potential difference that produces ion migration within the electrical field. (In Chapter 6 the active electrode was defined as the smaller of the two electrodes that has the greater current density. When using iontophoresis, the **active electrode** is defined as the one that is being used to carry the ion into the tissues.) Current density may be altered either by increasing or decreasing current intensity or by changing the size of the electrode. Increasing the size of the electrode will decrease current density under that electrode. It has been recommended that the current density be reduced at the cathode or negative electrode. The accumulation of positively charged ions in a small area creates an alkaline reaction that is more likely to produce tissue damage than an accumulation of negatively charged ions that produces an acidic reaction. Thus it has been recommended that the negative electrode should be larger, perhaps twice the size of the positive electrode to reduce current density.[16,53] This size relationship should remain the same even when the negative electrode is the active electrode. However, it should be added that this is not usually the case with current electrodes for iontophoresis, which are more likely to be the same size (Fig. 7-1).

Skin and fat are poor conductors of electrical current, offering greater resistance to current flow. Higher current intensities are necessary to create ion movement in areas where the skin and fat layers are thick, further increasing the likelihood of burns particularly around the negative electrode. However, the presence of sweat glands decreases impedance, thus facilitating the flow of direct current as well as ions. The sweat ducts are the primary paths by which ions move through the skin.[33] As the skin becomes more saturated with an electrolyte and blood flow increases to the area during treatment, overall skin impedance will decrease under the electrodes.[16] Iontophoresis should be considered a relatively superficial treatment, with the medication penetrating no more than 1.5 cm over a 12- to 24-hour period but only 1–3 mm during the duration of the average treatment.

The quantity of ions transferred into the tissues through iontophoresis is determined by the intensity of the current or current density at the active electrode, the duration of the current flow, and the concentration of ions in solution.[16] The number of ions absorbed is directly proportional to the current density. In addition, the longer the current flows, the greater the number of ions transferred to the tissues. Therefore, ion transfer may be increased by increasing the intensity and duration of the treatment. Unfortunately as treatment duration increases, the skin impedance decreases, thus increasing the likelihood of burns. Even though ion concentration affects ion transfer,

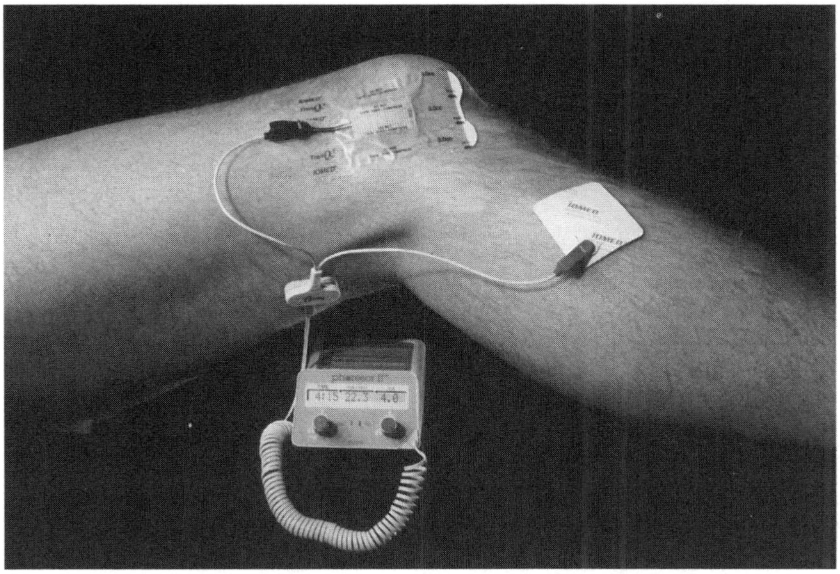

alkaline reaction The accumulation of positive ions under the negative electrode that produces sodium hydroxide.

•**Figure 7-1** The Phoresor is an example of a generator that produces continuous direct current that is specifically used for iontophoresis.

CASE STUDY 7-1
IONTOPHORESIS (1)

Background: A 56-year-old man developed pain in the region inferior to the right patella subsequent to a fall onto the knee while playing tennis. There was immediate mild, localized swelling, which resolved with ice and rest. The acute pain subsided after about 7 days, but the patient then noted significant stiffness following rest, localized tenderness, and pain with climbing stairs, squatting, and kneeling. The physical examination was benign except for mild swelling and point tenderness of the infrapatellar tendon, as well as creptius to palpation of the tendon during active knee extension.

Impression: Infrapatellar tendinitis.

Treatment Plan: In addition to rest and local ice application, a course of iontophoresis of dexamethasone was initiated. The area was prepared appropriately, and the cathode (negative polarity) was used as the delivery electrode. A total of 60 mA-min of current was delivered on an every-other-day schedule for a total of six treatments.

Response: There was a slight increase in the symptoms following the initial treatment, which persisted for approximately 12 hours following the second treatment. The signs and symptoms then began to diminish, and the patient was symptom-free following the fifth treatment. A progressive increase in physical activity was initiated, and the patient returned to preinjury function four weeks later.

Discussion Questions

- What tissues were injured/affected?
- What symptoms were present?
- What phase of the injury-healing continuum did the patient present for care in?
- What are the physical agent modality's biophysical effects (direct/indirect/depth/tissue affinity)?
- What are the physical agent modality's indications/contraindications?
- What are the parameters of the physical agent modality's application/dosage/duration/frequency in this case study?
- What other physical agent modalities could be utilized to treat this injury or condition? Why? How? What is the pathophysiology of tendinitis?
- What is the mechanism of action of the dexamethasone?
- What is the polarity of the dexamethasone molecule?
- What are the required and ideal characteristics for a molecule to be introduced via iontophoresis?
- What are the advantages and disadvantages of iontophoresis as compared to a needle injection?
- Why did the symptoms increase initially?

The rehabilitation professional employs physical agent modalities to create an optimum environment for tissue healing while minimizing the symptoms associated with the trauma or condition.

---

concentrations greater than 1–2 percent are not more effective than medications at lower concentrations.[60,62]

Once the ions have passed through the skin, they recombine with existing ions and free radicals floating in the bloodstream, thus forming the necessary new compounds for favorable therapeutic interactions.[53]

IONTOPHORESIS EQUIPMENT AND TREATMENT TECHNIQUES

TYPE OF CURRENT REQUIRED

Continuous direct current has traditionally been used for iontophoresis. Direct current insures the unidirectional flow of ions that cannot be accomplished using a bidirectional or alternating current. However, a recent study has shown that drugs can be delivered by AC iontophoresis. Iontophoresis using alternating current avoids electrochemical burns, and delivery of the drug increases with duration of application.[39] Neither high-voltage direct currents nor interferential currents may be used for iontophoresis since the current is interrupted and the current duration is too short to produce

Iontophoresis generators produce continuous DC current.

significant ion movement. It should be added, however, that modulated pulsed currents have been used with some success in in vivo and in vitro studies on laboratory animals for transdermal delivery of drugs.[3,74,84]

IONTOPHORESIS GENERATORS

There are a variety of current generators available on the market that produce continuous direct current and are specifically used for iontophoresis (Fig. 7-1). It should be emphasized that any generator that has the capability of producing continuous direct current may be used for iontophoresis. Some generators are driven by batteries, others by alternating current. Many generators produce current at a constant voltage that gradually reduces skin impedance, consequently increasing current density and thus increasing the risk of burns. The generator should deliver a constant voltage output to the patient by adjusting the output amperage to normal variations that occur in tissue impedance, thereby reducing the likelihood of burns. For safety purposes the generator should automatically shut down if the skin impedance decreases to some preset limit.

The generator should have some type of current intensity control that can be adjusted between 1 and 5 mA. There should also be an adjustable timer that can be set up to 25 minutes. Polarity of the terminals should be clearly marked, and a polarity reversal switch is desirable. The lead wires connecting the electrodes to the terminals should be well insulated and should be checked regularly for damage or breakdown.

CURRENT INTENSITY

Low-amperage currents appear to be more effective as a driving force than currents with higher intensities.[41,53,58] Higher-intensity currents tend to reduce effective penetration into the tissues. Recommended current amplitudes used for iontophoresis range between 3 and 5 mA.[8,17,34,53] When initiating the treatment, the current intensity should always be increased very slowly until the patient reports feeling a tingling or prickly sensation. If pain or a burning sensation is elicited, the intensity is too great and should be decreased. Likewise when terminating the treatment, current intensity should be slowly decreased to zero before the electrodes are disconnected.

It has been recommended that the maximum current intensity be determined by the size of the active electrode (Fig. 7-2).[59] Current amplitude is usually set so that the current density falls between 0.1 and 0.5 mA/cm^2 of the active electrode surface.[16]

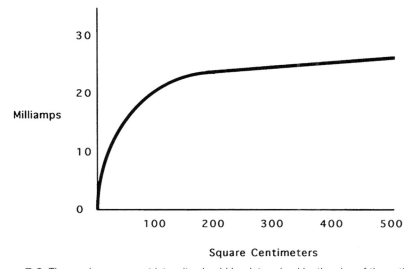

•**Figure 7-2** The maximum current intensity should be determined by the size of the active electrode. Current amplitude is usually set so that the current density falls between 0.1 and 0.5 mA/cm^2 of the active electrode surface.

TREATMENT DURATION

Recommended treatment durations range between 10 and 20 minutes, with 15 minutes being an average.[2] During this 15-minute treatment, the patient should be comfortable with no reported or visible signs of pain or burning. The therapist should check the patient's skin every 3–5 minutes during treatment, looking for signs of skin irritation. Since skin impedance usually decreases during the treatment, it may be necessary to decrease current intensity to avoid pain or burning.

It should be added that the medicated electrode can be left in place for 12–24 hours to enhance the initial treatment.[2]

DOSAGE OF MEDICATION

An iontophoresis dose of medication delivered during treatment is expressed in milliampere-minutes (mA-min). An mA-min is a function of current and time. The total drug dose delivered (mA-min) = current × treatment time. For example:

$$40 \text{ mA-min dose} = 4.0 \text{ mA}$$
$$\text{current} \times 10 \text{ minutes treatment time}$$
$$\text{OR}$$
$$30 \text{ mA-min dose} = 2.0 \text{ mA}$$
$$\text{current} \times 15 \text{ minutes treatment time}$$

A typical iontophoretic drug delivery dose is 40 mA-min but can vary from 0 to 80 mA-min depending on the medication.

ELECTRODES

The continuous direct electrical current must be delivered to the patient through some type of electrode. Many different electrodes are available to the therapist, ranging from those "borrowed" from other electrical stimulators to those that are commercially manufactured ready-to-use disposable electrodes made specifically for iontophoresis.[8,35]

The more traditional electrodes are made of tin, copper, lead, aluminum, or platinum backed by rubber and completely covered by a sponge, towel, or gauze that is in contact with the skin. The absorbent material is soaked with the ionized solution to be driven into the tissues. If the ions are contained in an ointment, it should be rubbed into the skin over the target zone and covered by some absorbent material soaked in water or saline before the electrode is applied.

The commercially produced electrodes are sold with most iontophoresis systems. These electrodes have a small chamber, in which the ionized solution is housed, that is covered by some type of semipermeable membrane. The electrode self-adheres to the skin (Fig. 7-3). This type of electrode has eliminated the "mess and hassles" that have been associated with electrode preparation for iontophoresis in the past.

Regardless of the type of electrode used, to ensure maximum contact of the electrodes, the skin should be shaved and cleaned prior to attachment of the electrodes. Care should be taken not to excessively abrade the skin during cleaning because damaged skin has a lower resistance to the current so that a burn may more easily occur. Also, caution should be used when treating areas that for one reason or another have reduced sensation.

active electrode The electrode is used to drive ions into the tissues.

Once this electrode has been prepared, it then becomes the active electrode, and the lead wire to the generator is attached such that the polarity of the wire is the same as the polarity of the ion in solution. A second electrode, the dispersive electrode, is prepared with water, gel, or some other conductive material as recommended by the manufacturer. Both electrodes must be securely attached to the skin such that uniform skin contact and pressure is maintained under both electrodes to minimize the risk of burns. Electrodes via the lead wires should not be connected to the generator unless

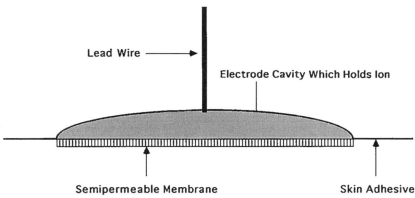

•**Figure 7-3** The commercially produced self-adhering electrodes used with most iontophoresis systems have a small chamber, in which the ionized solution is housed, that is covered by some type of semipermeable membrane.

both the generator and the amplitude or intensity control are turned off. At the end of the treatment, the intensity control should be returned to zero and the generator turned off before the electrodes are detached from the patient.

The size and shape of the electrodes can cause a variation in current density and affect the size of the area treated.[28] Smaller electrodes have a higher current density and should be used to treat a specific lesion. Larger electrodes should be used when the target treatment area is not well defined.

Recommendations for spacing between the active and dispersive electrodes seem to be variable. They should be separated by at least the diameter of the active electrode. One source has recommended spacing them at least 18 inches apart.[16] As spacing between the electrodes increases, the current density in the superficial tissues will decrease, perhaps minimizing the potential for burns.

SELECTING THE APPROPRIATE ION

It is critical that the therapist be knowledgeable in the selection of the most appropriate ions for treating specific conditions. In order for a compound to penetrate a membrane such as the skin it must be soluble in both fat and water. It must be water soluble if it is to remain in an ionized state in solution. However, human skin is relatively impervious to water ions, which are soluble only in water and do not diffuse in the tissues.[10] They must be fat soluble to permeate the tissues of the body.[35] Penetration is relatively superficial and is generally less than 1 mm.[34] The majority of the ions deposited in the tissues are found primarily at the site of the active electrode, where they are stored as either a soluble or insoluble compound. They may be used locally as a concentrated source or transported by the circulating blood, producing more systemic effects.[53]

The tendency of some ions to form insoluble precipitates as they pass into the tissues inhibits their ability to penetrate. This is particularly true with heavy metal ions, including iron, copper, silver, and zinc.[22]

Negative ions accumulating at the positive pole or anode produce an acidic reaction through the formation of hydrochloric acid. Negative ions are sclerotic and produce hardening of the tissues by increasing protein density. In addition, some negative ions can also produce an analgesic effect (salicylates).

The majority of the ions used for iontophoresis are positively charged. Positive ions that accumulate at the negative pole produce an alkaline reaction with the formation of sodium hydroxide. Positive ions are sclerolytic, thus they produce softening of the tissues by decreasing protein density. This is useful in treating scars or adhesions.

The **negative electrode** should be larger than the positive.

Indications and Contraindications for Iontophoresis

Indications
Inflammation
Analgesia
Muscle spasm
Ischemia
Edema
Calcium deposits
Scar tissue
Hyperhidrosis
Fungi
Open skin lesions
Herpes
Allergic rhinitis
Gout
Burns
Reflex sympathetic dystrophy

Contraindications
Skin sensitivity reactions
Sensitivity to aspirin (salicylates)
Gastritis or active stomach ulcer (hydrocortisone)
Asthma (mecholyl)
Sensitivity to metals (zinc, copper, magnesium)
Sensitivity to seafood (iodine)

TABLE 7-1	Recommended Ions for Use By Therapists[42]
POSITIVE	

Antibiotics, gentamycin sulfate (+), 8 mg/mL, for suppurative ear chondritis.

Calcium (+), from calcium chloride, 2% aqueous solution, believed to stabilize the irritability threshold in either direction, as dictated by the physiologic needs of the tissues. Effective with spasmodic conditions, tics, and "snapping fingers" (joints).

Copper (+), from a 2% aqueous solution of copper sulfate crystals; fungicide, astringent, useful with intranasal conditions, e.g., allergic rhinitis or "hay fever," sinusitis, and also dermatophytosis or "athlete's foot."

Hyaluronidase (+), from Wydase crystals in aqueous solution as directed; for localized edema.

Lidocaine (+), from XYLOCAINE 5% ointment, anesthetic/analgesic, especially with acute inflammatory conditions (e.g., bursitis, tendinitis, tic doloreux, and TMJ pain).

Lithium (+), from lithium chloride or carbonate, 2% aqueous solution, effective as an exchange ion with gouty tophi and hyperuricemia.

Magnesium (+), from magnesium sulfate ("Epsom Salts"), 2% aqueous solution, an excellent muscle relaxant, good vasodilator, and mild analgesic.

Mecholyl (+), familiar derivative of acetylcholine, 0.25% ointment, is a powerful vasodilator, good muscle relaxant, and analgesic. Used with discogenic low back radiculopathies and sympathetic reflex dystrophy.

Priscoline (+), from benzazoline hydrochloride, 2% aqueous solution, reported effective with indolent ulcers.

Zinc (+), from zinc oxide ointment, 20%, a trace element necessary for healing, especially effective with open lesions and ulcerations.

NEGATIVE

Acetate (−), from acetic acid, 2% aqueous solution; dramatically effective as a sclerolytic exchange ion with calcific deposits.

Chlorine (−), from sodium chloride, 2% aqueous solution, good sclerolytic agent. Useful with scar tissue, keloids, and burns.

Citrate (−), from potassium citrate, 2% aqueous solution, reported effective in rheumatoid arthritis.

Dexamethasone (−), from Decadron, used for treating musculoskeletal inflammatory conditions.

Iodine (−), from "Iodex" ointment, 4.7%, an excellent sclerolytic agent, as well as bacteriocidal, fair vasodilator. Used successfully with adhesive capsulitis ("frozen shoulder"), scars, etc.

Salicylate (−), from "Iodex with methyl salicylate," 4.8% ointment, a general decongestant, sclerolytic, and anti-inflammatory agent. If desired without the iodine, may be obtained from MYOFLEX ointment (trolamine salicylate 10%) or a 2% aqueous solution of sodium salicylate powder. Used successfully with frozen shoulder, scar tissue, warts, and other adhesive or edematous conditions.

EITHER

Ringer's solution (+/−), with alternating polarity for open decubitus lesions.

Tap water (+/−), usually administered with alternating polarity and sometimes with glycopyrronium bromide in hyperhidrosis.

Table 7-1, modified from a list compiled by Kahn, lists the ions most commonly used with iontophoresis.[49]

CLINICAL APPLICATIONS FOR IONTOPHORESIS

A relatively long list of conditions for which iontophoresis is an appropriate treatment technique has been cited in the literature.[5] Clinically, iontophoresis is most often used in the treatment of inflammatory musculoskeletal conditions.[21] It may also be used for analgesic effects, scar modification, wound healing, and in treating edema, calcium deposits, and hyperhidrosis. Many of these published studies are case reports that attempt to establish the clinical efficacy of iontophoresis in treating various conditions.[28] Table 7-2 provides a list of studies that have treated various conditions using iontophoresis.

Table 7-2   **Conditions Treated with Iontophoresis**

Condition	Ions Used in Treatment	Condition	Ions Used in Treatment
INFLAMMATION		Abell et al. 1974[1]	
Bertolucci 1982[8]	Hydrocortisone, salicylate	Shrivastava, Sing 1977[79]	
Kahn 1982[49]	Dexamethasone	Grice et al. 1972[29]	
Chantraine et al. 1986[12]		Hill 1976[38]	
Harris 1982[34]		Stolman 1987[83]	
Hasson 1991[36]			
Hasson et al. 1992[37]		**FUNGI**	
Delacerda 1982[17]		Kahn 1991[45]	Copper
Glass et al. 1980[27]		Haggard 1939[33]	
Zawislak et al. 1996[89]			
McEntaffer et al. 1996[57]		**OPEN SKIN LESIONS**	
Banta 1995[6]		Cornwall 1981[14]	Zinc
Petelenz et al. 1992[66]		Jenkinson et al. 1974[42]	
Panus et al. 1999[63]	Ketoprofen	Balogun et al. 1990[4]	
ANALGESIA		**HERPES**	
Evans et al. 2001[20]		Gangarosa et al. 1989[25]	
Schaeffer et al. 1971[76]	Lidocaine, magnesium		
Russo et al. 1980[73]		**ALLERGIC RHINITIS**	
Gangarosa 1974[24]		Kahn 1991[45]	Copper
Gangarosa 1993[23]			
Garzione 1978[26]		**GOUT**	
Pellecchia et al. 1994[64]		Kahn 1982[48]	Lithium
Reid et al. 1993[70]			
Schultz 2002[77]		**BURNS**	
		Rapperport et al. 1965[69]	Antibiotics
SPASM		Rigano et al. 1992[71]	
Kahn 1975[52]	Calcium, magnesium	Driscoll et al. 1999[19]	
Kahn 1985[47]			
		REFLEX SYMPATHETIC DYSTROPHY	
ISCHEMIA		Bonezzi et al. 1994[9]	Guanethidine
Kahn 1991[45]	Magnesium, mecholyl, iodine		
		LATERAL EPICONDYLITIS	
EDEMA		Demirtas et al. 1998[18]	Sodium salicylate
Kahn 1991[45]	Magnesium, mecholyl		Sodium diclofenac
Boone 1969[11]	Hyaluronidase, salicylate	Baskurt 2003[7]	Naproxen
Magistro 1964[56]			
Schwartz 1955[78]		**PLANTAR FASCIITIS**	
		Gudeman et al. 1997[30]	Dexamethasone
CALCIUM DEPOSITS		Gulick 2000[32]	Acetic acid
Ciccone 2003[13]			
Weider 1992[88]	Acetic acid	**PATELLAR TENDINITIS**	
Kahn 1977[48]		Huggard et al. 1999[40]	Dexamethasone
Psaki 1955[68]			
Kahn 1996[44]		**ROTATOR CUFF**	
Perron et al. 1997[65]		Preckshot 1999[67]	Dexamethasone
Tygiel 2003[86]			Lidocaine
SCAR TISSUE		**PLANTAR WARTS**	
Tannenbaum 1980[85]	Chlorine, iodine, salicylate	Soroko et al. 2002[82]	Sodium salicylate
Kahn 1985[47]			
		EPICONDYLITIS	
HYPERHIDROSIS		Nirschl 2003[61]	Dexamethazone
Kahn 1973[53]	Tap water		
Levit 1968[55]			

CASE STUDY 7-2
IONTOPHORESIS (2)

Background: A 28-year-old woman has a 3-week history of bilateral wrist pain and nocturnal paresthesia in the palmar aspect of the thumb, index, and long fingers. The symptoms started 2 weeks after starting a new job working on the trim line of an automobile manufacturing plant. The job involves repetitive motions with both hands, and a great deal of squeezing to seat weatherstripping in the doors. The paresthesia is provoked with driving, and holding objects, such as a telephone, blow dryer, or newspaper. She attempts to relieve the paresthesia by shaking the hand (flick sign). She has pain with passive wrist and finger extension and resisted finger flexion, and paresthesia is produced with compression over the carpal tunnel for 15 seconds. She has a positive Tinel sign over the median nerve at the distal wrist crease, and a positive Phalen test at 30 seconds. Crepitus is noted on the anterior wrist with finger flexion.

Impression: Tenosynovitis of the flexor digitorum tendons, with acute carpal tunnel syndrome.

Treatment Plan: The patient was instructed to use resting hand splints at night, and a course of iontophoresis was initiated for the right wrist only. In addition, work restrictions were placed on the patient, to avoid repetitive motion and gripping activities. Dexamethasone was delivered from the cathode (negative polarity), which was placed over the carpal tunnel, with the anode placed over the dorsum of the wrist. A total of 45 mA-min of current were delivered 3 days per week for 2 weeks.

Response: The patient's symptoms diminished in both hands over the 2-week period; however, she continued to have a positive carpal compression test, a positive Phalen test, and a positive Tinel sign only on the left. She returned to the trim line with instructions for a 2-week ramp-up period; however, the pain and paresthesia returned in the left wrist. She subsequently underwent a surgical decompression of the left carpal tunnel, and was able to return to work without restrictions following 6 weeks off work and a second 2-week ramp-up period.

Discussion Questions:
- What tissues were injured or affected?
- What symptoms were present?
- What phase of the injury-healing continuum did the patient present for care in?
- What are the physical agent modality's biophysical effects (direct, indirect, depth, and tissue affinity)?
- What are the physical agent modality's indications and contraindications?
- What are the parameters of the physical agent modality's application, dosage, duration, and frequency in this case study?
- What other physical agent modalities could be used to treat this injury or condition? Why? How?
- What is the significance of the Tinel sign?
- What is the significance of the Phalen test?
- Why does compression over the carpal tunnel reproduce the symptoms?
- Why does the patient experience nocturnal paresthesia rather than during work?
- What is another potential source of the patient's symptoms?
- If the patient also had cervical pain, would you anticipate a different treatment approach?
- Would electrophysiologic testing be appropriate for this patient? What findings would you anticipate?

The rehabilitation professional employs physical agent modalities to create an optimum environment for tissue healing while minimizing the symptoms associated with the trauma or condition.

TREATMENT PRECAUTIONS AND CONTRAINDICATIONS

Problems that might potentially arise from treating a patient using iontophoresis techniques may be avoided for the most part if the therapist (1) has a good understanding of the existing condition to be treated; (2) uses the most appropriate ions to accomplish the treatment goal; and (3) uses appropriate treatment parameters and equipment set-up. Poor treatment technique on the part of the therapist is most often responsible for adverse reactions to iontophoresis.

TREATMENT OF BURNS

Perhaps the single most common problem associated with iontophoresis is a chemical burn, which usually occurs as a result of the direct current itself and not as a result of the ion being used in treatment.[59] Passing a continuous direct electrical current through the tissues creates migration of ions, which alters the normal pH of the skin. The normal pH of the skin is between 3 and 4. In an **acidic reaction** the pH falls below 3, whereas in an **alkaline reaction** the pH is greater than 5. Although chemical burns may occur under either electrode, they most typically result from the accumulation of sodium hydroxide at the cathode. The alkaline reaction causes sclerolysis of local tissues. Initially, the burn lesion is pink and raised but within hours becomes a grayish, oozing wound.[53] Decreasing current density by increasing the size of the cathode relative to the anode can minimize the potential for chemical burn.

Heat burns may occur as a result of high resistance to current flow created by poor contact of the electrodes with the skin. Poor contact results when the electrodes are not moist enough; when there are wrinkles in the gauze or paper towels impregnated with the ionic solution; or when there is space between the skin and electrode around the perimeter of the electrode. The patient should not be treated with body weight resting on top of the electrode since this is likely to create some ischemia (reduced circulation) under the electrode. Instead, the electrode should be held firmly in place with adhesive tape, elastic bands, or lightweight sand bags. It is recommended that both chemical burns and heat burns should be treated with sterile dressings and antibiotics.[53]

Treatment Tip
To minimize the likelihood of a burn the size of the cathode relative to the anode can be increased and the current density can be decreased. Also, increasing the spacing between the electrodes will decrease current intensity, thus minimizing the chances of a chemical burn.

SENSITIVITY REACTIONS TO IONS

Sensitivity reactions to ions rarely occur; however, they may potentially be very serious. The therapist should routinely question the patient about known drug allergies prior to initiating iontophoresis treatment. During the treatment the therapist should closely monitor the patient, looking for either abnormal localized reactions of the skin or systemic reactions.

Patients who have sensitivity to aspirin may have a reaction when using salicylates. Hydrocortisone may adversely affect individuals with gastritis or an active stomach ulcer. In cases of asthma, mecholyl should be avoided. Patients who are sensitive to metals should not be treated with copper, zinc, or magnesium. Iodine iontophoresis should not be used with individuals who have allergies to seafood or those who have had a bad reaction to intravenous pyelograms.[53]

Treatment Tip
Dexamethasone should be placed under the positive electrode since it is a positively charged ion. Current intensity should be set between 3 and 5 mA. Treatment time should be 15 minutes. The therapist should check the skin every 3–5 minutes for a reaction.

SUMMARY

1. Iontophoresis is a therapeutic technique that involves the introduction of ions into the body tissues by means of a direct electrical current.

2. The manner in which ions move in solution forms the basis for iontophoresis. Positively charged ions are driven into the tissues from the positive pole and negatively charged ions are introduced by the negative pole.

3. The force that acts to move ions through the tissues is determined by both the strength of the electrical field and the electrical impedance of tissues to current flow.

4. The quantity of ions transferred into the tissues through iontophoresis is determined by the intensity of the current or current density at the active electrode, the duration of the current flow, and the concentration of ions in solution.

5. Continuous direct current must be used for iontophoresis, thus ensuring the unidirectional flow of ions that cannot be accomplished using a bidirectional or alternating current.

6. Electrodes may be either reusable or commercially produced, self-adhering, prepared electrodes that must be securely attached to the skin.

7. It is critical that the therapist be knowledgeable in the selection of the most appropriate ions for treating specific conditions.

8. Clinically, iontophoresis is used in the treatment of inflammatory musculoskeletal conditions, for analgesic effects, scar modification, wound healing, and in treating edema, calcium deposits, and hyperhidrosis.

9. Perhaps the single most common problem associated with iontophoresis is a chemical burn, which usually occurs as a result of the direct current itself and not because of the ion being used in treatment.

REVIEW QUESTIONS

1. What is iontophoresis and how may it be used?
2. What is the difference between iontophoresis and phonophoresis?
3. How do ions move in solution?
4. What determines the quantity of ions transferred through the tissues during iontophoresis?
5. Why must continuous direct current be used for iontophoresis?
6. What types of electrodes can be used with iontophoresis and how should they be applied?
7. What characteristics should be considered when selecting the appropriate ion for an iontophoresis treatment?
8. What are the various clinical uses for iontophoresis in athletic training?
9. What treatment precautions must be taken when using iontophoresis?

REFERENCES

1. Abell, E., Morgan, K.: Treatment of idiopathic hyperhidrosis by glycopyrronium bromide and tap water iontophoresis, Br. J. Dermatol. 91:87, 1974.

2. Anderson, C.R., Morris, R.I., Boeh, S.D., et al.: Effects of iontophoresis current magnitude and duration on dexamethasone deposition and localized drug retention, Phys. Ther. 83(2): 161–170, 2003.

3. Bagniefski, T., Burnette, R.: A comparison of pulsed and continuous current iontophoresis, J. Control. Rel. 11:113–122, 1990.

4. Balogun, J., Abidoye, A., and Akala, E.: Zinc iontophoresis in the management of bacterial colonized wounds: a case report, Physiother. Can. 42(3):147–151, 1990.

5. Banga, A.K., Panus, P.C.: Clinical applications of iontophoretic devices in rehabilitation medicine, Crit. Rev. Phys. Rehabil. Med. 10(2):147–179, 1998.

6. Banta, C.: A prospective nonrandomized study of iontophoresis, wrist splinting, and antiinflammatory medication in the treatment of early mild carpal tunnel syndrome, J. Orthop. Sports Phys. Ther. 21(2):120, 1995.

7. Baskurt, F.: Comparison of effects of phonophoresis and iontophoresis of naproxen in the treatment of lateral epicondylitis, Clin. Rehabil. 17(1):96–100, 2003.

8. Bertolucci, L.: Introduction of anti-inflammatory drugs by iontophoreses: a double-blind study, J. Orthop. Sports Phys. Ther. 4(2):103, 1982.

9. Bonezzi, C., Miotti, D., and Bettagilo, R.: Electromotive administration of guanethidine for treatment of reflex sympathetic dystrophy, J. Pain Sympt. Manage. 9(1):39–43, 1994.

10. Boone, D.: Applications of iontophoresis. In Wolf, S., editor. Electrotherapy, New York, 1981, Churchill Livingstone.

11. Boone, D.: Hyaluronidase iontophoresis, J. Am. Phys. Ther. Assoc. 49:139–145, 1969.

12. Chantraine, A., Lundy, J., and Berger, D.: Is cortisone iontophoresis possible? Arch. Phys. Med. Rehab. 67:380, 1986.

13. Ciccone, C.D.: Evidence in practice… Does acetic acid iontophoresis accelerate the resorption of calcium deposits in calcific tendinitis of the shoulder? Phys. Ther. 83(1):68–74, 2003.

14. Cornwall, M.: Zinc oxide iontophoresis for ischemic skin ulcers, Phys. Ther. 61(3):359, 1981.

15. Costello, C., Jeske, A.: Iontophoresis: applications in transdermal medication delivery, Phys. Ther. 75(6):554–563, 1995.

16. Cummings, J.: Iontophoresis. In Nelson, R.M., Currier, D.P., editors. Clinical electrotherapy, Norwalk, CT, 1991, Appleton & Lange.

17. Delacerda, F.: A comparative study of three methods of treatment for shoulder girdle myofascial syndrome, J. Orthop. Sports Phys. Ther. 4(1):51–54, 1982.

18. Demirtas, R.N., Oner, C.: The treatment of lateral epicondylitis by iontophoresis of sodium salicylate and sodium diclofenac, Clin. Rehabil. 12(1):23–29, 1998.

19. Driscoll, J.B., Plunkett, K., and Tamari, A.: The effect of potassium iodide iontophoresis on range of motion and scar maturation following burn injury, Phys. Ther. Case Rep. 2(1):13–18, 1999.

20. Evans, T., Kunkle, J., and Zinz, K.: The immediate effects of lidocaine iontophoresis on trigger-point-pain, J. Sport Rehabil. 10(4):287, 2001.

21. Federici, P.: Injury management update. Treating iliotibial band friction syndrome using iontophoresis, Athl. Ther. Today 2(5):22–23, 1997.

22. Gadsby, P.: Visualization of the barrier layer through iontophoresis of ferric ions, Med. Instrum. 13:281, 1979.

23. Gangarosa, L.: Iontophoresis in pain control, Pain Digest 3:162–174, 1993.

24. Gangarosa, L.: Iontophoresis for surface local anesthesia, J. Am. Dent. Assoc. 88:125, 1974.

25. Gangarosa, L., Payne, L., and Hayakawa, K.: Iontophoretic treatment of herpetic whitlow, Arch. Phys. Med. Rehabil. 70(4):336–340, 1989.

26. Garzione, J.: Salicylate iontophoresis as an alternative treatment for persistent thigh pain following hip surgery, Phys. Ther. 58 (5):570–571, 1978.

27. Glass, J., Stephen, R., and Jacobsen, S.: The quantity and distribution of radiolabeled dexamethasone delivered to tissues by iontophoresis, Int. J. Dermatol. 19:519, 1980.

28. Glick, E., Synder-Mackler, L.: Iontophoresis. In Snyder-Mackler, L., Robinson, A., editors. Clinical electrophysiology and electrophysiologic testing, Baltimore, MD, 1989, Williams & Wilkins.

29. Grice, K., Sattar, H., and Baker, H.: Treatment of idiopathic hyperhidrosis with iontophoresis of tap water and poldine methosulphate, Br. J. Dermatol. 86:72, 1972.

30. Gudeman, S.D., Eisele, S.A., Heidt, R.S. Jr., et al.: Treatment of plantar fasciitis by iontophoresis of 0.4% dexamethasone: a randomized, double-blind, placebo-controlled study, Am. J. Sports Med. 25(3):312–316, 1997.

31. Guffey, J.S., Rutherford, M.J., Payne, W., and Phillips, C.: Skin pH changes associated with iontophoresis, J. Orthop. Sports Phys. Ther. 29(11):656–660, 1999.

32. Gulick, D.T.: Effects of acetic acid iontophoresis on heel spur reabsorption, Phys. Ther. Case Rep. 3(2):64–70, 2000.

33. Haggard, H., Strauss, M., and Greenberg, L.: Fungus infections of hand and feet treated by copper iontophoresis, JAMA 112:1229, 1939.

34. Harris, P.: Iontophoresis: clinical research in musculoskeletal inflammatory conditions, J. Orthop. Sports Phys. Ther. 4(2): 109–112, 1982.

35. Harris, R.: Iontophoresis. In Licht, S., editor. Therapeutic electricity and ultraviolet radiation, Baltimore, MD, 1967, Waverly.

36. Hasson, S.: Exercise training and dexamethsone intophoresis in rheumatoid arthritis: a case study, Physiotherapy (Can.) 43:11, 1991.

37. Hasson, S., Wible, C., and Reich, M.: Dexamethasone iontophoresis: effect on delayed muscle soreness and muscle function, Can. J. Sport Sci. 17:8–13, 1992.

38. Hill, B.: Poldine iontophoresis in the treatment of palmar and plantar hyperhidrosis, Aust. J. Dermatol. 17:92, 1976.

39. Howard, J., Drake, T., and Kellogg, D.: Effects of alternating current iontophoresis on drug delivery, Arch. Phys. Med. Rehabil. 76(5):463–466, 1995.

40. Huggard, C., Kimura, I., and Mattacola, C.: Clinical efficacy of dexamethasone iontophoresis in the treatment of patellar tendinitis in college athletes: a double blind study, J. Athl. Train. 34(2):S-70, 1999.

41. Jacobson, S., Stephen, R., and Sears, W.: Development of a new drug delivery system (iontophoresis), University of Utah, Salt Lake City, Utah, 1980.

42. Jenkinson, D., McEwan, J., and Walton, G.: The potential use of iontophoresis in the treatment of skin disorders, Vet. Rec. 94:8 Arch. Phys. Med. Rehabil. 12, 1974.

43. Johnson, C., Shuster, S.: The patency of sweat ducts in normal looking skin, Br. J. Dermatol. 83:367, 1970.

44. Kahn, J.: Acetic acid iontophoresis, Phys. Ther. 76(5):S68, 1996.

45. Kahn, J.: Practices and principles of electrotherapy, New York, 1991, Churchill Livingstone.

46. Kahn, J.: Non-steroid iontophoresis, Clin. Manage. Phys. Ther. 7(1):14–15, 1987.

47. Kahn, J.: Clinical electrotherapy, ed. 4, Syosset, New York, 1985, J. Kahn.

48. Kahn, J.: A case report: lithium iontophoresis for gouty arthritis, J. Orthop. Sports Phys. Ther. 4:113, 1982.

49. Kahn, J.: Iontophoresis with hydrocortisone for Peyronie's disease, JAPTA 62(7):995, 1981.

50. Kahn, J.: Iontophoresis: practice tips. Clin. Manage. 2(4):37, 1981.

51. Kahn, J.: Acetic acid iontophoresis for calcium deposits, JAPTA 57(6):658, 1977.

52. Kahn, J.: Calcium iontophoresis in suspected myopathy, JAPTA 55(4):276, 1975.

53. Kahn, J.: Tap-water iontophoresis for hyperhidrosis. Reprinted in Medical Group News, August, 1973.

54. LeDuc, S.: Electric ions and their use in medicine, Liverpool, 1903, Rebman.

55. Levit, R: Simple device for treatment of hyperhidrosis by iontophoresis, Arch. Dermatol. 98:505–507, 1968.

56. Magistro, C.: Hyaluronidase by iontophoresis in the treatment of edema: a preliminary clinical report, Phys. Ther. 44:169, 1964.

57. McEntaffer, D., Sailor, M.: The effects of stretching and iontophoretically delivered dexamethasone on plantar fasciitis, Phys. Ther. 76(5):S68, 1996.

58. Mandleco, C.: Research: iontophoresis, University of Utah, Salt Lake City, 1978, Institute for Biomedical Engineering.

59. Molitor, H.: Pharmacologic aspects of drug administration by ion transfer, The Merck Report: 22–29, January, 1943.

60. Murray, W., Levine L., and Seifter E.: The iontophoresis of C2 esterified glucocorticoids: preliminary report, Phys. Ther. 43:579, 1963.

61. Nirschl, R.P.: Iontophoretic administration of dexamethasone sodium phosphate for acute epicondylitis: a randomized, double-blind, placebo-controlled study, Am. J. Sports Med. 31(2):189–195, 2003.

62. O'Malley, E., Oester, Y.: Influence of some physical chemical factors on iontophoresis using radioisotopes, Arch. Phys. Med. Rehabil. 36:310, 1955.

63. Panus, P.C., Ferslew, K.E., Tober-Meyer, B., and Kao, R.L.: Ketoprofen tissue permeation in swine following cathodic iontophoresis, Phys. Ther. 79(1):40–49, 1999.

64. Pellecchia, G., Hamel, H., and Behnke, P.: Treatment of infrapatellar tendinitis: a combination of modalities and transverse friction massage versus iontophoresis, J. Sport Rehabil. 3(2):135–145, 1994.

65. Perron M., Malouin, F.: Acetic acid iontophoresis and ultrasound for the treatment of calcifying tendinitis of the shoulder: a randomized control trial, Arch. Phys. Med. Rehabil. 78(4):379–384, 1997.

66. Petelenz, T., Buttke, J., and Bonds, C.: Iontophoresis of dexamethasone: laboratory studies, J. Control. Rel. 20:55–66, 1992.

67. Preckshot, J.: Iontophoresis with lidocaine and dexamethasone for treating rotator cuff injury in a hockey player, Int. J. Pharm. Compounding 3(6):441, 1999.

68. Psaki, C., Carol, J.: Acetic acid ionization: a study to determine the absorptive effects upon calcified tendinitis of the shoulder, Phys. Ther. Rev. 35:84, 1955.

69. Rapperport, A.: Iontophoresis—a method of antibiotic administration in the burn patient, Plast. Reconstr. Surg. 36(5):547–552, 1965.

70. Reid, K., Sicard-Rosenbaum, L., and Lord, D.: Iontophoresis with normal saline versus dexamethasone and lidocaine in the treatment of patients with internal disc derangement of the temporomandibular joint, Phys. Ther. 73(6):S20, 1993.

71. Rigano, W., Yanik, M., and Barone F.: Antibiotic iontophoresis in the management of burned ears, J. Burn Care Rehabil. 13(4):407–409, 1992.

72. Roberts, D.: Transdermal drug delivery using iontophoresis and phonophoresis, Orthop. Nurs. 18(3):50–54, 1999.

73. Russo, J., Lipman, A., and Comstock, T.: Lidocane anesthesia: comparison of iontophoresis, injection and swabbing, Am. J. Hosp. Pharm. 37:843–847, 1980.

74. Sabbahi, M., Costello, C., and Emran, A.: A method for reducing skin irritation from iontophoresis, Phys. Ther. 74:S156, 1994.

75. Sakurai, T.: Iontophoretic administration of prostaglandin E1 in peripheral arterial occlusive disease, Ann. Pharmacother. 37(5):747, 2003.

76. Schaeffer, M., Bixler, D., and Yu, P.: The effectiveness of iontophoresis in reducing cervical hypersensitivity, J. Peridontol. 42:695, 1971.

77. Schultz, A.A.: Safety, tolerability, and efficacy of iontophoresis with lidocaine for dermal anesthesia in ED pediatric patients, Journal of Emergency Nursing 28(4):289–196, 2002.

78. Schwartz, M.: The use of hyaluronidase by iontophoresis in the treatment of lymphedema, Arch. Intern. Med. 95:662, 1955.

79. Shrivastava, S., Sing, G.: Tap water iontophoresis in palm and plantar hyperhidrosis, Br. J. Dermatol. 96:189, 1977.

80. Singh, P., Mailbach, H.: Transdermal iontophoresis: pharmakokinetic considerations, Clin. Pharmacakinet. 26:327–334, 1994.

81. Smutok, M.A., Mayo, M.F., and Gabaree, C.L.: Failure to detect dexamethasone phosphate in the local venous blood postcathodic iontophoresis in humans, J. Orthop. Sports Phys. Ther. 32(9):461–468, 2002.

82. Soroko, Y.T., Repking, M.C., Clemment, J.A., et al.: Treatment of plantar verrucae using 2% sodium salicylate iontophoresis, Phys. Ther. 82(12):1184–1191, 2002.

83. Stolman, L.: Treatment of excess sweating of the palms by iontophoresis, Arch. Dermatol. 123:893, 1987.

84. Su, M., Srinivasan, V., and Ghanem, A.: Quantitative in vivo iontophoretic studies, J. Pharm. Sci. 83:12–17, 1994.

85. Tannenbaum, M.: Iodine iontophoresis in reduction of scar tissue, Phys. Ther. 60(6):792, 1980.

86. Tygiel, P.P.: On "Does acetic acid iontophoresis accelerate the resorption of calcium deposits in calcific tendinitis of the shoulder?" Phys. Ther. 83(7):667–670, 2003.

87. Van Herp, G.: Iontophoresis: a review of the literature, N.Z. J. Physiother. 25(2):16–17, 1997.

88. Weider, D.: Treatment of traumatic myositis ossificans with acetic acid iontophoresis, Phys. Ther. 72(2):133–137, 1992.

89. Zawislak, D., Rau, C., and Lee, M.: The effects of dexamethasone iontophoresis on acute inflammation using a sports model of treatment, Phys. Ther. 76(5):5–17, 1966.

SUGGESTED READINGS

Abramowitsch, D., Neoussikine, B.: Treatment by ion transfer, New York, 1946, Grune & Stratton.

Abramson, D.: Physiologic and clinical basis for histamine by ion transfer, Arch. Phys. Med. Rehabil. 48:583–592, 1967.

Agostinucci, J., Powers, W.: Motoneuron excitability modulation after desensitization of the skin by iontophoresis of lidocaine hydrochloride, Arch. Phys. Med. Rehabil. 73(2):190–194, 1992.

Akins, D., Meisenheimer, I., and Dobson, R.: Efficacy of the Drionic unit in the treatment of hyperhidrosis, J. Am. Acad. Dermatol. 16:828, 1987.

Brumett, A., Comeau, M.: Local anesthesia of the tympanic membrane by iontophoresis, Trans. Am. Acad. Otolaryngol. 78:453, 1974.

Cady, D., Zawislak, J., and Rau, C.: The effects of dexamethasone iontophoresis on acute inflammation using a sports model of treatment, Phys. Ther. 76(5):S17, 1996.

Comeau, M.: Anesthesia of the human tympanic membrane by iontophoresis of a local anesthetic, Laryngoscope 88:277–285, 1978.

Comeau, M.: Local anesthesia of the ear by iontophoresis, Arch. Otolaryngol. 98:114–120, 1973.

Chein, Y., Banga, A.: Iontophoretic (transdermal) delivery of drugs: overview of historical development, J. Pharm. Sci. 78:353–354, 1989.

Dellagatta, E., Thompson, E.: Changes in skin resistance produced by continuous direct current stimulation utilizing methyl nicotinate, Phys. Ther. 74(5):S12, 1994.

Falcone, A., Spadaro, J.: Inhibitory effects of electrically activated silver material on cutaneous wound bacteria, Plast. Reconstr. Surg. 77:455, 1986.

Fay, M.: Indications and applications for iontophoresis, Today's OR Nurse 11(4):10–16, 29–31, 1989.

Gangarosa, L., Park, N., and Fong, B.: Conductivity of drugs used for iontophoresis, J. Pharm. Sci. 67:1439–1443, 1978.

Gordon, A.: Sodium salicylate iontophoresis in the treatment of plantar warts, Phys. Ther. Rev. 49:869–870, 1969.

Haggard, H., Strauss, M., and Greenberg, L.: Copper, electrically injected, cures fungus diseases. Reprinted in Science Newsletter, May 6, 1939.

Hasson, S.: Exercise training and dexamethasone intophoresis in rheumatoid arthritis: a case study, Physiotherapy (Can.) 43:11, 1991.

Henley, J.: Transcutaneous drug delivery: iontophoresis, phonophoresis, Phys. Med. Rehabil. 2:139, 1991.

Jarvis, C., Voita, D.: Low voltage skin burns, Pediatrics 48:831, 1971.

Kahn, J.: Iontophoresis (video tape). AREN, Pittsburgh, PA, 1988.

Kahn, J.: Phoresor adaptation, Clin. Manage. Phys. Ther. 5(4):50–51, 1985.

Kahn, J.: Iontophoresis in clinical practice, Stimulus (APTA-SCE) 8(3), May, 1983.

Kahn, J.: Iontophoresis and ultrasound for post-surgical TMJ trismus and paresthesia, JAPTA 60(3):307, 1982.

LaForest, N., Confrancisco, C.: Antibiotic iontophoresis in the treatment of ear chondritis, JAPTA 58:32, 1978.

Langley, P.: Iontophoresis to aid in releasing tendon adhesions, Phys. Ther. 64(9):1395, 1984.

Lemming, M., Cole, R., and Howland, W.: Low voltage direct current burns, JAMA 214:1681, 1970.

McFadden, E.: Iontophoresis for pain management, J. Pediatr. Nurs. 10(5):331, 1995.

Nightingale, A.: Physics and electronics in physical medicine, London, 1959, F. Bell.

Nimmo, W.: Novel delivery systems: electrotransport, J. Pain Sympt. Manage. 7(3):160–162, 1992.

Panus, P., Campbell, J., and Kulkami, S.: Transdermal iontophoretic delivery of ketoprofen through human cadaver skin and in humans, Phys. Ther. 76(5):S67, 1996.

Phipps, J., Padmanabhan, R., and Lattin G.: Iontophoretic delivery of model inorganic and drug ions, J. Pharm. Sci. 78:365–369, 1989.

Puttemans, F., Massart, D., and Gilles, F.: Iontophoreses: mechanism of action studied by potentiometry and x-ray fluorescence, Arch. Phys. Med. Rehabil. 63:176–180, 1982.

Sawyer, C.: Cystic fibrosis of the pancreas: a study of sweat electrolyte levels in thirty-six families using pilocarpine iontophoresis, So. Med. J. 59:197–202, 1966.

Shapiro, B.: Insulin iontophoresis in cystic fibrosis, Soc. Exp. Biol. Med. 149:592–593, 1975.

Shriber, W.: A manual of electrotherapy, ed. 4, Philadelphia, PA, 1975, Lea & Febiger.

Sisler, H.: Iontophoresis local anesthesia for conjunctival surgery, Ann. Ophthalmol. 10:597, 1978.

Stillwell, G.: Electrotherapy. In Kottke, F., Stillwell, G., and Lehman, J., editors. Handbook of physical medical and rehabilitation, Philadelphia, PA, 1982, W.B. Saunders.

Tregear, R.: The permeability of mammalian skin to ions, J. Invest. Dermatol. 46:16–23, 1966.

Trubatch, J., Van Harrevel, A.: Spread of iontophoretically injected ions in a tissue, J. Theor. Biol. 36:355, 1972.

Waud, D.: Iontophoretic applications of drugs, J. Appl. Physiol. 28:128, 1967.

Zankel, H., Cress, R., and Kamin, H.: Iontophoreses studies with radioactive tracer, Arch. Phys. Med. Rehabil. 40:193–196, 1959.

GLOSSARY

acidic reaction The accumulation of negative ions under the positive pole that produces hydrochloric acid.

active electrode The electrode that is used to drive ions into the tissues.

alkaline reaction The accumulation of positive ions under the negative electrode that produces sodium hydroxide.

electrolytes Solutions in which ionic movement occurs.

electrophoresis The movement of ions in solution.

ionization A process by which soluble compounds such as acids, alkaloids, or salts dissociate or dissolve into ions that are suspended in some type of solution.

ions Positively or negatively charged particles.

iontophoresis A therapeutic technique that involves the introduction of ions into the body tissues by means of a direct electrical current.

ion transfer A technique of transporting chemicals across a membrane using an electrical current as a driving force.

LAB ACTIVITY

IONTOPHORESIS

DESCRIPTION:

Iontophoresis is the use of direct current electricity to introduce various drugs to subcutaneous tissues without using invasive means. Although there are many drugs that may be used, various corticosteroids and local anesthetics are the most commonly used drugs.

It is not possible to use any form of electrical current other than direct current to achieve movement of the drug; the misnamed "high-voltage galvanic stimulators" are not capable of phoresing a drug owing to the very low pulse charge. Because of the possibility of producing an electrolytic burn with direct current, it is recommended that the current amplitude remain below 0.7 mA × number of cm^2 of electrode.

There are many different electrodes available for iontophoresis. The most rudimentary is to use alligator clips to attach the cables to a tin or aluminum conductor, and use a paper towel soaked with the drug between the electrode and the patient. More commonly, electrodes developed by the manufacturer of the stimulator are used.

It is mandatory that the drug be in an ionic form; otherwise, the electrical current will not be able to move the drug. Many drugs come in both ionized forms and as a suspension. If in doubt, a PDR should be consulted.

PHYSIOLOGIC EFFECTS:

Depends on the drug

THERAPEUTIC EFFECTS:

Depends on the drug; generally, decreased inflammation and local anesthesia

INDICATIONS:

The primary indication is for the control of inflammation and/or pain.

CONTRAINDICATIONS:

- Pregnancy
- Implanted electrical pacing devices (e.g., cardiac pacemaker, bladder stimulator)
- Cardiac arrhythmia
- Over the carotid sinus area
- Hypersensitivity (i.e., the patient who has a strong aversion to electricity, or the patient with certain types of catheters or shunts)
- Known problems with medication used in treatment

ELECTRICAL STIMULATION: IONTOPHORESIS

PROCEDURE	EVALUATION		
	1	2	3
1. Check supplies.			
a. Obtain towels or sheets for draping, conductant.			
b. Check stimulator, electrodes, and cables for charged battery, broken or frayed insulation, and so on.			
c. Verify that the intensity control is at zero.			
2. Question patient.			
a. Verify identity of patient (if not already verified).			
b. Verify the absence of contraindications.			
c. Ask about previous exposure to electrotherapy.			

PROCEDURE	EVALUATION		
	1	2	3
3. Position patient.			
a. Place patient in a well-supported, comfortable position.			
b. Expose body part to be treated.			
c. Drape patient to preserve patient's modesty, protect clothing, but allow access to body part.			
4. Inspect body part to be treated.			
a. Check light touch perception.			
b. Assess function of body part (e.g., ROM, irritability).			
5. Apply electrical stimulation for iontophoresis.			
a. Prepare electrodes according to manufacturer's instructions, secure electrodes to patient. Electrode location will vary depending on the drug being phoresed; anionic drugs are repelled from the cathode, cations are repelled from the anode.			
b. Remind the patient to inform you when they feel something. Do not tell the patient what they will feel; for example, do not say "Tell me when you feel a burning or stinging."			
c. Turn on the stimulator, and increase the amplitude slowly. Monitor the patient's response, not the stimulator.			
d. After the patient reports the onset of the stimulus, adjust the amplitude to the appropriate intensity.			
e. Continue to monitor the patient during the duration of the treatment.			
6. Complete treatment.			
a. When the treatment time is over, turn the generator off, and turn the intensity control to zero; remove conductant with a towel.			
b. Remove material used for draping, assist the patient in dressing as needed.			
c. Have the patient perform appropriate therapeutic exercise as indicated.			
d. Clean the treatment area and equipment according to normal protocol.			
7. Assess treatment efficacy.			
a. Ask the patient how the treated area feels.			
b. Visually inspect the treated area for any adverse reactions.			
c. Perform functional tests as indicated.			

CHAPTER 8 EIGHT

BIOFEEDBACK

WILLIAM E. PRENTICE

OBJECTIVES

Following completion of this chapter, the student therapist will be able to:

- ✓ Define biofeedback and identify its uses in a clinical setting.
- ✓ Contrast the various types of biofeedback instruments.
- ✓ Explain physiologically how the electrical activity generated by a muscle contraction can be measured using an electromyograph (EMG).
- ✓ Break down how the electrical activity picked up by the electrodes is amplified, processed, and converted to meaningful information by the biofeedback unit.
- ✓ Differentiate between visual and auditory feedback.
- ✓ Outline the equipment setup and clinical applications for biofeedback.

Electromyographic biofeedback is a modality that seems to be gaining increased popularity in clinical settings. It is a therapeutic procedure that uses electronic or electromechanical instruments to accurately measure, process, and feed back reinforcing information via auditory or visual signals.[26] In clinical practice, it is used to help the patient develop greater voluntary control in terms of either neuromuscular relaxation or muscle reeducation following injury.

ELECTROMYOGRAPHY AND BIOFEEDBACK

Electromyography (EMG) is a clinical technique that involves recording of the electrical activity generated in a muscle for diagnostic purposes. It involves a sophisticated electrodiagnostic study performed in an EMG laboratory, which uses either surface or needle electrodes for measuring not only electrical activity in muscle but also various aspects of nerve conduction. An *electromyogram* is a graphic representation of those electrical currents associated with muscle action. Electromyography is widely used by physical therapists in the diagnosis of a variety of neuromuscular disorders. Certainly electromyography would not be considered a therapeutic modality.

The small portable biofeedback units that will be discussed in this chapter also measure electrical activity in the muscle and are in fact small electromyographs. The discussion in this chapter will be limited to the information on electromyography necessary for the therapist to understand, to be able to effectively incorporate biofeedback techniques into clinical practice.

THE ROLE OF BIOFEEDBACK

The term "biofeedback" should be familiar because all therapists routinely serve as instruments of biofeedback when teaching a therapeutic exercise or in coaching a movement pattern. Using feedback can help the patient to regain function of a muscle that may have been lost or forgotten following injury.[12] Feedback includes information related to the sensations associated with movement itself as well as information related to the result of the action relative to some goal or objective. Feedback refers to the intrinsic information inherent to movement, including kinesthetic, visual, cutaneous, vestibular, and auditory signals collectively termed as response-produced feedback. However, it also refers to extrinsic information or some knowledge of results that is presented verbally, mechanically, or electronically to indicate the outcome of some movement performance. Therefore, feedback is ongoing, in a temporal sense, occurring before, during, and after any motor or movement task. Feedback from some measuring instrument that provides moment-to-moment information about a biologic function is referred to as **biofeedback**.[22]

Perhaps the biggest advantage of biofeedback is that it provides the patient with a chance to make appropriate small changes in performance that are immediately noted and rewarded so that eventually larger changes or improvements in performance can be accomplished. The goal is to train the patient to perceive these changes without the use of the measuring instrument so that he or she can practice independently. Therefore, the patient learns early in the rehabilitation process to do something for him- or herself and not to totally rely on the therapist. This will help him or her to build confidence and increase feelings of self-efficacy. Treatments using biofeedback are useful, particularly in a patient who has difficulty in perceiving the initial small correct responses or who may have a faulty perception of what he or she is doing. Hopefully, the rehabilitating patient will be motivated and encouraged by seeing early signs of slight progress; thus relieving feelings of helplessness and reducing injury-related stress to some extent.[22]

To process feedback information, the patient makes use of a complicated series of interrelated feedback loops involving very complex anatomic and neurophysiologic components.[35] An in-depth discussion of these components is well beyond the scope of this text. Thus, our focus will be oriented toward how biofeedback may best be incorporated in a treatment program.

biofeedback Information provided from some measuring instrument about a specific biologic function.

BIOFEEDBACK INSTRUMENTATION

Biofeedback instruments are designed to monitor some physiologic event, objectively quantify these monitorings, and then interpret the measurements as meaningful information.[27] There are several different types of biofeedback modalities available for use in rehabilitation. These biofeedback units cannot directly measure a physiologic event. Instead they record some aspect that is highly correlated with the physiologic event. Thus the biofeedback reading should be taken as a convenient indication of a physiologic process but should not be confused with the physiologic process itself.[27]

The most commonly used instruments include those that record *peripheral skin temperatures*, indicating the extent of vasoconstriction or vasodilation; *finger phototransmission units (photoplethysmograph)*, which also measure vasoconstriction and vasodilation; units that record *skin conductance activity*, indicating sweat gland activity; and units that measure *electromyographic activity*, indicating amount of electrical activity during muscle contraction.

There are other types of biofeedback units available also, including electroencephalographs (EEGs), pressure transducers, and electrogoniometers.

Biofeedback instruments measure
- Peripheral skin temperature
- Finger phototransmission
- Skin conductance activity
- Electromyographic activity

PERIPHERAL SKIN TEMPERATURE

Peripheral skin temperature is an indirect measure of the diameter of peripheral blood vessels. As vessels dilate, more warm blood is delivered to a particular area, thus increasing

CASE STUDY 8-1
BIOFEEDBACK

Background: A 10-year-old female subluxed her left patella while jumping rope at school. There was immediate pain and a localized effusion which resolved with the use of an immobilizer, intermittent ice packs, and rest over a 7-day period. Her pediatrician requested the initiation of quadriceps rehabilitation 2 weeks later after the patient reported no pain, minimal swelling but with a residual stiffness and sensation of weakness in the knee joint. The physical examination was unremarkable except for limited ROM of 10–110 degrees and the inability of the patient to successfully initiate and sustain an isometric contraction of her quadriceps musculature.

Impression: Quadriceps inhibition secondary to injury and immobilization.

Treatment Plan: In addition to the initiation of therapeutic exercise—static stretching and active-assistive ROM exercise for the knee joint; biofeedback was initiated for the quadriceps mechanism. Using the vastus medialis muscle as the target muscle, the skin was cleansed and electrodes placed in alignment with the fibers of the muscle. A microvolt threshold of detection slightly above the patient's ability to maximize auditory and visual feedback was chosen. The patient was encouraged to perform isometric quadriceps setting exercises of 6–10 seconds duration attempting to "max out" feedback for the chosen threshold level. The threshold was advanced and the process repeated.

Response: Over the course of the initial rehabilitation session, the patient advanced several threshold levels and "reacquired" the ability to initiate and sustain an isometric quadriceps muscle contraction comparable to her uninvolved extremity. She was rapidly transitioned to limited range dynamic exercise and a functional closed-chain exercise sequence with emphasis on terminal range knee stability. She returned to unrestricted playground activities several weeks later.

Discussion Questions

- What tissues were injured/affected?
- What symptoms were present?
- What phase of the injury-healing continuum did the patient presented for care in?
- What are the physical agent modality's biophysical effects (direct/indirect/depth/tissue affinity)?
- What are the physical agent modality's indications/contraindications?
- What are the parameters of the physical agent modality's application/dosage/duration/frequency in this case study?

The rehabilitation professional employs physical agent modalities to create an optimum environment for tissue healing while minimizing the symptoms associated with the trauma or condition. What other physical agent modalities could be utilized to treat this injury or condition? Why? How?

---

the temperature in that area. This effect is easily seen in the fingers and toes where the surrounding tissue warms and cools rapidly. Variations in skin temperature seem to be correlated with affective states, with a decrease occurring in response to stress or fear. Temperature changes are usually measured in degrees Fahrenheit.[27]

FINGER PHOTOTRANSMISSION

The degree of peripheral vasoconstriction can also be measured indirectly using a photoplethysmograph. This instrument monitors the amount of light that can pass through a finger or toe, reflect off a bone, and pass back through the soft tissue to a light sensor. As the volume of blood in a given area increases, the amount of light detected by the sensor decreases, thus giving some indication of blood volume. Only changes in blood volume can be detected, because there are no standardized units of measure. These instruments are used most often to monitor pulse.[17]

SKIN CONDUCTANCE ACTIVITY

Sweat gland activity can be indirectly measured by determining electrodermal activity, most commonly referred to as the "galvanic skin response." Sweat contains salt that increases electrical conductivity. Thus sweaty skin is more conductive than dry skin. This instrument applies a very small electrical voltage to the skin, usually on the palmar surface of the hand or the volar surface of the fingers where there are a lot of sweat glands, and measures the impedance of the electrical current in micro-ohm units. Measuring skin conductance is a technique useful in objectively assessing psychophysiologic arousal and is most often used in "lie detector" testing.[27]

ELECTROMYOGRAPHIC BIOFEEDBACK

Electromyographic biofeedback is certainly the most typically used of all the biofeedback modalities in a clinical setting. Muscle contraction results from the more or less synchronous contraction of individual muscle fibers that compose a muscle. Individual muscle fibers are innervated by nerves that collectively comprise a motor unit. The axon of that motor unit conducts an action potential to the neuromuscular junction where a neurotransmitter substance (acetylcholine) is released. As this neurotransmitter binds to receptor sites on the sarcolemma, depolarization of that muscle fiber occurs, moving in both directions along the muscle fiber, creating movement of ions and thus an electrochemical gradient around the muscle fiber. Changes in potential difference or voltage associated with depolarization can be detected by an electrode placed in close proximity (Fig. 8-1).

electromyographic biofeedback A therapeutic procedure that uses electronic or electromechanical instruments to accurately measure, process, and feed back reinforcing information via auditory or visual signals.

MOTOR UNIT RECRUITMENT

The amount of tension developed in a muscle is determined by the number of active motor units. As more motor units are recruited and the frequency of discharge increases, muscle tension increases.

The pattern of motor unit recruitment varies depending on the inherent properties of specific motor neurons, the force required during the activity, and the speed of contraction. Smaller motor units are recruited first and are somewhat limited in their ability to generate tension. Larger motor units generate greater tension because more muscle fibers are recruited.

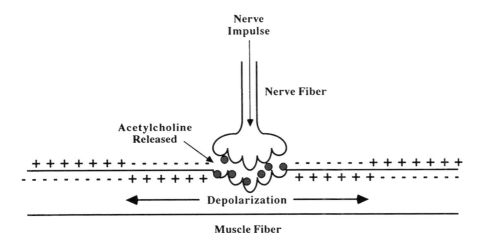

•**Figure 8-1** The nerve fiber conducts an impulse to the neuromuscular junction where acetylcholine binds to receptor sites on the sarcolemma, inducing a depolarization of the muscle fiber that creates movement of ions and thus an electrochemical gradient around the muscle fiber.

Motor units are recruited based on the force required in an activity and not on the type of contraction performed. Thus the firing rate and recruitment of the motor units are dependent on the external force required. The speed of contraction also influences motor unit recruitment. Fast contractions tend to excite larger and depress smaller motor units.

MEASURING ELECTRICAL ACTIVITY

Despite the fact that biofeedback is used to determine muscle activity, it does not measure muscle contraction directly. Instead it measures electrical activity associated with muscle contraction. Movement of ions across the membrane creates a depolarization of the muscle membranes, resulting in a reversal in polarity, followed by repolarization. The various stages of membrane activity generate a triphasic electrical signal.[4] Electrical activity of the muscle is measured in volts, or more precisely, microvolts (1 V = 1,000,000 μV).

Measurement of electrical activity is made in standard quantitative units. Monitoring is useful in detecting changes in electrical activity, although changes cannot be quantified. The advantage of measurement over monitoring is that an objective scale is used; therefore, comparisons can be made between different individuals, occasions, and instruments. Measurement allows *procedures* to be replicated.

Unfortunately, with biofeedback units there is no universally accepted standardized measurement scale. Each brand of biofeedback unit serves as its own reference standard. Different brands of biofeedback equipment may give different readings for the same degree of muscle contraction. Consequently, biofeedback readings can be compared only when the same equipment is used for all readings.[27]

The biofeedback unit receives small amounts of electrical energy generated during muscle contraction through an electrode. It then separates or filters this electrical energy from other extraneous electrical activity on the skin and amplifies the electrical energy. The amplified activity is then converted to information that has meaning to the user. Figure 8-2 is a diagram of the various components of a biofeedback unit.

Separation and Amplification of Electromyographic Activity

Once the electrical activity is detected by the electrodes, the extraneous electrical activity, or "**noise**," must be eliminated before the electrical activity is amplified and subsequently objectified. This is accomplished by using two **active electrodes** and a single ground or **reference electrode** in a **bipolar arrangement** to create three separate pathways from the skin to the biofeedback unit (Fig. 8-3). The active electrodes should be placed in close proximity to one another, whereas the reference electrode may be placed anywhere on the body. Typically in biofeedback, the reference electrode is placed between the two active electrodes.

The active electrodes pick up electrical activity from motor units firing in the muscles beneath the electrodes. The magnitude of the small voltages detected by each active electrode will differ with respect to the reference electrode, creating two separate signals. These two signals are then fed to a **differential amplifier** that basically subtracts the signal of one active electrode from the other. This, in effect, cancels out or rejects any components that the two signals have in common coming from the active electrodes, thus amplifying the difference between the signals. The differential amplifier uses the reference electrode to compare the signals of the two active or recording electrodes (see Fig. 8-3).

There will always be some degree of extraneous electrical activity created by power lines, motors, lights, appliances, and so on, that is picked up by the body and eventually detected by the surface electrodes on the skin. Assuming that this extraneous "noise" is detected equally by both active electrodes, the differential amplifier will subtract the noise detected by one active electrode from the noise detected by the other, leaving only the true difference between the active electrodes. The ability of the differential amplifier to eliminate the common noise between the active electrodes is called the **common mode rejection ratio (CMRR)**.

biofeedback Measures electrical activity of muscle, not muscle contraction.

Treatment Tip
Biofeedback units do not directly measure muscle contraction. Instead, they measure only the electrical activity associated with a muscle contraction. Thus the patient should understand that the electrical activity implies some information about the quality of a muscle contraction but does not measure the strength of that muscle contraction specifically.

Most biofeedback units use surface electrodes.

noise Extraneous electrical activity that may be produced by any source other than the contracting muscle.

reference electrode Also referred to as the ground electrode, serves as a point of reference to compare the electrical activity recorded by the active electrodes.

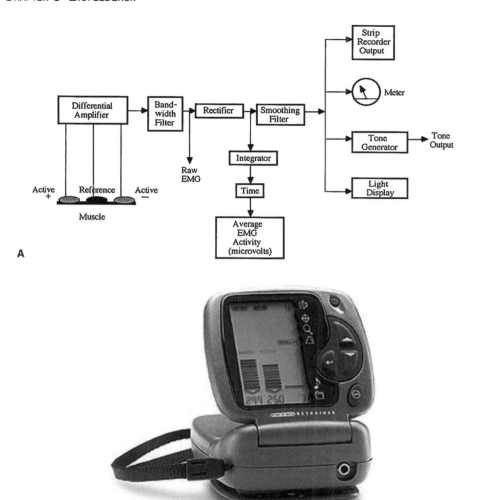

A

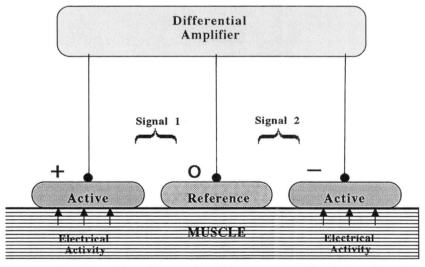

B

•Figure 8-2 A. Diagram of a typical biofeedback unit. B. Biofeedback unit. (Courtesy EMG Retraiver.)

•Figure 8-3 The differential amplifier monitors the two separate signals from the active electrodes and amplifies the difference, thus eliminating extraneous noise.

External noise can be reduced further by using **filters** that essentially make the amplifier more sensitive to some incoming frequencies and less sensitive to others. Therefore, the amplifier will pick up signals only at those frequencies produced by electrical activity in the muscle within a specific frequency range or **bandwidth**. In general, the wider the bandwidth, the higher the noise readings.

It must be noted that the therapist is interested in measuring the electrical activity within the muscle. An excessive external noise that is not eliminated by the biofeedback instrument will mask true electrical activity and will significantly decrease the reliability of the information being generated by that device.

CONVERTING ELECTROMYOGRAPHIC ACTIVITY TO MEANINGFUL INFORMATION

After amplification and filtering, the signal is indicative of the true electrical activity within the muscles being monitored. This is referred to as "raw" activity. **Raw activity** is an alternating voltage that means that the direction or polarity is constantly reversing (Fig. 8-4A). The amplitude of the oscillations increases to a maximum then diminishes. Biofeedback measures the overall increase and decrease in electrical activity. To obtain this measurement, the deflection toward the negative pole must be flipped upward toward the positive pole; otherwise the sum total of their deflections would cancel out

Raw electrical activity may be
- Rectified
- Smoothed
- Integrated

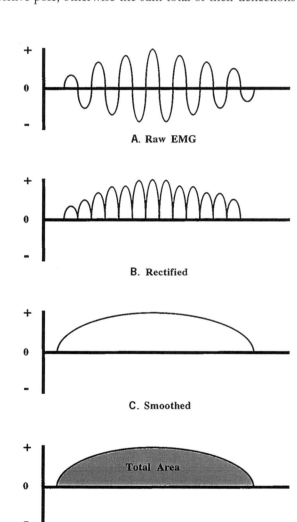

•**Figure 8-4** Processing an EMG signal involves taking **A.** raw EMG, **B.** rectifying, **C.** smoothing, and **D.** integrating it so that the information can be presented in some meaningful format.

one another (Fig. 8-4B). This process, referred to as **rectification**, essentially creates a pulsed direct current (DC).

Processing the Electromyographic Signal

The rectified signal can be smoothed and integrated. **Smoothing** the signal means eliminating the peaks and valleys or eliminating the high-frequency fluctuations that are produced with a changing electrical signal (Fig. 8-4C). Once the signal has been smoothed, the signal may be integrated by measuring the area under the curve for a specified period of time. **Integration** forms the basis for quantification of EMG activity (Fig. 8-4D).

BIOFEEDBACK EQUIPMENT AND TREATMENT TECHNIQUES

It is imperative that the therapist have some understanding of how biofeedback units monitor and record the electrical activity being produced in a muscle before attempting to set up and use the biofeedback unit in the treatment of a patient. Specific treatment protocols involve skin preparation, application of electrodes, selection of feedback or output modes, and selection of sensitivity settings, all of which have been previously discussed. Once these are complete, the therapist should choose to have the patient sitting, lying, or occasionally standing in a comfortable position, depending on the treatment objectives. Generally the therapist should begin with easy tasks and progressively make the activities more difficult. Teaching the patient how to appropriately use the biofeedback unit and briefly explaining what is being measured are essential. In most cases, it is recommended that the therapist attach the biofeedback unit to him or herself and then demonstrate to the patient exactly what will be done during the treatment.[20]

Electrodes

Skin-surface electrodes are most often used in biofeedback. Fine-wire indwelling electrodes may also be used that permit localized highly accurate measurement of electrical activity. However, these electrodes must be inserted percutaneously and thus are relatively impractical in a clinical setting.

Various types of surface electrodes are available for use with biofeedback units. Electrodes are most often made of stainless steel or nickel-plated brass recessed in a plastic holder. These less expensive electrodes are effective in EMG biofeedback applications. More expensive electrodes made of gold or silver/silver chloride also have been used.[34]

The size of the electrodes may range from 4 mm in diameter for recording small muscle activity to 12.5 mm for use with larger muscle groups. Increasing the size of the electrode will not cause an increase in the amplitude of the signal.[20]

Regardless of whether or not electrodes are disposable, some type of conducting gel, paste, or cream with high salt content is necessary to establish a highly conductive connection with the skin. Disposable electrodes come with the appropriate amount of gel and an adhesive ring already applied so that the electrode can be easily connected to the skin. Nondisposable electrodes need to have a double-sided adhesive ring applied. Then enough conducting gel must be added so that it is level with the surface of the adhesive ring before the electrode is applied to the skin.

Skin Preparation

Prior to attachment of the surface electrodes, the skin must be appropriately prepared by removing oil and dead skin along with excessive hair from the surface to reduce skin impedance. Scrubbing with an alcohol-soaked prep pad is recommended.[34] However, if the skin is cleaned until it becomes irritated, it may interfere with biofeedback recording.

Indications and Contraindications for Biofeedback

Indications
Muscle reeducation
Regaining neuromuscular control
Increasing isometric and isotonic strength of a muscle
Relaxation of muscle spasm
Decreasing muscle guarding
Pain reduction
Psychologic relaxation

Contraindications
Any musculoskeletal condition in which a muscular contraction might exacerbate that condition.

Some surface electrodes are permanently attached to cable wires, whereas others may snap onto the wire. Some biofeedback units include a set of three electrodes pre-placed on a Velcro band that may be easily attached to the skin.

Electrode Placement

The electrodes should be placed as near to the muscle being monitored as possible to minimize recording extraneous electrical activity. They should be secured with the body part in the position in which it will be monitored so that movement of the skin will not alter the positioning of the electrodes over a particular muscle (Fig. 8-5).[34]

The electrodes should be parallel to the direction of the muscle fibers to ensure that a better sample of muscle activity is monitored while reducing extraneous electrical activity.

Spacing of the electrodes is also a critical consideration. Electrodes generally detect measurable signals from a distance equal to that of the interelectrode spacing. Therefore, as the distance between the electrodes increases, the signal will include electrical activity not only from muscles directly under the electrodes but also from other nearby muscles.[4]

DISPLAYING THE INFORMATION

At this point it is necessary to take this rectified, smoothed, and integrated signal and display the information in a form that has some meaning. Biofeedback units generally provide either visual or auditory feedback relative to the quantity of electrical activity. Some biofeedback units can provide both visual and auditory feedback, depending on the output mode selected.

Visual Feedback

Raw activity is usually displayed visually on an oscilloscope. On most biofeedback units, integrated electrical activity is visually presented, either as a line traveling across a monitor, as a light or series of lights that go on and off, or as a bar graph that changes dimension in response to the incoming integrated signal. Some of the newer biofeedback units have incorporated video games as part of their visual feedback system. If a

Biofeedback information may be visual or auditory or both.

active electrode An electrode attached directly to the skin over a muscle that picks up the electrical activity produced by a muscle contraction.

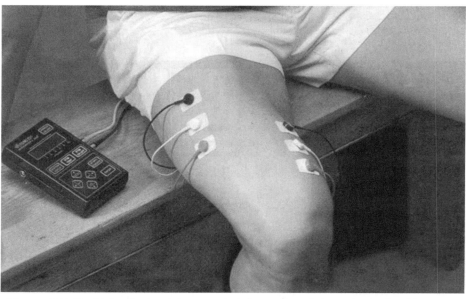

•**Figure 8-5** The biofeedback unit is connected via a series of electrodes to the skin over the contracting muscle.

CASE STUDY 8-2
BIOFEEDBACK

Background: A 19-year-old male suffered a twisting injury to the right knee during football practice. There was immediate pain, effusion, joint line tenderness, and hamstring muscle spasm that prevented full extension of the knee. Initial treatment involved the use of an immobilizer, intermittent application of ice packs, elevation, and rest over the first 24 hours postinjury. Referral for rehabilitation was immediate and the patient reported to the clinic with residual pain and minimal swelling but with residual hamstring muscle guarding that prevented full active or passive knee extension.

Impression: Hamstring muscle spasm secondary to injury.

Treatment Plan: Therapeutic exercise, PNF contract-relax, was initiated for the knee joint musculature—primarily the hamstrings; biofeedback was also initiated for the hamstring muscles. Using the semimembranosus/semitendinosus muscles as the targets, the skin was cleansed and electrodes placed in alignment with the fibers of the muscles. A microvolt threshold of detection at the level of the patient's current muscle spasm activity was chosen with continuous auditory feedback. The patient was encouraged to isometrically contract his hamstring muscles, then consciously think of relaxing the muscles and reducing the level of auditory feedback. When auditory silence was achieved for the chosen microvolt level, the threshold was reduced and the process repeated. The patient was then encouraged to actively and passively extend the knee.

Response: Over the course of the initial rehabilitation session, the patient was able to reduce the threshold level and "relax" the hamstring muscles to achieve full active and passive knee extension comparable to his uninvolved extremity. He was rapidly transitioned to dynamic exercise and a functional closed-chain exercise sequence with emphasis on terminal range knee stability. He returned to football activities several weeks later.

Discussion Questions

- What tissues were injured/affected?
- What symptoms were present?
- What phase of the injury-healing continuum did the patient present for care in?
- What are the physical agent modality's biophysical effects (direct/indirect/depth/tissue affinity)?
- What are the physical agent modality's indications/contraindications?
- What are the parameters of the physical agent modality's application/dosage/duration/frequency in this case study?
- What other physical agent modalities could be utilized to treat this injury or condition? Why? How?

Further Discussion Questions

- How would biofeedback assist in this patient's course of rehabilitation?
- What would the goal of the treatment session be?
- How long would you continue the use of biofeedback with this patient?
- Describe how you would integrate PNF techniques with biofeedback.

The rehabilitation professional employs physical agent modalities to create an optimum environment for tissue healing while minimizing the symptoms associated with the trauma or condition.

---

biofeedback unit uses some type of meter, it may either be calibrated in objective units such as microvolts, or it may simply give some relative scale of measure.[34]

Meters also may be either analog or digital. Analog meters have a continuous scale and a needle that indicates the level of electrical activity within a particular range. Digital meters display only a number. They are very simple and easy to read. However, the disadvantage of a digital meter is that it is more difficult to tell where the signal falls in a given range.

signal gain Determines the signal sensitivity. If a high gain is chosen the biofeedback unit will have a high sensitivity for the muscle activity signal.

Audio Feedback

On some biofeedback units, raw activity can be listened to and is one type of audio feedback. The majority of biofeedback units have audio feedback that produces some tone, buzzing, beeping, or clicking. An increase in the pitch of a tone, buzz, or beep, or an increase in the frequency of clicking indicates an increase in the level of electrical activity. This would be most useful for individuals who need to strengthen muscle contractions. Conversely, decreases in pitch or frequency indicating a decrease in electrical activity would be most useful in teaching patients to relax.

Setting Sensitivity

Signal sensitivity or **signal gain** may be set by the therapist on many biofeedback units. If a high gain is chosen, the biofeedback unit will have a high sensitivity for the muscle activity signal. Sensitivity may be set at 1, 10, or 100 µV. A 1-µV setting is sensitive enough to detect the smallest amounts of electrical activity and thus has the highest signal gain. High sensitivity levels should be used during relaxation training. Comparatively lower sensitivity levels are more useful in muscle reeducation, during which the patient may produce several hundred microvolts of EMG activity. Generally, when adjusting the sensitivity range it should be set at the lowest level that does not elicit feedback at rest.

CLINICAL APPLICATIONS FOR BIOFEEDBACK

There are a number of clinical conditions for which biofeedback would be useful as a therapeutic modality. The primary applications for using biofeedback include muscle reeducation, which involves regaining neuromuscular control and increasing muscle strength; relaxation of muscle spasm or muscle guarding; and pain reduction.

MUSCLE REEDUCATION

The goal in muscle reeducation is to provide feedback that will reestablish neuromuscular control or promote the ability of a muscle or group of muscles to contract. It may also be used to regain normal agonist/antagonist muscle action and for postural control retraining. Biofeedback is used to indicate the electrical activity associated with that muscle contraction.[16]

When biofeedback is being used to elicit a muscle contraction, the sensitivity setting should be chosen by having the patient perform a maximum isometric contraction of the target muscle. Then the gain should be adjusted such that the patient will be able to achieve the maximum on about two-thirds of the muscle contractions. If the patient cannot produce a muscle contraction, the therapist should attempt to facilitate a contraction by stroking or tapping the target muscle. It is also helpful to have the patient look at the muscle when trying to contract. It may be necessary to move the active electrodes to the contralateral limb and have the patient "practice" the muscle contraction you hope to achieve on the opposite side.

The patient should maximally contract the target muscle isometrically for 6–10 seconds. During this contraction, the visual or auditory feedback should be at a maximum and should be closely monitored by both the therapist and patient. Between each contraction the patient should be instructed to completely relax the muscle such that the feedback mode returns to baseline or zero prior to initiating another contraction. A period of 5–10 minutes working with a single muscle or muscle group is most desirable because longer periods tend to produce fatigue and boredom, neither of which is conducive to optimal learning.[19]

As increases in electrical activity occur, the patient should develop the ability to rapidly activate motor units. This can be accomplished by setting the sensitivity level to 60–80 percent of maximum isometric activity and instructing the patient to reach that level as many times as possible during a given time period (i.e., 10 or 30 sec). Again, total relaxation must occur between contractions.

It is essential that the treatment be functionally relevant to the patient. Attention to mobility and muscle power cannot be neglected in favor of biofeedback therapy.[19] The therapist should have the patient perform functional movements while observing body mechanics and the related electrical activity. Then recommendations can be

Treatment Tip
The therapist should set the signal gain on the biofeedback unit at a high-sensitivity setting whenever the goal is relaxation, whereas a low-sensitivity setting should be used with muscle reeducation.

Treatment Tip
Biofeedback electrodes should be placed as close to the muscle as possible to minimize "noise." They should be placed parallel to the direction of the muscle fibers. The spacing should be close enough to monitor activity from a specific muscle. If spaced too far apart, then electrical activity from other anatomically close muscles may also be detected.

made as to how movements can be altered to elicit normal responses.[8] Biofeedback is useful in patients who perform poorly on manual muscle tests. If the patient can only elicit a fair, trace, or zero grade, then biofeedback should be incorporated. Stronger muscles generally should be given resistive exercises rather than biofeedback, although biofeedback has been recommended for increasing the strength of healthy muscle.[10,19]

RELAXATION OF MUSCLE GUARDING

Often in a clinical setting, patients demonstrate a protective response in muscle that occurs owing to pain or fear of movement that is most accurately described as **muscle guarding**.

Muscle guarding must be differentiated from those neuromuscular problems arising from central nervous system deficits that result in a clinical condition known as muscle spasticity. For the therapist treating patients exhibiting muscle guarding, the goal is to induce relaxation of the muscle by reducing electrical activity through the use of biofeedback.[19]

Because muscle guarding most often involves fear of pain that may result when the muscle moves, perhaps the most important goal in treatment is to modulate pain. This is best accomplished through the use of other modalities such as ice or electrical stimulation.

Biofeedback treatments should be designed so that the patient experiences success from the first treatment. The patient is now attempting to reduce the visual or auditory feedback to zero. Initially, positioning of the patient in a comfortable relaxed position is critical to reduction of muscle guarding. A high sensitivity setting should be selected so that any electrical activity in the muscle will be easily detected.

During relaxation training, the patient should be given verbal cues that will enhance relaxation of either individual muscles, muscle groups, or body segments. For example, with individual muscles or small muscle groups, the patient may be instructed to contract then relax a specific muscle or to imagine a feeling of warmth within the muscle. For larger muscle groups, using mental imagery or deep-breathing exercises may be useful.

As relaxation progresses, the spacing between the electrodes should be increased. Also, the sensitivity setting should move from low to high. Both of these changes will require the patient to relax more muscles, thus achieving greater relaxation. The patient must then apply this newly learned relaxation technique in different positions that are potentially more uncomfortable. Again, the goal is to eliminate muscle guarding during functional activities.[19]

Treatment Tip

With biofeedback units there is no universally accepted or standardized measurement scale. Different machines are likely to give different readings for the same degree of muscle contraction. Each manufacturer has its own reference standards for a particular unit. Thus, information provided from two different units cannot be compared.

PAIN REDUCTION

A number of therapeutic modalities discussed in this text are used for the purpose of reducing or modulating pain. As mentioned in the section on muscle guarding, biofeedback can be used to relax muscles that are tense secondary to fear of pain on movement. If the muscle can be relaxed, then chances are that pain will also be reduced by breaking the "pain-guarding-pain" cycle. It has been experimentally demonstrated to reduce pain in headaches and low back pain.[2,7–9,25,31] Pain modulation is often associated with techniques of imagery and progressive relaxation.

Treating Neurologic Conditions

Biofeedback has been identified as an effective technique for treating a variety of neurologic conditions, including hemiplegia following stroke, spinal cord injury, spasticity, cerebral palsy, fascial paralysis, and urinary and fecal incontinence.[1,3,5,6,15,18,23,28,29,32,33]

SUMMARY

1. Biofeedback is a therapeutic procedure that uses electronic or electromechanical instruments to accurately measure, process, and feed back reinforcing information by using auditory or visual signals.

2. Perhaps the biggest advantage of biofeedback is that it provides the patient with a chance to make correct small changes in performance that are immediately noted and rewarded so that eventually larger changes or improvements in performance can be accomplished.

3. Several different types of biofeedback modalities are available for use in rehabilitation, with biofeedback being the most widely used in a clinical setting.

4. A biofeedback unit measures the electrical activity produced by depolarization of a muscle fiber as an indicator of the quality of a muscle contraction.

5. The biofeedback unit receives small amounts of electrical energy generated during muscle contraction through active electrodes, then separates or filters extraneous electrical energy via a differential amplifier before it is processed and subsequently converted to some type of information that has meaning to the user.

6. Biofeedback information is displayed either visually using lights or meters or auditorily using tones, beeps, buzzes, or clicks.

7. High sensitivity levels should be used during relaxation training, whereas comparatively lower sensitivity levels are more useful in muscle reeducation.

8. In a clinical setting, biofeedback is most typically used for muscle reeducation, to decrease muscle guarding, or for pain reduction.

REVIEW QUESTIONS

1. What is biofeedback and how can it be used in injury rehabilitation?

2. What are the various types of biofeedback instruments that are available to the therapist?

3. How can the electrical activity generated by a muscle contraction be measured using biofeedback?

4. What are the important considerations for attaching biofeedback electrodes?

5. How is the electrical activity picked up by the electrodes amplified, processed, and converted to meaningful information by the biofeedback unit?

6. What are the advantages and disadvantages of using visual and auditory feedback?

7. How should sensitivity settings be changed during relaxation training versus during muscle reeducation?

8. What are the most common uses for biofeedback in a rehabilitation setting?

REFERENCES

1. Amato, A., Hermomeyer, C., and Kleinman, K.: Use of electromyographic feedback to increase control of spastic muscles, Phys. Ther. 53:1063, 1973.

2. Arena, J., Bruno, G., and Hannah, S.: A comparison of frontal electromyographic biofeedback training, trapezius electromyographic biofeedback training, and progressive muscle relaxation therapy in the treatment of tension headache, Headache 35(7):411–419, 1995.

3. Asato, H., Twiggs, D., and Ellison, S.: EMG biofeedback training for a mentally retarded individual with cerebral palsy, Phys. Ther. 61:1447–1451, 1981.

4. Basmajian, J.: Description and analysis of EMG signal. In Basmajian, J., Deluca, C., editors. Muscles alive. Their functions revealed by electromyography, Baltimore, MD, 1985, Williams & Wilkins.

5. Brown, D., Nahai, F., and Wolf, S.: Electromyographic feedback in the re-education of fascial palsy, Am. J. Phys. Med. 57:183–190, 1978.

6. Brucker, B., Bulaeva, N.: Biofeedback effect on electromyography responses in patients with spinal cord injury, Arch. Phys. Med. Rehabil. 77(2):133–137, 1996.

7. Budzynski, D.: Biofeedback strategies in headache treatment. In Basmajian J., editor. Biofeedback: principles and practice for clinicians, Baltimore, MD, 1989, Williams & Wilkins.

8. Bush, C., Ditto, B., and Feuerstein, M.: Controlled evaluation of paraspinal EMG biofeedback in the treatment of chronic low back pain, Health Psychol. 4:307–321, 1985.

9. Chapman, S.: A review and clinical perspective on the use of EMG and thermal biofeedback for chronic headaches, Pain 27:1, 1986.

10. Croce, R.: The effects of EMG biofeedback on strength aquisition, Biofeedback Self Regul. 9:395, 1986.
11. Davlin, C.D., Holcomb, W.R., and Guadagnoli, M.A.: The effect of hip position and electromyographic biofeedback training on the vastus medialis oblique: vastus lateralis ratio, J. Athl. Train. 34(4):342–349, 1999.
12. Draper, V.: Electromyographic feedback and recovery in quadriceps femoris muscle function following anterior cruciate ligament reconstruction, Phys. Ther. 70:25, 1990.
13. Draper, V., Lyle, L., and Seymour, T.: From the field, EMG biofeedback versus electrical stimulation in the recovery of quadriceps surface EMG, Clin. Kinesiol. 51(2):28–32, 1997.
14. Draper, V., Lyle, L., and Seymour, T.: EMG biofeedback versus electrical stimulation in the recovery of quadriceps surface EMG, Clin. Kinesiol. 51(2):28–32, 1997.
15. Engardt, M.: Term effects of auditory feedback training on relearned symmetrical body weight distribution in stroke patients. A follow-up study, Scand. J. Rehabil. Med. 26(2): 65–69, 1994.
16. Fogel, E.: Biofeedback-assisted musculoskeletal therapy and neuromuscular re-education. In Schwartz, M.S., editor. Biofeedback: a practitioner's guide, New York, 1987, The Guilford Press.
17. Jennings, J., Tahmoush, A., and Redmond, D.: Non-invasive measurement of peripheral vascular activity. In Martin, I., Venables, P.H., editors. Techniques in psychophysiology, New York, 1980, Wiley.
18. Klose, K., Needham, B., and Schmidt, D.: An assessment of the contribution of electromyographic biofeedback as a therapy in the physical training of spinal cord injured persons, Arch. Phys. Med. Rehabil. 74(5):453–456, 1993.
19. Krebs, D.: Neuromuscular re-education and gait training. In Schwartz, M., editor. Biofeedback: a practitioner's guide, New York, 1987, The Guilford Press.
20. LeCraw, D., Wolf, S.: Electromyographic biofeedback (EMGBF) for neuromuscular relaxation and re-education, In Gersh, M., editor. Electrotherapy in rehabilitation, Philadelphia, PA, 1992, F.A. Davis Company.
21. Linsay, K.A.: Electromyographic biofeedback, Athl. Ther. Today 2(4), 1997, 49.
22. Miller, N.: Biomedical foundations for biofeedback as a part of behavioral medicine. In Basmajian, J., editor. Biofeedback: principles and practice for clinicians, Baltimore, MD, 1989, Williams & Wilkins.
23. Moreland, J., Thompson, M.: Efficacy of EMG biofeedback compared with conventional physical therapy for upper extremity function in patients following stroke: a research overview and meta-analysis, Phys. Ther. 74(6):534–543, 1994.
24. Moreland, J.D., Thomson, M.A., Fuoco, A.R.: Electromyographic biofeedback to improve lower extremity function after stroke: a meta-analysis, Arch. Phys. Med. Rehabil. 79(2): 134–140, 1998.
25. Nouwen, A., Bush, C.: The relationship between paraspinal EMG and chronic low back pain, Pain 20:109–123, 1984.
26. Olson, R.: Definitions of biofeedback. In Schwartz, M., editor. Biofeedback: a practitioner's guide, New York, 1987, The Guilford Press.
27. Peek, C.: A primer of biofeedback instrumentation. In Schwartz, M., editor. Biofeedback: a practitioner's guide, New York, 1987, The Guilford Press.
28. Regenos, E., Wolf, S.: Involuntary single motor unit discharges in spastic muscles during EMG biofeedback training, Arch. Phys. Med. Rehabil. 60:72–73, 1979.
29. Schleenbaker, R., Mainous, A.: Electromyographic biofeedback for neuromuscular reeducation in the hemiplegic stroke patient: a meta-analysis, Arch. Phys. Med. Rehabil. 74(12): 1301–1304, 1993.
30. Shinopulos, N.M., Jacobson, J.: Relationship between health promotion lifestyle profiles and patient outcomes of biofeedback therapy for urinary incontinence, Urol. Nurs. 19(4): 249–253, 1999.
31. Studkey, S., Jacobs, A., and Goldfarb, J.: EMG biofeedback training, relaxation training, and placebo for the relief of chronic back pain, Percept. Mot. Skills 63:1023, 1986.
32. Sugar, E., Firlit, C.: Urodynamic feedback: a new therapeutic approach for childhood incontinence/infection, J. Urol. 128: 1253, 1982.
33. Whitehead, W.: Treatment of fecal incontinence in children with spina bifida: comparison of biofeedback and behavior modification, Arch. Phys. Med. Rehabil. 67:218, 1986.
34. Wolf, S.: Treatment of neuromuscular problems, treatment of musculoskeletal problems. In Sandweiss, J., editor. Biofeedback: review seminars, Los Angeles, CA, 1982, University of California, 1982.
35. Wolf, S., Binder-Macleod, S.: Electromyographic feedback in the physical therapy clinic. In Basmajian, J.V., editor. Biofeedback: principles and practice for clinicians, Baltimore, MD, 1989, Williams & Wilkins.
36. Wolf, S., Binder-Macleod, S.: Neurophysiological factors in electromyographic feedback for neuromotor disturbances. In Basmajian, J.V., editor. Biofeedback: principles and practice for clinicians, Baltimore, MD, 1989, Williams & Wilkins.
37. Wong, A.M.K., Lee, M., Chang, W.H., and Tang, F.: Clinical trial of a cervical traction modality with electromyographic biofeedback, Am. J. Phys. Med. Rehabil. 76(1):19–25, 1997.

SUGGESTED READINGS

Baker, M., Hudson, J., and Wolf, S.: "Feedback" cane to improve the hemiplegic patient's gait: suggestion from the field, Phys. Ther. 59:170, 1979.

Baker, M., Regenos, E., and Wolf, S.: Developing strategies for biofeedback: applications in neurologically handicapped patients, Phys. Ther. 57:402–408, 1977.

Balliet, R., Levy, B., and Blood, K.: Upper extremity sensory feedback therapy in chronic cerebrovascular accident patients with impaired expressive aphasia and auditory comprehension, Arch. Phys. Med. Rehabil. 67:304, 1986.

Basmajian, J.: Biofeedback: principles and practice for clinicians, Baltimore, MD, 1989, Williams & Wilkins.

Basmajian, J: Biofeedback in rehabilitation: a review of principles and practice, Arch. Phys. Med. Rehabil. 62:469, 1981.

Basmajian, J.: Learned control of single motor units. In Schwartz, G.E., Beatty, J., editors. Biofeedback: theory and research, New York, 1977, Academic Press.

Basmajian, J., Blumenthal, R.: Electroplacement in electromyographic biofeedback. In Basmajian, J.V., editor. Biofeedback: principles and practice for clinicians, ed. 3, Baltimore, MD, 1989, Williams & Wilkins.

Basmajian, J., et al.: Biofeedback treatment of foot drop after stroke compared with standard rehabilitation technique: effects on voluntary control and strength, Arch. Phys. Med. Rehabil. 56:231–236, 1975.

Basmajian, J., Regenos, E., and Baker, M.: Rehabilitating stroke patients with biofeedback, Geriatrics 32:85, 1977.

Basmajian, J., Samson, J.: Special review: standardization of methods in single motor unit training, Am. J. Phys. Med. 52:250–256, 1973.

Beal, M., Diefenbach, G., and Allen, A.: Electromyographic biofeedback in the treatment of voluntary posterior instability of the shoulder, Am. J. Sports Med. 15:175, 1987.

Bernat, S., Wooldridge, P., and Marecki, M.: Biofeedback-assisted relaxation to reduce stress in labor, J. Obstet. Gynecol. Neonatal Nurs. (4):295–303, 1992.

Biedermann, H.: Comments on the reliability of muscle activity comparisons in EMG biofeedback research with back pain patients, Biofeedback Self Regul. 9:451–458, 1984.

Biedermann, H., McGhie, A., and Monga, T.: Perceived and actual control in EMG treatment of back pain, Behav. Res. Ther. 25:137–147, 1987.

Bowman, B., Baker, L., and Waters, R.: Positional feedback and electrical stimulation. An automated treatment for the hemiplegic wrist, Arch. Phys. Med. Rehabil. 60:497, 1979.

Brudny, J., Grynbaum, B., and Korein, J.: Spasmodic torticollis: treatment by feedback display of EMG, Arch. Phys. Med. Rehabil. 55:403–408, 1974.

Burke, R.: Motor unit recruitment: what are the critical factors? In Desmedt, J., editor. Progress in clinical neurophysiology, vol. 9, Basel, 1981, Karger.

Burnside, I., Tobias, H., and Bursill, D.: Electromyographic feedback in the remobilization of stroke patients: a controlled trial, Arch. Phys. Med. Rehabil. 63:1393, 1983.

Burnside, I., Tobias, H., and Bursill, D.: Electromyographic feedback in the rehabilitation of stroke patients: a controlled trial, Arch. Phys. Med. Rehabil. 63:217, 1982.

Carlsson, S.: Treatment of temporo-mandibular joint syndrome with biofeedback training, J. Am. Dent. Assoc. 91:602–605, 1975.

Christie, D., Dewitt, R., and Kaltenbach, P.: Using EMG biofeedback to signal hyperactive children when to relax, Except. Child. 50:547–548, 1984.

Cox, R., Matyas, T.: Myoelectric and force feedback in the facilitation of isometric strength training: a controlled comparison, Psychophysiology, 20:35–44, 1983.

Crow, J., Lincoln, N., and De Weerdt, N.: The effectiveness of EMG biofeedback in the treatment of arm function after stroke, Intern. Disabil. Stud. 11(4):155–160, 1989.

Cummings, M., Wilson, V., and Bird, E.: Flexibility development in sprinters using EMG biofeedback and relaxation training, Biofeedback Self Regul. 9:395–405, 1984.

Debacher, G.: Feedback goniometers for rehabilitation. In Basmajian, J., editor. Biofeedback: principles and practice for clinicians, Baltimore, MD, 1983, Williams & Wilkins.

Deluca, C.: Apparatus, detection, and recording techniques. In Basmajian, J., Deluca, C., editors. Muscles alive: their functions revealed by electromyography, Baltimore, MD, 1985, Williams & Wilkins.

Draper, V.: Electromyographic biofeedback and recovery of quadriceps femoris muscle function following anterior cruciate ligament reconstruction, Phys. Ther. 70(1):11–17, 1990.

Draper, V., Ballard, L.: Electrical stimulation versus electromyographic biofeedback in the recovery of quadriceps femoris muscle function following anterior cruciate ligament surgery, Phys. Ther. 71(6):455–464, 1991.

Dursun, N.: Electromyographic biofeedback-controlled exercise versus conservative care for patellofemoral pain syndrome; Arch. Phys. Med. and Rehabil. 82(12):1692–1695, 2001.

English, A., Wolf, S.: The motor unit: anatomy and physiology, Phys. Ther. 62:1763, 1982.

Fagerson, T.L., Krebs, D.E.: Biofeedback. In O'Sullivan SB et al.: Physical rehabilitation: assessment and treatment, Philadelphia, PA, 2001, F.A. Davis Company.

Fields, R.: Electromyographically triggered electric muscle stimulation for chronic hemiplegia, Arch. Phys. Med. Rehabil. 68: 407–414, 1987.

Flom, R., Quast, J., and Boller, J.: Biofeedback training to overcome poststroke footdrop, Geriatrics 31:47–51, 1976.

Flor, H., Haag, G., and Turk, D.: Long-term efficacy of EMG biofeedback for chronic rheumatic back pain, Pain 27:195–202, 1986.

Flor, H. et al.: Efficacy of EMG biofeedback, pseudotherapy, and conventional medical treatment for chronic rheumatic back pain, Pain 17:21–31, 1983.

Gaarder, K., Montgomery, P.: Clinical biofeedback: a procedural manual, Baltimore, MD, 1977, Williams & Wilkins.

Gallego, J., Perez de la Sota, A., and Vardon, G.: Electromyographic feedback for learning to activate thoracic inspiratory muscles, Am. J. Phys. Med. Rehabil. 70(4):186–190, 1991.

Goodgold, J., Eberstein, A.: Electrodiagnosis of neuromuscular diseases, Baltimore, MD, 1972, Williams & Wilkins.

Green, E., Walters, E., and Green, A.: Feedback technology for deep relaxation, Psychophysiology 6:371–377, 1969.

Hijzen, T., Slangen, J., and van Houweligen, H.: Subjective, clinical and EMG effects of biofeedback and splint treatment, J. Oral Rehabil. 13:529–539, 1986.

Hirasawa, Y., Uchiza, Y., and Kusswetter, W.: EMG biofeedback therapy for rupture of the extensor pollicis longus tendon, Arch. Orthop. Trauma Surg. 104:342, 1986.

Honer, L., Mohr, T., and Roth, R.: Electromyographic biofeedback to dissociate an upper extremity synergy pattern: a case report, Phys. Ther. 62:299–303, 1982.

Howard, P.: Use of EMG biofeedback to reeducate the rotator cuff in a case of shoulder impingement, JOSPT 23(1):79, 1996.

Ince, L., Leon, M.: Biofeedback treatment of upper extremity dysfunction in Guillain-Barre syndrome, Arch. Phys. Med. Rehabil. 67:30–33, 1986.

Ince, L., Leon, M., and Christidis, D.: EMG biofeedback with upper extremity musculature for relaxation training: a critical review of the literature, J. Behav. Ther. Exp. Psychiatry 16:133–137, 1985.

Ince, L., Leon, M., and Christidis, D.: Experimental foundations of EMG biofeedback with the upper extremity: a review of the literature, Biofeedback Self Regul. 9:371–383, 1984.

Inglis, J., Donald, M., and Monga, T.: Electromyographic biofeedback and physical therapy of the hemiplegic upper limb, Arch. Phys. Med. Rehabil. 65:755–759, 1984.

Johnson, H., Garton, W.: Muscle reeducation in hemiplegia by use of electromyographic device, Arch. Phys. Med. Rehabil. 54: 322–323, 1973.

Johnson, H., Hockersmith, V.: Therapeutic electromyography in chronic back pain. In Basmajian, J.V., editor. Biofeedback: principles and practice for clinicians, ed. 2, Baltimore, MD, 1983, Williams & Wilkins.

Johnson, R., Lee, K.: Myofeedback: a new method of teaching breathing exercise to emphysematous patients, J. Am. Phys. Ther. Assoc. 56:826–829, 1976.

Kasman, G.: Long-term rehab. Using surface electromyography: a multidisciplinary tool, sEMG can be a valuable asset to the rehab professional's muscle assessment arsenal, Rehabil. Manage. 14(9):56–59, 76, 2002.

Kelly, J., Baker, M., and Wolf, S.: Procedures for EMG biofeedback training in involved upper extremities of hemiplegic patients, Phys. Ther. 59:1500, 1979.

King, A., Ahles, T., and Martin, J.: EMG biofeedback-controlled exercise in chronic arthritic knee pain, Arch. Phys. Med. Rehabil. 65:341–343, 1984.

King, T.: Biofeedback: a survey regarding current clinical use and content in occupational therapy educational curricula, Occ. Ther. J. Res. 12(1):50–58, 1992.

Kleppe, D., Groendijk, H., and Huijing, P.: Single motor unit control in the human mm. abductor pollicis brevis and mylohyoideus in relation to the number of muscle spindles, Electromyogr. Clin. Neurophysiol. 22:21–25, 1982.

Krebs, D.: Biofeedback in neuromuscular reeducation and gait training. In Schwartz, M. editor. Biofeedback: a practitioner's guide, New York, 1987, The Guilford Press.

Large, R.: Prediction of treatment response in pain patients: the illness self-concept repertory grid and EMG feedback, Pain 21: 279–287, 1985.

Large, R., Lamb, A.: Electromyographic (EMG) feedback in chronic musculoskeletal pain: a controlled trial, Pain 17:167–177, 1983.

Lucca, J., Recchiuti, S.: Effect of electromyographic biofeedback on an isometric strengthening program, Phys. Ther. 63:200–203, 1983.

Mandel, A., Nymark, J., and Balmer, S.: Electromyographic versus rhythmic positional biofeedback in computerized gait retraining with stroke patients, Arch. Phys. Med. Rehabil. 71(9): 649–654, 1990.

Marinacci, A., Horande, M.: Electromyogram in neuromuscular reeducation, Bull. Los Angeles Neurol. Soc. 25:57–67, 1960.

Mims, H.: Electromyography in clinical practice, So. Med. J. 49:804, 1956.

Morasky, R., Reynolds, C., and Clarke, G.: Using biofeedback to reduce left arm extensor EMG of string players during musical performance, Biofeedback Self Regul. 6:565–572, 1981.

Morris, M., Matyas, T., and Bach, T.: Electrogoniometric feedback: its effect on genu recurvatum in stroke, Arch. Phys. Med. Rehabil. 73(12):1147–1154, 1992.

Mulder, T., Hulstijn, W.: Delayed sensory feedback in the learning of a novel motor task, Psychol. Res. 47:203–209, 1985.

Mulder, T., Hulstijn, W., and van der Meer, J.: EMG feedback and the restoration of motor control. A controlled group study of 12 hemiparetic patients, Am. J. Phys. Med. 65:173–188, 1986.

Nafpliotis, H.: EMG feedback to improve ankle dorsiflexion, wrist extension and hand grasp, Phys. Ther. 56:821–825, 1976.

Nord, S.: Muscle learning therapy—efficacy of a biofeedback based protocol in treating work-related upper extremity disorders, J. Occupational Rehabil. 11(1):23–31, 2001.

Nouwen, A.: EMG biofeedback used to reduce standing levels of paraspinal muscle tension in chronic low back pain, Pain 17:353–360, 1983.

Pages, I.: Comparative analysis of biofeedback and physical therapy for treatment of urinary stress incontinence in women, Am. J. Phys. Med. Rehabil. 80(7):494–502, 2001.

Petrofsky, J.S.: The use of electromyogram biofeedback to reduce Trendelenburg gait, Eur. J. Appl. Physiol. 85(5):135–140, 2001.

Poppen, R., Maurer, J.: Electromyographic analysis of relaxed postures, Biofeedback Self Regul. 7:491–498, 1982.

Pulliam, C.B.: Biofeeback 2003: its role in pain management, Crit. Rev. Rehabil. Med. 15(1):65–82, 2003.

Russell, G., Woolbridge, C.: Correction of a habitual head tilt using biofeedback techniques—a case study, Physiother. Can. 27: 181–184, 1975.

Saunders, J., Cox, D., and Teates, C.: Thermal biofeedback in the treatment of intermittent claudication in diabetes: a case study, Biofeedback Self Regul. 19(4):337–345, 1994.

Smith, D., Newman, D.: Basic elements of biofeedback therapy for pelvic muscle rehabilitation, Urol. Nurs. 14(3):130–135, 1994.

Soderback, I., Bengtsson, I., and Ginsburg, E.: Video feedback in occupational therapy: its effect in patients with neglect syndrome, Arch. Phys. Med. Rehabil. 73(12):1140–1146, 1992.

Swaan, D., van Wiergen, P., and Fokkema, S.: Auditory electromyographic feedback therapy to inhibit undesired motor activity, Arch. Phys. Med. Rehabil. 55:251, 1974.

Winchester, P.: Effects of feedback stimulation training and cyclical electrical stimulation on knee extension in hemiparetic patients, Phys. Ther. 63:1097, 1983.

Wolf, S.: Biofeedback. In Currier, D.P., Nelson, R.M., editors. Clinical electrotherapy, ed. 2, Norwalk, CT, 1991, Appleton & Lange.

Wolf, S.: Fallacies of clinical EMG measures from patients with musculoskeletal and neuromuscular disorders. Paper presented at the 14th annual meeting of the Biofeedback Society of America, Denver, CO, 1983.

Wolf, S.: Electromyographic biofeedback in exercise programs, Phys. Sports Med. 8:61–69, 1980.

Wolf, S.: EMG biofeedback application in physical rehabilitation: an overview, Physiother. Can. 31:65, 1979.

Wolf, S.: Essential considerations in the use of EMG biofeedback, Phys. Ther. 58:25, 1978.

Wolf, S., Baker, M., and Kelly, J.: EMG biofeedback in stroke: a 1-year follow-up on the effect of patient characteristics, Arch. Phys. Med. Rehabil. 61:351–355, 1980.

Wolf, S., Baker, M., and Kelly, J.: EMG biofeedback in stroke: effect of patient characteristics, Arch. Phys. Med. Rehabil. 60:96–102, 1979.

Wolf, S., Binder-Macleod, S.: Electromyographic biofeedback applications to the hemiplegic patient. Changes in lower extremity neuromuscular and functional status, Phys. Ther. 63:1404–1413, 1983.

Wolf, S., Binder-Macleod, S.: Electromyographic biofeedback applications to the hemiplegic patient: Changes in upper extremity neuromuscular and functional status, Phys. Ther. 63:1393, 1983.

Wolf, S., Edwards, D., and Shutter, L.: Concurrent assessment of muscle activity (CAMA): a procedural approach to assess treatment goals, Phys. Ther. 66:218, 1986.

Wolf, S., Hudson, J.: Feedback signal based upon force and time delay: modification of the Krusen limb load monitor: suggestion from the field, Phys. Ther. 60:1289, 1980.

Wolf, S., LeCraw, D., and Barton, L.: A comparison of motor copy and targeted feedback training techniques for restitution of upper extremity function among neurologic patients, Phys. Ther. 69:719, 1989.

Wolf, S., Nacht, M., and Kelly, J.: EMG feedback training during dynamic movement for low back pain patients, Behav. Ther. 13:395, 1982.

Wolf, S., Regenos, E., and Basmajian, J.: Developing strategies for biofeedback applications in neurologically handicapped patients, Phys. Ther. 57:402–408, 1977.

Young, M.: Electromyographic biofeedback use in the treatment of voluntary posterior dislocation of the shoulder a case study, JOSPT 20(3):173–175, 1994.

GLOSSARY

active electrode An electrode attached directly to the skin over a muscle that picks up the electrical activity produced by a muscle contraction.

bandwidth A specific frequency range in which the amplifier will pick up signals produced by electrical activity in the muscle.

bipolar arrangement Two active recoding electrodes placed in close proximity to one another.

common mode rejection ratio (CMRR) The ability of the differential amplifier to eliminate the common noise between the active electrodes.

differential amplifier A device that monitors the two separate signals from the active electrodes and amplifies the difference, thus eliminating extraneous noise.

electromyographic biofeedback A therapeutic procedure that uses electronic or electromechanical instruments to accurately measure, process, and feed back reinforcing information via auditory or visual signals.

filters Devices that help to reduce external noise that essentially make the amplifier more sensitive to some incoming frequencies and less sensitive to others.

integration An EMG signal-processing technique that measures the area under the curve for a specified period of time, thus forming the basis for quantification of EMG activity.

muscle guarding A protective response in muscle that occurs owing to pain or fear of movement.

noise Extraneous electrical activity that may be produced by any source other than the contracting muscle.

raw EMG A form in which the electrical activity produced by muscle contraction may be displayed and/or recorded before the signal is processed.

rectification A signal-processing technique that changes the deflection of the waveform from the negative to the positive pole, essentially creating a pulsed direct current.

reference electrode Also referred to as the ground electrode; serves as a point of reference to compare the electrical activity recorded by the active electrodes.

signal gain Determines the signal sensitivity. If a high gain is chosen, the biofeedback unit will have a high sensitivity for the muscle activity signal.

smoothing An EMG signal-processing technique that eliminates the high-frequency fluctuations that are produced with a changing electrical signal.

LAB ACTIVITY

BIOFEEDBACK

DESCRIPTION

Biofeedback utilizes the body's self-generated motor unit action potentials (MUAP). These signals are recorded by surface electrodes, amplified, then processed and converted into audio or visual signals to allow an individual to monitor various psychophysiologic processes and recognize appropriate responses.

PHYSIOLOGIC EFFECTS

Increase level of motor unit activation
Decrease level of motor unit activation

THERAPEUTIC EFFECTS

Increase level of muscle activation (muscle reeducation)
Decrease level of muscle activation (reduce spasticity)
General body muscular relaxation

INDICATIONS

Biofeedback is primarily employed by the therapist as an adjunct in the reeducation of muscle function following injury, immobilization, or surgery or as an aid to identifying unwanted levels of muscle activity (spasticity) that may be interfering with the athlete's recovery. Sometimes biofeedback is used as a tool to assess the body's general neuromuscular status as an aid in relaxation to reduce pain and anxiety.

CONTRAINDICATIONS

- Possible skin irritation at electrode site from coupling gel or adhesives

BIOFEEDBACK

PROCEDURE	EVALUATION		
	1	2	3
1. Check supplies.			
a. Obtain biofeedback unit, coupling gel, and tape.			
b. Insure that batteries in unit are fresh.			
2. Question patient.			
a. Verify identity of patient and review previous treatment notes.			
b. Verify the absence of contraindications.			
3. Position patient.			
a. Place patient in a well-supported, comfortable position.			
b. Select and expose appropriate muscle or group to monitor.			
c. Drape patient to preserve patient's modesty, and protect clothing, but allow access to muscle or group.			
4. Select appropriate electrode.			
5. Prepare the electrode site.			
a. Clean the skin surface with alcohol or soap and water.			

PROCEDURE	EVALUATION		
	1	2	3
6. Apply the electrodes.			
a. Secure with tape or wrap.			
7. Explain the procedure to patient.			
8. Begin the indicated procedure.			
a. Muscle reeducation			
i. Adjust unit to lowest threshold (μV) that picks up any activity (MUAPs).			
ii. Adjust audio and visual feedback.			
iii. Have patient contract target muscle to produce maximum audio and visual feedback.			
iv. Facilitate target muscle contraction as necessary by tapping, stroking, or contracting opposite like muscle.			
v. When maximum feedback is obtained for selected threshold, advance threshold and attempt again.			
vi. Advance muscle or limb to other positions.			
vii. Continue muscle contractions for 10–15 minutes per training session or until maximal muscle activation is obtained.			
b. Spasticity inhibition			
i. Adjust unit to sensitivity threshold (μV) that picks up maximal activity (MUAPs).			
ii. Adjust audio or visual feedback.			
iii. Have patient relax target muscle to produce minimum audio or visual feedback.			
iv. Facilitate target muscle relaxation as necessary by tapping, stroking, or contracting opposite like muscle.			
v. When minimum feedback is obtained for selected threshold, reduce threshold and attempt relaxation again.			
vi. Advance muscle or limb to other functional positions.			
vii. Continue muscle relaxation for 10–15 minutes per training session or until muscle relaxation is obtained.			
viii. Complete the treatment.			
9. Remove the electrodes.			
a. Thoroughly clean electrode site.			
b. Record results of session.			
c. Assess treatment efficacy.			
10. Instruct the patient in any indicated exercise.			
11. Return equipment to storage after cleaning.			

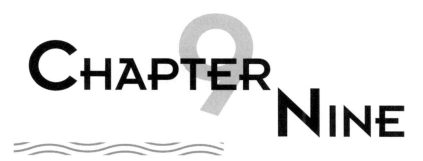

CHAPTER NINE

PRINCIPLES OF ELECTROPHYSIOLOGIC EVALUATION AND TESTING

JOHN HALLE and
DAVID GREATHOUSE

OBJECTIVES

Following completion of this chapter, the student therapist will be able to:

✓ Define and describe the anatomic and physiologic basis of clinical electrophysiologic testing (neural conduction and electromyographic studies).

✓ Given a patient with a neuromuscular dysfunction, evaluate the appropriateness of requesting clinical electrophysiologic testing (neural conduction and electromyographic studies), and describe the specific additional information that would be provided by this testing, if ordered.

✓ Describe the basic role of each of the following pieces of equipment in routine electrophysiologic testing:

- Electrodes (needle, reference, and ground)
- Differential amplifiers
- Oscilloscope
- Audio speakers
- Stimulator
- Electrophysiologic processing unit
- Printer

✓ Discuss why nerve conduction studies (NCS) assess both sensory and motor fibers within a nerve, the information obtained from these tests, and the reason why sensory studies are typically assessed in microvolts (μV), while motor studies are typically assessed in millivolts (mV).

✓ Explain the role of latency, shape, amplitude, and nerve conduction velocity (NCV) in a nerve conduction study. Within this explanation, compare and contrast the information provided by normal and abnormal findings.

✓ Describe a "central conduction study" (F-wave) physiologically and what information is provided by this portion of the examination.

✓ An H-wave (Hoffman's reflex) can only be elicited in select sites in the upper and lower extremity. Explain why this testing procedure cannot be applied universally, identify the specific regions where this test is appropriate, and discuss the additional information that it provides to the clinical electrophysiologist.

✓ Identify the type of nerve conduction evaluation that is particularly useful with conditions affecting the neuromuscular junction, such as myasthenia gravis and Lambert-Eaton syndrome. For each of these conditions, describe the anticipated neurophysiologic results.

✓ List and describe the four basic components of the electromyographic study (needle evaluation) outlined in this chapter. Within the description, identify the type of information that can be obtained from each component.

✓ While pathologic states often represent conditions that cause some damage to both myelin and axons, the pattern of damage is often predominantly demyelinating or axonal. Compare and contrast the electrophysiologic findings demonstrated in a primarily demyelinating condition (e.g., entrapment syndrome such as carpal tunnel syndrome) with a primarily axonal condition (e.g., radiculopathy).

✓ Describe the specific electrophysiologic parameters associated with positive sharp waves (PSWs) and fibrillation potentials, and discuss what these abnormal spontaneous electrical potentials represent physiologically.

✓ Given a patient that is suspected of having a myopathic disease (e.g., dermatomyositis), describe the type of electrophysiologic findings that would be present if this muscle disease was validated.

✓ List and discuss four potential limitations associated with electrophysiologic testing.

✓ Explain the purpose of somatosensory evoked potential (SEP) testing and the additional data that this form of testing can provide.

✓ Given electrophysiologic test results (neural conduction and electromyographic studies), describe how this information could be used to assist in diagnosis, tailor treatment plans, and guide patient prognosis.

INTRODUCTION

Electrophysiologic testing can be an important adjunct to a good physical examination. The physical examination is stressed as a key element obtained prior to electrophysiologic testing because it forms the basis for the subsequent assessment performed during electrophysiologic testing for neuromuscular problems. As such, the role that electrophysiologic testing takes is somewhat analogous to an ordered magnetic resonance imaging (MRI) examination or some other procedure that assists in forming the medical diagnosis. Electrophysiologic testing potentially provides objective findings that are used to corroborate or refute the working hypothesis developed from the initial subjective and physical examination. When coupled with a good physical examination, this form of testing often permits clear identification of the specific neuromuscular problem and provides insight regarding the mechanisms associated with findings such as numbness or weakness.[31,57,82] Additionally, the initial physical examination and detailed history dictates the key elements that will be evaluated during the electrophysiologic examination. To an extent, each electrophysiologic evaluation is customized to the needs of the individual being evaluated, based on the findings presented during the history and physical examination.

The electrophysiologic testing referred to above typically consists of some combination of three procedures: (1) Nerve conduction studies **(NCS)**, (2) **electromyography (EMG)**, and (3) Somatosensory evoked potentials **(SEPs)**.[57] Nerve conduction studies basically evaluate the function of peripheral nerves, the neuromuscular junction, and the collective muscle fibers innervated by the nerve being examined. These studies look at elements like the speed of conduction and the size of the collective action potential generated to make a determination about the health of the aforementioned structures.[7,93] The EMG examination evaluates the electrical activity of the muscles and the muscle action potentials (APs) monitored from a small sample of muscle fibers through the use of a small gauge needle electrode inserted into a specific muscle. While more detail will be provided later, this portion of the electrophysiologic examination monitors the muscle at rest and during various states of voluntary contraction, and evaluates the overall function of the muscle fibers located near the tip of the needle.[9,18] From the shape, size, duration, and presence or absence of the muscle action potentials generated, judgments can be made on the health or dysfunction of both the nerves that innervate these muscle fibers and the muscle itself.[10,101] The combination of NCS and EMG testing provides an excellent way of directly evaluating the peripheral nervous system (PNS) and its constituent parts. While an excellent evaluative tool for the PNS, the two procedures listed above have limited utility for evaluating the brain and spinal cord, or central nervous system (CNS).[32] Since not all pathologies are isolated to the PNS, the third procedure of SEPs has some capability of evaluating elements of the CNS such as specific tracts within the spinal cord.[59,84,96] Apart from specialized electrophysiologic testing practices, however, the vast majority of electrophysiologic testing is limited to the first two procedures outlined, the NCS and the EMG. Most electrophysiologic evaluations are limited to the PNS and the constituent parts of a motor unit that include the anterior horn cell and one or more synapses located between **afferent** and **efferent** neurons, which are technically part of the CNS.[4,73]

ELECTROPHYSIOLOGIC TESTING EQUIPMENT AND SETUP

After obtaining the patient history and performing the physical evaluation, the electrophysiologic examination is constructed to evaluate any suspected areas of neuromuscular dysfunction. To perform this portion of the examination, specialized equipment is required that permits the objective evaluation of nerves, neuromuscular junctions, muscle fibers, and other elements associated with the PNS. The basic elements of this type of a system are electrodes (to couple to the patient), differential amplifiers (to boost the signal), a way to monitor the signal generated (an oscilloscope to see the signal and/or speakers to hear the signal), a processing unit of some type (typically a computer or laptop that has word processing capabilities), and a way of eliciting a response from a patient (a stimulus electrode capable of stimulating the patient or a needle electrode inserted into the muscle and monitored during insertion, at rest, and during a voluntary contraction).[27] This "system" is then combined with a printer so that reports can be generated, and if desired, examples of particular findings can be recorded and placed into the patient's records (Fig. 9-1).

Electrodes

From a patient's perspective, this is the part of the equipment that they actually come into contact with during a NCV study (Fig. 9-2). There are three electrodes that are attached to the individual:

1. Active (pickup) electrode
2. Reference electrode
3. Ground electrode—filters out background noise (Fig. 9-2A)

The electrodes are typically reusable with silver/silver chloride contacts that are coupled to the patient with an electrode gel that decreases the resistance across the skin and is taped into place, or disposable electrodes that are pregelled, and self-adhesive. In either case, the skin must be clean and free of any agents that would create a barrier to the transfer of an electrical signal (such as hand lotion).

Specific types of electrodes for NCV studies:

1. Stimulation electrodes (Fig. 9-2B)
2. Sensory ring electrodes (Fig. 9-2C)
3. Bar electrodes (Fig. 9-2D)
4. Clip

size of the compound motor unit action potential (CMAP), so the EMG is a more sensitive procedure for this type of problem. In any case, these two examples illustrate that while the NCS and EMG procedures most commonly used are described as capable of testing only the PNS, there are select elements of the CNS such as the alpha motor neurons that can also be evaluated.

Two other terms need to be introduced because they relate directly to the ability of peripheral nerves to function as these nerves are assessed with electrodiagnostic testing. The first is **demyelination**, and it is related to some type of damage to the myelin sheath that is synthesized by Schwann cells. Myelinated nerves conduct an action potential via saltatory (node to node) conduction at a faster rate than nonmyelinated nerves. When myelin is damaged, regardless of the causative agent, the speed by which an action potential can travel down an axon is reduced. Therefore, demyelinating conditions result in a slowed conduction velocity, in both afferent and efferent axons. Two conditions that may have a significant demyelinating component are long-standing diabetes mellitus and carpal tunnel syndrome. The second major type of problem is an **axonopathy**. An axonopathy is found when a portion of the potential pools of axons available no longer function. In this case, the speed of conduction is largely preserved, since the remaining axons conduct normally. What is affected is the amplitude of the summed synchronous depolarization of the muscle fibers innervated by the depolarized nerve and the stability of the sarcolemma of the muscle fibers. The decreased stability of the muscle membrane is the earliest finding, with abnormal spontaneous electrical activity to needle EMG that was described in the preceding paragraph. After significant axonal loss has occurred, a smaller sensory nerve action potential (SNAP) or CMAP amplitude will be observed in the response to stimulation of a motor or sensory nerve. The previously mentioned loss of anterior horn cells with the subsequent loss of axons is one example of an axonopathy. As will be seen in the subsequent sections, many of the dysfunctions encountered will have demyelinating components, characteristics of axonopathy, or some combination of both.

ANATOMY OF THE SPINAL NERVE AND NEUROMUSCULAR JUNCTION

Starting at the periphery and working proximally, the typical spinal nerve consists of the following elements (Fig. 9-3B): (1) specialized sensory receptor that functions as a transducer to transform one type of energy (e.g., touch, temperature, pain, etc.) into a sensory action potential, (2) at least one synapse within the CNS that links the afferent neuron to efferent neurons, (3) the alpha motor neurons located in the anterior (ventral) horn of the spinal cord and their respective axons in the PNS, (4) the neuromuscular junction, and (5) the muscle fibers innervated by the nerve being investigated.[47]

The sensory neuron is functionally a combination of the specialized sensory receptor and the afferent axon or first-order neuron with its cell body located in the posterior (dorsal) root ganglion—as such, they will be considered together.[3] The cell body type is a pseudounipolar neuron and it projects into the CNS where the first synapse occurs. A key point to be made here is that this afferent neuron is one cell, often with an axon over a meter in length, with the cell body representing the metabolic center of the cell. If there is any problem with the nerve anywhere along its length, the most distal aspects of the afferent neuron will normally manifest signs of the problem first.

Sensory Receptor and Size of the Axon

The specific sensory receptor associated with this receptor neuron is not really important for the NCS/EMG evaluations, apart from the fact that some receptors are linked with large diameter axons (e.g., muscle spindles have Ia and group II fibers, both of which are large and fast conducting), and the loss of a given modality (e.g., light touch) is often what brings the patient into the clinic. The size of the afferent axon is important, however, because when an electrical signal is evoked by an external stimulus, the time measured from one point to another is only representative of the fastest conducting fibers. The large diameter axons are the ones that are preferentially affecting this time measurement and the speed by which impulses are conducted in humans varies tremendously, from a slow speed of approximately 0.3 m/sec for unmyelinated fibers to 60 or 70 m/sec for large, myelinated fibers.[1,22,105] Additionally, there are some nerves, such as the superficial radial nerve in the forearm and sural nerve in the leg that are predominantly sensory nerves (they may also contain a few visceral motor fibers, but these are functionally ignored). Thus, the integrity of these afferent axons can be directly assessed through electrophysiologic testing.

Synapse

The second part needed for a reflex arc is at least one synapse that occurs within the CNS to link the afferent action potential to the generation of an action potential by the alpha motor neuron. The functioning of this synapse can be assessed by a procedure known as an H-reflex (to be discussed in more detail later).

Alpha Motor Neuron

The alpha motor neuron with its axon is responsible for the motor signal projected from the spinal cord to the periphery. Alpha motor neurons vary in size, with the largest neurons going to extrafusal (skeletal) muscle fibers associated with group II or fast twitch fibers. Conversely, the smallest alpha motor neurons are those that go to the group I or slow twitch fibers.[14,55] As was the case with the afferent axons, any time measurements taken due to an external stimulus are measuring only the fastest conducting fibers and thus are preferentially biased toward the axons supplying the fast twitch fibers.

Neuromuscular Junction

The neuromuscular junction is the space that links the efferent action potential with the muscle fibers that it innervates. This is a chemically gated channel that has many receptors sensitive to the release of acetylcholine (ACh) embedded within a membrane with numerous folds to increase its surface area.[54] With conduction of an action potential down an efferent neuron, ACh is released into the neuromuscular junction, and if sufficient in quantity, the neurotransmitter will bind with the receptor and gates will open to begin the conduction of an action potential along a muscle fiber. Normally, the "quantal" release of ACh in response to an efferent action potential is more than sufficient to achieve this opening of the gates on the muscle fiber and the conduction of a motor action potential. However, there are conditions such as myasthenia gravis (postsynaptic problem) and Lambert-Eaton syndrome (presynaptic problem), where the neuromuscular junction can be implicated as the cause of the weakness that a patient is experiencing.[88,97]

Muscle Fiber

The muscle fibers themselves are the effector organs that the efferent fibers are acting on. When individuals volitionally contract a muscle, they are sending a signal from the CNS and activating a population of alpha motor neurons that transmit action potentials down the efferent axons, across the neuromuscular junction, resulting in contraction of skeletal muscle. When done through external stimulation, the process is the same except that the action potential begins at the point along the nerve where stimulation is provided, and an action potential travels away from that site in both directions (**orthodromic** conduction if in the direction that the axon normally conducts, and antidromic conduction if in the direction opposite that of normal action potential conduction).[39,92] As mentioned earlier, because electrical current follows the path of least resistance, the largest axons are preferentially activated first and the first muscle fibers to respond to electrical stimulation are the fast twitch fibers.[14] Normally, the external activation of a nerve is done supramaximally, to attempt to activate all the muscle fibers innervated by that peripheral nerve. When supramaximal stimulation is achieved, judgments can be made regarding the entire population of muscle fibers activated.

THE ELEMENTS OF THE SPINAL NERVE

While the typical spinal nerve and its associated elements provide a good starting point to examine what can and cannot be reasonably evaluated through electrophysiologic testing, a few comments are needed. First, the typical spinal nerve represented in Fig. 9-3B appears to have both afferent and efferent fibers that pass directly from or directly to the periphery, without mixing with other nerves. This may roughly be the case for the simple segmental nerves represented by the intercostal nerves of the thorax. For virtually all other afferent and efferent fibers, they are integrated through a plexus (or mixing), as is the case with the brachial, cervical, lumbar, or sacral plexuses. The examiner needs to be aware of the actual course taken by the axons being evaluated in order to be able to make potential judgments about where a problem may be occurring. Additionally, the typical spinal nerve shows two major branches traveling to the periphery, the anterior (ventral) primary rami and the posterior (dorsal) primary rami. The anterior primary rami are what supply the vast majority of the muscles and areas of cutaneous sensation for the limbs and anterior body wall, and the axons contained within it are what merge together in the various plexuses. The posterior primary rami, on the other hand, supply three structures: (1) skin of the back, (2) the true back muscles (erector spinae, transversospinalis, interspinalis, intertransversarii, and levator costarum), and (3) the facet (zygapophyseal) joints.[73] To evaluate both the anterior and posterior primary rami and some of the structures innervated, muscles representative of both these regions need to be assessed. Second, the typical spinal nerve as has been drawn in Fig. 9-3B has been taken from the thoracic level of the spinal cord. As such, the cell bodies associated with the presynaptic sympathetic neurons are evident in the intermediolateral cell column of the spinal cord, and the sympathetic chain ganglia are also included adjacent to the anterior primary rami. This serves as a reminder that peripheral nerves contain some autonomic (e.g., sympathetic nervous system [SNS] fibers) components and many injuries reflect this contribution through physical manifestations such as altered sweating or skin color changes.[50,74] There are no parasympathetic nervous system fibers found in peripheral nerves of the extremities.[73] While these autonomic fibers are part of virtually every peripheral nerve, there is currently not a good way to selectively evaluate the function of these specific fibers. Therefore, the autonomic nervous system is not currently evaluated in the typical electrophysiologic test. This is an area of investigation, and in the future, it may be possible to quantify function of portions of the autonomic nervous system.[13,49,86,99]

Structurally, there are other elements of the typical spinal nerve that need to be considered that are not readily apparent from Fig. 9-3. All nerves are located below the skin, either in the subcutaneous tissue (some of the cutaneous nerves), or at a deeper level. Because of the nerve's physical location, any stimulation or detection of the action potential traveling across the nerve has to pass through both the skin and any fat in the region.[73] Since fat is a reasonably good insulator, this creates a potential barrier to easy stimulation or identification of the evoked response. Additionally, the collection of axons that make up a peripheral nerve is organized in a bundle. Starting at the level of the axon, the connective tissue surrounding a given axon is termed the endoneurium. A collection of axons grouped together makes up a fasciculi, the next larger layer, with the connective tissue enclosing this bundle termed the perineurium.[89] Finally, the collection of fasciculi are grouped together and surrounded by more connective tissue, termed the epineurium. Each of these connective tissue layers assist in giving the peripheral nerve strength, but they also create additional barriers to the direct electrical evaluation of the axons of interest.

TESTING PROCEDURES

Once the clinician has an understanding of the equipment and pertinent anatomy, electrophysiologic evaluation may begin. There is no particular order for this portion of the examination, with some clinicians preferring to collect NCS data prior to proceeding with the EMG evaluation that requires inserting needle electrodes into select muscles. Other clinicians prefer to determine what they can from the EMG first and use this to assist them in designing the rest of the examination. In reality, different disorders lend themselves to suggesting one element as particularly advantageous to perform first, so given clinicians may adjust the order of testing to optimize the evaluation in terms of time and the number of elements of each test that the patient is exposed to. Recognizing that the order of testing is an arbitrary choice, this overview of the basic procedures will begin with the NCS and then cover the EMG evaluation. Following this, a brief overview of the much less frequently used SEP test will be provided.

LIMB TEMPERATURE AND AGE CONSIDERATIONS

The examiner performing these electrophysiologic tests additionally needs to be aware of other factors that will impact on the results obtained. Two of the most important are temperature of the limb being examined and age. Numerous studies have demonstrated that there is an inverse correlation between temperature of the region being studied and the speed of the action potential.[48,90] A cold limb will conduct electrical impulses slower than a limb of normal temperature. To control for this variable, skin temperature is monitored during the examination and if the temperature drops too low, it is warmed prior to continuing with the examination. For the upper extremities, the surface temperature of the hand should be at least 30°C, with 32°C preferred.[45] For the feet, the temperature should be at least 30°C, although these values do vary between electrophysiologic laboratories.[58,83] To promote an optimal environment for this type of testing, the room should also be maintained at a temperature of at least 25°C.[83] Due to the importance of temperature in obtaining valid results, the temperature of the limb being evaluated should be indicated on any report published. Additionally, individuals that are young (under 16) or are over 50 years of age may have action potentials that conduct at a speed different than adults between the ages of 18 and 50.[58,83] Most nerves mature by the age of 4, but this varies and some elements of the PNS may not be fully mature until approximately 14–16 years of age. A nerve that is not fully mature typically conducts slower than would be expected and the normative tables that have been constructed for this younger age group take this factor into consideration. On the other end of the spectrum, individuals older than 40 years of age begin to see slight slowing in nerve conduction velocity. By the age of 50, this 1 or 2 m/sec per decade slowing that begins over the age of 40 is enough that a separate set of normative values are available for individuals over the age of 50.[58,83] After the age of 70, the slowing becomes much more significant.[58,83] Due to the inverse correlation between aging and nerve conduction velocity, the aging process also needs to be factored in when performing this type of testing.

NERVE CONDUCTION STUDY

The family of tests commonly performed and grouped under the label of NCS includes the following: (1) sensory nerve studies, (2) motor nerve studies, (3) reflex studies (Hoffman's reflex and central conduction studies), and (4) repetitive stimulation testing. Each of these tests has a common characteristic of stimulating a nerve with an evoked (or generated) potential, then picking up the response at some other location. By providing a known stimulus, and knowing other factors such as the distance between the point of stimulation and the time required for the response to occur, factors such as speed of conduction and the size of the sensory or motor nerve action potential can be measured.

Sensory Nerve Studies

The general premise of a sensory nerve conduction study is that the examiner is introducing an action potential along a peripheral nerve and picking up that action potential at a second site. Action potentials travel in both directions from the point of stimulation.

In sensory testing, if the active recording electrode is placed proximal to the point of stimulation, the conduction is orthodromic (in the direction that sensory fibers normally conduct an action potential, with afferent fibers conducting toward the central nervous system). Conversely, if the active recording electrode is placed along the nerve distal to the point of stimulation, then the conduction is antidromic (opposite the direction that sensory fibers normally conduct an action potential). In some cases an antidromically generated action potential will be larger or easier to elicit than one obtained orthodromically. An orthodromic latency may be slightly shorter than one obtained antidromically; however, Dumitru states that antidromic and orthodromic latencies are equivalent if the distance between the active and directive electrodes is 4 cm apart.[37,83] Because there are advantages to both methods, both are options commonly used by clinical electrophysiologists, with the direction used usually noted in the written report.

The setup for a typical sensory nerve conduction study is illustrated in Fig. 9-4 for an orthodromically generated action potential of the 2digit-(index finger) wrist segment of the median nerve. In this case, stimulating ring electrodes have been placed on the index finger spanning the course of the nerve, with the cathode (negative pole that is responsible for depolarization of the nerve) placed proximally and the anode placed distally. At a given distance proximal to the cathode, typically 14 cm for this type of study, the active electrode is positioned on the skin of the wrist over the course of the nerve. The reference electrode is similarly placed along the course of the nerve, several centimeters proximal to the active electrode. The ground electrode is positioned on the same extremity, typically on the opposite side of the limb between the point of stimulation and point of pickup. Recall that the skin has to be clean prior to the positioning of the electrodes, and conduction gel is used to maximize conduction

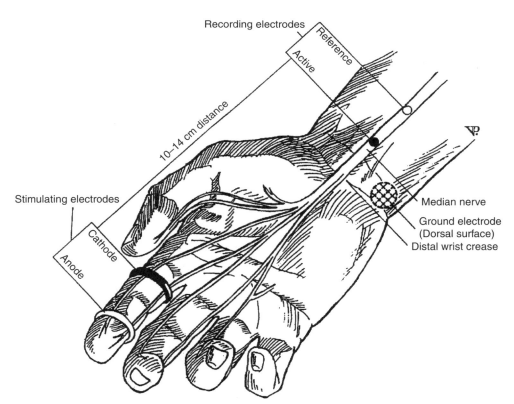

•**Figure 9-4** Setup for a typical sensory nerve conduction study for an orthodromically generated action potential of the 2digit-wrist segment of the median nerve. (*Source*: Nestor, D.E., Nelson, R.M.: Performing motor and sensory neuronal conduction studies in adult humans—a NIOSH technical manual. DHHS (NIOSH) Publication No. 89-XXX, 1987, Morgantown, WV, Division of Safety Research, National Institute for Occupational Safety and Health.)

at the site of the stimulation. Conduction gel is also used for the other electrodes if they are reusable metal electrodes and they are taped into place. If disposable electrodes are used, then the self-adhering gel fixes the electrodes onto the extremity being tested. Recall also that other probes may also be placed on the limb, such as the surface temperature probe discussed earlier, to monitor and record the temperature of the limb at the time of testing.

When the examiner triggers or activates the stimulating electrode, a single brief monophasic square wave is created. This "electrical shock" results in a sudden and rapid alteration of the axons contained within the collective peripheral nerve being examined, resulting in some or all of those fibers being depolarized past the point of threshold. If the stimulus intensity is not sufficient to activate all of the axons, then a submaximal SNAP has been generated. Because factors such as the size of the potential are reflective of the number of axons activated, a submaximal SNAP is not what is sought. With adequate stimulus intensity, all of the axons within the nerve being investigated will be activated and a supramaximal SNAP will be obtained. Because each individual action potential is "all or none," the summed responses of all the action potentials traveling down the peripheral nerve create a representative picture of the function of this nerve. The signal being monitored along the course of the nerve does not involve either the neuromuscular junction or the innervated muscle, so the SNAP is primarily reflective of the contribution of sensory axons because they are the largest and fastest conducting fibers.[49]

Specific parameters measured in association with a SNAP are the following (see Fig. 9-5): (1) amplitude or the size of the potential, measured in μV, (2) shape of the action potential, that is usually biphasic with a phase on each side of the baseline, (3) latency, or the time that it takes from stimulus to the response over a predetermined distance, measured in msec, and (4) NCV, the speed by which a nerve conducts an action potential, measured in m/sec. (Note that latency and NCV are both based on the same information, with latency reflecting a measure of time over a given distance, and NCV reflecting speed. If one is known, the other can be calculated.)

Amplitude

Amplitude is reflective of the summed action potentials within the peripheral nerve assessed in an environment where there is some resistance due to skin, subcutaneous

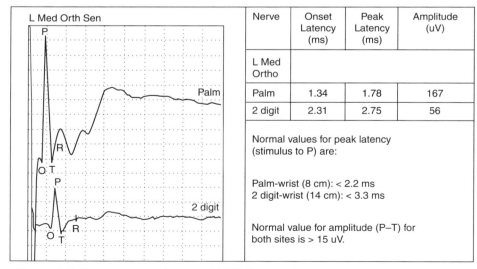

•**Figure 9-5** Sensory nerve action potential (SNAP)—associated parameters include (a) Amplitude: Measured in microvolts (μV), from peak to trough, (b) latency: measured from stimulus onset to peak of the negative potential, and (c) shape: biphasic potential with initial negative then positive phase (small positive phase in this case) is typical.

tissue (fat), and connective tissue elements. For sensory fibers, it is defined as the distance from the peak of the negative phase to the peak of the positive phase (see Fig. 9-5). By convention, electrophysiologists have named the deflection below the isopotential baseline as a positive deflection, while a deflection above this baseline is considered to be a negative deflection. While this positive and negative phase notation is reversed compared to the construction of a typical y-axis on a two-dimensional plot, it is the standard that is used. Another way of saying the same thing is that the amplitude is measured from the peak (top of the negative deflection) to the trough (peak of the positive deflection). The size of the amplitude of the SNAP provides the examiner with information regarding the function of the axons within that segment. A relatively large amplitude SNAP is good, and charts are available that give minimum normative values for a variety of sensory nerves being evaluated. If the amplitude of the SNAP is smaller than these values, or a SNAP cannot be elicited, this suggests some type of compromise of the axons within that segment of the nerve. These amplitude values are obtained with the oscilloscope using a fairly large gain and measured in μV, since the size of the potential obtained from a SNAP is small when compared to the CMAP that is measured in mV. (For conversion, 1000 μV = 1 mV.)

Shape

Prior to discussing latency, it is necessary to clarify what is meant in the paragraph above by a waveform that is described as having one or more positive and negative phases. For a SNAP, the phase simply means that as the collective depolarizing waveform travels down the nerve, the individual axons that have been brought to threshold are conducting an action potential along their length. Since these axons vary in both type (myelinated and unmyelinated) and size (large axons conduct faster than similarly structured smaller diameter axons), the cumulative waveform represents the contribution of all of the axons contained within the peripheral nerve. Recall that the site where the action potential is being picked up has two electrodes in place, an active electrode (sometimes referred to as electrode-1 [E1]) and a reference electrode (sometimes referred to as electrode-2 [E2]). The reference electrode is plugged into an inverting port on the differential amplifier, so that any signal that it receives will be inverted and then added to the signal detected by the active electrode.[26] This functional subtraction of one electrode potential from the other (inverting and adding is the same as subtraction) provides a flat baseline at rest and a potential that is typically biphasic when stimulated. Prior to any stimulation, both the active and reference electrodes are measuring the nerve at rest and are at essentially the same voltage level, producing a baseline of zero volts. Immediately after the stimulus has been delivered, the resting potential of the nerve under the active and reference electrodes remains unaffected, and the isopotential line remains flat, or unchanged. With time, however, this elicited waveform will travel down the nerve and the leading edge (fastest conducting axons) will begin to depolarize in the vicinity of the active electrode. At this moment in time, a potential difference will be observed between the electrical potentials recorded by the active and reference electrodes. As the collective waveform continues to progress down the length of the nerve, more axons will have their action potentials reach the active electrode and contribute to this potential electrical difference. Since the obtained SNAP measured on the oscilloscope is the difference between the active and reference electrodes (differential amplifier amplifies the difference in potential), and the reference electrode measures this collective waveform with a slight temporal delay because it is further along the nerve, a biphasic potential is generated. This biphasic potential simply reflects the potential difference between the active and reference electrodes as the collective waveform is moving under them along the course of the nerve. Normally, the initial deflection associated with a SNAP is a negative deflection, followed by a positive deflection—these two phases thus create a biphasic potential. Once the evoked waveform has moved past the two electrodes assessing any potential difference, the resting baseline of zero potential difference is reestablished. Since a given nerve's action potential is approximately 0.5 msec in duration within the nerve and approximately 2.0–3.0 msec at the surface of the skin, this is the typical duration of a SNAP.[26]

Since this SNAP is assessing simultaneously what is measured at the active and reference electrodes, the waveform could be inverted by reversing the electrode leads into the differential amplifier. While this would break with convention since measurements are typically made to the peak of the negative deflection of a SNAP (see section on latency), it has been mentioned here to illustrate that the deflections are not fixed and are simply reflective of potential differences between two electrode sites. For completeness, it should also be noted that the changes in potential at any one site (either the active or reference electrode) are really physiologically triphasic within the nerve. The observed biphasic potential is a product of the differential amplifier measuring equivalent voltage changes separated temporally.[26] Thus, there may be some SNAP waveforms that have triphasic morphology, typically positive–negative–positive phase, if the reference electrode is not placed directly along the path of the nerve being assessed and the two electrodes are not measuring equivalent voltage changes.

Latency

The latency measurement associated with a SNAP is the time that it takes from a stimulus to the peak of the negative response, over a predetermined distance, measured in msec (see Fig. 9-5). For a number of common clinical conditions, such as a distal median neuropathy with slowing at or distal to the wrist (carpal tunnel syndrome), this may be the most sensitive and earliest indicator of a clinically significant problem.[38,49] Since the latency measurement is a given time, irrespective of the size of the individual, it is based on known distances and the normative values are available in tables.

The latency value obtained is reflective only of the function of the fastest conducting fibers (e.g., the large diameter, myelinated fibers). Recall from the discussion above that the collective waveform contains some contribution from all of the axons that make up the nerve being examined. Since the latency is from the point of the stimulation to the peak of the negative phase of the waveform, the fastest conducting axons will be the ones that are responsible for the latency assessed. In a condition that is typified by demyelination of a nerve, such as carpal tunnel syndrome, a prolonged latency (slowing) would be observed because the large, myelinated axons will be involved. On the other hand, in a condition such as a cervical radiculopathy where select axons have been damaged somewhere along their course, but most axons remains intact, the latency value will remain unchanged. The reason that the latency value will remain unchanged is that the intact axons still present in the nerve are conducting as fast as they ever have and this preserves the overall speed of the nerve.

These **distal sensory latencies** (DSL) are typically obtained on the most peripheral (or distal) aspect of the nerve under investigation. The DSL may involve several segments of a sensory nerve, such as a palm to wrist segment and a digit to wrist segment of a nerve like the median. Or, the DSL may involve simply one segment of the nerve, such as with the sural in the leg or the lateral cutaneous nerve of the forearm (lateral antebrachial cutaneous nerve). In either case, since the distal aspect of the nerve is located farthest from the cell body that lives in the posterior (dorsal) root ganglion, this segment is sensitive to either a proximal problem affecting overall neuron functioning of multiple axons or to a distal problem such as peripheral compression or microcirculation ischemia. A 5digit-(little finger) wrist orthodromic stimulation setup is shown in Fig. 9-6A, while an antidromic stimulation setup for the superficial branch of the radial nerve is shown in Fig. 9-6B.

Nerve Conduction Velocity

While the most common procedure performed with sensory nerve fibers is that of DSL determination just described, there are occasionally times when a sensory nerve conduction velocity will be sought. An example of where this might be employed is if the examiner wanted to test the speed of conduction over a particular segment of a nerve, such as where the ulnar nerve passes under the medial epicondyle of the humerus (normally done with a motor nerve study but can be done with a sensory latency). The procedure

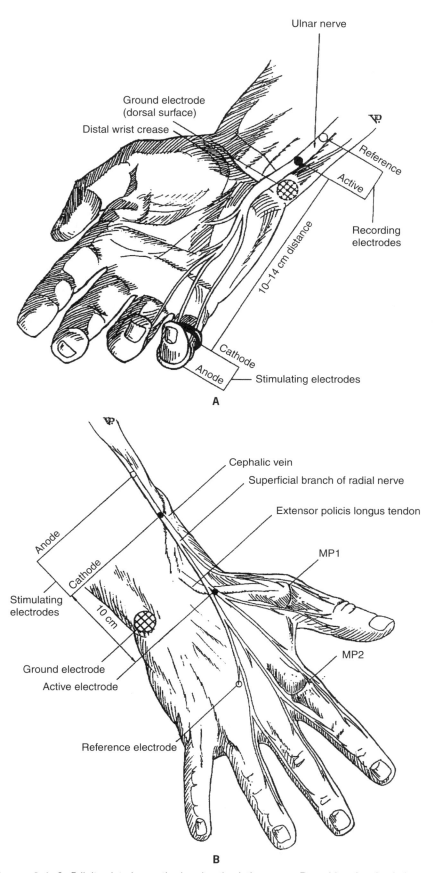

Ulnar nerve

Ground electrode
(dorsal surface)

Distal wrist crease

Reference

Active

Recording
electrodes

10–14 cm distance

Cathode

Anode — Stimulating electrodes

A

Cephalic vein

Superficial branch of radial nerve

Extensor policis longus tendon

MP1

Anode

Cathode

10 cm

Stimulating
electrodes

Ground electrode

Active electrode

MP2

Reference electrode

B

•**Figure 9-6 A.** 5digit-wrist ulnar orthodromic stimulation setup. **B.** antidromic stimulation setup for the superficial branch of the radial nerve. (*Source:* Nestor, D.E., Nelson, R.M.: Performing motor and sensory neuronal conduction studies in adult humans—a NIOSH technical manual. DHHS (NIOSH) Publication No. 89-XXX, 1987, Morgantown, WV, Division of Safety Research, National Institute for Occupational Safety and Health.)

   b. Ulnar nerve

   (1) DML of the ulnar nerve

   (2) NCV of the ulnar nerve (both below elbow-wrist and above elbow-below elbow segment) (e.g., forearm and across the elbow)

   3. F-wave of the ulnar nerve

   The sensory and motor nerve studies outlined above provide the examiner with some information about the function of the three major nerves of the upper extremity: the median, ulnar, and radial. The DSL studies, often more sensitive than the motor studies for early problems, provide data about the ability of the distal afferent axons to conduct.[38,57,82] The DML studies provide equivalent information about the status of the distal efferent axons to conduct and additionally test the neuromuscular junction and the innervated muscle fibers. Nerve conduction velocities of specific segments of both the median and ulnar nerves are assessed, as is the total length of the nerve through the use of the F-wave. All of the data collected need to be compared against normative values, known conduction velocities, expected amplitudes, and so forth. Tables of normal values for NCS measurements should be developed for each clinical electrophysiologic laboratory. Based on this evaluation, the examiner performing the examination can add other specialized tests to look at a given area in more detail, or proceed to the electromyographic portion of the examination. (Several case studies have been provided to illustrate how the data obtained with the above NCS testing can be used to formulate clinical conclusions.)

THE ELECTROMYOGRAPHIC EXAMINATION

The EMG portion of the examination involves inserting a sterile needle electrode into a muscle to provide the examiner with information regarding the spontaneous and voluntary electrical activity of the muscular tissue. The general setup for this procedure is diagrammed in Fig. 9-11 and contains the same basic elements used to monitor action potentials during the neural conduction studies. A ground electrode is used on the limb being examined, and there is an active electrode and a reference electrode. The two key differences with this setup are that the active electrode is a needle electrode placed within

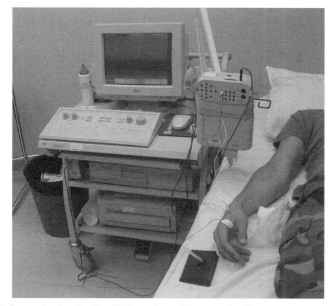

•**Figure 9-11** General setup for the EMG portion of the examination.

the muscle, and there is no externally supplied electrical stimulus. All activity monitored is from the muscle at rest, or due to the insertion of the needle, movement of the needle, or the patient's prompted voluntary activity. The needle electrode is typically coated with a material like Teflon to both insulate all portions of the needle except the very tip and minimize discomfort during insertion. The active tip monitors the few muscle fibers located within approximately 0.5 mm of the noninsulated region.[21] It has been estimated that at any one time, the electrical activity of 1–12 muscle fibers is being evaluated by this small active region on the needle electrode.[21] It is therefore necessary to move the needle slightly over the course of the examination of a muscle to increase the pool of potential muscle fibers that are observed. Due to the combination of potential discomfort associated with inserting the needle, moving the needle slightly, and asking the patient to contract the muscle while the needle electrode remains in the muscle, this portion of the examination is typically, but not always, performed following neural conduction studies. Good communication with the patient is essential to prepare them for this portion of the examination and to solicit their cooperation during the course of the evaluation.

Prior to providing an overview of a basic EMG examination, it may be beneficial to provide a rationale for why this portion of the examination is performed. Direct observation of the spontaneous and voluntary activity of muscle fibers can provide a great deal of information regarding the efferent portion of the neuromuscular system, from the anterior horn cell to the muscle fibers themselves. For example, if an anterior horn cell has become diseased, then the axon associated with that structure dies and the muscle fibers associated with that axon become denervated. This creates a situation where the muscle fibers and muscle fiber membrane are "irritable" and prone to abnormal spontaneous electrical activity (e.g., positive sharp waves and fibrillation potentials) during needle movement and at rest. A second potential site of entrapment is where a nerve root exits the intervertebral foramina. If the root is compromised at this site, the axons passing through this space can become damaged, again resulting in abnormal spontaneous electrical activity. Identification of a nerve root compression at a specific level is done by sampling a variety of muscles, noting which ones have evidence of abnormal electrical activity, and correlating this with the root levels that supply the muscles sampled. For example, a patient with findings in the right pronator teres (median nerve, C6-7), extensor carpi radialis brevis (posterior interosseous nerve of radial, C7-8) triceps brachii (radial nerve, C6-8), and the flexor carpi ulnaris (ulnar nerve, C7-8) have common findings in the C7 nerve root contributions to all of these different nerves. If this is coupled with normal hand intrinsics (median and ulnar nerves, C8-T1), normal biceps brachii (musculocutaneous, C5-6), normal deltoid (axillary, C5-6), and normal supraspinatus (suprascapular nerve, C5-6), the examination suggests that the C5, C6, C8, and T1 root levels are not involved. The single most probable site for this type of a finding is at the C7 intervertebral foramina where the nerve root could be compressed as it exits this space. The final piece of the puzzle is to test the lower cervical paraspinals, thus sampling the muscles supplied by the posterior (dorsal) primary rami of the C7 nerve root (review previous section on the typical spinal nerve, Fig. 9-3). If the cervical paravertebral muscles (PVM) also demonstrates abnormal electrical findings and these findings correlate with the patient's physical examination, the implication is quite strong that the problem is occurring proximal to the point where the posterior (dorsal) and anterior (ventral) primary rami split and contribute to the brachial plexus and the true muscles of the back. This would be strong evidence in support of a C7 cervical radiculopathy. Practically, the EMG examination is the most useful aspect of the electrophysiologic examination to detect radiculopathies, and it is a valuable adjunct to collaborate the findings of magnetic resonance imaging or other specialized imaging tests. A third potential site of a neuromuscular problem is within the muscle itself, with myopathic diseases such as Duchene muscular dystrophy. With diseases affecting the muscle fibers themselves, the electrical potentials generated are unusual in aspects such as their size and duration. This information in the hands of an experienced clinician can be used to aid in the diagnosis of the underlying pathology.

The three examples provided in the paragraph above were not meant to suggest that this is the range of disorders that can be identified with EMG testing, but rather provide illustrative examples of locations within the efferent neuromuscular chain where problems can be identified. While three simple examples were provided here, there are literally hundreds of conditions that manifest themselves in different ways with signs evident during an EMG examination. It takes significant skill, experience, as well as an excellent understanding of anatomy and the pathophysiology of disease to provide a linkage between the patient's problem and the mechanism underlying the condition. The range of problems that can be evaluated with EMG testing is very broad and beyond the scope of what can be provided in this chapter. As has been referenced previously, the specific approach used for any one patient will be customized by the practitioner based on the patient's particular findings during the physical examination and history. Recognizing this need to customize examinations and the range of specific pathologies, there are common elements to the basic approach to this portion of the examination used during most EMG examinations. The generic EMG information provided below deals with the elements commonly examined during the evaluation of one muscle. For the interested reader desiring more detail on specialized techniques or ways of modifying this type of examination, see some of the excellent texts on this topic written by Oh, Kimura, and Dumitru.

Clinical EMG Procedures

The routine EMG examination does not have a set format, nor are there a set number of muscles that need to be examined. The judgment regarding which distal and proximal muscles to test, the number of muscles that should be examined, and whether or not the paraspinals (innervated by posterior [dorsal] primary rami) should be evaluated, is based on the clinician's experience and to some extent on the insurance companies' willingness to reimburse. The four steps of the evaluation typically performed on each muscle examined are as follows. The first step comprises insertion activity, the spontaneous electrical activity due to the insertion of the EMG needle electrode.[60] Additionally, the needle electrode is moved slightly to sample different regions and different depths of the muscle, to assess muscle membrane irritability, and look for abnormal spontaneous electrical activity. The second step includes identifying any abnormal spontaneous electrical potentials while the muscle is at rest. The normal muscle is electrically silent at rest. If any spontaneous electrical activity is observed, it is recorded. The third step of the EMG examination includes observation of the muscle fibers during voluntary contraction. The patient is asked to contract the muscle, first at a very low level to allow the observation of single motor units, then with increasing intensity to examine for an orderly recruitment from the smaller, type I muscle fibers, to the larger, type II muscle fibers. Ultimately, with a full contraction the oscilloscope screen should be completely "filled" when examining a normal muscle. Synthesis of the information obtained in steps 1–3 provides a summary of the EMG testing and is the fourth and final step. A more detailed explanation of each of these four steps is provided below.

Insertion

The insertion activity assesses the electrical response of a sample of muscle fibers to the insertion and moving of the needle electrode within a resting muscle. When a needle electrode is placed within a muscle or is moved, it is normal for electrical activity to be observed on the oscilloscope screen lasting from 50–230 msec.[34,60] Since the tip of the needle typically samples the muscle action potential of less than 12 muscle fibers, it needs to be moved to provide a representative sample of the muscle under investigation. One recommended scheme is to move the needle to "the four corners of a small box," and repeat this three times assessing a different depth of the muscle with each series of sampling.[21] After each needle movement, the electrical activity of the muscle is assessed. This provides data from 12 samples of the muscle and increases the likelihood of identifying any abnormal electrical activity, if it exists. When abnormal spontaneous electrical activity is observed that persists longer than 230 msec following cessation of needle movement, this is abnormal and the particular characteristics of that activity are described. Additionally, if no electrical activity is observed with the needle movement, this is also considered to be abnormal. The increased abnormal electrical activity associated with insertion and needle movement is associated with conditions such as denervation, myotonic disorders, and some myogenic disorders (myositis).[60,106] When reduced electrical activity is observed, this is suggestive of chronic muscle changes and a muscle that is subject to fatty or fibrotic degeneration. In this case, there may be an abnormal feel or resistance to movement of the needle, such as if the needle were being moved through a bag of sand. These examples are intended to illustrate that with insertion of a needle, increased or decreased electrical activity can be observed in addition to normal insertional activity. Additionally, with movement of the needle in the relaxed muscle, other abnormal spontaneous electrical activities can be observed beyond the 230-msec reflective of normal muscle fiber activity.

Several of the more common examples of abnormal spontaneous electrical activity at rest are provided below. This very abridged list include the following.

Fibrillation Potentials

This represents the electrical activity associated with the spontaneous contraction of a single muscle fiber. Since the contraction of a single muscle fiber is too small to either be felt or observed visually, the only way to assess for this condition is through EMG needle electrode examination. The origin of fibrillation potentials is from membrane instability due to loss of axonal innervation of the individual muscle fibers that collectively make up a motor unit. These denervated fibers become irritable and, in a response to encourage reinnervation by another axon, begin to have their resting membrane potential oscillate toward the level of threshold.[26] As this threshold level is reached, the single muscle fiber will spontaneously fire, or fibrillate. These fibrillation potentials have a characteristic shape, with an initial positive deflection, typically two to three phases, and are of a very short duration of a few milliseconds (less than 5 msec). Additionally, they emit a characteristic high-pitched sound that has been described as "rain on a tin roof" when heard through a loudspeaker.[26] The amplitude of these potentials can vary from a few hundred μV's to over one mV, with fibrillation potential amplitude more prominent in acute denervation compared to chronic denervation.[20] Fig. 9-12A is an illustration of a typical fibrillation potential.

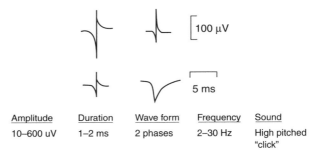

Amplitude	Duration	Wave form	Frequency	Sound
10–600 uV	1–2 ms	2 phases	2–30 Hz	High pitched "click"

A. Fibrillation potentials

Amplitude	Duration	Wave form	Frequency	Sound
30–4,000 uV	2–10 ms	2 phases	2–100 Hz	Dull "thud"

B. Positive sharp waves

•**Figure 9-12** Figure that demonstrates: **A.** Fibrillation potentials. **B.** Positive sharp waves. (*Source*: Nestor, D.E., Nelson, R.M.: Performing motor and sensory neuronal conduction studies in adult humans—a NIOSH technical manual. DHHS (NIOSH) Publication No. 89-XXX, 1987, Morgantown, WV, Division of Safety Research, National Institute for Occupational Safety and Health.)

Positive Sharp Waves

PSWs are biphasic, positive then negative, potentials recorded in response to needle movement with a muscle at rest. These potentials, like the previously described fibrillation potentials, are representative of muscle denervation. The basic etiology of these PSWs is believed to be similar to fibrillation potentials, in that they indicate membrane instability secondary to the loss of axonal innervation.[26] The true origin of these PSWs has not been clearly identified, but it is clear that these potentials represent an unstable muscle fiber membrane. The shape of these potentials is characteristic, with an initial positive deflection and two phases, a regular firing rate of between 1 and 50 Hz, amplitudes that range from 100 to 1000 µV, and a duration that can vary from several to 100 msec.[26] When amplified on a speaker system, these potentials sound like a dull thud or plop. These potentials are often seen mixed in with fibrillation potentials, and are found with a variety of pathologic conditions ranging from denervation to polymyositis, progressive muscular dystrophy, and motor neuron diseases. Fig. 9-12B provides an example of PSWs mixed in with fibrillation potentials.

Grading Fibrillation Potentials and PSWs

In a patient's records, the presence of fibrillation potentials and/or PSWs will be quantified through the use of the following notations used by the Mayo Clinic[15,28]: (1) 0 indicates the absence of either of these two potentials, (2) 1+ indicates that the potential being quantified persisted for over 1 second in at least two of the 12 areas examined, (3) 2+ indicates one or both of these potentials persisted over 1 second in many but not all areas, (4) 3+ indicates observation of one or both of these potentials in all areas, but the potentials were intermittent, and (5) 4+ indicates continuous abnormal electrical activity observed in all areas examined. From a prognostic standpoint, 1+ findings are less severe than 3+ or 4+ fibrillation potentials and/or PSWs, that are indicative of a more widespread or severe pathology.

Myotonic Discharges

These are variations on the theme discussed above with fibrillation potentials and PSWs, with myotonic discharges representing a sustained run of potentials that resemble PSWs. A difference here is that the potentials wax and wane, sounding over a loud speaker like a motorcycle, dive-bomber, or chainsaw.[12,28] Potentials of this type are observed in conditions such as myotonia congenita, myotonia dystrophia, paramyotonia congenital, and hyperkalemic periodic paralysis.[12,28] Myotonic discharges have an initial positive deflection, two phases, fire at a rate of 20–100 Hz, have an amplitude of 10–1000 µV, and have a very short duration of approximately 2 –5 msec.[12,28]

Other Potentials

The three types of potentials noted above (fibrillation potentials, PSWs, and myotonic discharges) are not the only types of abnormal electrical activity observed with needle insertion and movement, but they are the most common. Other types of abnormal potentials such as complex repetitive discharges and myokymic discharges can be seen across a variety of patient conditions. The above potentials are illustrative of the more common abnormal findings that might be observed in a patient's records with significant EMG results. For additional information, see the excellent EMG texts on this topic by Oh,[82] Kimura,[57,58] and Dumitru.[31]

Rest

With a needle electrode inserted into a muscle and the muscle at rest, the isoelectric line should remain stable and the loud speaker should be silent. There are exceptions to this electrical silence that occur in normal muscle, such as the detection of the random release of a quanta of ACh at the neuromuscular junction (miniature end-plate potential) or the detection of a spontaneous nonpropagated potential occurring at the neuromuscular junction (end-plate potential). While these are exceptions found in normal muscle, they are relatively easily identified by their size, shape, and sound, and are eliminated by moving the needle to a new site. Exceptions to electrical silence that can occur within a muscle at rest include all of the previously discussed potentials in the section above on insertional activity (fibrillation potentials, PSWs, myotonic discharges, complex repetitive discharges, etc.), as well as fasciculations.

A fasciculation potential is the potential associated with the random and spontaneous activation of a group of muscle fibers or all of the muscle fibers originating from a motor unit. Everyone has experienced fasciculation potentials, such as when the eyelid "twitches" at the end of the day when an individual is fatigued. This is generally thought to be due to the abnormal discharge of an alpha motor neuron, resulting in contraction of all the muscle fibers innervated by the motor unit. Because a single alpha motor neuron innervates up to several thousand muscle fibers in muscles like the soleus in the leg,[28,57] these contractions can be both felt by the individual and observed by a clinician. In a pathologic state, their etiology is not as clear and it has been shown that the fasciculation potential can originate from the anterior horn cell, the peripheral nerve, or the terminal nerve membrane.[21] A general rule of thumb is that fasciculations are known by the company that they keep. In other words, since everyone experiences fasciculations on occasion when particularly fatigued or stressed, they are not in and of themselves pathognomic of a neuromuscular problem. Fasciculations occurring in normal muscle and those associated with disease visually appear to be identical. However, when they occur in the presence of clinical findings such as atrophy and unexplained loss of strength, the "company" that they are associated with is less than ideal and the importance of noting their regular appearance is greatly increased. The clinician looking for fasciculation potentials will normally observe a muscle at rest from one to several minutes and count the number of fasciculation potentials observed. Abnormal fasciculation potentials are graded on a scale from 1+ to 4+. A 1+ finding indicates that fasciculations were observed in two samples, occurring at a rate of between 2 and 10 per minute. A 4+ finding means that these potentials were observed in all areas sampled, and the fasciculations were occurring at a rate of over 60 per minute.[71] The 2+ and 3+ grades are simply levels expressing findings between these two ends of the grading scale. This provides one more bit of information that may assist in making a diagnosis, because abnormal fasciculation potentials are associated with anterior horn cell disease, metabolic disturbances, and other disorders such as primary muscular atrophy and syringomyelia.[21]

Voluntary Activity

The next step in the evaluation is to have the patient initiate a voluntary contraction. Initially, a very slight contraction is sought that will cause the activation of only a few motor units. This type of slight contraction provides the examiner with the information needed to examine the summated activity of the muscle fibers from a single motor unit that are volitionally activated. Recall from the previous discussion of normal recruitment patterns of motor neurons, the smallest motor neurons innervating slow twitch (Type I) fibers will be recruited initially.[25] With increasing levels of voluntary activation, larger motor units will be recruited. The examiner is looking for an orderly recruitment of motor units suggesting this small-to-large pattern, and also identifying at least 12 motor units to characterize in each muscle examined. The elements typically used to characterize a motor unit are the following: (1) shape, that typically has two to three phases (areas above and below the isoelectric baseline); (2) amplitude, that normally ranges from 300 to 5000 μV (5 mV, with the amplitude of some normal intrinsic hand muscles in the 10,000 μV range), with the motor units associated with the earlier recruited type I fibers having the smaller amplitudes; (3) duration, representing the time involved from the departure of the potential from the baseline until the baseline is reestablished and that normally varies between 3 and 15 msec; and (4) sound of the motor unit. A healthy motor unit with the needle electrode positioned near it will have a sharp, crisp sound. The first three of these traits are often characterized by the acronym SAD (shape, amplitude, and duration).

Shape

A normal MUAP and a MUAP with too many phases (polyphasic potential) are both presented in Fig. 9-13. A normal MUAP has two to three phases typically. A polyphasic potential has five or more phases. A phase is that portion of the action potential that

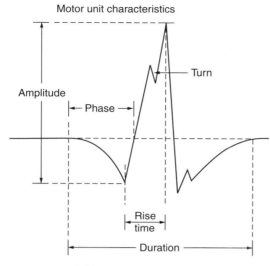

Motor unit characteristics

A. Motor unit characteristics

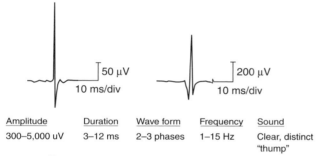

Amplitude	Duration	Wave form	Frequency	Sound
300–5,000 uV	3–12 ms	2–3 phases	1–15 Hz	Clear, distinct "thump"

B. Normal motor unit action potentials

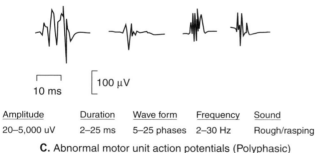

Amplitude	Duration	Wave form	Frequency	Sound
20–5,000 uV	2–25 ms	5–25 phases	2–30 Hz	Rough/rasping

C. Abnormal motor unit action potentials (Polyphasic)

Source: Nestor (NIOSH)

•**Figure 9-13** Motor units. **A.** Motor unit characteristics. **B.** Normal motor unit action potentials. **C.** Abnormal motor unit action potentials (polyphasic). (*Source*: Nestor, D.E., Nelson, R.M.: Performing motor and sensory neuronal conduction studies in adult humans—a NIOSH technical manual. DHHS (NIOSH) Publication No. 89-XXX, 1987, Morgantown, WV, Division of Safety Research, National Institute for Occupational Safety and Health.)

occurs on one side of the baseline. Thus, a biphasic potential may have an initial positive deflection that ends when the potential returns to the baseline, and a negative deflection that is the continuation of the upward sweep of the waveform to a peak, returning again to the baseline that completes the second phase.

Polyphasic potentials are often found in tissue that has been denervated and is in the process of regeneration.[28] While the presence of polyphasic potentials can be collaborative of denervation, interpretation solely on the basis of observing these potentials is problematic, because it has been shown that normal muscle can have polyphasic potentials that range from 12 to 35 percent.[26] Having said that, low amplitude and long-duration polyphasic potentials may be suggestive of nascent (from Latin, meaning *to be born*) potentials that are observed during early states of reinnervation of muscle.[20] Identification of potentials with an abnormal number of phases may assist in understanding what is occurring in the muscle tissue.

A related issue associated with the topic of phases is turns. Turns are the change in direction of a portion of the MUAP (in either a positive or negative direction) that does not continue to the point where the baseline is encountered (see Fig. 9-13). The typical normal MUAP does not have turns, but these small changes in direction of the waveform increase with age.[52] A few turns without other findings are not indicative of pathology. If they are noted in a patient's record, then the minimal excursion required to be classified as a turn should be specified.[20]

Amplitude

The amplitude is the size of the MUAP, measured from peak to peak[75] (see Fig. 9-13). Normal MUAPs range from 300 to 5000 μV (5 mV),[40,43,67,77,78] with distal muscles occasionally normally exhibiting larger amplitudes that may range up to 10 mV. The type I (slow twitch) MUAPs should have an amplitude that ranges from 300 to 1000 μV, while the type II (fast twitch) MUAPs normally range from 1000 to 5000 μV. Deviations of amplitude size from this range of normal values may be a clue in a pathologic process. For example, many motor unit action potentials that are reduced below normal values (300 μV or less) are often observed in patients with myopathies.[44,62,67] Additionally, small amplitude motor units may be present during early axonal regeneration, indicating ongoing recovery from a nerve injury. On the other hand, extremely large amplitude MUAPs are indicative of a neuropathic process where axonal sprouting has occurred. For example, in a patient with anterior horn cell disease, axons are dying and muscle fibers are losing their innervation. Early in this cycle, the denervated muscle fibers will attract axonal sprouts from neurons that are still relatively healthy, creating a motor unit with more than its typical contingent of muscle fibers. This "giant motor unit" will have an amplitude that exceeds the normal range, thus providing collaborative information that a neuropathic process is present. The amplitude of a MUAP will often provide the examiner with important information regarding the underlying state of aspects of the motor unit.

Duration

The duration of a MUAP is the length of time, expressed in milliseconds, from the onset of the potential until a normal baseline is reestablished (see Fig. 9-13). Normal MUAP durations range from 3 to 15 msec. Duration deviations from this range of normal values provide additional important information regarding the status of the motor unit. A duration of less than 3 msec is suggestive of a myopathic process and is the most consistent motor unit morphologic parameter[30] (recall from the paragraph above, that a myopathic process will also typically have a small amplitude of less than 300 μV). On the other hand, a duration that exceeds 15 msec is suggestive of a neuropathic process. This can be seen when considering several elements discussed previously that accompany axonal loss. As muscle fibers become denervated and seek axonal sprouts from healthy axons, the newly configured motor unit has more muscle fibers innervated (giant motor unit). In addition to having an enhanced amplitude, this new motor unit will also tend to have more phases to the MUAP (e.g., polyphasic) resulting in a longer lasting potential that exceeds 15 msec. In this way, the examiner can use this element of the MUAPs appearance to deduce the mechanistic cause of the patient's problem.

Sound

The sound emitted from the loud speaker system is an important tool that assists the examiner in making determinations regarding both what is occurring and their technique. For the observation of MUAPs shape, amplitude, and duration, the examiner attempts to locate the needle close to the motor unit being characterized. This is aided by listening to the sound emitted and moving the needle to elicit a sharp, crisp sound. If the sound is dull, then the MUAP is distant and the examiner should work to reposition the needle closer to the MUAP being assessed.

Contraction Level

The description of the shape, amplitude, duration, and sound provided above was all performed at a reasonably low level of contraction where individual MUAPs could be characterized. As the patient is instructed to increase the level of contraction, other factors such as the orderly recruitment of MUAPs from small to large, the rate of firing and the overall ability to "fill the screen" with a near maximal contraction, a greater number of MUAPs are observed. The rate of firing of the MUAPs first recruited is about 2–3 Hz with a stable firing rate achieved by approximately 5–7 Hz. The first recruited, smaller motor units will increase their firing rate with an increasing level of voluntary contraction. Additionally, as the contraction level continues to increase, additional motor units will be recruited. Thus, at one point in time, several MUAPs may be observed, with one firing at 5 Hz, a second at 10 Hz, and a third at 15 Hz.[19,28] When several MUAPs have been recruited, their firing rate may increase up to 20 Hz. The key point here is that the recruitment should be orderly and progressive. If only large motor units are observed with an initial recruitment and they are firing at a rate clearly in excess of 10 Hz, this suggests that MUAPs have been lost to denervation and that the muscle is trying to compensate by increasing the demands on the remaining fibers (e.g., firing faster and recruiting units associated with type II fibers described earlier). This potential loss of both type I and type II motor units may be confirmed during a strong muscle contraction, if the interference pattern expressed on the oscilloscope is not relatively uniform and full (see Fig. 9-14 for an example of a normal interference pattern). A strong muscle contraction is the summed responses of all the available MUAPs and this normally fills the oscilloscope screen, creating a normal interference pattern. If the interference pattern is less than full with the observed motor units firing at a rapid rate, it is described as representing only single units, or partial screen fill. Loss of motor units and the resulting less-than-optimal screen fill can be indicative of neuropathic conditions.[62]

Summarizing the voluntary contraction part of the examination, the patient will be asked to contract minimally, increase the level of contraction from mild to strong, and then relax the muscle. The minimal contraction permits identification of the MUAP characteristics outlined above. The increase in level of contraction permits examination of recruitment order, the overall amplitude of the largest units, and the ability to achieve a full, smooth contraction (e.g., complete screen fill or normal interference pattern). Finally, the patient needs to relax and the muscle should be monitored until the normal rest state is reestablished.

The number of muscles that should be assessed in a given examination is the prerogative of the examiner. While in some cases this is limited due to reimbursement issues, the examiner is tasked with ensuring that enough muscles have been sampled

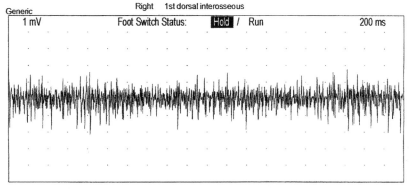

•**Figure 9-14** Interference pattern with normal motor units.

with EMG that the question that brought the patient into the clinic can be answered and reasonable alternative explanations can be addressed. This typically entails selecting a sample of muscles that span both the nerve levels of interest (e.g., C5-T1 for an upper extremity problem where some element of the brachial plexus or its derivative elements may be suspected—this includes the nerve roots, the trunks, the divisions, and the cords), and the terminal elements of the named nerve branches. Additionally, if a nerve root impingement is suspected, the examination should include a sample of the posterior (dorsal) primary rami that supply the true muscles of the back (e.g., erector spinae, transversospinalis muscles, and others).[73] See the introduction of this section on EMG for one example of a possible screen for the upper extremity.

Drawing Information from the EMG Examination (Information Synthesis)

As stated earlier, conclusions are drawn based on the collaborative findings from all the clinical electrophysiologic testings performed. Beginning with the physical examination and any clinical abnormal finding of weakness, sensory alteration, reflex change, atrophy, or any other unusual presentation, the findings from the NCS and EMG examination are analyzed and synthesized. Two examples are provided below that may be illustrative of how this information can be pulled together.

Sensitivity and Specificity of the NCS/EMG Examination

Given a patient with either a positive or negative finding from the collective NCS/EMG examination, what is the likelihood that they actually have the problem identified or ruled out by this examination? As is the case with virtually all diagnostic tests, there is the potential for some false positives or false negatives to occur with this type of testing. Sensitivity and specificity values are often used for interpreting the results of diagnostic tests. Test sensitivity is representative of the proportion of patients with the condition that have a positive test result, so a sensitive test is one that recognizes a problem when a problem is actually present. Test specificity, on the other hand, is the ability to recognize when the condition is absent.[42] Each of these measures can have values up to 100 percent, and higher values are better than lower values. Thus, the ideal is to have a test that has both a high level of sensitivity and specificity. Unfortunately, few tests possess both high sensitivity and specificity.[42]

Sensitivity and specificity values will also depend on the region of the body being investigated, because the electrophysiologic techniques work better in some areas than in others. As an example, for the distal median nerve, sensitivity of composite electrophysiologic measures have ranged between 49 and 84 percent.[5,53,57] Specificity values associated with the median nerve have typically been even better, yielding values of 95 percent or higher[38,66] for a variety of electrodiagnostic tests. When looking at other pathologies that are more readily identified by the EMG portion of the examination (e.g., radiculopathies), studies have shown that the sensitivity of EMG alone is limited, although the specificity remains relatively high.[9,17,102] Note that values like those reported above are not based on only one finding, but on the collaborative picture that emerges from the complete electrophysiologic examination. The range of findings is not surprising because sensitivity and specificity are examined across a wide variety of conditions and the criteria used to make a clinical judgment can be markedly different. Recognizing that electrophysiologic testing is based on a strong physical examination, when there are more clinical findings (e.g., abnormal history, weakness, sensory changes, changes in muscle stretch reflexes [MSRs]), the percentage of patients with abnormal findings also increases. In a recent study, abnormal EMG was found in 90 percent of subjects with three clinical signs, 59 percent with two signs, and only 10 percent with one sign.[72] In another report examining the sensitivity and specificity of 19 separate parameters for carpal tunnel syndrome, the collective presence of nine parameters permitted a specificity of 97 percent in the electrodiagnosis of this problem.[66] While these are excellent sensitivity and specificity values, they are not perfect and false positive electrophysiologic findings have been reported.[87]

If individual parts rather than collaborative findings of the electrophysiologic examination are examined, the results in terms of sensitivity and specificity may appear to be markedly different. For example, in patients with carpal tunnel syndrome, the sensory nerve conduction studies are more frequently abnormal than the motor nerve conduction studies.[66] Or, some aspects of the examination such as the central conduction study (F-wave), by itself, can have a high sensitivity yet low specificity and be of little value when considered alone.[66] Thus, the above findings underscore two key elements associated with electrophysiologic testing: (1) these procedures can yield high sensitivity and specificity based on collaborative findings across the physical examination, NCS and EMG studies, and (2) the findings identified by electrophysiologic testing will be higher in patients with abnormal findings on the physical examination.[76] At the risk of being redundant, it is important to realize that this type of testing is based on an accurate and complete physical examination.

Limitations Associated with the NCS/EMG Process

Electrophysiologic testing has an advantage over some forms of medical testing, in that the methodology employed permits direct evaluation of the functional status of nerves, and to a degree neuromuscular synapses and muscle fibers. This is in contrast to other procedures such as MRIs and x-rays that identify structure rather than function. While the functional approach of electrophysiologic testing is an important adjunctive procedure to delineate a problem suggested by clinical examination or other testing procedures such as MRI, this procedure like all tests has clear limitations. The following abridged list identifies some of the limitations that health care practitioners sending patients for electrodiagnostic testing or interpreting the obtained results should take into consideration. Limitations include the following.

1. By itself, the electrophysiologic examination is not diagnostic, but provides information that the health care practitioner who is overseeing the patient's care can consider when making a medical diagnosis.

2. Not all nerves and muscles lend themselves to electrophysiologic testing. Significant technical difficulties are present when attempting to obtain nerve conduction values from nerves that are not superficially situated or found in individuals with a significant amount of fat. Thus, not all procedures will be obtainable on all individuals. This also holds true for select muscles, where the risk of performing an EMG might outweigh the potential benefit. For example, obtaining an EMG of an internal intercostal muscle might be technically possible, but the risk of having the needle pierce the parietal pleura and creating a pneumothorax is too great. Therefore, these procedures are not routinely performed.

3. As mentioned in the section above on sensitivity and specificity, the findings from a NCS/EMG examination are not perfect. Rather, they are reflective of the functional state of the structures sampled at a moment in time and the skill of the individual both performing and interpreting the examination. Therefore, the findings need to be considered in light of all the medical examination procedures performed to form an appropriate picture of the patient's condition.

4. As alluded to in the point above, there are a number of technical pitfalls that can be confusing to an inexperienced electrophysiologic examiner. Daniel Dumitru in his excellent text states, "Lack of medical training, lack of expertise in the operation of electrophysiologic instruments, and inability to collect electrodiagnostic data accurately are a prescription for potential misdiagnoses and hence possible patient harm. This is likely the most common pitfall in electrodiagnostic medicine consultations".[37]

5. All the procedures that have been discussed thus far are limited to basically evaluating the PNS, synapses directly involved with the PNS (including some at the segmental level of the spinal cord in the case of an H-reflex), and muscle fibers. Thus, the electrophysiologic testing typically performed provides collaborative information that aids in making a diagnosis and the information obtained is largely limited to the peripheral nervous system. There are special tests, such as the somatosensory evoked potentials discussed below that can be used to evaluate some elements of the central nervous system.

SOMATOSENSORY EVOKED POTENTIALS

In the procedures outlined thus far, the only nerve elements that could be examined directly with stimulation at one site and picking up a signal at a second site, were either the efferent (motor) or afferent (sensory) fibers distal to the spinal cord. The obtained latencies and amplitudes formed the basis of the motor and sensory nerve conduction studies described previously. Somatosensory evoked potentials (SEPs) on the other hand, expand the structures that can be assessed by this form of stimulation and pickup. With pickup sites at various locations along the spinal cord (lumbosacral region and cervical region), portions of the brainstem (e.g., medulla), and also for cortical structures (e.g., thalamus and central sulcus of the cortex), these other structures can also be evaluated. It should be noted here that the tracts in the spinal cord and brainstem leading up to the cortex that are assessed with this technique are sensory tracts. Therefore, SEPs are reflective of only sensory neurons and the action potentials traveling along them. The two major pathways that carry sensory information in the central nervous system are (1) the anterolateral system (a composite reference to the individual tracts of the spinothalamic, spinomesencephalic, and spinoreticular tracts) carrying the modalities of pain, temperature, and crude touch and (2) the dorsal column system, carrying the modalities of two-point discrimination, light touch, vibration, and proprioception.[103,104]

While the equipment and specific setups are beyond the scope of this text, the basic premise of SEPs is the following. A stimulator is used to generate an action potential that involves the largest, myelinated axons within a peripheral sensory nerve.[59] This stimulation intensity is typically adjusted by increasing the intensity until a twitch response is noted in the adjacent musculature and using an intensity slightly greater than the onset of the observed twitch. It is believed that this intensity of stimulation will be picked up by these large, myelinated axons since the externally applied current will flow to them preferentially due to their decreased internal resistance (e.g., current will flow along the path of least resistance in accordance with Ohm's law, as described earlier in the chapter). With an elicited SNAP, the action potential is carried into the spinal cord and transmitted up to the thalamus via either the anterolateral system or the dorsal column system. From the thalamus, the information being conveyed by a later generation neuron of the original action potential is conveyed to the cortex. If the multiple neuron pathway from the periphery to the cortex is healthy, there will be characteristic positive or negative deflection potentials that can be obtained. This information can then be used to assert that the sensory neurons within the central nervous system (spinal cord and brain) are conducting normally. If, however, there is a problem in a specific tract in the spinal cord, brainstem, or cortex, the expected deflection potential may be smaller than normal or not obtainable, or it may have a prolonged latency (e.g., be slowed), or it may demonstrate some other type of unusual characteristic. This basic type of assessment can be used to examine the anterolateral system with conditions like syringomyelia and the dorsal columns in disease states such as multiple sclerosis.[59] In these and a host of other conditions, the obtained information can be used in association with other medical tests performed (e.g., MRIs, laboratory tests, etc.) to attempt to localize the lesion and provide an explanation for the patient's symptoms.

Several other points need to be made in this very brief overview. First, because only sensory fiber tracts are involved and the collective action potentials are typically being picked up by surface electrodes (epidural needle electrodes can be used in the lumbosacral region), the size of any one obtained potential is too small to be observed. To correct this potential limitation, numerous stimuli are given and averaged together. The theory here is that time-locked phenomena will build on themselves while random noise will cancel out during the averaging process. Depending on the latency component of the potential under investigation, the number of stimuli may vary from 200 to 4000 that are averaged together. The rate of stimulation typically varies from once per second to four times per second. With modern computers, the averaging and subsequent processing can be done to provide a set of positive and negative potentials that can be interpreted by an expert in these types of studies. Second, there can be numerous pickup electrodes positioned over the scalp, brainstem, cervical region, or other area, and they can record simultaneously. When mapping of the cortex is desired, electrodes are placed on 16–32 sites for monitoring.[59] For most clinical procedures, two to four electrodes at preestablished scalp sites will usually suffice. Clinicians that perform these procedures have a universal system that adapts to skulls of varying size and permits evaluation of areas of suspected pathology. As the above description implies, the nomenclature used to describe the many types and locations of potentials and their associated latencies and amplitudes is confusing. This is an area where consultation with an expert in the field is warranted. Third, because the sensory systems cross the neuraxis prior to reaching the cortex, if unilateral monitoring is done, the stimulation of an extremity will be contralateral to the skull site being evaluated. With today's modern computer systems, bilateral stimulation and monitoring can be done, in addition to unilateral evaluation. Fourth, the most common sites of stimulation are the median nerve at the wrist for the upper extremities and the tibial nerve at the ankle for the lower extremities. Other nerves that are frequently used include the ulnar nerve, fibular nerve, and the pudendal nerve. Fifth, the stability of the obtained SEPs is related to the stimulation site, with action potentials evoked from the upper extremities providing a more stable response than those obtained from the lower extremities. There is also a strong correlation of obtained latencies with the height of the individual. This is to be expected, because taller individuals have a longer tract pathway from the periphery to the cortex and this creates a longer latency response. Additionally, body temperature affects latency, because nerves conduct faster as temperature increases. The examiner performing these tests needs to consider these and other factors when making judgments regarding the obtained findings.

This brief description of SEPs has been provided to make the point that while the most commonly used NCS/EMG procedures described earlier in the chapter evaluate predominantly the peripheral nervous system, there are methodologies that permit examination of the less accessible areas of the spinal cord, brainstem, thalamus, and cortex. Somatosensory-evoked potentials do this for sensory fibers. There is a related technique of motor-evoked potentials that can be used to evaluate portions of the voluntary motor system. These techniques are not performed in all electrophysiologic laboratories, and they require a practitioner with significant experience with this type of testing. Having said that, these adjunctive techniques are used with patient categories ranging from bowel, bladder, and sexual dysfunction, to the impact of diabetes within the central nervous system, to Charcot-Marie Tooth and subacute combined degeneration.[59] Thus, SEPs is a procedure that may be employed with a patient referred for electrophysiologic evaluation.

OTHER ELECTROPHYSIOLOGIC TESTING PROCEDURES

Electrophysiologic testing is a specialty area. The NCS/EMG examinations outlined in this chapter are routinely performed and with some education and experience, readily interpreted. The aforementioned SEPs and many other forms of testing that can be done in an electrophysiologic laboratory do not lend themselves to interpretation without significant time, education, and experience in this field. Therefore, while there are many other procedures such as single fiber techniques, motor evoked potentials, intraoperative monitoring,[68,94] magnetic stimulation of the central and peripheral nervous system, to name just a few, they are beyond the scope of this chapter. (The interested reader is referred to the excellent texts by Dumitru,[31] Oh,[82] and Kimura.[57] The intent of the description provided in this chapter was to simply provide general information regarding basic NCS and EMG procedures, along with the type of clinical information that they provide.)

REQUESTING NCS/EMG EXAMINATIONS

If requesting an NCS/EMG examination, the following is suggested:

1. Based on a good physical examination.
2. Specific clinical findings are highlighted and a working hypothesis put forth.

Nerve conduction studies and EMG examinations are appropriate for patients that require information beyond that regularly available from a clinical examination or imaging studies, regarding the status of their neuromuscular system. Since the information that will be provided from the NCS/EMG examination will be collaborative with the clinical examination and imaging studies, this information should be provided along with the consult. A key point stressed throughout this chapter is that the NCS/EMG examination is based on a good physical examination. Therefore, the referring clinician should ideally obtain a good subjective (history) and complete a thorough objective (physical) examination. A working hypothesis should be formulated based on the specific findings of the history and physical examinations. This working hypothesis or referring diagnosis will assist the clinical electrophysiologist in developing and implementing the NCS and EMG examinations. In the presence of a completely normal physical examination, it is the exception rather than the rule that electrophysiologic testing will reveal any additional information.

It is not appropriate to send patients for NCS/EMG examinations as a method of screening the neuromuscular system when the physical examination is completely normal. This is because the tests are relatively expensive, involve some discomfort and risk due to the insertion of needle electrodes and electrical shocks, and have a relatively low yield in patients without physical findings. However, with signs and symptoms such as sensory changes, weakness, atrophy, reflex changes, and easy fatigability, the likelihood of identifying abnormal electrophysiologic parameters increases dramatically. This collaborative information is then used along with the previously obtained information to make a clear diagnosis and provide the basis from which a logical treatment program can be developed. Thus, a consult for this type of evaluation should be based on a good physical examination and be as specific as is reasonable.

CONCLUSION

Nerve conduction studies and the electromyographic examination provide a great deal of information regarding the functional status of nerves, neuromuscular junctions, and muscle. As such, they are excellent adjunctive procedures to complement the findings by either a clinical physical examination or other special tests such as MRIs or x-rays. Strengths associated with this form of testing include the fact that they are minimally invasive, very safe, and provide information that is a direct assessment of the functional status of the structures under examination. Limitations include the fact that some aspects of the examination are technically difficult, significant skill and sophisticated equipment need to be possessed by the examiner, and the primary region that is investigated with the typical NCS/EMG examination is the peripheral nervous system, synapse, and muscle. While other regions of the nervous system such as the brain and spinal cord can be examined, this is beyond the scope of all but the most specialized practitioners, and these tests are consequently not as frequently performed. The findings from these tests are typically provided back to the referral source in language that describes what was observed electrophysiologically. This information then gives the health care practitioner additional information on which a diagnosis can be developed.

It is hoped that the information provided on basic neurophysiology and an overview of the generic NCS/EMG procedures used has shed some insight on the application of these procedures. While the chapter has been written to provide a basic understanding of the process, it is not intended to provide the information needed to perform these procedures. The electrophysiologic testing is an area of specialization that requires advanced didactic and clinical experience.

SUMMARY

1. Electrophysiologic testing is an extension of a good physical examination and normally consists of

   (a) Nerve function evaluation (integrity, speed, and the size of obtained potentials)

   (b) Electromyography (use of a needle assessing muscle action potentials) and less frequently

   (c) SEPs that are capable of evaluating some central nervous system components

2. Specialized equipment is needed to perform an electrophysiologic evaluation. The basic components involved include the following:

   (a) Electrodes (to couple the equipment to the patient to obtain an electrical signal)

   (b) An amplifier to boost the normally small natural change in voltage potentials

   (c) An oscilloscope to observe the response

   (d) A computer to quantify the response

   (e) A stimulator to provide an electrical current to elicit a response

   (f) Speakers to permit audio assessment of the response

   (g) A printer to document findings. Depending on the testing performed, these and potentially other equipment will be used to test the integrity of specific portions of the nervous system.

3. The typical NCS and EMG evaluation primarily focuses on evaluating the PNS, the neuromuscular synapse, and function of muscle fibers. In addition to these peripheral structures, the function of anterior horn cells located in the gray matter of the anterior horn of the spinal cord, and thus technically part of the CNS, can also be evaluated. (As stated in #1 above, specialized testing with additional techniques such as SEPs are needed if more CNS evaluation is required.)

4. Not all nerves conduct with equal speed and the environment that they exist in can affect their function. Nerve conduction velocity tests evaluate the fastest conducting fibers and generally these fibers conduct faster in the upper extremity than in the lower extremity. Additionally, the speed of nerve function is influenced by other factors such as temperature (nerves that are cold conduct slower) and age (the nerves of young and old individuals typically conduct slower than those of young adults).

5. The typical elements of a NCS are:

   (a) Sensory nerve studies that assess the time it takes for a signal to pass over a known distance or latency. This is evaluating the fastest conducting sensory fibers of a segment of a nerve and the small signal is typically measured in μV. In addition to the latency, the size (amplitude), shape, and nerve conduction velocity of the sensory nerve action potential is assessed.

   (b) Motor nerve studies, assessing the ability of the fastest conducting motor axons to conduct to the neuromuscular junction, cross the junction, and activate the innervated muscle fibers. Because this is the combined signal of numerous muscle fibers, the assessed response is much larger than a sensory potential and is measured in mV. Some of the factors evaluated in these studies include latency, amplitude, rise time, duration, shape, and nerve conduction velocity.

   - Other complementary tests can also be performed, such as central conduction studies and H-waves that assess the integrity of the nerve along its entire length, up to the level of the spinal cord and back.

6. The electromyographic evaluation consists of placing some type of small diameter, sterile needle electrode (these vary) into a muscle and obtaining a signal. Abnormal responses during the insertion, examination of the muscle at rest, or during voluntary contraction are noted and correlated with the patient's complaint and physical examination. This portion of the examination is very useful for a wide variety of conditions, including those that result

in abnormal axon function (axonopathy) or in diseases affecting muscle function (myopathies).

7. A NCS/EMG evaluation is a reasonably sensitive and specific test for problems involving anterior horn cells, the peripheral nervous system, the neuromuscular junction, and innervated muscle fibers. The sensitivity and specificity improve when the physical examination provides more than one clinical finding. While reasonable tests, these evaluation procedures are not perfect and false positive electrophysiologic findings have been reported.

8. Electrophysiologic testing is a valuable adjunct to the physical examination, but it does not lend itself to all nerves and muscles. Some nerves and muscles are too technically difficult to assess routinely (e.g., the intercostal nerves and muscles in close proximity to the lungs). The electrophysiologic examination, by itself, is not diagnostic. The electrophysiologic examination confirms the information assessed during the subjective physical examination and provides information the health care provider overseeing an individual's care can consider when making a medical diagnosis.

9. Electrophysiologic testing is a specialty area that requires considerable training, anatomical and physiologic knowledge, and experience.

REVIEW QUESTIONS

1. What are the characteristics of patients that make them prime referral candidates for a NCS/EMG evaluation?

2. In examining the portions of the typical electrophysiologic evaluation (NCS/EMG), what portion of the examination and findings suggest a problem that is predominantly due to the loss of myelin?

3. In examining the portions of the typical electrophysiologic evaluation (NCS/EMG), what portion of the examination and findings suggest a problem that is predominantly due to damage or loss of axons (axonopathy)?

4. Within the context of a nerve conduction study, what is the general principle behind a sensory nerve study compared to a motor nerve study?

5. Two measurements of speed of conduction are latency and nerve conduction velocity. How are these two variables related, how do they differ, and on what are they based?

6. If a patient has a suspected problem with the neuromuscular junction, how will the NCS/EMG examination be modified to address this particular area of the neuromuscular system?

7. How does the duration, shape, and size of motor unit action potentials compare between an individual with normally innervated muscle and an individual with a myopathy?

8. What do the following findings suggest, both in terms of altered function and potential disease processes?

   a. Positive sharp waves

   b. Fibrillations

   c. Fasciculations

   d. Interference pattern that is not uniform and full (dropped motor units)

   e. Myotonic discharges

9. During voluntary contraction of muscle, what is the normally expected order of recruitment of motor units? Why?

10. What are five limitations associated with electrophysiolgical testing, as outlined in the chapter?

REFERENCES

1. Aidley, D., editor: Electrical properties of the nerve axon. In The physiology of excitable cells, New York, 1989, Cambridge University Press, pp. 30–53.

2. Aidley, D., editor: Neuromuscular transmission. In The physiology of excitable cells, ed. 3, New York, 1989, Cambridge University Press, pp. 110–138.

3. Aidley, D., editor: The organization of sensory receptors. In The physiology of excitable cells, New York, 1989, Cambridge University Press, pp. 346–365.

4. Amaral, D.: The anatomical organization of the central nervous system. In Kandel, E., Schwartz, J., and Jessell, T., editors. Principles of neural science, ed. 4, New York, 2000, McGraw-Hill, pp. 317–336.

5. American Association of Electrodiagnostic Medicine: Practice parameter for electrodiagnostic studies in carpal tunnel syndrome: summary statement, Muscle Nerve 16:1390–1391, 1993.

6. Ayotte, K., Boswell, L., and Hansen, D.: A comparison of orthodromic and antidromic sensory neural conduction latencies and amplitudes for the palmar branch of the median and ulnar nerves in healthy subjects, J. Clin. Electrophysiol. 4:12–18, 1992.

7. Bahrami, M., Rayegani, S., and Zare, A.: Studying nerve conduction velocity and latency of accessory nerve motor potential in normal persons, Electromyogr. Clin. Neurophysiol. 44:11–14, 2004.

8. Bawa, P., Binder, M., Ruenzel, P., and Henneman, E.: Recruitment order of motoneurons in stretch reflexes is highly correlated with their axonal conduction velocity, J. Neurophysiol. 52:410–420, 1984.

9. Blijham, P., Hengstman, G., Ter Laak, H., Van Engelen, B., and Zwarts, M.: Muscle-fiber conduction velocity and electromyography as diagnostic tools in patients with suspected inflammatory myopathy: a prospective study, Muscle Nerve 29:46–50, 2004.

10. Boon, A., Harper, C.: Needle EMG of abductor hallicis and peroneus tertius in normal subjects, Muscle Nerve 27:752–756, 2003.

11. Brown, P.: The Electrochemical basis of neuronal integration. In Haines, D., editor. Fundamental neuroscience, New York, 1997, Churchill Livingstone, pp. 31–50.

12. Brumlik, J., Drechsler, B., and Vannin, T.: The myotonic discharge in various neurological syndromes: a neurophysiologic analysis, Electromyography 10:369–383, 1970.

13. Burke, D.: Microneurography, impulse conduction, and paresthesias, Muscle Nerve 16:1025–1032, 1993.

14. Clamann, H., Henneman, E.: Electrical measurement of axon diameter and its use in relating motoneuron size to critical firing level, J. Neurophysiol. 39:844–851, 1976.

15. Daube, J.A.: AAEM minimonograph #11: needle examination in electromyography, Rochester, MN, 1979, AAEM.

16. Davidoff, R.: Skeletal muscle tone and the misunderstood stretch reflex, Neurology 42:951–963, 1992.

17. Dillingham, T.: Electrodiagnostic approach to patients with suspected radiculopathy, Phys. Med. Rehabil. Clin. N. Am. 14:567–588, 2003.

18. Dobner, J., Nitz, A.: Postmeniscectomy tourniquet palsy and functional sequelae, Am. J. Sports Med. 10:211–214, 1982.

19. Dorfman, L., Howard, J., and McGill, K.: Motor unit firing rates and firing variability in the detection of neuromuscular disorders, Electroenceph. Clin. Neurophysiol. 73:215–224, 1989.

20. Dumitru, D., editor: AAEM glossary of terms. In Electrodiagnostic medicine, Philadelphia, PA, 1995, Hanley & Belfus, pp. 1172–1208.

21. Dumitru, D.: Needle electromyography. In Electrodiagnostic medicine, Philadelphia, PA, 1995, Hanley & Belfus, pp. 211–248.

22. Dumitru, D., editor: Nerve and muscle anatomy and physiology. In Electrodiagnostic medicine, Philadelphia, PA, 1995, Hanley & Belfus, pp. 3–28.

23. Dumitru, D., editor: Nerve conduction studies. In Electrodiagnostic medicine, Philadelphia, PA, 1995, Hanley & Belfus, pp. 111–176.

24. Dumitru, D., editor: Neuromuscular junction disorders. In Electrodiagnostic medicine, Philadelphia, PA, 1995, Hanley & Belfus, pp. 929–1030.

25. Dumitru, D., editor: Special nerve conduction techniques. In Electrodiagnostic medicine, Philadelphia, PA, 1995, Hanley & Belfus, pp. 177–209.

26. Dumitru, D., editor: Volume conduction. In Electrodiagnostic medicine, Philadelphia, PA, 1995, Hanley & Belfus, pp. 29–64.

27. Dumitru, D., Instrumentation. In Dumitru, D., Amato, A., and Zwarts, M., editors. Electrodiagnostic medicine, ed. 2, Philadelphia, PA, 2002, Hanley & Belfus, pp. 69–97.

28. Dumitru, D. editor: Needle electromyography. In Dumitru, D., Amato, A., and Zwarts, M., editors. Electrodiagnostic medicine, Philadelphia, PA, 2002, Hanley & Belfus, pp. 257–291.

29. Dumitru, D., editor: Special nerve conduction techniques. In Electrodiagnostic medicine, Philadelphia, PA, 2002, Hanley & Belfus, pp. 225–256.

30. Dumitru, D., Amato, A.: Introduction to myopathies and muscle tissue's reaction to injury. In Dumitru, D., Amato, A., and Zwarts, M., editors. Electrodiagnostic medicine, ed. 3, Philadelphia, PA, 2002, Hanley & Belfus, pp. 1229–1264.

31. Dumitru, D., Amato, A., and Zwarts, M.: Electrodiagnostic medicine, ed. 2. Philadelphia, PA, 2002, Hanley & Belfus.

32. Dumitru, D., Amato, A., and Zwarts, M.: Nerve conduction studies. In Dumitru, D., Amato, A., and Zwarts, M., editors. Electrodiagnostic medicine, ed. 2, Philadelphia, PA, 2002. Hanley & Belfus, pp. 159–223.

33. Dumitru, D., Gitter, A.: Nerve and muscle anatomy and physiology. In Dumitru, D., Amato, A., and Zwarts, M., editors. Electrodiagnostic medicine, ed. 2, Philadelphia, PA, 2002, Hanley & Belfus, pp. 3–26.

34. Dumitru, D., King, J., and Stegeman, D.: Normal needle electromyographic insertional activity morphology: a clinical and simulation study, Muscle Nerve 21:910–920, 1998.

35. Dumitru, D., Robinson, L., and Zwarts, M.: Somatosensory evoked potentials. In Dumitru, D., Amato, A., and Zwarts, M., editors. Electrodiagnostic medicine, ed. 2, Philadelphia, PA, 2002, Hanley & Belfus, pp. 357–414.

36. Dumitru, D., Stegeman, D., and Zwarts, M.: Electrical sources and volume conduction. In Dumitru, D., Amato, A., and Zwarts M., editors. Electrodiagnostic medicine, ed. 2, Philadelphia, PA, 2002, Hanley & Belfus, pp. 27–53.

37. Dumitru, D., Zwarts, M.: Electrodiagnostic medicine pitfalls. In Dumitru, D., Amato, A., and Zwarts, M., editors. Electrodiagnostic medicine, ed. 2, Philadelphia, PA, 2002, Hanley & Belfus, pp. 541–577.

38. Dumitru, D., Zwarts M.: Focal peripheral neuropathies. In Dumitru, D., Amato, A., and Zwarts, M., editors. Electrodiagnostic medicine, ed. 2, Philadelphia, PA, 2002, Hanley & Belfus, pp. 1043–1126.

39. Ellenberg, M., Gardin, H., Hyman, S., and Chodoroff, G.: Orthodromic vs. antidromic latencies, Arch. Phys. Med. Rehabil. 72:431–432, 1991.

40. Finsterer, J., Fuglsang-Frederiksen, A.: Concentric-needle versus macro EMG. II. Detection of neuromuscular disorders, Clin. Neurophysiol. 112:853–860, 2001.

41. Fisher, M.: F response latency determination, Muscle Nerve 5:730–734, 1982.

42. Fritz, J., Wainner, R.: Examining diagnostic tests: an evidence-based perspective, Phys. Ther. 81:1546–1564, 2001.

43. Goodgold, J., Eberstein, A.: The normal electromyogram. In Goodgold, J., Eberstein, A., editors. Electrodiagnosis of neuromuscular diseases, Baltimore, MD, 1972, Williams & Wilkins, pp. 60–73.

44. Goodgold, J., Eberstein, A.: Myopathy. In Goodgold, J., Eberstein, A., editors. Electrodiagnosis of neuromuscular diseases, Baltimore, MD, 1972,Williams & Wilkins, pp. 116–138.

45. Greathouse, D.G., Halle, J.S.: Neural conduction study guidelines—laboratory values. Electrophysiology Laboratory, 2004, Blanchfield Army Community Hospital.

46. Guyton, A.: Textbook of medical physiology, ed. 8, Philadelphia, PA, 1991, W.B. Saunders, pp. 38–50.

47. Haines, D., Mihailoff, G., and Yezierski, R.: The spinal cord. In Haines, D., editor. Fundamental neuroscience, New York, 1997, Churchill Livingstone, pp. 129–141.

48. Halle, J., Scoville, C., and Greathouse, D.: Ultrasound's effect on the conduction latency of the superficial radial nerve in man, Phys. Ther. 61:345–350, 1981.

49. Hanson, P., Deltombe, T.: Preliminary study of large and small peripheral nerve fibers in Charcot-Marie-Tooth disease, type I, Am. J. Phys. Med. Rehabil. 77:45–48, 1998.

50. Hassantash, S., Afrakhteh, M., and Maier, R.: Causalgia: a meta-analysis of the literature, Arch. Surg. 138:1226–1231, 2003.

51. Howard, F.J.: The electromyogram and conduction velocity studies in peripheral nerve trauma, Clin. Neurosurg. 17:63–75, 1970.

52. Howard, J., McGill, K., and Dorfman, L.: Age effects on properties of motor unit action potentials: ADEMG analysis, Ann. Neurol. 24:207–213, 1988.

53. Jablecki, C., Andary, M., and So, Y.: Literature review of the usefulness of nerve conduction studies and electromyography for the evaluation of patients with carpal tunnel syndrome, Muscle Nerve 16:1392–1414, 1993.

54. Kandel, E., Siegelbaum, S.: Signaling at the nerve-muscle synapse: directly gated transmission. In Kandel, E., Schwartz, J., and Jessell, T., editors. Principles of neural science, ed. 4, New York, 2000, McGraw-Hill, pp. 187–206.

55. Kawamura, Y., Okazaki, H., O'Brien, P., and Dych, P.: Lumbar motoneurons of man: I) number and diameter histogram of alpha and gamma axons of ventral root, J. Neuropathol. Exp. Neurol. 36:853–860, 1977.

56. Kimura, J.: Proximal versus distal slowing of motor nerve conduction velocity in the Guillain-Barre syndrome, Ann. Neurol. 3:344–350, 1978.

57. Kimura, J.: Electrodiagnosis in diseases of nerve and muscle, ed. 2, Philadelphia, PA, 1989, F.A. Davis.

58. Kimura, J., editor: Principles of nerve conduction studies. In Electrodiagnosis in diseases of nerve and muscle, Philadelphia, PA, 1989, F.A. Davis, pp. 78–102.

59. Kimura, J., editor: Somatosensory and motor evoked potentials. In Electrodiagnosis in diseases of nerve and muscle, ed. 2, Philadelphia, PA, 1989, F.A. Davis, pp. 375–426.

60. Kimura, J., editor: Techniques and normal findings. In Electrodiagnosis in diseases of nerve and muscle: principles and practice, ed. 2, Philadelphia, PA, 1989, F.A. Davis, pp. 227–248.

61. Kimura, J., editor: The F wave. In Electrodiagnosis in diseases of nerve and muscle: principles and practice, ed. 2, Philadelphia, PA, 1989, F.A. Davis, pp. 332–355.

62. Kimura, J., editor: Types of abnormality. In Electrodiagnosis in diseases of nerve and muscle: principles and practice, ed. 2, Philadelphia, PA, 1989, F.A. Davis, pp. 249–274.

63. Kimura, J., Butzer, J.: F-wave conduction velocity in Guillain-Barre syndrome: assessment of nerve segment between axilla and spinal cord, Arch. Neurol. 32:524–529, 1975.

64. Kimura, J., Yamada, T., and Stevland, N.: Distal slowing of motor nerve conduction velocity in diabetic polyneuropathy, J. Neurol. Sci. 42:291–302, 1979.

65. Knaflitz, M., Merletti, R., and De Luca, C.: Inference of motor unit recruitment order in voluntary and electrically elicited contractions, J. Appl. Physiol. 68:1657–1667, 1990.

66. Kuntzer, T.: Carpal tunnel syndrome in 100 patients: sensitivity, specificity on multi-neurophysiological procedures and estimation of axonal loss of motor, sensory and sympathetic median nerve fibers, J. Neurol. Sci. 20:221–229, 1994.

67. LaHoda, F., Russ, A., and Issel, W., editors: Electromyography. In EMG primer, Berlin, GE, 1974, Springer-Verlag, p. 16.

68. Lopez, J.: The use of evoked potentials in intraoperative neurophysiologic monitoring, Phys. Med. Rehabil. Clin. N. Am. 15:63–84, 2004.

69. Lundborg, G., Dahlin, L.: Pathophysiology of nerve compression. In Szabo, R., editor. Nerve compression syndromes: diagnosis and treatment, Thorofare, NJ, 1989, Slack Incorporated, pp. 15–39.

70. Magladery, J., McDougal, D.J.: Electrophysiological studies of nerve and reflex activity in normal man, Bull. Johns Hopkins Hosp. 86:265–290, 1950.

71. Mayo Clinic: Mayo Clinic EMG Laboratory Procedure Manual, Rochester, MN, 1992, Mayo Clinic.

72. Miller, T., Pardo, R., and Yaworski, R.: Clinical utility of reflex studies in assessing cervical radiculopathy, Muscle Nerve 22:1075–1079, 1999.

73. Moore, K., Dalley, A.: Clinically oriented anatomy, Philadelphia, PA, 1999, Lippincott Williams & Wilkins.

74. Naftel, J., Hardy, S.: Visceral motor pathways. In Haines, D., editor. Fundamental neuroscience, New York, 1997, Churchill Livingstone, pp. 417–430.

75. Nandedkar, S., Stalberg, E., and Sanders, D.: Quantitative EMG. In Dumitru, D., Amato, A., and Zwarts, M., editors. Electrodiagnostic medicine, ed. 2, Philadelphia, PA, 2002, Hanley & Belfus, pp. 293–356.

76. Nardin, R., Patel, M., Gudas, T., Rutkove, S., and Raynor, E.: Electromyography and magnetic resonance imaging in the evaluation of radiculopathy, Muscle Nerve 22:149–150, 1999.

77. Nelson, R., Nestor, D.: Electrophysiological evaluation: an overview. In Nelson, R., Currier, D., editors. Clinical electrotherapy, Norwalk, CT, 1991, Appleton & Lange, pp. 331–384.

78. Nelson, R., Shedlock, M., Kaczmarek, C., Gahrs, J., and MacLaughlin, H.: Comparison of motor unit action potentials using monopolar vs. concentric needle electrodes in the middle deltoid and abductor digiti minimi muscles, Electromyogr. Clin. Neurophysiol. 43:459–464, 2003.

79. Nestor, D.E., Nelson, R.M.: Performing motor and sensory neuronal conduction studies in adult humans—A NIOSH technical manual. DHHS (NIOSH) Publication No. 89-XXX. 1987, Morgantown, WV, Division of Safety Research, National Institute for Occupational Safety and Health.

80. Ochoa, J., Danta, G., and Fowler, T.: Nature of the nerve lesion caused by a pneumatic tourniquet, Nature 233:265–266, 1971.

81. Ochoa, J., Fowler, T., and Gilliatt, R.: Anatomical changes in peripheral nerves caused by a pneumatic tourniquet, J. Anat. 113:433–455, 1972.

82. Oh, S.: Clinical electromyography—nerve conduction studies, ed. 2, Baltimore, MD, 1993, Williams & Wilkins.

83. Oh, S., editor: Physiological factors affecting nerve conduction. In Clinical electromyography—nerve conduction studies, ed. 2, Baltimore, MD, 1993, Williams & Wilkins, pp. 297–313.

84. Oh, S., editor: Somatosensory evoked potentials in peripheral nerve lesions. In Clinical electromyograph—nerve conduction studies, ed. 2, Baltimore, MD, 1993, Williams & Wilkins, pp. 447–478.

85. Preston, D., Shapiro, B.: Needle electromyography: fundamentals, normal and abnormal patterns, Neurol. Clin. 20:361–396, 2002.

86. Prout, B.: Independence of the galvanic skin reflex from the vasoconstrictor reflex in man, J. Neurol. Neurosurg. Psychiatr. 30:319–324, 1967.

87. Redmond, M., Rivner, M.: False positive electrodiagnostic tests in carpal tunnel syndrome, Muscle Nerve 11:511–518, 1988.

88. Richman, D., Agius, M.: Treatment of autoimmune myasthenia gravis, Neurology 61:1652–1661, 2003.

89. Ross, M., Kaye, G., and Pawlina, W., editors: Nerve tissue. In Histology: a text and atlas, ed. 4, Baltimore, MD, 2003, Lippincott Williams & Wilkins, pp. 282–325.

90. Rutkove, S.: Effects of temperature on neuromuscular electrophysiology, Muscle Nerve 24:867–882, 2001.

91. Seddon, H.: Three types of nerve injury, Brain 66:237–288, 1943.

92. Seror, P.: The medial antebrachial cutaneous nerve: antidromic and orthodromic conduction studies, Muscle Nerve 26:421–423, 2002.

93. Shakir, A., Micklesen, P., and Robinson, L.: Which motor nerve conduction study is best in ulnar neuropathy at the elbow? Muscle Nerve 29:585–590, 2004.

94. Slimp, J.: Electrophysiologic intraoperative monitoring for spine procedures, Phys. Med. Rehabil. Clin. N. Am. 15:85–105, 2004.

95. Stevens, J.: AAEM minimonograph #26: the electrodiagnosis of carpal tunnel syndrome, Muscle Nerve 20:1477–1486, 1997.

96. Storm, S., Kraft, G.: The clinical use of dermatomal somatosensory evoked potentials in lumbosacral spinal stenosis, Phys. Med. Rehabil. Clin. N. Am. 15:107–115, 2004.

97. Takamori, M., Komai, K., and Iwasa, K.: Antibodies to calcium channel and synaptotagmin in Lambert-Eaton myasthenic syndrome, Am. J. Med. Sci. 319:204–208, 2000.

98. Tasaki, I.: Electric stimulation and the excitatory process in the nerve fiber, Am. J. Physiol. 125:395, 1939.

99. Torebjork, E.: Human microneurography and intraneural microstimulation in the study of neuropathic pain, Muscle Nerve 19:1483, 1993.

100. Troni, W.: The value and limits of the H reflex as a diagnostic tool in S1 root compression, Electromyogr. Clin. Neurophysiol. 23:471–480, 1983.

101. Ulas, U., Cengiz, B., Alanoglu, E., Ozdag, M., Odabasi, Z., and Vural, O.: Comparison of sensitivities of macro EMG and concentric needle EMG in L4 radiculopathy, Neurol. Sci. 24:258–260, 2003.

102. Wainner, R., Fritz, J., Irrgang, J., Boninger, M., Delitto, A., and Allison, S.: Reliability and diagnostic accuracy of the clinical examination and patient self-report measures for cervical radiculopathy, Spine 28:52–62, 2003.

103. Warren, S., Capra, N., and Yezierski, R.: The somatosensory system II: nondiscriminative touch, temperature, and nociception. In Haines, D., editor. Fundamental neuroscience, New York, 1997, Churchill Livingstone, pp. 237–254.

104. Warren, S., Yezierski, R., and Capra, N.: The Somatosensory system I: discriminative touch and position sense. In Haines, D., editor. Fundamental neuroscience, New York, 1997, Churchill Livingstone, pp. 219–236.

105. Waxman, S.G., Foster, R.E.: Ionic channel distribution and heterogeneity of the axon membrane in myelinated fibers, Brain Res. Rev. 2:205–234, 1980.

106. Wiechers, D.: Mechanically provoked insertional activity before and after nerve section in rats, Arch. Phys. Med. Rehabil. 58:402–405, 1977.

107. Wiechers, D., Stow, R., and Johnson, E.: Electromyographic insertional activity mechanically provoked in the biceps brachii, Arch. Phys. Med. Rehabil. 58:573–578, 1977.

108. Wilbourn, A.: Sensory nerve conduction studies, J. Clin. Neurophysiol. 11:584–601, 1994.

Afferent Axons from neurons carrying a signal toward the spinal cord (a sensory fiber).

Amplitude The size of the potential. In a sensory nerve assessment, this represents the summed action potential traveling across one point of that nerve. In a motor nerve assessment, this represents the summed action potentials traveling across the collective muscle fibers under the pickup electrode. Motor amplitudes are typically much larger than sensory action potentials.

Anterior (ventral) primary rami A branch of a mixed spinal nerve emanating from the spinal cord that carries both motor and sensory axons. The anterior primary rami are the origin of the fibers that make up the various plexi and named peripheral nerves.

Antidromic An electrical signal conducted in a direction that is opposite of normal. For example, for sensory neurons, an antidromic conduction would be toward the periphery.

Axonopathy Disease or pathology involving an axon.

Biphasic A nerve potential with two phases.

Compound motor action potential (CMAP) The action potential generated by stimulating a nerve that innervates the muscle under investigation. This CMAP represents the collective action potentials passing across all of the muscle fibers under the pickup electrode.

Demyelination Damage or removal of the myelin sheath that covers myelinated nerves. This results in slowed or blocked conduction of an electrical signal along individual axons and the collective nerve.

Differential amplifier The action potentials passing across nerves or over muscle fibers are small and need to be amplified to seen, heard, and measured. A differential amplifier boosts the signal strength and subtracts out the portions of the signal that are common to both the active and reference electrodes.

Distal motor latency (DML) The time that it takes from stimulation of a motor nerve to pick-up of the action potentials traveling across the appropriately innervated muscle fibers. Note that this action potential travels down to the distal end of the nerve, crosses the neuromuscular junction, and elicits a contraction of the muscle under investigation. Since this is a latency value, the time is compared to a table of normal values, for that known measured distance.

Distal sensory latency (DSL) The time that it takes from stimulation to pick-up of a peripheral sensory nerve, measured in milliseconds. Since this is a latency value, the time is compared to a table of normal values for that known measured distance.

Duration The length of time that the compound motor action potential persists, measured in milliseconds.

Efferent Axons from neurons carrying a signal away from the spinal cord (a motor fiber).

Electromyographic studies The needle electrode portion of the examination that typically involves four steps: needle insertion, observation of electrical activity at rest, observation of electrical activity during voluntary contraction ranging from minimal to maximal, and information synthesis.

Erb's point A stimulation point where the brachial plexus can be activated. The point of stimulation is located supraclavicularly at the midportion of the clavicle.

Fasciculation potential The potential associated with the random and spontaneous activation of a group of muscle fibers or all of the muscle fibers originating from a motor unit. These are large enough to be felt, such as an "eyelid twitch" when an individual is tired. Cause can be something as innocent as fatigue or it may be indicative of a serious problem.

Fibrillation potential Represents the electrical activity associated with the spontaneous contraction of a single muscle fiber.

F-wave (central conduction study) An electrically stimulated action potential that travels antidromically to the spinal cord (anterior horn cells) and then is bounced back orthodromically to elicit a secondary contraction of the muscle under investigation. This central conduction study provides a way of looking at the entire loop from the point of stimulation, to the spinal cord, and back again. Through the obtained latency values, clinical judgments can be made.

Henneman size principle A skeletal muscle consists of potentially hundreds of motor units of different sizes. Voluntary recruitment in the central nervous system of the spinal cord occurs in an orderly manner, recruiting the different size units from small to large. Functionally, this recruits the smaller neurons associated with slow twitch, high endurance muscle fibers prior to recruiting the larger motor neurons associated with the more easily fatigable fast twitch muscle fibers.

Hoffman's reflex (H-wave) An electrically stimulated reflex that is a physiologic example of the normal reflex arc (entering the spinal cord by way of afferent neurons and exiting via efferent motor neurons). This reflex can only be elicited in a few muscles (such as the calf muscles) but has clinical utility in conditions like an S1 radiculopathy.

Latency The time that it takes from the stimulus to the response over a predetermined distance, measured in milliseconds.

Myopathic An acquired or congenital disease that clinically presents with either focal or diffuse muscular weakness. A myopathic process is characterized electrophysiologically by short duration and low amplitude motor action potentials.

Myotonic discharges A sustained run of potentials that wax and wane, sounding over a loud speaker like a "dive bomber." Visually, these resemble either or both fibrillation potentials and positive sharp waves. These discharges are found in conditions like myotonic dystrophy.

Nerve conduction studies Studies that evaluate the ability of a nerve to conduct an electrical signal. These are performed in ways that assess the sensory fibers within a nerve, specific segments of a nerve (either sensory or motor fibers), or the combined contribution of the neuromuscular junction and the innervated muscle fibers of the nerve under investigation.

Nerve conduction velocity (NCV) The speed by which an action potential travels down a peripheral nerve, measured in meters/second (distance/latency = NCV). This measures only the fastest conducting fibers, because the measured response is the first detected arrival of the action potential at the pickup electrode.

Neuromuscular junction The junction between the distal end of a nerve fiber and the muscle fibers that it innervates. Communication at this junction site is done via the neurotransmitter acetylcholine.

NONTHERMAL EFFECTS

Pulsed shortwave diathermy has also been used for its nonthermal effects in the treatment of soft-tissue injuries and wounds.[22]

The mechanism of its effectiveness has been theorized to occur at the cellular level, relating specifically to cell membrane potential.[24] Damaged cells undergo depolarization, resulting in cell dysfunction that might include loss of cell division and proliferation and loss of regenerative capabilities. Pulsed shortwave diathermy has been said to repolarize damaged cells, thus correcting cell dysfunction.[33]

It has also been suggested that sodium tends to accumulate in the cell because of a decrease in activity of the sodium pump during the inflammatory process, thus creating a negatively charged environment. When a magnetic field is induced, the sodium pump is reactivated, thus allowing the cell to regain normal ionic balance.[44]

SHORTWAVE DIATHERMY EQUIPMENT AND TREATMENT TECHNIQUES

A shortwave diathermy unit is basically a radio transmitter. **The Federal Communications Commission (FCC)** assigned three frequencies to shortwave diathermy units: the first is 27.12 MHz with a wavelength of 11 m; the second is 13.56 MHz with a wavelength of 22 m; and the third, although rarely used, is 40.68 MHz with a wavelength of 7.5 m (see Fig. 10-2).

SHORTWAVE DIATHERMY GENERATORS

The shortwave diathermy unit consists of a power supply that provides power to a radio frequency oscillator (Fig. 10-1). This radio frequency oscillator provides stable, drift-free oscillations at the required frequency. The power amplifier generates the power required to drive the different types of electrodes. The output resonant tank tunes in the patient as part of the circuit and allows maximum power to be transferred to the patient.

Figure 10-2 shows the control panel of a shortwave diathermy unit. The output intensity knob controls the percentage of maximum power transferred to the patient circuit. This is similar to the volume control on a radio. The tuning control adjusts the output circuit for maximum energy transfer from the radio frequency oscillator, which is similar to tuning in a station on a radio. The power output meter monitors only the current that is drawn from the power supply and not the energy being delivered to the patient. Thus, it is only an indirect measure of the energy reaching the patient.

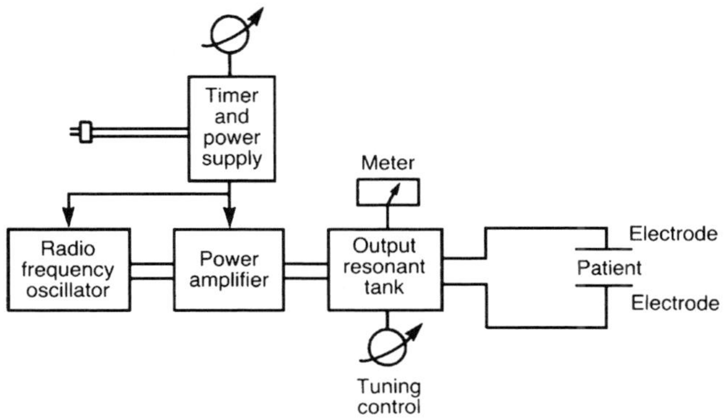

Pulsed Shortwave Diathermy
- Pulsed electromagnetic energy (PEME)
- Pulsed electromagnetic field (PEMF)
- Pulsed electromagnetic energy treatment (PEMET)

Pulsed shortwave diathermy = nonthermal effects

Treatment Tip
Pulsed shortwave diathermy is capable of heating a much larger area than ultrasound; the applicator is stationary so the heat applied to the area is more constant; the rate of temperature decay is slower following diathermy application allowing more time for stretching; using diathermy doesn't require constant monitoring.

Pulsed shortwave diathermy uses drum electrodes.

Federal Communications Commission (FCC) Federal agency charged with assigning frequencies for all radio transmitters, including diathermies.

•**Figure 10-1** The component parts of a shortwave diathermy unit.

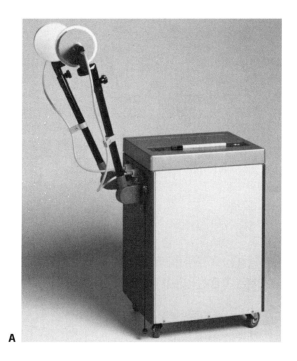

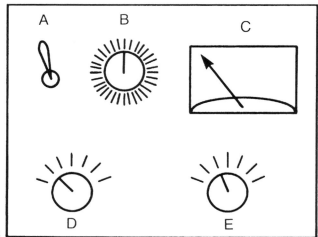

•**Figure 10-2 A.** Shortwave diathermy unit. **B.** Control panel of a shortwave diathermy unit: *A,* Power switch; *B,* timer; *C,* output power meter (monitors current drawn from power supply only and not in patient circuit); *D,* output intensity (controls the percentage of maximum power transferred to the patient); and *E,* tuning control (tunes the output circuit for maximum energy transfer from radio frequency oscillator).

specific absorption rate (SAR) Represents the rate of energy absorbed per unit area of tissue mass.

The power output of a shortwave diathermy unit should produce sufficient energy to raise the tissue temperature into a therapeutic range. The **specific absorption rate (SAR)** represents the rate of energy absorbed per unit area of tissue mass. Most shortwave units have a power output of between 80 and 120 W.

Some units are not capable of this, making them safe but ineffective. It is important to remember that the tissue temperature rise with diathermy units can be offset dramatically by an increase in blood flow, which has a cooling effect in the tissue being energized. Therefore, units should be able to generate enough power to provide for an excess of the SAR.

Patient sensation provides the basis for recommendations of continuous shortwave diathermy dosage and thus varies considerably with different patients.[29,44] The following dosage guidelines have been recommended.

Dose I (lowest): No sensation of heat
Dose II (low): Mild heating sensation
Dose III (medium): Moderate (pleasant) heating sensation
Dose IV (heavy): Vigorous heating that is tolerable below the pain threshold

Some older shortwave diathermy generators have manual tuning although the majority of new models do have automatic tuning devices. If the machine is not an automatically tuning type, it is necessary to tune the patient's circuit to resonance with the oscillating circuit of the unit. This is accomplished by placing the electrodes over the area to be treated and then setting the output intensity at 30–40 percent. Then, the variable capacitor in the generator's circuitry can be adjusted by using the meter on the generator to determine the peak tuning readings. These readings should not be confused as an indication of the power received by the patient. The tuning control should be adjusted until the output power meter moves to the maximum and then it should be adjusted down to patient tolerance, which is usually about 50 percent of maximum output. If more than 50 percent of the available power on the meter is used, then the patient's setup is out of tune or out of resonance. Shortwave diathermy units with automatic tuning turn off the power when the patient circuit is out of tune.

A shortwave diathermy unit that generates a high-frequency electrical current will produce both an **electrical field** and a **magnetic field** in the tissues.[14] The ratio of the electrical field to the magnetic field depends on the characteristics of the different units as well as on the characteristics of electrodes or applicators. Shortwave units with a frequency of 13.56 MHz tend to produce a stronger magnetic field than do units with the frequency of 27.12 MHz, which produces a stronger electric field. The majority of the new pulsed shortwave diathermy units use a drum electrode and produce a stronger magnetic field.

electrical field The lines of force exerted on charged ions in the tissues by the electrodes that cause charged particles to move from one pole to the other.

magnetic field Created when current is passed through a coiled cable affecting surrounding tissues by inducing localized secondary currents, called eddy currents within the tissues.

SHORTWAVE DIATHERMY ELECTRODES

Shortwave diathermy may be delivered to the patient via either capacitance or induction techniques. Each of these techniques can affect different biologic tissues, and selection of the appropriate electrodes is essential for effective treatment.

The shortwave diathermy uses several types of applicators or electrodes, including air space plates, pad electrodes, cable electrodes, or drum electrodes.

Capacitor Electrodes

The capacitance technique, using **capacitor electrodes**, creates a stronger electrical field than a magnetic field. As discussed in Chapter 7, within the body there are many free ions that are positively or negatively charged. A positively charged electrode or plate will repel positively charged ions and attract negatively charged ions. Conversely, the negative electrode will repel negative ions and attract positive ions (Fig. 10-3).

An electrical field is essentially the lines of force exerted on these charged ions by the electrodes that cause charged particles to move from one pole to the other (Fig. 10-4). The intensity of the electrical field is determined by the spacing of the electrodes and is greatest when they are close together. The center of this electrical field has a higher current density than regions at the periphery. When using capacitance electrodes, the patient is placed between two electrodes or plates and becomes part of the circuit. Thus, the tissue between the two electrodes is in a series circuit arrangement (see Chapter 5).

As the electrical field is created in the biologic tissues, the tissue that offers the greatest resistance to current flow tends to develop the most heat. Tissues that have a high fat content tend to insulate and resist the passage of an electrical field. These tissues, particularly subcutaneous fat, tend to overheat when an electrical field is used, which is characteristic of a capacitance type of electrode application.

Capacitor Electrodes
• Air space plates
• Pad electrodes

capacitor electrodes Air space plates or pad electrode that creates a stronger electrical field than a magnetic field.

Capacitor electrodes = strong electrical field

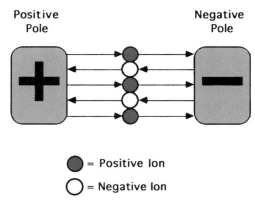

Positive Pole   Negative Pole

● = Positive Ion

○ = Negative Ion

•**Figure 10-3** A positively charged electrode or plate will repel positively charged ions and attract negatively charged ions. Conversely, the negative electrode will repel negative ions and attract positive ions.

Air Space Plates

Air space plates are an example of a capacitance (strong electrical field) technique or a capacitor electrode. This type of electrode consists of two metal plates with a diameter of 7.5–17.5 cm surrounded by a glass or plastic plate guard. The metal plates may be adjusted approximately 3 cm within the plate guard, thus changing the distance from the skin (Fig. 10-5).[24] Air space plates produce high-frequency oscillating current that is passed through each plate millions of times per second. When one plate is overloaded, it discharges to the other plate of the lower potential, and this is reversed millions of times per second.[16]

When air space plates are used, the area to be treated is placed between the electrodes and becomes part of the external circuit (Fig. 10-6). The sensation of heat tends to be in direct proportion to the distance of the plate from the skin. The closer the plate is to the skin, the better the energy transmission because there is less reflection of the energy. However, it should be remembered that the closer plate will also generate more

air space plate A capacitor type electrode in which the plates are separated from the skin by the space in a glass case. Used with shortwave diathermy.

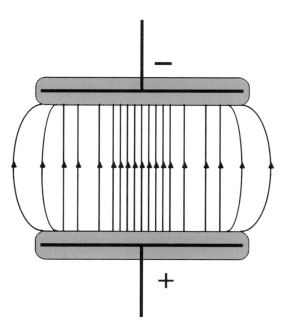

•**Figure 10-4** An electrical field is essentially the lines of force exerted on these charged ions by the electrodes that cause charged particles to move from one pole to the other. (Modified from Michlovitz, S.: Thermal agents in rehabilitation, Philadelphia, PA, 1990, F.A. Davis.)

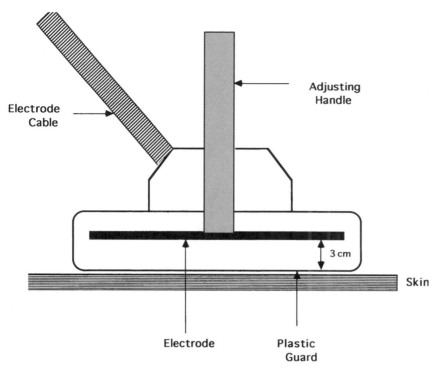

•**Figure 10-5** Air space plate electrodes consist of a metal plate enclosed in a glass or plastic plate guard. The metal plate may be adjusted approximately 3 cm within the plate guard, thus changing the distance from the skin.

surface heat in the skin and the subcutaneous fat in that area (Fig. 10-7). The greatest surface heat will be under the electrodes. Parts of the body that are low in subcutaneous fat content (e.g., hands, feet, wrists, and ankles) are best treated by this method. Patients who have a very low subcutaneous fat content can be effectively treated in other body areas.[15] This technique is also very effective for treating the spine and the ribs.

Pad Electrodes

Pad electrodes are seldom used in the clinical setting; however, they may be available for some units. They are true capacitor electrodes, and they must have uniform contact pressure on the body part if they are to be effective in producing deep heat, as well as in

pad electrodes Capacitor type electrode used with shortwave diathermy to create an electrical field.

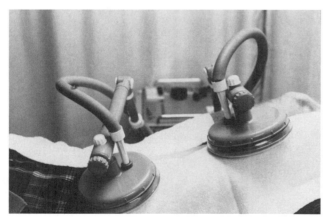

•**Figure 10-6** Treatment of the low back with air space plates. The patient is in a series setup.

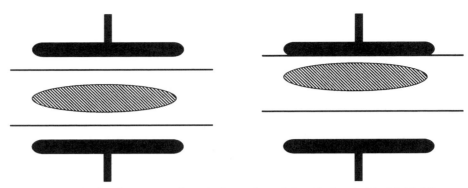

•**Figure 10-7** As the plate moves closer to the surface of the skin the electrical field shifts, generating more surface heat in the skin and the subcutaneous fat.

avoiding skin burns (Fig. 10-8). The patient is part of the external circuit. Several layers of toweling are necessary to make sure that there is sufficient space between the skin and the pads. The pads should be separated such that they are at least as far apart as the cross-sectional diameter of the pads. In other words, if the pads are 15 cm across, then there should be at least 15 cm between the pads. The closer the spacing of the pads, the higher the current density in the superficial tissues. Increasing the space between the pads will increase the depth of penetration in the tissues (Fig. 10-9). The part of the body to be treated should be centered between the pads.[14,16,19,27]

Induction Electrodes

The inductance technique, using **induction electrodes**, creates a stronger magnetic field than an electrical field. When the induction technique is used in shortwave diathermy, a cable or coil is either wrapped circumferentially around an extremity or it is coiled within an electrode. In either case, when current is passed through a coiled cable a magnetic field is generated that can affect surrounding tissues by inducing localized secondary currents, called **eddy currents**, within the tissues (Fig. 10-10).[24] Eddy currents are small circular electrical fields, and the **intermolecular oscillation (vibration)** of tissue contents causes heat generation.

In the induction technique, the patient is in a magnetic field and is not part of the circuit. The tissues are in a parallel circuit, thus the greatest current flow is through the tissues with least resistance (see Chapter 5). When a magnetic field is used with an

induction electrodes Cable electrodes or drum electrodes that create a stronger magnetic field than electrical field.

intermolecular vibration Movement between molecules that produces friction and thus heat.

eddy currents Small circular electrical fields induced when a magnetic field is created the result in intramolecular oscillation (vibration) of tissue contents, causing heat generation.

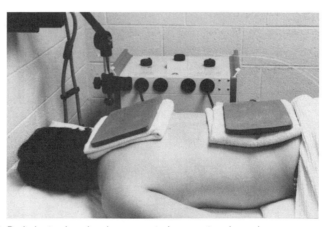

•**Figure 10-8** Pad electrodes showing correct placement and spacing.

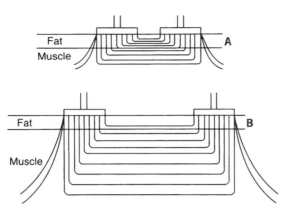

•**Figure 10-9** Pad electrodes should be separated by at least the diameter of the electrodes. **A.** Electrodes placed close together produce more superficial heating. **B.** As spacing increases, the current density increases in the deeper tissues.

induction-type setup, the fat does not provide nearly as much resistance to the flow of the energy. Therefore, tissues that are high in electrolytic content (i.e., muscle and blood) respond best to the magnetic field by producing heat. It is important to remember that if the energy is owing primarily to generation of a magnetic field, heating may not be as obvious to the patient because the magnetic field will not provide nearly as much sensation of warmth in the skin as an electrical field.

Cable Electrodes

The **cable electrode** is an induction electrode, which produces a magnetic field (Fig. 10-11). There are two basic types of arrangements: the pancake coil and the wraparound coil. If a pancake coil is used, the size of the smaller circle should be greater than 6 inches in diameter. In either arrangement, there should be at least 1 cm of toweling between the cable and the skin. Stiff spacers should be used to keep the coils or the turns of the pancake or the wraparound coil between 5 and 10 cm between turns of the cable, thus providing spacing consistency. Both the pancake coils and the wraparound coils often provide more even heating because they are able to follow the contours of the skin than are the drum or the air space plates. It is important that the cables not touch each other because they will short out and cause excessive heat buildup. Diathermy units that operate on a frequency of 13.56 MHz are probably best suited to cable electrode-type applications. This is primarily because the lower frequency provides better production of a magnetic field.[15]

cable electrodes An inductance type electrode in which the electrodes are coiled around a body part, creating an electromagnetic field.

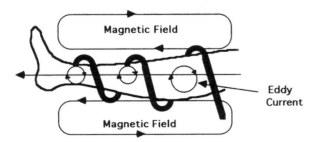

•**Figure 10-10** When current is passed through a coiled cable, a magnetic field is generated that can affect surrounding tissues by inducing localized secondary currents, called eddy currents, within the tissues. (Modified from Michlovitz, S.: Thermal agents in rehabilitation, Philadelphia, PA, 1990, F.A. Davis.)

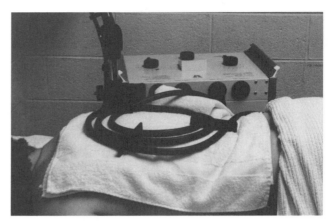

•**Figure 10-11** Pancake cable electrode.

Drum Electrodes

The **drum electrode** also produces a magnetic field. The drum electrode is made up of one or more monoplanar coils that are rigidly fixed inside some kind of housing (Fig. 10-12). If a small area is to be treated, particularly a small flat area, then a one-drum setup is fine. However, if the area is contoured, then two or more drums, which may be on a hinged apparatus or hinged arm, may be more suitable.

Penetration into the tissues tends to be on the order of 2–3 cm if the skin is no more than 1–2 cm away from the drum.[5] The magnetic field may be significant up to 5 cm away from the drum. A light towel must be kept in contact with the skin and between the drum and the skin. The towel is used to absorb moisture because an accumulation of water droplets would tend to overheat and cause hot spots on the surface.

drum electrodes Induction electrodes that produce a strong magnetic field. Primarily used with pulsed shortwave diathermy.

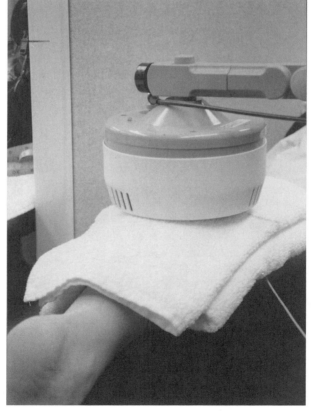

•**Figure 10-12** Drum electrode.

CASE STUDY 10-1
SHORTWAVE DIATHERMY

Background: A 22-year-old graduate student developed the gradual onset of lumbar paravertebral muscle spasm following a self-made move of his apartment contents. The symptoms were noted the day after the move upon arising and were described as a tightness and restriction of mobility in the low back. He reported no radiation of his symptoms into the buttocks or legs and no difficulty with bowel or bladder function. Physical examination revealed restriction in forward flexion and side rotation of the trunk with tenderness to palpation in the lumbar paravertebral musculature 1 week after the episode of extensive bending and lifting.

Impression: Lumbar paravertebral muscle strain, subacute.

Treatment Plan: The patient was initiated on a course of inductive shortwave diathermy to the lumbar paravertebral musculature, followed by active and active-assisted lumbar region range of motion exercise. Treatment was provided on an every-other-day basis for 2 weeks with increasing emphasis on mobilizing and strengthening the lumbar paravertebral musculature.

Response: The patient experience immediate, but short duration relief of his low back pain following the initial treatment and enthusiastically pursued his exercise

sequence. With each subsequent session, the duration of relief and improved trunk mobility increased. At the 2-week point in the treatment regimen, the patient was independent in the performance of his lumbar exercise regimen and scheduled to attend a back education class prior to discharge.

Discussion Questions
- What tissues were injured/affected?
- What symptoms were present?
- What phase of the injury-healing continuum did the patient present for care in?
- What are the physical agent modality's biophysical effects (direct/indirect/depth/tissue affinity)?
- What are the physical agent modality's indications/contraindications?
- What are the parameters of the physical agent modality's application/dosage/duration/frequency in this case study?
- What other physical agent modalities could be utilized to treat this injury or condition? Why? How?

The rehabilitation professional employs physical agent modalities to create an optimum environment for tissue healing while minimizing the symptoms associated with the trauma or condition.

If there is more than 2 cm of fat, there probably will be no great tissue temperature rise under the fat with a drum setup. The maximum penetration of shortwave diathermy with a drum electrode is 3 cm, provided there is no more than 2 cm of fat beneath the skin. For best absorption of energy, the housing of the drum should be in contact with the towel that is covering the skin.[15]

PULSED SHORTWAVE DIATHERMY

Pulsed shortwave diathermy, also referred to in the literature as pulsed electromagnetic energy (PEME), pulsed electromagnetic field (PEMF), or pulsed electromagnetic energy treatment (PEMET), is a relatively new form of diathermy.[20] Pulsed diathermy is created by simply interrupting the output of continuous shortwave diathermy at consistent intervals (Fig. 10-13). Energy is delivered to the patient in a series of high-frequency bursts or pulse trains. Pulse duration is short, ranging from 20 to 400 μsec with an intensity of up to 1000 W per pulse. The interpulse interval or off time depends on the pulse repetition rate, which ranges between 1 and 7000 Hz. The pulse repetition rate may be selected using the pulse-frequency control on the generator control panel.[24] Generally the off time is considerably longer than the on time. Therefore, even though the power output during the on time is sufficient to produce tissue heating, the long off time interval allows the heat to dissipate. This reduces the likelihood of any significant tissue temperature increase and reduces the patient's perception of heat.

pulsed shortwave diathermy Created by simply interrupting the output of continuous shortwave diathermy at consistent intervals, it is used primarily for nonthermal effects.

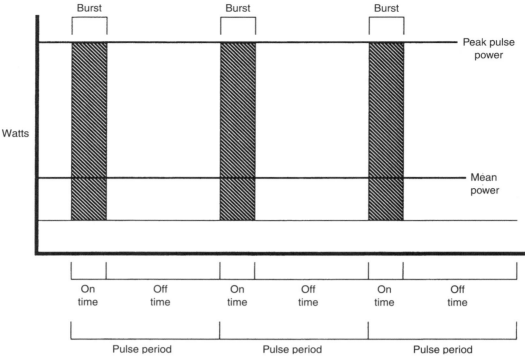

•**Figure 10-13** Pulsed diathermy is created by simply interrupting the output of continuous shortwave diathermy at consistent intervals.

Treatment Tip
Pulsed shortwave diathermy is capable of heating a much larger area than ultrasound; the applicator is stationary so the heat applied to the area is more constant; the rate of temperature decay is slower following diathermy application allowing more time for stretching; using diathermy doesn't require constant monitoring.

Pulsed Shortwave Diathermy uses drum electrodes.

Pulsed diathermy is claimed to have therapeutic value and to produce nonthermal effects with minimal thermal physiologic effects, depending on the intensity of the application. But pulsed shortwave diathermy can also have thermal effects.[40] When pulsed diathermy is used in intensities that create an increase in tissue temperature, its effects are no different from those of continuous shortwave diathermy. Successful treatments have largely resulted from the application of higher intensities and longer treatment times. Studies that use pulsed shortwave diathermy do not normally compare it with continuous shortwave diathermy but rather with a control group that has received no heat treatment.[28]

With pulsed shortwave diathermy, mean power provides a measure of heat production. Mean power may be calculated by dividing peak pulse power by the pulse repetition frequency to determine the pulse period (on time plus off time).

$$\text{Pulse period} = \frac{\text{peak pulse power (W)}}{\text{pulse repetition frequency (Hz)}}$$

The percentage on time is calculated by dividing the pulse duration by pulse period.

$$\text{Percentage on time} = \frac{\text{pulse duration (msec)}}{\text{pulse period (msec)}}$$

The mean power is then determined by dividing the peak pulse power by the percentage on time.

$$\text{Mean power} = \frac{\text{peak pulse power (W)}}{\text{percentage on time}}$$

With pulsed shortwave diathermy, the highest mean power output is usually lower than the power delivered with continuous shortwave diathermy.

Generators that deliver pulsed shortwave diathermy typically use a drum type of electrode (Fig. 10-14). As with continuous shortwave diathermy, the drum electrode is made of a coil wrapped in a flat circular spiral pattern and housed within a plastic case. The energy is induced in the treatment area via the production of a magnetic field.

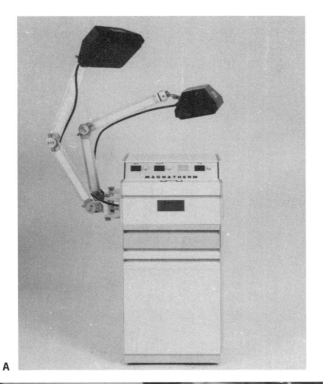

A

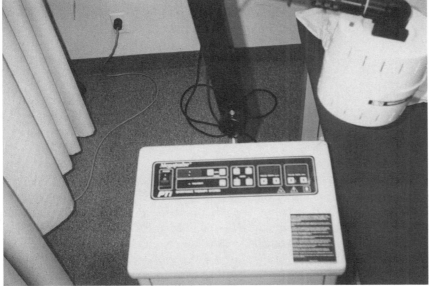

B

•**Figure 10-14 A.** The Magnatherm (*courtesy of International Medical Electronics*). **B.** The Mega-pulse (*courtesy of Physiotechnology*). Both are examples of generators capable of producing pulsed shortwave diathermy. Energy is delivered to the patient through a drum electrode.

TREATMENT TIME

Treatments lasting only 15 minutes have produced vigorous heating of the triceps surae muscle of humans.[9] A 20- to 30-minute treatment for one body area is probably all that is necessary to reach maximum physiologic effects.[15] The physiologic effects, particularly circulatory, seem to last about 30 minutes.

Treatments in excess of 30 minutes may create a circulatory rebound phenomenon in which the digital temperature may drop after the treatment because of reflex vasoconstriction. If a therapist finds that a diathermy unit has been left on in excess of

CASE STUDY 10-2
SHORTWAVE DIATHERMY

Background: A 79-year-old male with a documented history of right knee osteoarthritis, comes to your clinic with a history of increasing pain and swelling over the past 2 months. Gait endurance is beginning to decline. The referral was to initiate quadriceps strengthening, joint protection activities, and gait training as indicated.

Impression: Degenerative joint disease with concurrent muscle inhibition and atrophy.

Treatment Plan: The patient received 15 minutes of capacitive shortwave diathermy prior to initiating quadriceps exercise. He reported short-term relief, which allowed for the performance of his exercise program. Treatment was provided on a twice per week outpatient basis with the patient given specific instructions in the performance of home lower extremity closed-chain exercises two other times per week. At the tenth visit the patient was discharged as he was adequately self-managing his condition.

Response
Discussion Questions

- What tissues were injured/affected?
- What symptoms were present?

- What phase of the injury-healing continuum did the patient present for care in?
- What are the physical agent modality's biophysical effects (direct/indirect/depth/tissue affinity)?
- What are the physical agent modality's indications/contraindications?
- What are the parameters of the physical agent modality's application/dosage/duration/frequency in this case study?
- What other physical agent modalities could be used to treat this injury or condition? Why? How?

Further Discussion Questions

- Was the choice of SWD optimal for this patient's suspected injury?
- What other things would you counsel this patient to be aware of while undergoing diathermy treatment?

The rehabilitation professional employs physical agent modalities to create an optimum environment for tissue healing while minimizing the symptoms associated with the trauma or condition.

---

30 minutes, it would be wise to check the temperature of the toes or fingers, depending on which extremity has been treated. It was observed that pulsed shortwave diathermy administered to the triceps surae resulted in peak heating at only 15 minutes into the treatment, and the temperature actually dropped 0.3°C from the 15- to 20-minute mark.[9] Perhaps this can be explained by the increase in blood flow created by the thermal effects of diathermy. The increase in temperature and blood flow engages the body's natural cooling mechanism. Therefore, it may be more difficult to heat muscle tissue than the less vascular tendinous tissue. Perhaps tissue temperatures as high as 45°C, as postulated by other researchers, are too high for the body to tolerate.[9]

It is important to remember that as skin temperature goes up, impedance goes down. Therefore, the unit may need to be returned after 5–10 minutes of treatment.

MICROWAVE DIATHERMY

Microwave diathermy has two FCC-assigned frequencies in this country, 2456 and 915 MHz. Microwave has a much higher frequency and a shorter wavelength than shortwave diathermy. Microwave diathermy units generate a strong electrical field and relatively little magnetic field.

With appropriate setup of the microwave diathermy unit, less than 10 percent of the energy is lost from the machine as it is applied to the patient. The microwave

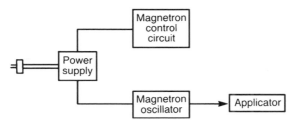

Microwave Diathermy Applicators
• Circular
• Rectangular

•**Figure 10-15** Component parts of a microwave diathermy unit.

applicator beams energy toward the patient, creating the potential for much of the energy to be reflected. Heating is caused by the intramolecular vibration of molecules that are high in polarity.[23] If subcutaneous fat is greater than 1 cm, the fat temperature will rise to a level that is too uncomfortable before there is a tissue temperature rise in the deeper tissues.[16] This is less of a problem if the microwave diathermy is of the frequency of 915 MHz. However, there are very few commercial units operating on that frequency. Almost all of the older units have the higher frequency of 2456 MHz. If the subcutaneous fat is 0.5 cm or less, microwave diathermy can penetrate and cause a tissue temperature rise up to 5 cm deep in the tissue. Bone tends to absorb more shortwave and microwave energy than any type of soft tissue.

MICROWAVE DIATHERMY GENERATORS

The microwave diathermy generator consists of a power supply that energizes the magnetron and timing circuitry. The magnetron control regulates output power by varying the magnetron operating voltage. The magnetron oscillator uses a magnetic field to produce high-frequency currents (Fig. 10-15).

Figure 10-16 represents the control panel of a microwave unit. The power output can be adjusted to patient tolerance. The output meter indicates the relative output in watts or the amount of transmitted and unabsorbed energy. There are two indicator lamps: the amber lamp indicates that the machine is still warming up, and the red lamp indicates that the machine is ready to output energy.

MICROWAVE DIATHERMY APPLICATORS

Electrodes for microwave diathermy are called **applicators**. The microwave energy can only be beamed to one surface at a time. The contour of that surface must be very flat, otherwise there will be considerable reflection of the energy.

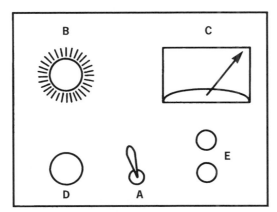

•**Figure 10-16** Control panel of a microwave diathermy unit. **A.** power switch; **B.** timer; **C.** output meter (indicates relative output in watts of transmitted energy); **D.** power output level; **E.** indicator lamps (amber, standby, magnetron accelerating; red, microwaves available for output).

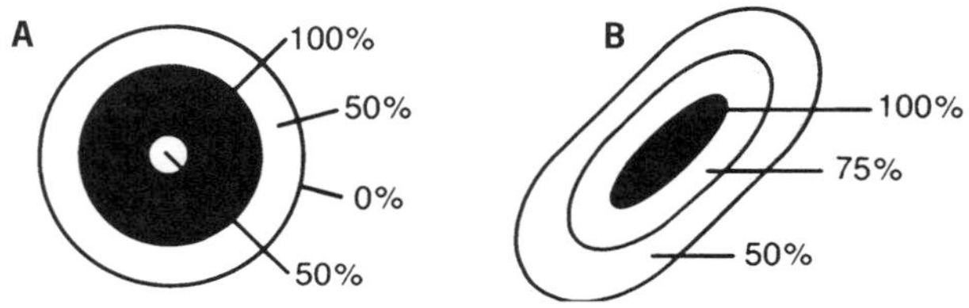

•**Figure 10-17 A.** Circular-shaped microwave electrode. **B.** Rectangular-shaped microwave electrode.

Those microwave diathermy units operating on the frequency 2456 MHz will have a specified air space required between the applicator and the skin. The manufacturer-suggested distances and power output should be followed closely. A directional antenna is attached to the applicator perpendicular to the face of the applicator to assure that spacing is correct and that the energy generated from the microwave unit is striking the target treatment area at the correct angle (cosine law). Units that operate on the higher frequency may have one or more applicators of various shapes and configurations.

There are two types of applicators that may be used with microwave diathermy: circular- and rectangular-shaped. The circular-shaped applicators are either 4 or 6 inches in diameter. With circular-shaped electrodes, the maximum temperature is produced at the periphery of each radiation field (Fig. 10-17A).

Rectangular-shaped applicators are either $4\frac{1}{2} \times 5$ inches or 5×21 inches and produce the maximum temperature at the center of the radiation field (Fig. 10-17B).

In units that have a frequency of 915 MHz, the applicators are placed at a distance of 1 cm from the skin, and the air space between the antenna and the skin is built into the applicator, thus minimizing energy reflection.[27]

MICROWAVE TREATMENT TECHNIQUE

Microwave diathermy units require a period of time to warm up. This is normally built into the circuitry so that the unit power cannot be turned on until the unit is sufficiently warmed. This warm-up time is a good time for the therapist to position the director and the patient (Fig. 10-18). The director should be located so that the maximum amount of energy will be penetrating at a right angle or perpendicular to the skin. Any angle greater or less than perpendicular will create reflection of the energy and significant loss of absorption (cosine law). Microwave diathermy is best used to treat conditions that exist in those areas of the body that are covered with low subcutaneous fat content. The tendons of the foot, hand, and wrist are well treated, as are the acromioclavicular and sternoclavicular joints, the patellar tendon, the distal tendons of the

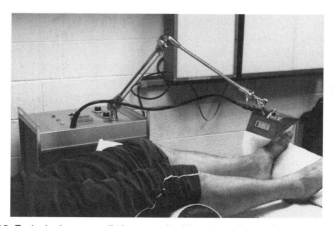

•**Figure 10-18** Typical microwave diathermy unit with rectangular applicator.

hamstrings, the Achilles tendon, and the costochondral joints and sacroiliac joints in lean individuals.

In review, there are some distinct differences between shortwave and microwave diathermy. Some of the major differences are as follows.

1. Microwave diathermy produces an electrical field that generates heat owing to dipole response within the cell membrane. Shortwave diathermy produces magnetic fields.

2. Microwave diathermy does not penetrate as deep as shortwave diathermy.

3. Microwave diathermy cannot penetrate the fat layer as well as shortwave diathermy. (Energy is collected by adipose tissue, rendering the effects at about one-third the depth of shortwave diathermy.)

4. No metal should be within 4 ft of microwave diathermy, because it will interfere with the signal.

5. Spacing is required between the skin and applicator with microwave diathermy, whereas the applicator on a shortwave unit can be placed in contact with the treatment area.

6. It appears that shortwave diathermy is much safer than microwave diathermy.

CLINICAL APPLICATIONS FOR DIATHERMY

For the most part, the clinical applications for the diathermies are similar to those of other physical agents that are capable of producing thermal effects resulting in a tissue temperature increase.[45] In addition to the diathermies, the infrared modalities discussed in Chapter 11 and ultrasound discussed in Chapter 12 are commonly used as heating modalities.

As with pulsed shortwave diathermy, there have been nonthermal effects documented with microwave diathermy; however, there does not appear to be any evidence that these nonthermal effects have any significant role in the medical application of microwave diathermy.[17,29]

The diathermies have been used in the treatment of a variety of musculoskeletal conditions, including muscle strains, contusions, ligament sprains, tendinitis, tenosynovitis, bursitis, joint contractures, myofascial trigger points, and osteoarthritis.[36]

Continuous shortwave and microwave diathermies are used most often for a variety of thermal effects, including inducing local relaxation by decreasing muscle guarding and pain; increasing circulation and improving blood flow to an injured area for the purpose of facilitating resolution of hemorrhage and edema as well as removal of the by-products of the inflammatory process; and in reducing both subacute and chronic pain.[24,28,34]

Diathermy has been used for selectively heating joint structures for the purpose of improving joint range of motion by decreasing stiffness and increasing the extensibility of the collagen fibers and the resilience of contracted soft tissues.[39] The role of diathermy in increasing range of motion and flexibility has been studied with mixed results. One study showed that diathermy and short-duration stretching were no more effective than short-duration stretching alone at increasing hamstring flexibility.[11] A second study indicated that pulsed shortwave diathermy used before prolonged long-duration static stretching appeared to be more effective than stretching alone in increasing flexibility over a 3-week period. After 14 treatments, prolonged long-duration stretching combined with pulsed shortwave diathermy followed by ice application caused greater immediate and net range-of-motion increases than prolonged long-duration stretching alone.[41]

The majority of recent clinical studies relative to diathermy have focused primarily on the efficacy of pulsed shortwave diathermy in facilitating tissue healing, and to date results have been inconclusive at best.[21,33] Various claims have been made as to the specific mechanisms that facilitate healing, including an increase in the number and activity of the cells in the area, reduced swelling and inflammation, resorption of hematoma, increased rate of collagen deposition and organization, and increased nerve growth and repair. These claims are based on a limited number of clinical studies and even fewer experimental studies.[22]

Indications and Contraindications for Shortwave and Microwave Diathermy

Indications
Postacute musculoskeletal injuries
Increased blood flow
Vasodilation
Increased metabolism
Changes in some enzyme reactions
Increased collagen extensibility
Decreased joint stiffness
Muscle relaxation
Muscle guarding
Increased pain threshold
Enhanced recovery from injury
Joint contractures
Myofascial trigger points
Improved joint range of motion
Increased the extensibility collagen
Increased circulation
Reduced subacute and chronic pain
Resorption of hematoma
Increased nerve growth and repair

Contraindications
Acute traumatic musculoskeletal injuries
Acute inflammatory conditions
Areas with ischemia
Areas of reduced sensitivity to temperature or pain
Fluid-filled areas or organs
Joint effusion
Synovitis
Eyes
Contact lenses
Moist wound dressings
Malignancies
Infection
Pelvic area during menstruation
Testes
Pregnancy
Epiphyseal plates in adolescents
Metal implants
Unshielded cardic pacemakers
Intrauterine devices
Watches or jewelry

There are a number of conditions that may potentially occur in clinical settings that would make diathermy the treatment of choice.

1. If for any reason the skin or some underlying soft tissue is very tender and will not tolerate the loading of a moist heat pack or pressure from an ultrasound transducer, then diathermy should be used.

2. Both continuous shortwave and microwave diathermies are more capable of increasing temperatures to a greater tissue depth than any of the infrared modalities.

3. When the treatment goal is to increase tissue temperatures in a large area (i.e., throughout the entire shoulder girdle, in the low back region), the diathermies should be used.[10]

4. In areas where subcutaneous fat is thick and deep heating is required, the induction technique using either cable or drum electrodes should be used to minimize heating of the subcutaneous fat layer. The capacitance technique with both shortwave diathermy and microwave diathermy is more likely to selectively heat more superficial subcutaneous fat.

5. The therapist should never underestimate the placebo effects that a treatment with any large machine may be capable of producing.

Therapists should take the opportunity to examine several different types of diathermy units, as well as the different applicators available with each unit. They should not only practice using the different applicators on healthy tissue, but they should also experience the sensation themselves. In particular, they should recognize or experience the difference between the energy flow with an induction-type application as opposed to the capacitor-type application.

DIATHERMY TREATMENT PRECAUTIONS AND CONSIDERATIONS

There are probably more treatment precautions and contraindications for the use of shortwave, and especially microwave diathermies, than for any of the other physical agents used in a clinical setting.[47]

A survey of over 42,000 physical therapists found a modest increase in the risk of miscarriage of pregnant therapists who were regularly exposed to microwave diathermy.[19,20] Regular exposure to shortwave diathermy during pregnancy, however, did not increase the risk of miscarriage. There are basic differences between microwave and shortwave diathermies that could explain the difference in miscarriage risk. Shortwave diathermy uses high-frequency currents generated at 27.12 MHz and is applied using either a capacitive or inductive applicator, sometimes requiring the patient to become part of the circuit. Microwave diathermy, however, uses higher frequencies of 2450 MHz, and electromagnetic waves are beamed or transmitted into the body by a reflector. Microwave diathermy does not require close contact between the applicator and the therapist, thus allowing some stray emissions.[20] Until further research in this area is performed, it is suggested that the pregnant therapist who treats patients with microwave diathermy first set up the microwave application and then leave the immediate area until the treatment is completed. At this time, however, there is no known risk of miscarriage by pregnant therapists who regularly employ shortwave diathermy.

SWD can be continuous or pulsed.

Diathermy is known to produce a tissue temperature rise and may be contraindicated in any condition where this increased temperature may produce negative or undesired effects, including traumatic musculoskeletal injuries with acute bleeding; acute inflammatory conditions; areas with reduced blood supply (ischemia); and areas with reduced sensitivity to temperature or pain.[13,24,26] It is important to keep in mind that the power meter on the diathermy units does not indicate the energy entering the tissues. Therefore, the therapist must rely on the sensation of pain for a warning that the patient's tolerance levels have been exceeded.[30]

Because diathermy selectively heats tissues that are high in water content, caution must be exercised when using diathermy over fluid-filled areas or organs. Joint effusion may be exacerbated by heating with diathermy. The increase in temperature may cause an increase in synovitis.[26] Because of the high fluid content, it should not be used around the eyes for any prolonged periods of time or for repeated treatments, nor should it be used with contact lenses.[25,46]

In most cases, toweling should be used to absorb perspiration.[15] A single layer of toweling should be used with both the drum and air space plates. However, with other types of applicators, such as pads and cables, the toweling should be more dense and thicker, up to 1 cm or more.[3] Toweling is not necessary with microwave diathermy. There should be no overlapping of skin surfaces. If the buttocks area is to be treated, a towel should be placed in the cleavage between the buttocks. If the shoulder area is to be treated, a towel should be placed between the skin folds in the axilla.

If clothing is permitted in the exposed area, the treatment should be closely monitored. In most cases, however, pulsed shortwave diathermy can be applied over some clothing such as a cotton T-shirt (Fig. 10-19). Be aware that many of the synthetic fabrics worn today allow for no evaporation of moisture, serving as a vapor barrier allowing moisture to accumulate. Similarly, moisture can accumulate in patients taped with adhesive tape or wearing compressive wraps or supportive braces. This moisture can create extreme hot spots with diathermy treatments.[42] Diathermy should not be used over moist wound dressings, again because of potential for rapid heating of moisture.[24]

Diathermy should not be applied to the pelvic area of the female who is menstruating, since this can increase blood flow.[26]

Exposure of the gonads to diathermy also should be avoided.[45] The testes are more superficial and thus are more susceptible to injury from microwave treatment than the ovaries. Minimal evidence exists that diathermy may potentially cause damage to the human fetus, and because research in this area is impossible, it is recommended that caution be used in treating the pregnant female.[48]

Caution should be used when using diathermy over bony prominences to avoid burning of the overlying soft tissue.[27] There should be no vigorous heating of the epiphysis in children.[26]

The patient should not come in contact with any of the cables connecting the generator with the air space plates, pad, cable, or drum electrodes. There should be no crossover of the lead cables with any electrode setup. At no time should the antenna within the microwave applicator ever come in contact with skin, because this would cause a buildup of energy sufficient to cause severe burns.

It is very important to use diathermy units at a safe distance from other types of medical electrical devices or equipment that is transistorized. Transcutaneous electrical nerve stimulation units and other low-frequency current units often have transistor-type circuits, and these can be damaged by the reflected or stray radiation that is produced by shortwave and microwave diathermy units.[26] Unshielded cardiac pacemakers may also be damaged by diathermy.[49]

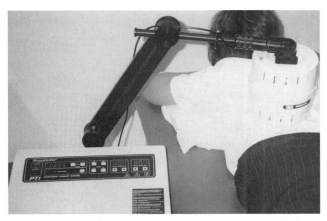

•**Figure 10-19** In most cases pulsed shortwave diathermy can be applied over some clothing such as a cotton T-shirt.

There should be no metal chairs or metal tables used to support the patient during treatment. The area being treated should also be free of metal implants. Women wearing intrauterine devices should not be treated in the low back or lower abdomen. There should be no watches or jewelry in the area because the electromagnetic energy will tend to magnetize the watch, and the electromagnetic energy may heat up the jewelry.[26]

The patient must remain in a reasonably comfortable position for the duration of the treatment so that the field does not change because of movement during treatment.

The skin should be inspected before and after a diathermy treatment. It is recommended that the part being treated either be horizontal or elevated during treatment.

COMPARING SHORTWAVE DIATHERMY AND ULTRASOUND AS THERMAL MODALITIES

The use of therapeutic ultrasound will be discussed in detail in Chapter 12. Ultrasound and pulsed shortwave diathermy are both clinically effective modalities for heating of both superficial and deep tissues; however, ultrasound is used much more frequently than shortwave diathermy. In surveys of physical therapists in both Canada and Australia, only 0.6 and 8 percent of respondents, respectively, used shortwave diathermy daily, yet 94 and 93 percent, respectively, used ultrasound daily.[31,32]

Recent research has demonstrated that shortwave diathermy may be more effective as a heating modality than ultrasound in treating certain conditions.[7,8] A study was done to determine the rate of temperature increase during pulsed shortwave diathermy and the rate of temperature decay postapplication. A 23-gauge thermistor was inserted 3 cm below the skin surface of the anesthetized left medial triceps surae muscle belly of 20 subjects (Fig. 10-20). Diathermy was applied to the muscle belly for 20 minutes at 800 Hz, a pulse duration of 400 μsec, and an intensity of 150 W. Temperature changes were recorded every 5 minutes during the treatment (Fig. 10-21). The mean baseline temperature was 35.8°C, and the temperature peaked at 39.8°C in 15 minutes, then dropped slightly (0.3°C) during the last 5 minutes of treatment. After the treatment terminated, intramuscular temperature dropped 1°C in 5 minutes and 1.8°C by the tenth minute. Based on these findings, it appears that shortwave diathermy compares

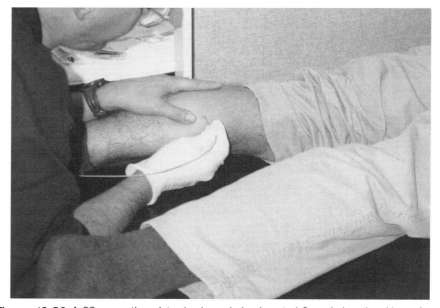

•**Figure 10-20** A 23-gauge thermistor is shown being inserted 3 cm below the skin surface of the anesthetized left medial triceps surae muscle belly.

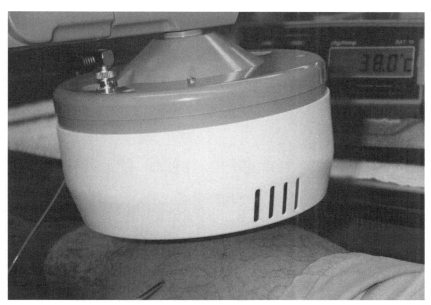

•**Figure 10-21** With the temperature probe in place, muscle temperature changes were measured during shortwave diathermy treatments (Courtesy, Sportsmedicine research laboratory, Brigham Young University, Provo, Utah).

favorably with heating rates of 1 MHz ultrasound (1 W/cm^2 for 12 min = a 4°C temperature increase at 3 cm intramuscularly) (Fig. 10-22).

Shortwave diathermy, however, may be a better modality than ultrasound in some situations, and it appears that there are several advantages of diathermy use over ultrasound.

1. Because the surface of the shortwave applicator drum is 25 times larger than a typical ultrasound treatment area, it heats a much larger area. (A standard drum heating area of the diathermy unit is 200 cm^2, or approximately 25 times that of ultrasound.)
2. Unlike ultrasound that causes a fluctuating tissue heating rate as the transducer is moved, diathermy's applicator is stationary so the heat applied to the area is more constant.
3. The rate of temperature decay is slower following diathermy application. Muscle heated with pulsed shortwave diathermy will retain heat over 60 percent longer than identical

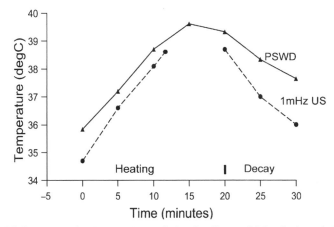

•**Figure 10-22** Intramuscular temperatures during heating and 10 minutes of decay resulting from 20 minutes of shortwave diathermy (PSWD; triangles) and 12 minutes of 1 MHz ultrasound (US; squares) application. This illustrates that shortwave diathermy and 1 MHz ultrasound have similar heating rates, yet muscle heated with shortwave diathermy will retain its heat two to three times longer.

muscle depths heated with 1 MHz ultrasound.[8,43] This is important because it provides the clinician more time for stretching, friction massage, and joint mobilization before the temperature drops to an ineffective level.

4. Application of diathermy does not require constant monitoring by the therapist, whereas ultrasound application requires constant monitoring. Thus, a therapist can work with another patient while one is receiving diathermy treatment. This enables the therapist to be more efficient.

GUIDELINES FOR THE SAFE USE OF DIATHERMY

Therapists who are knowledgeable in the physics and biophysics of diathermy, as well as its applications to a variety of cases, tend to achieve good results. Therapists who work with shortwave and microwave diathermy units must spend considerable time experimenting with equipment setup and the application of different types of electrodes on a variety of uninjured parts of the body if they are to develop the skills necessary to use diathermy safely and effectively on injured tissue.[42] The following guidelines will help ensure safety.

1. Question patient (contraindications and previous treatments).
2. Position patient (comfort, modesty).
3. Inspect part to be treated (check for rashes, infections, or open wounds).
4. If indicated, drape area with toweling.
5. Place electrode drum on treatment area.
6. Turn unit on.
7. Set pulse duration.
8. Set pulse frequency.
9. Adjust intensity.
10. Set treatment time (15–30 min).
11. Press start button.
12. Periodically ask patient if heating is too vigorous.
13. When timer shuts off, terminating the treatment, turn all dials to zero.
14. Assess treatment efficacy (inspect area; feedback from patient).
15. Record treatment parameters.

SUMMARY

1. Diathermy is the application of high-frequency electromagnetic energy that is primarily used to generate heat in body tissues. Diathermy as a therapeutic agent may be classified as two distinct modalities, shortwave diathermy and microwave diathermy. Shortwave diathermy may be continuous or pulsed.

2. The physiologic effects of continuous shortwave and microwave diathermies are primarily thermal, resulting from high-frequency vibration of molecules. Pulsed shortwave diathermy has been used for its nonthermal effects in the treatment of soft-tissue injuries and wounds.

3. A shortwave diathermy unit that generates a high-frequency electrical current will produce both an electrical field and a magnetic field in the tissues. The ratio of the electrical field to the magnetic field depends on the characteristics of the different units as well as on the characteristics of electrodes or applicators.

4. The capacitance technique, using capacitor electrodes (air space plates and pad electrodes), creates a strong electrical field that is essentially the lines of force exerted on charged ions by the electrodes that cause charged particles to move from one pole to the other.

5. The inductance technique, using induction electrodes (cable electrodes and drum electrodes), creates a strong magnetic field when current is passed through a coiled cable. It may affect surrounding tissues by inducing localized secondary currents, called eddy currents, within the tissues.

6. Pulsed diathermy is created by simply interrupting the output of continuous shortwave diathermy at consistent intervals. Generators that deliver pulsed shortwave diathermy typically use a drum type of electrode to induce energy in the treatment area via the production of a magnetic field.

7. Microwave diathermy units generate a strong electrical field and relatively little magnetic field through either circular- or rectangular-shaped applicators that beam energy to the treatment area.

8. The diathermies have been used in the treatment of a variety of musculoskeletal conditions, including muscle strains, contusions, ligament sprains, tendinitis, tenosynovitis, bursitis, joint contractures, and myofascial trigger points.

9. There are probably more treatment precautions and contraindications for the use of microwave diathermy than for any of the other physical agents used in a clinical setting.

10. Effective treatments using the diathermies require practice in application and adjustment of techniques to the individual patient.

11. Four advantages for the use of diathermy over ultrasound are larger heating area, more uniform heating, longer stretching window, and more clinician freedom.

REVIEW QUESTIONS

1. What is diathermy and what are the different types of diathermy?

2. What are the potential physiologic effects of using continuous shortwave, pulsed shortwave, or microwave diathermies?

3. What determines the ratio of the electrical field to the magnetic field in shortwave diathermy?

4. What are the differences between shortwave diathermy techniques that use capacitance or induction?

5. How is pulsed shortwave diathermy used, and what type of electrode is most typically used?

6. How should microwave diathermy be set up to achieve the most effective results?

7. What are the various clinical applications and indications for using continuous shortwave, pulsed shortwave, and microwave diathermies?

8. What are the most important treatment precautions for using the diathermies?

9. What are the major differences between microwave and shortwave diathermies?

10. What are the advantages and disadvantages of using diathermy or ultrasound as deep-heating modalities?

REFERENCES

1. Abramson, D.I., Burnett, C., Bell, Y., and Tuck, S.: Changes in blood flow, oxygen uptake and tissue temperatures produced by therapeutic physical agents, Am. J. Phys. Med. 47:51–62, 1960.

2. Behrens, B.J., Michlovitz, S.L.: Physical agents: theory and practice for the physical therapist assistant, Philadelphia, PA, 1996, F.A. Davis.

3. Brown, M., Baker, R.D.: Effect of pulsed shortwave diathermy on skeletal muscle injury in rabbits, Phys. Ther. 67(2):208–213, 1987.

4. Castel, J.C., Draper, D.O., Knight, K., Fujiwara, T., and Garrett, C.: Rate of temperature decay in human muscle after treatments of pulsed shortwave diathermy, J. Athl. Train. 32: S–34, 1997.

5. DeLateur, B.J., Lehmann, J.F., Stonebridge, J.B., et al.: Muscle heating in human subjects with 915 MHz microwave contact applicator, Arch. Phys. Med. 51:147–151, 1970.

6. Delpizzo, V., Joyner, K.H.: On the safe use of microwave and shortwave diathermy units, Aust. J. Physiother. 33(3):152–162, 1987.

7. Draper, D.O.: Current research on therapeutic ultrasound and pulsed short-wave diathermy. Presented at Physio Therapy Research Seminars Japan, Nov. 17, Sendai, Japan, 1996.

8. Draper, D.O., Castel, J.C., and Castel, D.: Rate of temperature increase in human muscle during 1 MHz and 3 MHz continuous ultrasound, J. Orthop. Sports Phys. Ther. 22:142–150, 1995.

9. Draper, D.O., Castel, J.C., Knight, K., et al.: Temperature rise in human muscle during pulsed short wave diathermy: does this modality parallel ultrasound? J. Athl. Train. 32:S–35, 1997.

10. Draper, D., Knight, K.L., and Fujiwara, T.: Temperature change in human muscle during and after pulsed shortwave diathermy, J. Orthop. Sports Phys. Ther. 29(1):13–18, 1999.

11. Draper, D., Miner, L., Kinght, K.: The carry-over effects of diathermy and stretching in developing hamstring flexibility, J. Athl. Train. 37(1):37–42, 2002.

12. Fenn, J.E.: Effect of pulsed electromagnetic energy (Diapulse) on experimental haematomas, Can. Med. Assoc. J. 100:251, 1969.

13. Fischer, C., Solomon, S.: Physiologic responses to heat and cold. In Licht, S., editor. Therapeutic heat and cold, New Haven, CT, 1965, Elizabeth Licht.

14. Griffin, J.E.: Update on selected physical modalities, Paper presented in Chicago, Dec., 1981.

15. Griffin, J.E., Karselis, T.C.: The diathermies. In Physical agents for physical therapists, ed. 2, Springfield, IL, 1982, Charles C Thomas.

16. Griffin, J.E., Santiesleban, A.J., and Kloth, L.: Electrotherapy for instructors, Paper presented in Lacrosse, WI, Aug. 1982.

17. Guy, A.W., Lehmann, J.F.: On the determination of an optimum microwave diathermy frequency for a direct contact applicator, Inst. Electric. Electron. Eng. Trans. Biomed. Eng. 13:76–87, 1966.

18. Hansen, T.I., Kristensen, J.H.: Effect of massage, shortwave diathermy and ultrasound upon ^{133}Xe disappearance rate from muscle and subcutaneous tissue in the human calf, Scand. J. Rehabil. Med. 5:179–182, 1973.

19. Health devices shortwave diathermy units, Proceedings of the Emergency Care Research Institute, Meeting in Plymouth, PA, June 1979, pp. 175–193.

20. Hellstrom, R.O., Stewart, W.F.: Miscarriages among female physical therapists who report using radio- and microwave-frequency electromagnetic radiation, Am. J. Epidemiol. 138 (10):775–785, 1993.

21. Hill, J.: Pulsed short-wave diathermy effects on human fibroblast proliferation, Arch. Phys. Med. Rehabil. 83(6)832–836, 2002.

22. Kitchen, S., Partridge, C.: A review of microwave diathermy, Physiotherapy 77(9):647–652, 1991.

23. Kitchen, S., Partridge, C.: Review of shortwave diathermy continuous and pulsed patterns, Physiotherapy 78(4):243–252, 1992.

24. Kloth, L., Ziskin, M.: Diathermy and pulsed electromagnetic fields. In Michlovitz, S.L., editor. Thermal agents in rehabilitation, ed. 2, Philadelphia, PA, 1990, F.A. Davis.

25. Konarska, I., Michneiwicz, L.: Shortwave diathermy of diseases of the anterior portion of the eye, Klin. Oczna. 25:185, 1955.

26. Lehmann, J.F.: Comparison of relative heating patterns produced in tissues by exposure to microwave energy with exposures at 2450 and 900 megacycles, Arch. Phys. Med. Rehabil. 46:307, 1965.

27. Lehmann, J.F.: Diathermy. In Krusen, F.H., editor. Handbook of physical medicine and rehabilitation, Philadelphia, PA, 1965, W.B. Saunders.

28. Lehmann, J.F.: Therapeutic heat and cold, ed. 4, Baltimore, MD, 1990, Williams & Wilkins.

29. Lehmann, J.F., deLateur, B.J.: Diathermy and superficial heat and cold. In Krusen, F.H., editor. Krusen's handbook of physical medicine and rehabilitation, ed. 3, Philadelphia, PA, 1982, W.B. Saunders.

30. Lehmann, J.F., Warren, C.G., and Scham, S.M.: Therapeutic heat and cold, Clin. Orthop. 99:207, 1974.

31. Lindsay, D.M., Dearness, J., and McGinley, C.C.: Electrotherapy usage trends in private physiotherapy practice in Alberta, Physiother. Can. 47(1):30–34, 1995.

32. Lindsay, D.M., Dearness, J., Richardson, C., et al.: A survey of electromodality usage in private physiotherapy practices, Aust. J. Physiother. 36(4):249–256, 1990.

33. Low, J.: Dosage of some pulsed shortwave clinical trials. Physiotherapy 81(10):611–616, 1995.

34. Low, J.: The nature and effects of pulsed electromagnetic radiations, N.Z. Physiother. 6:18, 1978.

35. Low, J., Reed, A.: Electrotherapy explained: principles and practice, London, 1990, Butterworth-Heinemann.

36. Marks, R., Ghassemi, M., Duarte, R., and Van Nguyen, J.P.: A review of the literature on shortwave diathermy as applied to osteo-arthritis of the knee, Physiotherapy 85(6):304–316, 1999.

37. Merrick, M.A.: Do you diathermy? Athletic therapy today 6(1):55–56, 2001.

38. Millard, J.B.: Effect of high frequency currents and infra-red rays on the circulation of the lower limb in man, Ann. Phys. Med. 6:45,1961.

39. Miner, L., Draper, D., and Knight, K.L.: Pulsed shortwave diathermy application prior to stretching does not appear to aid hamstring flexibility, J. Athl. Train. 35(2):S–48, 2000.

40. Murray, C.C., Kitchen, S.: Effect of pulse repetition rate on the perception of thermal sensation with pulsed shortwave diathermy, Physiother. Res. Int. 5(2):73–84, 2000.

41. Peres, S., Draper, D., and Knight, K.: Pulsed shortwave diathermy and long-duration stretching increase dorsiflexion range of motion more than identical stretching without diathermy, J. Athl. Train. 37(1):43–50, 2002.

42. Progress Report, American Physical Therapy Association, June, 1980.

43. Rose, S., Draper, D.O., Schulthies, S.S., and Durrant, E.: The stretching window part two: rate of thermal decay in deep muscle following 1 MHz ultrasound, J. Athl. Train. 31:139–143, 1996.

44. Sanseverino, E.G.: Membrane phenomena and cellular processes under the action of pulsating magnetic fields, Presented at the Second International Congress for Magneto Medicine, Rome, 1980.

45. Schliephake, E.: Carrying out treatment. In Thom, H., editor. Introduction to shortwave and microwave diathermy, ed. 3, Springfield, IL, 1966, Charles C Thomas.

46. Scott, B.O.: Effect of contact lenses on shortwave field distribution, Br. J. Opthalmol. 40:696, 1956.

47. Shields, N.: Short-wave diathermy: current clinical and safety practices, Physiother. Res. Int. 7(4):191–202, 2002.

48. Smith, D.W., Clarren, S.K., and Harvey, M.A.: Hyperthermia as a possible teratogenic agent, J. Pediatr. 92:878, 1978.

49. Smyth, H.: The pacemaker patient and the electromagnetic environment, JAMA 227:1412, 1974.

50. Van Demark, N.L., Free, M.J.: Temperature effects. In Johnson, A.D., editor. The testis, vol. 3, New York, 1973, Academic Press.

51. Wilson, D.H.: Treatment of soft tissue injuries by pulsed electrical energy, Br. Med. J. 2:269, 1972.

52. Wright, G.G.: Treatment of soft tissue and ligamentous injuries in professional footballers, Physiotherapy 59(12), 1973.

SUGGESTED READINGS

Abramson, D.I: Physiologic basis for the use of physical agents in peripheral vascular disorders, Arch. Phys. Med. Rehabil. 46: 216, 1965.

Abramson, D.I., Bell, Y., Rejal, H., et al.: Changes in blood flow, oxygen uptake and tissue temperatures produced by therapeutic physical agents, Am. J. Phys. Med. 39:87–95, 1960.

Abramson, D.I., Chu, L.S.W., Tuck, S., et al.: Effect of tissue temperature and blood flow on motor nerve conduction velocity, JAMA 198:1082–1088, 1966.

Adey, W.R.: Electromagnetic field effects on tissue, Physiol. Rev. 61(3):436–514, 1981.

Adey, W.R.: Physiological signaling across cell membranes and co-operative influences of extremely low frequency electromagnetic fields. In Frohlich, H., editor. Biological coherence and response to external stimuli, Heidelberg, 1988, Springer Verlag.

Allberry, J.: Shortwave diathermy for herpes zoster, Physiotherapy 60:386, 1974.

Aronofsky, D.: Reduction of dental post-surgical symptoms using non-thermal pulsed high-peak-power electromagnetic energy, Oral Surg. 32(5)688–696, 1971.

Babbs, C.F., Dewitt, D.P.: Physical principles of local heat therapy for cancer, Med. Instrument. USA 15:367–373, 1981.

Balogun, J., Okonofua, F.: Management of chronic pelvic inflammatory disease with shortwave diathermy: a case report, Phys. Ther. 68(10):1541–1545, 1988.

Bansal, P.S., Sobti, V.K., and Roy, K.S.: Histomorphochemical effects of shortwave diathermy on healing of experimental muscle injury in dogs, Ind. J. Exp. Biol. 28:766–770, 1990.

Barclay, V., Collier, R.J., and Jones, A.: Treatment of various hand injuries by pulsed electromagnetic energy, Physiotherapy 69(6):186–188, 1983.

Barker, A.T., Barlow, P.S., Porter, J., et al.: A double-blind clinical trial of low power pulsed shortwave therapy in the treatment of a soft tissue injury, Physiotherapy 71(12):500–504, 1985.

Barnett, M.: SWD for herpes zoster, Physiotherapy 61:217, 1975.

Bassett, C.: The development and application of pulsed electromagnetic fields (PEMFs) for united fractures and arthrodeses, Orthop. Clin. North Am. 15(10):61–89, 1984.

Benson, T.B., Copp, E.P.: The effect of therapeutic forms of heat and ice on the pain threshold of the normal shoulder, Pheumatol. Rehabil. 13:101–104, 1974.

Bentall, R.H., Eckstein, H.B.: A trial involving the use of pulsed electromagnetic therapy on children undergoing orchidopexy, Kinderchirugie 17(4):380–389, 1975.

Brown, M., Baker, R.D.: Effect of pulsed shortwave diathermy on skeletal muscle injury in rabbits, Phys. Ther. 67(2):208–214, 1987.

Brown-Woodnan, P.D.C., Hadley, J.A., Richardson, L., et al.: Evaluation of reproductive function of female rats exposed to radio frequency fields (27.12 MHz) near a shortwave diathermy device, Health Phys. 56(4):521–525, 1989.

Burr, B.: Heat as a therapeutic modality against cancer, Report 16, U.S. National Cancer Institute, Bethesda, M., 1974.

Cameron, B.M.: Experimental acceleration of wound healing, Am. J. Orthopaed. 3:336–343, 1961.

Cameron, M.H.: Diathermy for wound care, Adv. Dir. Rehabil. 12(1):71, 2003.

Chamberlain, M.A., Care, G., and Gharfield, B.: Physiotherapy in osteo-arthrosis of the knee, Ann. Rheum. Dis. 23:389–391, 1982.

Cole, A., Eagleston, R.: The benefits of deep heat: ultrasound and electromagnetic diathermy, Phys. Sportsmed. 22(2):76–78, 81–82, 84, 1994.

Constable, J.D., Scapicchio, A.P., and Opitz, B.: Studies of the effects of Diapulse treatment on various aspects of wound healing in experimental animals, J. Surg. Res. 11:254–257, 1971.

Coppell, R.: Survey of stray electromagnetic emissions from microwave and shortwave diathermy equipment, N.Z. J. Physiother. 16(3): 9–12, 14, 1988.

Currier, D.P., Nelson, R.M.: Changes in motor conduction velocity induced by exercise and diathermy, Phys. Ther. 49(2):146–152, 1969.

Daels, J.: Microwave heating of the uterine wall during parturition, J. Microwave Power 11:166, 1976.

de la Rosette, J., de Wildt, M., and Alivizatos, G.: Transurethral microwave thermotherapy (TUMT) in benign prostatic hyperplasia: placebo versus TUMT, Urology 44(1):58–63, 1994.

Department of Health: Evaluation report: shortwave therapy units, J. Med. Eng. Technol. 11(6):285–298, 1987.

Department of Health and Welfare (Canada): Canada wide survey of non-ionising radiation-emitting medical devices, 80-EHD-52, 1980.

Department of Health and Welfare (Canada): Safety code 25: Shortwave diathermy guidelines for limited radio frequency exposure, 80-EHD-98, 1983.

Doyle, J.R., Smart, B.W.: Stimulation of bone growth by shortwave diathermy, J. Bone Joint Surg. 45A:15, 1963.

Engel, J.P.: The effects of microwaves on bone and bone marrow and adjacent tissues, Arch. Phys. Med. Rehabil. 31:453, 1950.

Erdman, W.J.: Peripheral blood flow measurements during application of pulsed high frequency currents, Am. J. Orthopaed. 2:196–197, 1960.

Feibel, H., Fast, H.: Deepheating of joints: a reconsideration, Arch. Phys. Med. Rehabil. 57:513, 1976.

Fenn, J.E.: Effect of pulsed electromagnetic energy (Diapulse) on experimental haematomas, Can. Med. Assoc. J. 100:251–253, 1969.

Foley-Nolan, D., Barry, C., Coughlan, R.J., et al.: Pulsed high frequency (27MHz) electromagnetic therapy for persistent neck pain, Orthopaedics 13(4):445–451, 1990.

Foley-Nolan, D., Moore, K., and Codd, M.: Low energy high frequency pulsed electromagnetic therapy for acute whiplash injuries. A double blind randomized controlled study, Scand. J. Rehabil. Med. 24(1):51–59, 1992.

Foster, P.: Diathermy burns, Nursing RSA Verpleging 2(10):4–5, 7–9, 1987.

Frankenberger, L.: Making a comeback: diathermy is an effective therapeutic agent and should be part of every therapist's armamentarium, Adv. Dir. Rehabil. 10(5):43–46, 2001.

Gibson, T., Grahame, R., Harkness, J., et al.: Controlled comparison of shortwave diathermy treatment with osteopathic treatment in non-specific low back pain, Lancet 1:1258–1261, 1985.

Ginsberg, A.J.: Pulsed shortwave in the treatment of bursitis with calcification, Int. Rec. Med. 174(2):71–75, 1961.

Goldin, J.H., Broadbent, N.R.G., Nancarrow, J.D., and Marshall, T.: The effect of diapulse on healing of wounds: a double blind randomized controlled trial in man, Br. J. Plastic Surg. 34: 267–270, 1981.

Grant, A., Sleep, J., McIntosh, J., and Ashurst, H.: Ultrasound and pulsed electromagnetic energy treatment for peroneal trauma: a randomised placebo-controlled trial, Br. J. Obstet. Gynaecol. 96:434–439, 1981.

Guy, A.W.: Analyses of electromagnetic fields induced in biological tissues by thermographic studies on equivalent phantom models, IEEE Trans. Microwave Theory Tech. Vol. MTT 19:205, 1971.

Guy, A.W.: Biophysics of high frequency currents and electromagnetic radiation, In Lehmann, J.F., editor. Therapeutic heat and cold, ed. 4, Baltimore, MD, 1990, Williams & Wilkins.

Guy, A.W., Lehmann, J.F., and Stonebridge, J.B.: Therapeutic applications of electromagnetic power, Proc. Inst. Electric. Electr. Eng. 62:55–75, 1974.

Guy, A.W., Lehmann, J.F., Stonebridge, J.B., and Sorensen, C.C.: Development of a 915 MHz direct contact applicator for therapeutic heating of tissues, Inst. Electric. Electr. Eng. Microwave Theory Techn. 26:550–556, 1978.

Hall, E.L.: Diathermy generators, Arch. Phys. Med. Rehabil. 33:28, 1952.

Hansen, T.I., Kristensen, J.H.: Effect of massage, shortwave diathermy and ultrasound upon ^{133}Xe disappearance rate from muscle and subcutaneous tissue in the human calf, Scand. J. Rehabil. Med. 5:179–182, 1973.

Harris, R.: Effect of shortwave diathermy on radio-sodium clearance from the knee joint in the normal and in rheumatoid arthritis, Phys. Med. Rehabil. 42:241, 1961.

Hayne, R.: Pulsed high frequency energy: its place in physiotherapy, Physiotherapy 70(12):459–466, 1984.

Herrick, J.F., Jelatis, D.G., and Lee, G.M.: Dielectric properties of tissues important in microwave diathermy, Fed. Proc. 9:60, 1950.

Herrick, J.F., Krusen, F.H.: Certain physiologic and pathologic effects of microwaves, Elect. Eng. 72:239, 1953.

Hoeberlein, T., Katz, J., and Balogun, J.: Does indirect heating using shortwave diathermy over the abdomen and sacrum affect peripheral blood flow in the lower extremities? Phys. Ther. 76(5):S67, 1996.

Hollander, J.L.: Joint temperature measurement in evaluation of antiarthritic agents, J. Clin. Invest. 30:701, 1951.

Hutchinson, W.J., Burdeaux, B.D.: The effects of shortwave diathermy on bone repair, J. Bone Joint Surg. 33A:155, 1951.

Johnson, C.C., Guy, A.W.: Nonionizing electromagnetic wave effects in biological materials and systems, Proc. Inst. Electric. Electr. Eng. 66:692, 1972.

Jones, S.L.: Electromagnetic field interference and cardiac pacemakers, Phys. Ther. 56:1013, 1976.

Kantor, G.: Evaluation and survey of microwave and radio frequency applicators, J. Microwave Power (2)16:135, 1981.

Kantor, G., Witters, D.M.: The performance of a new 915 MHz direct contact applicator with reduced leakage—a detailed analysis, HHS Publication (FDA) S3-8199, April 1983.

Kaplan, E.G., Weinstock, R.E.: Clinical evaluation of Diapulse as adjunctive therapy following foot surgery, J. Am. Ped. Assoc. 58:218–221, 1968.

Kloth, L.C., Morrison, M., and Ferguson, B.: Therapeutic microwave and shortwave diathermy: a review of thermal effectiveness, safe use, and state-of-the-art-1984, Center for Devices and Radiological Health, DHHS, FDA 85-8237, Dec. 1984.

Krag, C., Taudorf, U., Siim, E., and Bolund, S.: The effect of pulsed electromagnetic energy (Diapulse) on the survival of experimental skin flaps, Scand. J. Plas. Reconstr. Surg. 13:377–380, 1979.

Landsmann, M.A.: Rehab products: equipment focus. Defending diathermy: recently fallen out of favor, this modality deserves a second look, Adv. Dir. Rehabil. 11(11):61–62, 2002.

Lehmann, J.F.: Microwave therapy: stray radiation, safety and effectiveness, Arch. Phys. Med. Rehabil. 60:578, 1979.

Lehmann, J.F.: Review of evidence for indications, techniques of application, contraindications, hazards and clinical effectiveness for shortwave diathermy, DHEW/FDA HFA510, Rockville, MD, 1974.

Lehmann, J.F., DeLateur, B.J., and Stonebridge, J.B.: Selective muscle heating by shortwave diathermy with a helical coil, Arch. Phys. Med. Rehabil. 50:117, 1969.

Lehmann, J.F., Guy, A.W., deLateur, B.J., et al.: Heating patterns produced by shortwave diathermy using helical induction coil applicators, Arch. Phys. Med. 49:193–198, 1968.

Lehmann, J.F., McDougall, J.A., Guy, A.W., et al.: Heating patterns produced by shortwave diathermy applicators in tissue substitute models, Arch. Phys. Med. Rehabil. 64:575–577, 1983.

Licht, S., editor. Therapeutic heat and cold, ed. 2, New Haven, CT, 1972, Elizabeth Licht.

Martin, C., McCallum, H., and Strelley, S.: Electromagnetic fields from therapeutic diathermy equipment: a review of hazards and precautions, Physiotherapy 77(1):3–7, 1991.

McDowell, A.D., Lunt, M.J.: Electromagnetic field strength measurements on Megapulse units, Physiotherapy 77(12):805–809, 1991.

McGill, S.N.: The effect of pulsed shortwave therapy on lateral ligament sprain of the ankle, N.Z. J. Physiother. 10:21–24, 1988.

McNiven, D.R., Wyper, D.J.: Microwave therapy and muscle blood flow in man, J. Microwave Power 11:168–170, 1976.

Michaelson, S.M.: Effects of high frequency currents and electromagnetic radiation. In Lehmann, H.F., editor. Therapeutic heat and cold, ed. 4, Baltimore, MD, 1990, Williams & Wilkins.

Millard, J.B.: Effect of high frequency currents and infrared rays on the circulation of the lower limb in man, Ann. Phys. Med. 6(2):45–65, 1961.

Morrissey, L.J.: Effects of pulsed shortwave diathermy upon volume blood flow through the calf of the leg: plethysmography studies, J. Am. Phys. Ther. Assoc. 46:946–952, 1966.

Mosely, H., Davison, M.: Exposure of physiotherapists to microwave radiation during microwave diathermy treatment, Clin. Phys. Physiol. Meas. No. 3. 2:217, 1981.

Nadasdi, M.: Inhibition of experimental arthritis by athermic pulsing shortwave in rats, Am. J. Orthopaed. 2:105–107, 1960.

Nelson, A.J.M., Holt, J.A.G.: Combined microwave therapy, Med. J. Aust. 2:88–90, 1978.

Nicolle, F.V., Bentall, R.M.: The use of radiofrequency pulsed energy in the control of post-operative reaction to blepharoplasty, Anaesth. Plast. Surg. 6:169–171, 1982.

Nielson, N.C., Hansen, R., and Larsen, T.: Heat induction in copper bearing IUDs during shortwave diathermy, Acta Obstet. Gynaecol. Scand. (Stockh.) 58:495, 1972.

Nwuga, G.B.: A study of the value of shortwave diathermy and isometric exercise in back pain management, Proceedings of the IXth International Congress of the WCPT, Legitimerader Sjukgymnasters Riksforbund, Stockholm, Sweden, 1982.

Oliver, D.: Pulsed electromagentic energy—what is it? Physiotherapy 70(12):458–459, 1984.

Osborne, S.L., Coulter, J.S.: Thermal effects of shortwave diathermy on bone and muscle, Arch. Phys. Ther. 38:281–284, 1938.

Paliwal, B.R.: Heating patterns produced by 434 MHz erbotherm UHF69, Radiology 135:511, 1980.

Pasila, M., Visuri, T., and Sundholm, A.: Pulsating shortwave diathermy: value in treatment of recent ankle and foot sprains, Arch. Phys. Med. Rehabil. 59:383–386, 1978.

Patzold, J.: Physical laws regarding distribution of energy for various high frequency methods applied in heat therapy, Ultrason. Biol. Med. 2:58, 1956.

Quirk, A.S., Newman, R.J., and Newman, K.J.: An evaluation of interferential therapy, shortwave diathermy and exercise in the treatment of osteo-arthrosis of the knee, Physiotherapy 71(2):55–57, 1985.

Rae, J.W., Herrick, J.F., Wakim, K.G., and Krusen, F.H.: A comparative study of the temperature produced by MWD and SWD, Arch. Phys. Med. Rehabil. 30:199, 1949.

Raji, A.M.: An experimental study of the effects of pulsed electromagnetic field (diapulse) on nerve repair, J. Hand Surg. 9B(2):105–112, 1984.

Reed, M.W., Bickerstaff, D.R., Hayne, C.R., et al.: Pain relief after inguinal herniorrhaphy: ineffectiveness of pulsed electromagnetic energy, Br. J. Clin. Pract. 41(6):782–784, 1987.

Religo, W., Larson, T.: Microwave thermotherapy: new wave of treatment for benign prostatic hyperplasia, J. Am. Acad. Phys. Assist. 7(4):259–267, 1994.

Richardson, A.W.: The relationship between deep tissue temperature and blood flow during electromagnetic irradiation, Arch. Phys. Med. Rehabil. 31:19, 1950.

Rubin, A., Erdman, W.: Microwave exposure of the human female pelvis during early pregnancy and prior to conception, Am. J. Phys. Med. 38:219, 1959.

Ruggera, P.S.: Measurement of emission levels during microwave and shortwave diathermy treatments, Bureau of Radiological Health Report, HHS Publication (FDA), 80–8119, 1980.

Schwan, H.P.: Interaction of microwave and radio frequency radiation with biological systems. In Cleary, S.F., editor. Biological effects and health implications of microwave radiation, U.S. Department of Health, Education and Welfare, Washington, DC, 1970.

Schwan, H.P., Piersol, G.M.: The absorption of electromagnetic energy in body tissues. Part I, Am. J. Phys. Med. 33:371, 1954.

Schwan, H.P., Piersol, G.M.: The absorption of electromagnetic energy in body tissues. Part II, Am. J. Phys. Med. 34:425, 1955.

Shields, N.: Short-wave diathermy and pregnancy: what is the evidence? Adv. Physiother. 5(1):2–14, 2003.

Silverman, D.R., Pendleton, L.A.: A comparison of the effects of continuous and pulsed shortwave diathermy on peripheral circulation, Arch. Phys. Med. Rehabil. 49:429–436, 1968.

Stuchly, M.A., Repacholi, M.H., Lecuyer, D.W., and Mann, R.D.: Exposure to the operator and patient during shortwave diathermy treatments, Health Phys. 42(3):341–366, 1982.

Svarcova, J., Trnavsky, K., and Zvarova, J.: The influence of ultrasound, galvanic currents and shortwave diathermy on pain intensity in patients with osteo-arthritis, Scand. J. Rheumatol. Suppl. 67:83–85, 1988.

Taskinen, H., Kyyronen, P., and Hemminki, K.: The effects of ultrasound, shortwaves and physical exertion on pregnancy outcome in physiotherapists, J. Epidemiol. Commun. Health 44:96–201, 1990.

Thom, H.: Introduction to shortwave and microwave therapy, ed. 3, Springfield, IL, 1966, Charles C Thomas.

Tzima, E., Martin, C.: An evaluation of safe practices to restrict exposure to electric and magnetic fields from therapeutic and surgical diathermy equipment, Physiol. Measure 15(2):201–216, 1994.

Vanharanta, H.: Effect of shortwave diathermy on mobility and radiological stage of the knee in the development of experimental osteo-arthritis, Am. J. Phys. Med. 61(2):59–65, 1982.

Van Ummersen, C.A.: The effect of 2450 MHz radiation on the development of the chick embryo. In Peyton, M.F., editor. Biological effects of microwave radiation, vol. 1, New York, 1961, Plenum Press.

Verrier, M., Falconer, K., and Crawford, J.S.: A comparison of tissue temperature following two shortwave diathermy techniques, Physiother. Can. 29(1):21–25, 1977.

Wagstaff, P., Wagstaff, S., and Downie, M.: A pilot study to compare the efficacy of continuous and pulsed magnetic energy (shortwave diathermy) on the relief of low back pain, Physiotherapy 72(11):563–566, 1986.

Ward, A.R.: Electricity fields and waves in therapy, Science Press, Australia, 1980, NSW.

Wilson, D.: Treatment of soft tissue injuries by pulsed electrical energy continuous and pulsed magnetic energy (shortwave diathermy) on the relief of low back pain, Physiotherapy 72(11):563–566, 1986.

Wilson, D.H.: The effects of pulsed electromagnetic energy on peripheral nerve regeneration, Ann. N.Y. Acad. Sci. 238:575, 1975.

Wilson, D.H.: Comparison of shortwave diathermy and pulsed electromagnetic energy in treatment of soft tissue injuries, Physiotherapy 60(10):309–310, 1974.

Wilson, D.H.: Treatment of soft tissue injuries by pulsed electrical energy, Br. Med. J. 2:269–270, 1972.

Wise, C.S.: The effect of diathermy on blood flow, Arch. Phys. Med. Rehabil. 29:17, 1948.

Witters, D.M., Kantor, G.: An evaluation of microwave diathermy applicators using free space electric field mapping, Phys. Med. Biol. 26:1099, 1981.

Worden, R.E.: The heating effects of microwaves with and without ischemia, Arch. Phys. Med. Rehabil. 29:751, 1948.

Wyper, D.J., McNiven, D.R.: Effects of some physiotherapeutic agents on skeletal muscle blood flow, Physiotherapy 63(3):83–85, 1976.

GLOSSARY

air space plate A capacitor-type electrode in which the plates are separated from the skin by the space in a glass case. Used with shortwave diathermy.

applicator The electrode used to transfer energy in microwave diathermy.

cable electrodes An inductance-type electrode in which the electrodes are coiled around a body part, creating an electromagnetic field.

capacitor electrodes Air space plates or pad electrode that creates a stronger electrical field than a magnetic field.

diathermy The application of high-frequency electrical energy that is used to generate heat in body tissues as a result of the resistance of the tissue to the passage of energy. It may also be used to produce nonthermal effects.

drum electrodes Induction electrodes that produce a strong magnetic field. Primarily used with pulsed shortwave diathermy.

eddy currents Small circular electrical fields induced when a magnetic field is created that results in intermolecular oscillation (vibration) of tissue contents, causing heat generation.

electrical field The lines of force exerted on charged ions in the tissues by the electrodes that cause charged particles to move from one pole to the other.

Federal Communications Commission (FCC) Federal agency charged with assigning frequencies for all radio transmitters, including diathermies.

induction electrodes Cable electrodes or drum electrodes that create a stronger magnetic than electrical field.

intermolecular vibration Movement between molecules that produces friction and thus heat.

magnetic field Created when current is passed through a coiled cable affecting surrounding tissues by inducing localized secondary currents, called eddy currents, within the tissues.

pad electrodes Capacitor-type electrode used with shortwave diathermy to create an electrical field.

pulsed shortwave diathermy Created by simply interrupting the output of continuous shortwave diathermy at consistent intervals, it is used primarily for nonthermal effects.

specific absorption rate (SAR) Represents the rate of energy absorbed per unit area of tissue mass.

LAB ACTIVITY

SHORTWAVE DIATHERMY

DESCRIPTION

Shortwave diathermy (SWD; *diathermy* means to heat through) uses an alternating current (most commonly 27.12 MHz) passed either through a coiled conductor or to a capacitor plate.

With the coil method, the patient is placed in the magnetic field that is generated when the current passes through the coil; the magnetic field then is absorbed by the molecules in the body, increasing the patient's internal energy. This method is referred to as inductive, because the body acts as a secondary coil, and the current in the body is induced by the current in the primary coil; the body never becomes part of the electrical circuit.

With the second method, there are two capacitor plates that are charged, and the body acts as a lower resistance conductor for the discharge of the capacitive current; thus the term capacitive shortwave diathermy. Again, the molecules of the body absorb the energy and have their internal energy increased. In capacitive SWD, the patient becomes part of the electrical circuit.

Because the motion of a molecule is dependent on its internal energy, when a molecule absorbs any type of energy, its motion increases. Temperature is a reflection of the average kinetic energy of a system, and the kinetic energy is by definition the random molecular motion. Therefore, when the molecular motion increases, the temperature increases. Although there are increased molecular collisions when the thermal energy of a system increases, these collisions do not produce any energy; they merely transfer the energy from one molecule to another. It is a misconception that the "friction" that occurs between the molecules causes the increased temperature.

Although electrical energy is used in SWD, action potentials are not induced in excitable tissue. At such high frequencies, the phase charge of the current is inadequate to alter the membrane voltage enough for the membrane to reach threshold. The amount of heat generated does follow Joule's law

$$Q = I^2Rt$$

where Q is heat, I is current, R is resistance, and t is time. The heat is generated in the tissue that absorbs the energy, and this varies according to the type of SWD used. Inductive SWD is absorbed mostly by tissues that have a high electrical conductivity, such as muscle. Capacitive SWD is absorbed mostly by tissues that have a low electrical conductivity, such as skin and fat. Because of this, capacitive SWD does not penetrate as deeply as inductive SWD, but does produce a more marked sensation of warmth in the patient. The general guideline for the depth of penetration of capacitive SWD is 1 cm, and 3–4 cm for inductive SWD.

PHYSIOLOGIC EFFECTS

Vasodilation
Decreased pain perception
Increased local metabolism
Increased connective tissue plasticity
Decreased isometric strength (transient)

THERAPEUTIC EFFECTS

Decreased pain
Increased soft tissue extensibility

INDICATIONS

Shortwave diathermy is a heating physical agent; therefore, the indications are the same as for any heating agent. However, the depth of penetration, at least for inductive SWD, is greater than for any of the infrared agents. Ultrasound has a deeper penetration than SWD, but SWD can be used to treat a much larger area.

CONTRAINDICATIONS

- Lack of normal temperature sensibility
- Peripheral vascular disease with compromised circulation
- Over tumors, the testes, open growth plates, acutely inflamed tissue, active hemorrhage, the eyes, or metallic objects
- Pregnancy
- In patients with implanted electrical stimulators (e.g., cardiac pacemakers, phrenic nerve stimulators)

Shortwave Diathermy

PROCEDURE	EVALUATION		
	1	2	3
1. Check supplies.			
a. Obtain sheet or towels for draping, timer, signaling device.			
b. Check SWD generator for frayed power cords, integrity cables and drum, shields, and so on.			
c. Verify that the output control is at zero.			
2. Question patient.			
a. Verify identity of patient (if not already verified).			
b. Verify the absence of contraindications.			
c. Ask about previous thermotherapy treatments; check treatment notes.			
3. Position patient.			
a. Place patient in a well-supported, comfortable position. This is particularly crucial, because the patient should not shift positions after the treatment starts.			
b. Expose body part to be treated; have patient remove all jewelry from the area.			
c. Drape patient to preserve modesty, protect clothing, but allow access to body part.			
4. Inspect body part to be treated.			
a. Check light touch perception.			
b. Check circulatory status (pulses, capillary refill). Assess function of body part (e.g., ROM, irritability).			
5. Apply SWD.			
a. Place a single layer of towel on the treatment area.			
b. Inductive: Position the drum containing the coil parallel to the body part and in contact with the towel. Capacitive: Position the plates parallel to the body part and about 2.5–7.5 cm away from the body.			
c. Turn on the SWD generator, allow to warm up if necessary.			
d. Inform the patient that he or she should feel only warmth; if it becomes hot, the patient should inform you immediately.			
e. Adjust intensity of SWD to the appropriate level. Set a timer for the appropriate treatment time and give the patient a signaling device. Make sure the patient understands how to use the signaling device.			
f. Check the patient's response after the first 5 minutes by asking how it feels.			

PROCEDURE	EVALUATION		
	1	2	3
6. Complete the treatment.			
a. When the treatment time is over, turn the intensity control to zero, and move the generator away from the patient; dry the area with a towel.			
b. Remove material used for draping, assist the patient in dressing as needed.			
c. Have the patient perform appropriate therapeutic exercise as indicated.			
d. Clean the treatment area and equipment according to normal protocol.			
7. Assess treatment efficacy.			
a. Ask the patient how the treated area feels.			
b. Visually inspect the treated area for any adverse reactions.			
c. Perform functional tests as indicated.			

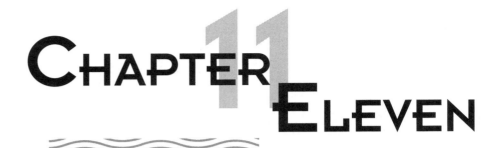

CHAPTER ELEVEN

INFRARED MODALITIES

GERALD W. BELL and
WILLIAM E. PRENTICE

OBJECTIVES

Following completion of this chapter, the student therapist will be able to:

✓ Explain how the infrared modalities are classified in the electromagnetic spectrum.
✓ Differentiate between the physiologic effects of therapeutic heat and cold.
✓ Describe the contemporary modalities of the infrared spectrum in thermotherapy and cryotherapy.
✓ Categorize the indications and contraindications for each infrared modality discussed.
✓ Select the most effective infrared modalities for a given clinical diagnosis.
✓ Explain how the therapist can use the infrared modalities to reduce pain.

infrared That portion of the electromagnetic spectrum associated with thermal changes; located adjacent to the red portion of the visible light spectrum.

Of the therapeutic modalities discussed in this text, perhaps none are more commonly used than **infrared** modalities. As indicated in Chapter 1, the infrared region of the electromagnetic spectrum falls between the microwave diathermy and the visible light portions of the spectrum in terms of wavelength and frequency. There is a great deal of misunderstanding among therapists regarding which of the modalities used in a clinical setting are actually classified as infrared. Traditionally, the term "infrared heating" conjures up visions of infrared lamps and bakers. However, it must be emphasized that most of the heat and cold modalities, such as hydrocollator packs, paraffin baths, hot and cold whirlpools, and ice packs, as well as infrared lamps, produce forms of radiant energy that have wavelengths and frequencies that fall into the infrared region (see Fig. 1-2). This chapter includes a discussion of all the modalities that fall into the infrared portion of the electromagnetic spectrum.

Mechanisms of Heat Transfer
• Conduction
• Convection
• Radiation
• Conversion

conduction Heat loss or gain through direct contact.

MECHANISMS OF HEAT TRANSFER

Easy application and convenience of use of hot and cold modalities provide the therapist with the necessary tools for primary care of injuries. Heat is defined as the internal vibration of the molecules within a body. The transmission of heat occurs by three mechanisms: **conduction**, **convection**, and **radiation**. A fourth mechanism of heat transfer, **conversion**, is discussed in Chapter 12.

TABLE 11-1 Mechanisms of Heat Transfer of the Various Modalities

Conduction	Convection	Radiation	Conversion
Ice massage	Hot whirlpool	Infrared lamps	Ultrasound
Cold packs	Cold whirlpool	Laser	Diathermy
Hydrocollator packs	Fluidotherapy	Ultraviolet light[a]	
Cold spray			
Ice immersion			
Contrast baths[b]			
Cryo-Cuff			
Cryokinetics			
Paraffin bath			

[a] Ultraviolet therapy does not involve a tissue temperature change, but the energy from the ultraviolet source radiates to the skin surface.
[b] Contrast baths could also involve convection if hot or cold whirlpools are being used.

Conduction occurs when the body is in direct contact with the heat or cold source. Convection occurs when particles (air or water) move across the body, creating a temperature variation. Radiation is the transfer of heat from a warmer source to a cooler source through a conducting medium, such as air (e.g., infrared lamps). The body may either gain or lose heat through any of these three processes of heat transfer. The infrared modalities discussed in this chapter use these three methods of heat transfer to effect a tissue temperature increase or decrease. Table 11-1 summarizes the mechanisms of heat transfer for the various modalities.

> Infrared modalities should be used primarily to provide analgesia and reduce pain.

APPROPRIATE USE OF THE INFRARED MODALITIES

Infrared modalities should not be used randomly by therapists without reviewing the benefits. Placing the patient in the whirlpool or a slush bucket of ice simply because these two modalities are available is not an acceptable treatment technique.

Heating techniques used for therapeutic purposes are referred to as **thermotherapy**. Thermotherapy is used when a rise in tissue temperature is the goal of treatment. The use of cold, or **cryotherapy**, is most effective in the acute stages of the healing process immediately following injury when a loss of tissue temperature is the goal of therapy. Cold applications can be continued into the reconditioning stage of injury management. Thermotherapy and cryotherapy are included in this section on the basis of their classification in the electromagnetic spectrum. The term **hydrotherapy** can be applied to any cryotherapy or thermotherapy technique that uses water as the medium for tissue temperature exchange.

> **cryotherapy** The use of cold in the treatment of pathology or diseases.

The electromagnetic spectrum has a relatively large region of radiations designated as infrared. The infrared wavelength provides the radiant energy used therapeutically (see Fig. 1-2). Penetration of the energy is dependent on the source but is generally considered to be a superficial form of treatment.

> **hydrotherapy** Cryotherapy and thermotherapy techniques that use water as the medium of heat transfer.

Although this chapter is concerned primarily with application of the infrared modalities and their physiologic effects, several other modalities discussed in this text (e.g., the diathermies and ultrasound) cause similar physiologic responses. Specifically, the effects of heat and cold therapy discussed in this chapter may be applied to any modality that alters tissue temperature.

Heating and cooling agents can be used successfully to treat injuries and trauma.[29] The therapist must know the injury mechanism and specific pathology, as well as the physiologic effects of the heating and cooling agents, to establish a consistent treatment schedule.

CLINICAL USE OF THE INFRARED MODALITIES

The physiologic effects of heat and cold discussed previously are rarely the result of direct absorption of infrared energy. There is general agreement that no form of infrared energy can have a depth of penetration greater than 1 cm.[1] Thus, the effects of the infrared modalities are primarily superficial and directly affect the cutaneous blood vessels and the cutaneous nerve receptors.[74]

Absorption of infrared energy cutaneously increases and decreases circulation subcutaneously in both the muscle and fat layers. If the energy is absorbed cutaneously over a long enough period of time to raise the temperature of the circulating blood, the hypothalamus will reflexively increase blood flow to the underlying tissue. Likewise, absorption of cold cutaneously can decrease blood flow via a similar mechanism in the area of treatment.[1]

Thus, if the primary treatment goal is a tissue temperature increase with a corresponding increase in blood flow to the deeper tissues, it is wiser perhaps to choose a modality, such as diathermy or ultrasound, that produces energy that can penetrate the cutaneous tissues and be directly absorbed by the deep tissues. If the primary treatment goal is to reduce tissue temperature and decrease blood flow to an injured area, the superficial application of ice or cold is the only modality capable of producing such a response.

Perhaps the most effective use of the infrared modalities should be to provide analgesia or reduce the sensation of pain associated with injury. The infrared modalities stimulate primarily the cutaneous nerve receptors. Through one of the mechanisms of pain modulation discussed in Chapter 4 (most likely the gate control theory), hyperstimulation of these nerve receptors by heating or cooling reduces pain. Within the philosophy of an aggressive program of rehabilitation, the reduction of pain as a means of facilitating therapeutic exercise is a common practice. As emphasized in the preface to this text, therapeutic modalities are perhaps best used as an adjunct to therapeutic exercise. Certainly, this should be a prime consideration when selecting an infrared modality for use in any treatment program.

Continued investigation and research into the use of heat and cold is warranted to provide useful data for the therapist. Heat and cold applications, when used properly and efficiently, will provide the therapist with the tools to enhance recovery and provide the patient with optimal health care management. Thermotherapy and cryotherapy are only two of the tools available to assist in the well-being and reconditioning of the injured patient.

EFFECTS OF TISSUE TEMPERATURE CHANGE ON CIRCULATION

Local application of heat or cold is indicated for **thermal** physiologic effects. The main physiologic effect is on superficial circulation because of the response of the temperature receptors in the skin and the sympathetic nervous system.

Circulation through the skin serves two major functions: nutrition of the skin tissues and conduction of heat from internal structures of the body to the skin so that heat can be removed from the body.[39] The circulatory apparatus is composed of *two major vessel types*: arteries, capillaries, and veins; and vascular structures for heating the skin. Two types of vascular structures are the subcutaneous venous plexus, which holds large quantities of blood that heat the surface of the skin, and the arteriovenous anastomosis, which provides vascular communication between arteries and venous plexuses.[27] The walls of the plexuses have strong muscular coats innervated by sympathetic vasoconstrictor nerve fibers that secrete norepinephrine. When constricted, blood flow is reduced to almost nothing in the venous plexus. When maximally dilated, there is an extremely rapid flow of blood into the plexuses. The arteriovenous anastomoses are found principally in the volar or palmar surfaces of the hands and feet, lips, nose, and ears.

When cold is applied directly to the skin, the skin vessels progressively constrict to a temperature of about 10°C (50°F), at which point they reach their maximum

thermotherapy The use of heat in the treatment of pathology or disease.

constrictions. This constriction results primarily from increased sensitivity of the vessels to nerve stimulation, but it probably also results at least partly from a reflex that passes to the spinal cord and then back to the vessels. At temperatures below 10°C (50°F), the vessels begin to dilate. This dilation is caused by a direct local effect of the cold on the vessels themselves, producing paralysis of the contractile mechanism of the vessel wall or blockage of the nerve impulses coming to the vessels. At temperatures approaching 0°C (32°F), the skin vessels frequently reach maximum vasodilation.

Skin plexuses are supplied with sympathetic vasoconstrictor innervation. In times of circulatory stress, such as exercise, hemorrhage, or anxiety, sympathetic stimulation of these skin plexuses forces large quantities of blood into internal vessels. Thus, the subcutaneous veins of the skin act as an important blood reservoir, often providing blood to serve other circulatory functions when needed.[39]

Three types of sensory receptors are found in the subepithelial tissue: cold, warm, and pain. The pain receptors are free nerve endings. Temperature and pain are transmitted to the brain via the lateral spinothalamic tract (see Chapter 4). The nerve fibers respond differently at different temperatures. Both cold and warm receptors discharge minimally at 33°C (91.4°F). Cold receptors discharge between 10 and 41°C (50–105.8°F), with a maximum discharge in the 37.5–40°C (99.5–104°F) range. Above 45°C (113°F), cold receptors begin to discharge again, and pain receptors are stimulated. Nerve fibers transmitting sensations of pain respond to the temperature extremes. Both warm and cold receptors adapt rapidly to temperature change; the more rapid the temperature change, the more rapid the receptor adaptation. The number of warm and cold receptors in any given small surface area is thought to be few. Therefore, small temperature changes are difficult to perceive in localized areas. Larger surface areas stimulate summation of thermal signals. These larger patterns of excitation activate the vasomotor centers and the hypothalamic center.[68,71] Stimulation of the anterior hypothalamus causes cutaneous vasodilation, whereas stimulation of the posterior hypothalamus causes cutaneous vasoconstriction.[39,102]

The cutaneous blood flow depends on the discharge of the sympathetic nervous system. These sympathetic impulses are transmitted simultaneously to the blood vessels for cutaneous vasoconstriction and to the adrenal medulla. Both norepinephrine and epinephrine are secreted into the blood vessels and induce vessel constriction.[39] Most of the sympathetic constriction influences are mediated chemically through these neural transmitters. General exposure to cold elicits cutaneous vasoconstriction, shivering, piloerection, and an increase in epinephrine secretion; therefore, vascular contraction occurs. Simultaneously, metabolism and heat production are increased to maintain the body temperature.[39]

Increased blood flow supplies additional oxygen to the area, explaining the analgesic and relaxation effects on muscle spasm. An increased proprioceptive reflex mechanism may explain these effects. Receptor end organs located in the muscle spindle are inhibited by heat temporarily, whereas sudden cooling tends to excite the receptor end organ.[68,71]

EFFECTS OF TISSUE TEMPERATURE CHANGE ON MUSCLE SPASM

Numerous studies deal with the effects of heat and cold in the treatment of many musculoskeletal conditions. Although it is true that the use of heat as a therapeutic modality has long been accepted and documented in the literature, it is apparent that most recent research has been directed toward the use of cold. There seems to be general agreement that the physiologic mechanisms underlying the effectiveness of heat and cold treatments in reducing muscle spasm lie at the level of the muscle spindle, Golgi tendon organs, and the gamma system.[98]

Heat is believed to have a relaxing effect on skeletal muscle tone.[33] Local application of heat relaxes muscles throughout the skeletal system by simultaneously lessening the stimulus threshold of muscle spindles and decreasing the gamma efferent firing rate. This suggests that the muscle spindles are easily excited. Consequently, the muscles

cryokinetics The use of cold and exercise in the treatment of pathology or disease.

contrast bath Hot (106°F) and cold (50°F) treatments in a combined sequence to stimulate superficial capillary vasodilation or vasoconstriction.

Treatment Tip
As long as the patient is not complaining of tenderness to touch, it is probably safe to switch from cold to some form of heat. When treating deeper tissues it is recommended that either ultrasound or shortwave diathermy be used since the depth of penetration of both is greater than any infrared modality.

Cold may be better for reducing muscle spasm.

may be electromyographically silent while at rest during the application of heat, but the slightest amount of voluntary or passive movement may cause the efferents to fire, thus increasing muscular resistance to stretch. If this is indeed the case, then it seems logical that decreasing the afferent impulses by raising the threshold of the muscle spindles might be effective in facilitating muscle relaxation, as long as there is no movement.

The rate of firing of both primary and secondary endings is directly proportional to temperature. Local applications of cold decrease local neural activity. Annulospiral, flower-spray (small fibers located in the muscle spindle that detect changes in muscle position), and Golgi tendon organ endings all fire more slowly when cooled. Cooling actually decreases the rate of afferent activity even more, with an increase in the amount of tension on the muscle. Thus, cold appears to raise the threshold stimulus of muscle spindles, and heat tends to lower it.[31] Although firing of the primary spindle afferents increases abruptly with the application of cold, a subsequent decrease in spindle afferent activity occurs and persists as the temperature is lowered.[72]

Simultaneous use of heat and cold in the treatment of muscle spasm has also been studied.[27] Local cooling with ice, although maintaining body temperature to prevent shivering, results in a significant reduction of muscle spasm, greater than that which occurs with the use of heat or cold independently. This effect was attributed to maintenance of body temperature, which decreases efferent activity, whereas local cooling decreases afferent activity. If the core temperature of the body is not maintained, the reflex shivering results in increased muscle tone, thus inhibiting relaxation.

There is a substantial reduction in the frequency of action potential (stimulus intensity necessary for firing muscle fibers) firing of the motor unit when the muscle temperature is reduced. Muscle spindle activity is most significantly reduced when the muscle is cooled, whereas normal body temperature is maintained.[82]

Miglietta[82] presented a slightly different perspective on the effect of cold in reducing muscle spasm. He performed an electromyographic analysis of the effects of cold on the reduction of clonus (increased muscle tone) or spasticity in a group of 15 patients. After immersion of the spastic extremity in a cold whirlpool for 15 minutes, it was observed that electromyographic activity dropped significantly and in some cases disappeared altogether. The cold was thought to induce an afferent bombardment of cold impulses, which modify the cortical excitatory state and block the stream of painful impulses from the muscle. Thus, relaxation of skeletal muscle is assumed to occur with the disappearance of pain.[120] It is not certain whether it is the excitability of the motor neurons or the hyperactivity of the gamma system, which is changed either at the muscle spindle level or at the spinal cord level, that is responsible for the reduction of spasticity. However, it is certain that cold is effective in reducing spasticity by reducing or modifying the highly sensitive stretch-reflex mechanism in muscle.

Another factor that may be important to the reduction of spasticity is reduction in the nerve conduction velocity as a result of the application of cold.[22] These changes may result from a slowing of motor and sensory nerve conduction velocity and a decrease of the afferent discharges from cutaneous receptors.

Several studies investigated the use of cold followed by some type of exercise in the treatment of various injuries to the musculotendinous unit.[36,60] Each of these studies indicated that the use of cold and exercise were extremely effective in the treatment of acute pathologies of the musculoskeletal system that produced restrictions of muscle action. However, if stretching was indicated, it has been stressed that stretching is more important for increasing flexibility than using either heat or cold.[30,115]

EFFECTS OF TEMPERATURE CHANGE ON PERFORMANCE

Several studies have examined the effects of altering tissue temperature on physical performance capabilities.

Changes in the ability to produce torque during isokinetic testing following the application of heat and cold have been demonstrated, although there appears to be some disagreement relative to the degree of change in concentric and eccentric torque

paraffin bath A combined paraffin and mineral oil immersion commonly used on the hands and feet for distal temperature gains in blood flow and temperature.

capabilities.[52] One study observed that the strength of an eccentric contraction was improved with the application of ice, whereas another indicated the ice helped to facilitate concentric but not eccentric strength.[21,105] This may be due to an increase in the ability to recruit additional motor neurons during and after cooling.[64] It also appears that higher torque values can be produced following the application of cold packs than hot packs.[16] The use of cryotherapy does not seem to effect peak torque but may increase endurance.[118] Cold appears to have some effect on muscular power; also, it has been shown that performance in vertical jumping is decreased following the application of cold.[34,37] Cold water immersion does not seem to affect range of motion.[17]

It seems that heating or cooling of an extremity has minimal or no effects on proprioception, joint position sense, and balance.[12,49,66,69,96,105,107,116,117,122,127] Thus, it follows that tissue temperature changes have no effect on agility or the ability to change direction.[31,57,108]

CRYOTHERAPY

Cryotherapy is the use of cold in the treatment of acute trauma and subacute injury and for the decrease of discomfort after reconditioning and rehabilitation.[54]

cryotherapy The use of cold in the treatment of pathology or diseases.

PHYSIOLOGIC EFFECTS OF TISSUE COOLING

The physiologic effects of cold are the opposite of those of heat for the most part, the primary effect being a local decrease in temperature. Cold has its greatest benefit in acute injury.[6,38,52,53,55,79] There is general agreement that the use of cold is the initial treatment for most conditions in the musculoskeletal system. The primary reason for using cold in acute injury is to lower the temperature in the injured area, thus reducing the metabolic rate with a corresponding decrease in production of metabolites and metabolic heat.[46] This helps the injured tissue survive the hypoxia and limits further tissue injury.[53,55] Cold has been demonstrated to be more effective when applied along with compression than using ice alone for reducing metabolism in injured tissue.[79,80] It is also used immediately after injury to decrease pain and promote local **vasoconstriction,** thus controlling hemorrhage and edema.[76,94] However, pre-exercise cooling does not affect the magnitude of muscle damage in response to eccentric exercise.[93] Cold is also used in the acute phase of inflammatory conditions, such as bursitis, tenosynovitis, and tendinitis, in which heat may cause additional pain and swelling.[71]

Cold is also used to reduce pain and the reflex muscle spasm and spastic conditions that accompany it.[79] Its analgesic effect is probably one of its greatest benefits.[28,72,98] One explanation of the analgesic effect is that cold decreases the velocity of nerve conduction, although it does not entirely eliminate it.[22,72,73] It is also possible that cold bombards central pain receptor areas with so many cold impulses that pain impulses are lost through the gate control theory of pain modulation. With ice treatments, the patient usually reports an uncomfortable sensation of cold followed by stinging or burning, then an aching sensation, and finally complete numbness.[56]

Cold also has been demonstrated to be effective in the treatment of **myofascial pain.**[120] This type of pain is referred from active myofascial trigger points with various symptoms, including pain on active movement and decreased range of motion. Trigger points may result from muscle strain or tension, which sensitizes nerves in a localized area. A trigger point may be palpated as a small nodule or as a strip of tense muscle tissue.[121]

It appears that cold is more effective in treating acute muscle pain as opposed to delayed-onset muscle soreness (DOMS), which occurs following exercise.[15] Ultrasound has been shown to be more effective than ice for treating DOMS.[81]

Cold depresses the excitability of free nerve endings and peripheral nerve fibers, and this increases the pain threshold.[62] This is of great value in short-term treatment. Cold applications can also enhance voluntary control in spastic conditions, and in acute traumatic conditions they may decrease painful spasms that result from local muscle irritability.[3]

Cold may be better for reducing muscle spasm.

Indications and Contraindications for Cryotherapy

Indications
During acute or subacute inflammation
Acute pain
Chronic pain
Acute swelling (controlling hemorrhage and edema)
Myofascial trigger points
Muscle guarding
Muscle spasm
Acute muscle strain
Acute ligament sprain
Acute contusion
Bursitis
Tenosynovitis
Tendinitis
Delayed onset muscle soreness

Contraindications
Impaired circulation
Peripheral vascular disease
Hypersensitivity to cold
Skin anesthesia
Open wounds or skin conditions (cold whirlpools and contrast baths)
Infection

hydrocollator A synthetic hot (170°F) or cold (0°F) gel used as an adjunctive modality to stimulate a rise or fall in tissue temperature.

hunting response A reflex increase in temperature that occurs in response to cold approximately 15 minutes into the treatment.

Cold treatments do not necessarily have as much of an effect in the deeper tissues relation to blood flow. Positron emission tomography is an imaging technique which can be used to directly quantify local blood flow in response to cold application. Using this technology, it has been shown that muscle tissue blood flow is reduced after a 20-minute ice treatment. However, this reduction only occurs in the most superficial layer, which may suggest that the therapeutic effects of ice application diminishes with tissue depth.[19]

Treatment Tip
Contrast baths produce little or no "pumping action" and are not very effective in treating swelling. A better alternative is to use cryokinetics, which involves cold followed by active muscle contractions and relaxation to help eliminate swelling.

Reduction in muscle guarding relative to acute trauma has been observed by all active therapists. The literature reviewed indicates various reasons behind reduced muscle guarding, with the common thought of decreased muscle spindle activity.[61]

The initial reaction to cold is local vasoconstriction of all smooth muscle by the central nervous system to conserve heat.[94] Localized vasoconstriction is responsible for the decrease in the tendency toward formation and accumulation of edema, probably as a result of a decrease in local hydrostatic pressure.[113] There is also a decrease in the amount of nutrients and phagocytes delivered to the area, thus reducing phagocytic activity.[113]

It has been hypothesized that when local temperature is lowered considerably for a period of about 30 minutes, intermittent periods of vasodilation occur, lasting 4–6 minutes. Then vasoconstriction recurs for a 15- to 30-minute cycle, followed again by vasodilation. This phenomenon is known as the **hunting response** and is necessary to prevent local tissue injury caused by cold.[14,18,70] The hunting response has been accepted for a number of years as fact; in reality, however, these investigations talked about measured temperature changes rather than circulatory changes. Thus, the hunting response is more likely a measurement artifact than an actual change in blood flow in response to cold.[2,56] Even if some cold-induced vasodilation occurs, the effects are negligible.[52]

If a large area is cooled, the hypothalamus (the temperature-regulating center in the brain) will reflexively induce shivering, which raises the core temperature as a result of increased production of heat. Cooling of a large area might also cause arterial vasoconstriction in other remote parts of the body, resulting in an increased blood pressure.[113] Because of the low thermal conductivity of underlying subcutaneous fat tissue, applications of cold for short periods of time probably are ineffective in cooling deeper tissues.[94] It has been shown also that using cold for too long may be detrimental to the healing process.[38]

The length of treatment time needed to cool tissue effectively depends on differences in subcutaneous tissue thickness.[90] Patients with thick subcutaneous tissue should be treated with cold applications for longer than 5 minutes to produce a significant drop in intramuscular temperature. Grant treated acute and chronic conditions of the musculoskeletal system and found that thin people require shorter icing periods and that response was more successful.[36] McMaster supported these findings.[76] Recommended treatment times range from direct contact of 5–45 minutes to obtain adequate cooling.

It has been recommended that in patients with differing subcutaneous adipose thickness the duration of cryotherapy treatment needed to produce a standard cooling effect must vary. To produce similar intramuscular temperature changes, treatment duration should be adjusted based on the subject's subcutaneous adipose thickness as determined through skin-fold measurements. A 25-minute treatment may be adequate for a patient with a skin-fold of 20 mm or less; however, a 40-minute application is required to produce similar results in a patient whose skin-fold is between 20 and 30 mm. A 60-minute treatment is required to produce similar results in a patient whose skin-fold is between 30 and 40 mm.[95]

It is generally believed that cold treatments are more effective in reaching deep tissue than most forms of heat. Cold applied to the skin is capable of significantly lowering the temperature of tissue at a considerable depth. The extent of this lowered tissue temperature is dependent on the type of cold applied to the skin, the duration of its application, the thickness of the subcutaneous fat, and the region of the body on which it is applied.

The application of cold decreases cell permeability, decreases cellular metabolism, and decreases accumulation of edema and should be continued in 5- to 45-minute applications for at least 72 hours after initial trauma.[52] Care should be taken to avoid aggressive cold treatment to prevent disruption of the healing sequence.

The physiologic effects of cold are summarized in Table 11-2.

TABLE 11-2	Physiologic Effects of Heat and Cold

EFFECTS OF HEAT

Increased local temperature superficially
Increased local metabolism
Vasodilation of arterioles and capillaries
Increased blood flow to part heated
Increased leukocytes and phagocytosis
Increased capillary permeability
Increased lymphatic and venous drainage
Increased metabolic wastes
Increased axon reflex activity
Increased elasticity of muscles, ligaments, and capsule fibers
Analgesia
Increased formation of edema
Decreased muscle tone
Decreased muscle spasm

EFFECTS OF COLD

Decreased local temperature, in some cases to a considerable depth
Decreased metabolism
Vasoconstriction of arterioles and capillaries (at first)
Decreased blood flow (at first)
Decreased nerve conduction velocity
Decreased delivery of leukocytes and phagocytes
Decreased lymphatic and venous drainage
Decreased muscle excitability
Decreased muscle spindle depolarization
Decreased formation and accumulation of edema
Extreme anesthetic effects

Frostbite

Frostbite is defined as freezing of a body part and occurs when tissue temperatures fall below 0°C (32°F). Symptoms of frostbite initially include tingling and redness from hyperemia, which indicate blood is still circulating to the superficial tissues, followed by pallor (a lack of color in the skin) and numbness, which indicate that vasoconstriction has occurred and blood is no longer circulating to the superficial tissues.

When using a cryotherapy technique the chances of frostbite are minimal if the recommended procedures are followed. However, if treatment time exceeds recommendations, of if the temperature of the modality is below what is recommended, the chances of frostbite will be increased. Certainly if there is circulatory insufficiency the chances of frostbite are also increased.

If frostbite is suspected, the body part should be immediately removed from the cold source and immersed in water at 38–40°C (100–104°F). It is also advisable to refer the patient to a physician.

CRYOTHERAPY TREATMENT TECHNIQUES

Tools of cryotherapy include ice packs, cold whirlpool, ice whirlpool, ice massage, commercial chemical cold spray, and contrast baths. Application of cryotherapy produces a three- to four-stage sensation. First, there is an uncomfortable sensation of cold followed by a stinging, then a burning or aching feeling, and finally numbness. Each stage is related to the nerve endings as they temporarily cease to function as a result of both decreased blood flow and decreased nerve conduction velocity. The time required for this sequence varies, but several authors indicate that it occurs within 5–15 minutes.[2,4,7,36,42,56,84,86,94] After 12–15 minutes the hunting response is sometimes demonstrated with intense cold (10°C [50°F]).[14,58,84,94] Thus, a minimum of 15 minutes are necessary to achieve extreme analgesic effects.

CASE STUDY 11-2
HYDROTHERAPY: COLD WHIRLPOOL

Background: A 32-year-old woman fell onto her outstretched left hand 12 weeks ago and sustained a comminuted fracture of the distal radius as well as a noncomminuted fracture of the scaphoid. She was treated with a closed reduction and external fixation (fiberglass cast) for 8 weeks, then a splint for 4 weeks. She has been referred for rehabilitation, to include mobilization, strengthening, and range-of-motion exercise. The radius demonstrates radiographic healing, and there is no evidence of aseptic necrosis. Her distal forearm, wrist, hand, and fingers remain markedly swollen, and she is experiencing significant pain at rest. She is unable to tolerate more than mild pressure on the wrist, making joint mobilization extremely difficult, and has severe pain with attempted active range of motion.

Impression: Posttraumatic pain and swelling, postimmobilization pain and loss of motion.

Treatment Plan: A small extremity hydrotherapy tank was filled with ice and water to achieve a water temperature of 17°C (63°F). The patient's left upper member was immersed in the water up to the level of the midforearm, and the turbine was used to direct water onto the wrist and hand. For the initial 5 minutes, the patient was instructed to gently move the wrist and hand actively. For the next 5 minutes, passive range of motion was conducted by the therapist; 5 minutes of joint mobilization followed the passive range of motion. The total treatment time in the cold whirlpool was 15 minutes. She was instructed in a home exercise program to gain motion and strength.

Response: The patient was treated with the cold whirlpool 3 days per week for 3 weeks, at which time the swelling had subsided to a minimal amount. Her range of motion was approximately 50 percent that of the right wrist and hand. The cold whirlpool was discontinued after 9 sessions, and other physical agents were used to facilitate a return to function. After an additional 12 sessions, the patient was discharged to a home program, with her left wrist and hand motion and strength approximately 80 percent that of the right wrist and hand.

Discussion Questions
- What tissues were injured or affected?
- What symptoms were present?
- What phase of the injury-healing continuum did the patient present for care in?
- What are the physical agent modality's biophysical effects (direct, indirect, depth, and tissue affinity)?
- What are the physical agent modality's indications and contraindications?
- What are the parameters of the physical agent modality's application, dosage, duration, and frequency in this case study?
- What other physical agent modalities could be used to treat this injury or condition? Why? How?
- What is aseptic necrosis? Are particular areas more vulnerable? What areas? What is the mechanism of the disorder?
- What does the abbreviation "FOOSH" stand for? What types of injuries would you anticipate in a patient who had experienced a "FOOSH"?
- If the cold whirlpool was helpful in achieving the therapeutic goals, why was the cold whirlpool discontinued after nine sessions? Why was a cold whirlpool selected for this patient?
- What disadvantages are there in using a whirlpool to assist in the resolution of the soft tissue swelling? Advantages?
- If the patient had coexisting cardiovascular pathology (e.g., heart failure, peripheral vascular disease), would the ideal treatment have been different? Why or why not?
- What effect does the water driven by the turbine have on the ability of the patient to tolerate the aggressive stretching? What is the mechanism for this effect?

The rehabilitation professional employs physical agent modalities to create an optimum environment for tissue healing while minimizing the symptoms associated with the trauma or condition.

effect of the water flow. Removal of the part being treated from the whirlpool will necessitate a review of the skin surface and an assessment of edema in the extremities. If total body immersion is used, care should be taken for the intensity and duration of the whirlpool and for protection of the genitals from direct water flow. Applications can be repeated following rewarming of the body segment after sensation has

congestion Presence of an abnormal amount of blood in the vessels resulting from an increase in blood flow or obstructed venous return.

returned. If the cold application is administered before practice, it should be done before the application of preventive strapping. Enough time should also be allowed for sensation to return before taping. Studies have indicated that the reflex vasodilation lasts up to 2 hours. A patient could practice, then return to the training room and receive additional treatment without additional edema created by **congestion** as a result of vascular and capillary insufficiency occurring during the healing process. Increased heart rate and blood pressure are associated with cold application. Conditioned patients should not have a problem with dizziness after cold applications, but care should be taken when transferring the patient from the whirlpool area. Whirlpool cultures of the tank and jet should be taken monthly to keep bacterial growth under control.

Whirlpool Maintenance

Safety considerations for using both cold and hot whirlpools have been discussed previously. It is equally important to mention the importance of maintaining the cleanliness of the whirlpools in a clinical setting.

It is not uncommon for several individuals to use a whirlpool between cleanings. This practice is certainly not recommended and in fact is contrary to the standards of most health regulatory agencies in many states.

It is recommended that the whirlpool be drained and cleaned after each treatment to minimize the potential risks of spreading fungal, viral, or bacterial infections, especially in those individuals who have open lesions. Whirlpools should be cleaned by filling the basin above the level of the turbine, adding a commercial antibiotic solution, disinfecting agent, or chlorine bleach, and then running the turbine for at least 1 minute. The turbine and drain filter should be scrubbed and the tub thoroughly rinsed. The outside surface of the whirlpool should be cleaned daily.

To keep bacterial and fungal growth in check, whirlpool cultures should be taken monthly.

Cold Spray

Cold sprays, such as Fluori-Methane, do not provide adequate deep penetration, but they do provide adjunctive therapy for acupressure techniques to reduce muscle spasm. Physiologically this is accomplished by stimulating the A fibers involved in the gate control theory. The primary action of a cold spray is reduction of the pain spasm sequence secondary to direct trauma. However, it will not reduce hemorrhage because it works on the superficial nerve endings to reduce the spasm via the stimulation of A fibers to reduce the so-called painful arc. Cold spray is an extremely effective technique in the treatment of myofascial trigger points. Precautions concerning the use of cold spray include protecting the patient's face from the fumes and spraying the skin at an acute rather than a perpendicular angle.[119] Cold spray is indicated when stretching of an injured part is desired along with cold treatment.

Equipment Needed

1. Fluori-Methane.
2. Toweling.
3. Padding.

Treatment

The area to be treated should be sprayed and then stretched.
Spasm should be reduced.
Treatment should be distal to proximal.
A quick jetstream spray or stroking motion should be used.
Cooling should be superficial; no frosting should occur.

Cold sprays may be used in conjunction with acupressure. Treatment time should be set according to body segment.

Physiologic Responses

Muscle spasm is reduced.
Golgi tendon organ response is facilitated.
Muscle spindle response is inhibited.
Musculoskeletal structures may be stimulated.

Considerations

Both the acute and the subacute response should be positive.
The room should be well ventilated to avoid the accumulation of fumes.
Patient comfort should be considered at all times.

Application

The application of Fluori-Methane is typical of the application of other cold sprays (Fig. 11-6). The following application procedures apply specifically to Fluori-Methane, but they provide an outline of the procedures, indications, and precautions applicable to all cold sprays. The therapist should follow the manufacturer's instructions in the use of any cold spray.

Fluori-Methane is a topical vapocoolant that acts as a counterirritant to block pain impulses of muscles in spasm. When used in conjunction with the "spray-and-stretch" technique, Fluori-Methane can break the pain cycle, allowing the muscle to be stretched to its normal length (pain-free state). The application of the "spray-and-stretch" technique is a therapeutic modality that involves three stages: evaluation, spraying, and stretching. The therapeutic value of "spray-and-stretch" becomes most effective when the practitioner has mastered all stages and applies them in the proper sequence.

Evaluation

During the evaluation phase the cause of pain is determined as local spasm or an irritated trigger point. The method of applying "spray-and-stretch" to a muscle spasm differs slightly from application to a trigger point. The trigger point is a deep hypersensitive localized spot in a muscle that causes a referred pain pattern. With trigger points the source of pain is seldom the site of the pain. A trigger point may be detected by a snapping

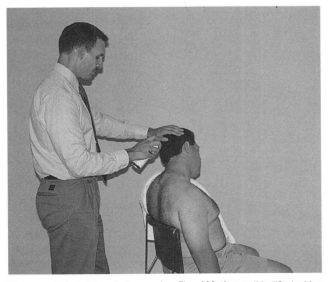

•**Figure 11-6** "Spray-and-stretch" technique using Fluori-Methane. (Modified with permission of the Gebauer Chemical Company, Cleveland, OH, 44104, (800) 321-9348; Ohio (216) 271-5252.)

palpation over the muscle, causing the muscle in which the irritated trigger point is situated to "jump." In the case of muscle spasm, the source and site of pain are identical. A trigger point may also be effectively treated using ultrasound and electrical stimulation.[67]

Spraying

The following steps should be followed to apply Fluori-Methane.

1. The patient should assume a comfortable position.
2. Take precautions to cover the patient's eyes, nose, and mouth if spraying near the face.
3. Hold the spray can or spray bottle (upside down) 12–18 inches away from the treatment surface, allowing the jetstream of vapocoolant to meet the skin at an acute angle.
4. Apply the spray in one direction only—not back and forth—at a rate of 4 inches (10 cm) per second. Three or four sweeps of the spray in one direction only are sufficient to treat the trigger point or to overcome painful muscle spasms. The skin must not be frosted. It is possible but not very likely that the intense cold (15°C) of the Fluori-Methane can freeze the skin, causing frostbite, and result in superficial tissue necrosis. Certainly the chances of this occurring are not nearly as likely as when using ethyl chloride. In the case of trigger point, spray should be applied from the trigger point to the area of referred pain. If there is no trigger point, the spray should be applied from the affected muscle to its insertion. The spray should be applied in an even sweep. About two to four parallel, but not overlapping, sweeps of spray should be enough to cover this skin representation of the affected muscle.

Stretching

The static stretch should begin as you start spraying from the origin to the insertion (simple muscle spasm pain) or from the trigger point to the referred pain when the trigger point is present. Spray-and-stretch until the muscle reaches its maximal or normal resting length. You will usually feel a gradual increase in range of motion. The spraying and stretching may require two to four spray applications to achieve the therapeutic results in any treatment session. A patient may have multiple treatment sessions in any 1 day.

The spray-and-stretch technique outlined in the preceding must be considered a therapeutic system. The practitioner should spend some time each day practicing until the technique is mastered.

Composition

Fluori-Methane is a combination of two chlorofluorocarbons—15 percent dichlorodifluoromethane and 85 percent trichloromonofluoromethane. The combination is not flammable and at room temperature is only volatile enough to expel the contents from the inverted container. Fluori-Methane is supplied in amber Dispenseal bottles that emit a jetstream from a calibrated nozzle.

Indications

Fluori-Methane is a vapocoolant intended for topical application in the management of myofascial pain, restricted motion, and muscle spasm. Clinical conditions that may respond to spray-and-stretch include low back pain (caused by muscle spasm), acute stiff neck, torticollis, acute bursitis of shoulder, muscle spasm associated with osteoarthritis, ankle sprain, tight hamstring, masseter muscle spasm, certain types of headache, and referred pain from trigger points.

Precautions

Federal law prohibits dispensing without a prescription. Although Fluori-Methane is safe for topical application to the skin, care should be taken to minimize inhalation of vapors, especially when it is being applied to the head or neck. Fluori-Methane is not intended for production of local **anesthesia** and should not be applied to the point of frost formation. Freezing can occasionally alter pigmentation.

Contrast Bath

Contrast baths are used to treat subacute swelling, gravity-dependent swelling, and vasodilation-vasoconstriction response. Both contrast baths and cold whirlpools have

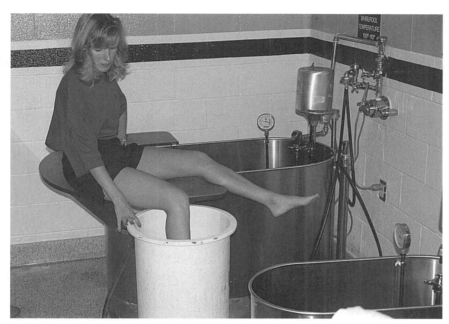

•**Figure 11-7** Contrast bath using a warm whirlpool and ice immersion cylinder.

been demonstrated to be effective in treating delayed-onset muscle soreness.[65] A contrast-therapy technique using hot and cold packs has been shown to have little or no effect on deep muscle temperatures.[88]

Equipment Needed (Fig. 11-7)

1. Two containers. One container is used to hold cold water (50–60°F), and the other is used to hold warm water (104–106°F). Whirlpools may be used for one or both containers.
2. Ice machine.
3. Towels.
4. Chair.

Treatment

Hot and cold immersions are alternated. Treatment time should be at least 20 minutes. Treatments should consist of five 1-minute cold immersions and five 3-minute warm immersions, although the exact ratio of cold to hot treatment is highly variable.

Physiologic Responses

Vasoconstriction and vasodilation occur.
There is a reduction of necrotic cells at the cellular level.
Edema is decreased.

Considerations

The temperatures of the baths must be maintained.
A large area is required for treatment.
Patient comfort must be considered at all times.

Application

After the area is set up, a whirlpool can be used for either hot or cold application, with the opposite method of treatment contained in a bucket or sterile container. The temperatures of these immersion baths must be maintained (cold at 50–60°F, hot at 98–110°F) by adding ice or warm water. It is generally easier to use a large whirlpool for the warm water application and a bucket for the cold water application. There has

Treatment Tip
Contrast baths produce little or no "pumping action" and are not very effective in treating swelling. A better alternative is to use cryokinetics, which involves cold followed by active muscle contractions and relaxation to help eliminate swelling.

vasoconstriction Narrowing of the blood vessels.

CASE STUDY 11-3
HYDROTHERAPY: CONTRAST BATH

Background: A 29-year-old police officer sustained a laceration of the right posterior forearm as a result of a struggle with an individual using a knife. There was a partial laceration of the extensor carpi radialis longus and brevis, and the extensor digitorum (communis), no arterial damage, no motor nerve damage, but a complete transection of the superficial radial nerve. The laceration was sutured primarily, and a splint applied to prevent stress on the repair. The patient is now 12 weeks postinjury, and has full wrist and hand motion and near-normal strength. However, he has developed extreme sensitivity to any stimulus over the dorsal-radial aspect of the wrist and hand, which is disabling. The patient guards the area by holding the right forearm with his left hand, and experiences severe pain when anything touches the area (including a breeze). The area innervated by the superficial radial nerve is glossy in appearance, and is now hairless (as compared to the left forearm and hand). He has been referred for pain management and desensitization.

Impression: Complex regional pain syndrome (CRPS) type II (also known as causalgia).

Treatment Plan: Two basins large enough to immerse the entire forearm were filled with water, one at 40°C (104°F) and the other at 14°C (57°F). The patient's forearm was immersed in the warm water for 2 minutes, then removed and immersed in the cold water for 1 minute. The sequence was repeated six times, for a total treatment duration of 18 minutes. Immediately after the final immersion, the patient was encouraged to brush the painful area with his left hand, and to tap over the mid- and distal-radius, along the course of the superficial radial nerve.

Response: After the initial treatment, the patient noted little improvement, and was unable to tolerate the desensitization. The treatment was repeated the next day, and he was able to tolerate a few seconds of desensitization. He was treated in the clinic daily for a total of four sessions, and, he was then instructed to continue the

contrast bath treatment on a home program, with weekly rechecks. He completed twice-daily sessions at home, and noted very gradual increases in the duration of the increased tolerance to touch and tapping, as well as an ability to tolerate more vigorous touch. Two months later, there was no hypersensitivity in the superficial radial nerve distribution, and the skin had returned to a normal appearance.

Discussion Questions

- What tissues were injured or affected?
- What symptoms were present?
- What phase of the injury-healing continuum did the patient present for care in?
- What are the physical agent modality's biophysical effects (direct, indirect, depth, and tissue affinity)?
- What are the physical agent modality's indications and contraindications?
- What are the parameters of the physical agent modality's application, dosage, duration, and frequency in this case study?
- What other physical agent modalities could be used to treat this injury or condition? Why? How?
- What is CRPS type II?
- What is the difference between CRPS type I and CRPS type II?
- Is it likely that CRPS could have been prevented in this patient? How?
- If the patient's fingertips had become very pale during the immersion in the cold water, and the patient had complained of severe pain in the fingertips, what would have been your response? What pathology would you suspect?

The rehabilitation professional employs physical agent modalities to create an optium environment for tissue healing while minimizing the symptoms associated with the trauma or condition.

been considerable controversy regarding the use of contrast baths to control swelling. Contrast baths are most often indicated when changing the treatment modality from cold to hot to facilitate a mild tissue temperature increase. The use of a contrast bath allows for a transitional period during which a slight rise in tissue temperature may be effective for increasing blood flow to an injured area without causing the accumulation of additional edema. The theory that contrast baths induce a type of pumping action by alternating vasoconstriction with vasodilation has little or no credibility.

Contrast baths probably cause only a superficial capillary response, resulting from inability of the larger deep blood vessels to constrict and dilate in response to superficial heating.[87,111]

Thus, it is recommended that during the initial stages of contrast bath treatment the ratio of hot to cold treatment begins with a relatively brief period in the hot bath, gradually increasing the length of time in the hot bath during subsequent treatments. Recommendations as to specific lengths of time are extremely variable. However, it would appear that a 3:1 ratio (3 min in hot, 1 min in cold) or 4:1 ratio for 19–20 minutes is fairly well accepted. Whether the treatment is ended with cold or hot depends to some extent on the degree of tissue temperature increase desired. Other therapists prefer to use the same ratios of 3:1 or 4:1, beginning with cold. The technique may certainly be modified to meet specific needs. Since the extremity is in the gravity-dependent position, once the injured part is removed from the contrast bath, skin sensation and the amount of edema accumulation should be assessed to make sure that the treatment has not actually increased the amount of edema.[5]

Cryo-Cuff

The Cryo-Cuff is a device that uses both cold and compression simultaneously. The Cryo-Cuff is used both acutely following injury and postsurgically. Originally developed by Aircast, it is made of a nylon sleeve that connects via a tube to a 1-gallon cooler/jug. Cold water flows into the sleeve from the cooler. As the cooler is raised, the pressure in the cuff is increased. During the treatment, the water warms and can be rechilled by lowering the cooler to drain the cuff, mixing the warmer water with the colder water, and then again raising the jug to increase pressure in the cuff. The only drawback to this simple yet effective piece of equipment is that you must continually rechill the water in the cuff. However the Cryo-Cuff is portable, easy to use, and inexpensive.[52]

Ice Immersion

Ice buckets allow ease of application for the therapist. Again, a wet area should be selected (where spilled water is not a concern), with the patient positioned for comfort. The immersion, like the contrast bath, should be maintained until desired results are reached. If cryokinetics are part of the treatment, then the container should be large enough to allow for the movement of the body segment. Although ice immersion has been shown to be effective in controlling posttraumatic edema,[25] ice immersion is similar to cold whirlpool in that the body segment may be subject to gravity-dependent positions. Cold pain may be worse during ice immersion than during cold pack application.[59]

Cryokinetics

Cryokinetics is a technique that combines cryotherapy or the application of cold with exercise.[52,53] The goal of cryokinetics is to numb the injured part to the point of analgesia and then work toward achieving normal range of motion through progressive active exercise. Using cryokinetics does not seem to delay the onset of fatigue.[9]

The technique begins by numbing the body part via ice immersion, cold packs, or ice massage. Most patients will report a feeling of numbness within 12–20 minutes. If numbness is not perceived within 20 minutes, the therapist should proceed with exercise regardless. The numbness usually will last for 3–5 minutes, at which point ice should be reapplied for an additional 3–5 minutes until numbness returns. This sequence should be repeated five times.

Exercises are performed during the periods of numbness. The exercises selected should be pain-free and progressive in intensity, concentrating on both flexibility and strength.[97] Changes in the intensity of the activity should be limited by both the nature of the healing process and individual patient differences in perception of pain. However, progression always should be encouraged within the framework of those limiting factors, the ultimate goal being a return to full activity.[53]

cryokinetics The use of cold and exercise in the treatment of pathology or disease.

CASE STUDY 11-4
CRYO-CUFF

Background: A 28-year-old woman sustained blunt trauma to her right forefoot when she dropped a full box of copy paper on it while attempting to remove the box from a shelf. She reported to an occupational health clinic and after having an x-ray taken to rule out fracture, she was referred to you for emergent care. The forefoot was noted to be visibly swollen and discolored. Circumferential measure taken at MTI heads was increased by 1 cm over the uninvolved side measure. You quickly repositioned the patient with her foot elevated above heart level and continued your examination. Both PD and TP were intact, and there was no medial or lateral ankle ligament tenderness. Attempts at assessing AROM/PROM were abandoned secondary to the patient's complaints of forefoot pain.

Impression: Soft tissue contusion with acute soft tissue edema formation right forefoot.

Treatment Plan: You apply a moistened cotton stockingnette to the right foot and ankle followed by the application of a Cryo-Cuff ankle sleeve. The sleeve was filled from the ice water reservoir until full. Treatment with the cold, mild compression and elevation lasted approximately 20 minutes. Immediately following the completion of the initial cold, compression, and elevation treatment, the patient was instructed in crutch walking, nonweight-bearing right lower extremity, and the use of the Cryo-Cuff once each waking hour along with attention to maintaining the limb in an elevated position. The patient was advised to return to the clinic first thing the next morning.

Response: The patient tolerated cold compression and elevation very well and reported immediate pain relief in the forefoot. Upon return to the clinic the next morning, the patient was noted to have no further increase in forefoot edema. Gentle passive- and active-assistive range of motion exercise for digits and ankle were initiated.

Weight-bearing as tolerated with crutches was attempted. By treatment day 5 strengthening exercises were added to the program. Between treatments the patient was placed in a compression stocking and walker boot. One week after the injury, the patient was able to wear a shoe without discomfort and return to full work status.

Discussion Questions

- What tissues were injured/affected?
- What symptoms were present?
- What phase of the injury-healing continuum did the patient present for care in?
- What are the physical agent modailty's biophysical effects (direct/indirect/depth/tissue affinity)?
- What are the physical agent modality's indications/contraindications?
- What are the parameters of the physical agent modality's application/dosage/duration/frequency in this case study?

The rehabilitation professional employs physical agent modalities to create an optimum environment for tissue healing while minimizing the symptoms associated with the trauma or condition.

- What other physical agent modalities could be utilized to treat this injury or condition? Why? How?

Further Discussion Questions

- What other techniques could have been used to provide pain management/acute edema control?
- What are the physiologic mechanisms for the pain relief/acute edema control?
- Why was it necessary to elevate the foot above the level of the heart?
- What effect might the Cryo-Cuff have on the properties of the forefoot soft tissues?

THERMOTHERAPY

PHYSIOLOGIC EFFECTS OF TISSUE HEATING

Local superficial heating (infrared heat) is recommended in subacute conditions for reducing pain and **inflammation** through analgesic effects. Superficial heating produces lower tissue temperatures at the site of the pathology (injury) relative to the higher temperatures in the superficial tissues, resulting in **analgesia**. During the later stages of injury healing, a deeper heating effect is usually desirable; it can be achieved by using the diathermies or ultrasound. Heat dilates blood vessels, causing the patent capillaries to open up and increase circulation. The skin is supplied with sympathetic vasoconstrictor fibers that secrete norepinephrine at their endings (especially evident in feet, hands, lips, nose, and ears). At normal body temperature, the sympathetic vasoconstrictor nerves keep vascular anastomoses almost totally closed, but when the superficial tissue is heated, the number of sympathetic impulses is greatly reduced so that the anastomoses dilate and allow large quantities of blood to flow into the venous plexuses. This increases blood flow about twofold, which can promote heat loss from the body.[39]

The **hyperemia** created by heat has a beneficial effect on injury. This is based on increases of blood flow and pooling of blood during the metabolic processes. Recent hematomas (blood clots) should never be treated with heat until resolution of bleeding is completed. Some therapists have advocated never using heat during any therapeutic modality application.[47,52,53,58]

hyperemia Presence of an increased amount of blood in part of the body.

The rate of metabolism of tissues depends partly on temperature. The metabolic rate has increased approximately 13 percent for each 1°C (1.8°F) increase in temperature.[47] A similar decrease in metabolism has been demonstrated when temperatures are lowered.

A primary effect of local heating is an increase in the local metabolic rate with a resulting increase in the production of **metabolites** and additional heat. These two factors lead to an increased intravascular hydrostatic pressure, causing arteriolar **vasodilation** and increased capillary blood flow.[113] However, with increased hydrostatic pressure, there is a tendency toward formation of edema, which may increase the time required for rehabilitation of a particular injury. Increased capillary blood flow is important with many types of injury in which there is mild or moderate inflammation, because it causes an increase in the supply of oxygen, antibodies, leukocytes, and other necessary **nutrients** and enzymes, along with an increased clearing of metabolites. With higher heat intensities, vasodilation and increased blood flow will spread to remote areas, causing increased metabolism in the unheated area. This is known as **consensual heat vasodilation** and may be useful in many conditions where local heating is contraindicated.[33]

vasodilation Dilation of the blood vessels.

vasoconstriction Narrowing of the blood vessels.

consensual heat vasodilation Vasodilation and increased blood flow will spread to remote areas, causing increased metabolism in the unheated area.

The application of heat can produce an analgesic effect, resulting in a reduction in the intensity of pain. The analgesic effect is the most frequent **indication** for the use.[113] Although the mechanisms underlying this phenomenon are not well understood, it is related in some way to the gate control theory of pain modulation. Heat has been shown to reduce pain associated with delayed onset muscle soreness following a 30-minute treatment.[114]

Heat is applied in musculoskeletal and neuromuscular disorders, such as sprains, strains, articular (joint-related) problems, and muscle spasms, which all describe various types of muscle pain.[33] Heat generally is considered to produce a relaxation effect and a reduction in guarding in skeletal muscle. It also increases the elasticity and decreases the viscosity of connective tissue, which is an important consideration in postacute joint injuries or after long periods of immobilization. This may also be important during a warm-up activity prior to exercise for increasing intramuscular temperatures.[112] However, it has also been demonstrated that heat alone without stretching has little or no effect in improving flexibility.[8,106] It appears that a deep heating treatment using ultrasound may be more effective for increasing range of motion than using a more superficial heating technique.[51]

Many therapists empirically believe that heat has little effect on the disease itself but serves rather to facilitate further treatment by producing relaxation in these types of disorders.[33] This is accomplished by relieving pain, lessening hypertonicity of muscles, producing sedation (which decreases spasticity, tenderness, and spasm), and decreasing tightness in muscles and related structures.

THERMOTHERAPY TREATMENT TECHNIQUES

Heat is still used as a universal treatment for pain and discomfort. Much of the benefit is derived from the treatment simply feeling good. However, in the early stages after injury, heat causes increased capillary blood pressure and increased cellular permeability; this results in additional swelling or **edema** accumulation.[2,13,33,56,128] *No patient with edema should be treated with any heat modality until the reasons for the edema are determined.* It is in the best interest of the therapist to use cryotherapy techniques to reduce the edema before applying heat. Superficial heat applications seem to feel more comfortable for complaints of the neck, back, low back, and pelvic areas and may be most appropriate for the patient

edema Excessive fluid in cells.

that patient. A haphazard approach to the use of infrared modalities will only reflect a disregard for the health care of the patient.

Questioning, thinking therapists will determine which procedure is best and most appropriate clinically. They will take responsibility for seeing that the most appropriate therapeutic modality is applied to enhance the patient's reconditioning and rehabilitation. Regardless of which infrared modality therapists choose, they should be aware of (1) the physiologic implications relative to circulation; (2) the ease of application; and (3) the short- and long-term benefits of treatment.

Additional areas of concern relate to (1) benefits of the infrared modality application, whether cryotherapy or thermotherapy; (2) economy of modality application; and (3) repeatability of applications. Common sense in the application of these modalities will provide optimum injury management and modality usage for tissue healing of athletic trauma.

SUMMARY

1. Any modality that radiates energy with wavelengths and frequencies that fall into the infrared region of the electromagnetic spectrum are referred to as infrared modalities.
2. When infrared modalities are applied to connective tissue or muscle and soft tissue, they will cause either a tissue temperature decrease or tissue temperature increase.
3. The primary physiologic effect of heat is vasodilatation of capillaries with increased blood flow, increased metabolic activity, and relaxation of muscle spasm.
4. The primary physiologic effects of cold are vasoconstriction of capillaries with decreased blood flow, decreased metabolic activity, and analgesia with reduction of muscle spasm.
5. The infrared energies have a depth of penetration of less than 1 cm, thus the physiologic effects are primarily superficial and directly affect the cutaneous blood vessels and nerve receptors.
6. Examples of thermotherapy are whirlpools, moist heat packs, infrared lamps, heating pads, and fluidotherapy.
7. Examples of cryotherapy are ice packs, ice massage, commercial ice packs, ice whirlpools, and cold sprays.

REVIEW QUESTIONS

1. What is the definition of an infrared modality and how are they classified within the electromagnetic spectrum?
2. What are the two basic therapeutic clinical uses for the infrared modalities?
3. What is the depth of penetration into the tissues of the infrared modalities?
4. What are the effects of changing temperatures on circulation?
5. How does changing tissue temperature affect muscle spasm?
6. What are the physiologic effects of both therapeutic heat and cold?
7. What are the differences between the terms *cryotherapy*, *thermotherapy*, and *hydrotherapy*?
8. What are the various cryotherapy techniques that can be used by the therapist?
9. What are the various thermotherapy techniques that can be used by the therapist?

REFERENCES

1. Abramson, D., Tuck, S., and Lee, S.: Vascular basis for pain due to cold, Arch. Phys. Med. Rehabil. 47:300–305, 1966.
2. Baker, R., Bell, G.: The effect of therapeutic modalities on blood flow in the human calf, JOSPT 13:23, 1991.
3. Basset, S., Lake, B.: Use of cold applications in management of spasticity, Phys. Ther. 38(5):333–334, 1958.
4. Behnke, R.: Cold therapy, Athl. Train. 9(4):178–179, 1974.
5. Bibi, K.W., Dolan, M.G., and Harrington, K.: Effects of hot, cold, contrast therapy whirlpools on non-traumatized ankle volumes, J. Athl. Train. 34(2):S–17, 1999.
6. Bierman, W., Friendiander, M.: The penetrative effect of cold, Arch. Phys. Med. Rehabil. 21:585–592, 1940.
7. Braswell, S., Frazzini, M., and Knuth, A.: Optimal duration of ice massage for skin anesthesia, Phys. Ther. 74(5):S156, 1994.
8. Burke, D., Holt, L., and Rasmussen, R.: The effect of hot or cold water immersion and proprioceptive neuromuscular facilitation on hip joint range of motion, J. Athl. Train. 36(1):16–19, 2001.
9. Campbell, H., Cordova, M., and Ingersoll, C.: A cryokinetics protocol does not affect quadriceps muscle fatigue, J. Athl. Train. (Suppl.) 38 (2S):S-48, 2003.
10. Chambers, R.: Clinical uses of cryotherapy, Phys. Ther. 49(3): 145–149, 1969.
11. Chung, J.M., Lee, K.H., Hori, Y., and Willis, W.D.: Effects of capsaicin applied to a peripheral nerve on the responses of primate spinothalamic tract cells, Brain Res. 329(1–2):27–38, 1985.
12. Clarke, D.: Effect of immersion in hot and cold water upon recovery of muscular strength following fatiguing isometric exercise, Arch. Phys. Med. Rehabil. 44:565–568, 1963.
13. Clarke, D., Stelmach, G.: Muscle fatigue and recovery curve parameters at various temperatures, Res. Quart. 37(4): 468–479, 1966.
14. Clarke, R., Hellon, R., and Lind, A.: Vascular reactions of the human forearm to cold, Clin. Sci. 17:165–179, 1958.
15. Clark, R., Lephardt, S., and Baker, C.: Cryotherapy and compression treatment protocols in the prevention of delayed onset muscle soreness, J. Athl. Train. 31(2):S33, 1996.
16. Clemente, F., Frampton, R., and Temoshenka, A.: The effects of hot and cold packs on peak isometric torque generated by the back extensor musculature, Phys. Ther. 74(5):S70, 1994.
17. Comeau, M.J., Potteiger, J.A.: The effects of cold water immersion on parameters of skeletal muscle damage and delayed onset muscle soreness, J. Athl. Train. 35(2):S–46, 2000.
18. Cote, D., Prentice, W., and Hooker, D.: A comparison of three treatment procedures for minimizing ankle edema, Phys. Ther. 68(7):1072–1076, 1988.
19. Coulombe, B., Swanik, C., and Raylman, R.: Quantification of musculoskeletal blood flow changes in response to cryotherapy using positron emission tomography, J. Athl. Train. (Suppl.) 36(2S):S-49, 2001.
20. Curl, W.W., Smith, B.P., Marr, A., et al.: The effect of contusion and cryotherapy on skeletal muscle microcirculation, J. Sports Med. Phys. Fitness 37(4):279–286, 1997.

21. Cutlaw, K., Arnold, B., and Perrin, D.: Effect of cold treatment on concentric and eccentric force velocity relationship of the quads, J. Athl. Train. 30(2):S31, 1995.
22. Dejong, R., Hershey, W., and Wagman, I.: Nerve conduction velocity during hypothermia in man, Anesthesiology 27:805–810, 1966.
23. Dervin, G.F., Taylor, D.E., and Keene, G.C.: Effects of cold and compression dressings on early postoperative outcomes for the athroscopic ACL reconstruction patient, J. Orthop. Sports Phys. Ther. 27(6):403–411, 1998.
24. Dolan, M.G., Mendel, F.M., and Teprovich, J.M.: Effects of dependent positioning and cold water immersions on nontraumatized ankle volumes, J. Athl. Train. 34(2):S–17, 1999.
25. Dolan, M.G., Thornton, R.M., and Fish, D.R.: Effects of cold water immersion on edema formation after blunt injury to the hind limbs of rats, J. Athl. Train. 32(3):233–237, 1997.
26. Dolan, M., Thornton, R., and Mendel, F.: Cold water immersion effects on edema formation following impact injury to hind limbs of rats, J. Athl. Train. 31(2):S48, 1996.
27. Dontigny, R., Sheldon, K.: Simultaneous use of heat and cold in treatment of muscle spasm, Arch. Phys. Med. Rehabil. 43:235–237, 1962.
28. Downer, A.: Physical therapy procedures, ed. 3, Springfield, IL, 1978, Charles C Thomas.
29. Downey, J.: Physiological effects of heat and cold, J. Am. Phys. Ther. Assoc. 44(8):713–717, 1964.
30. Dufresne, T., Jarzabski, K., and Simmons, D.: Comparison of superficial and deep heating agents followed by a passive stretch on increasing the flexibility of the hamstring muscle group, Phys. Ther. 74(5):S70, 1994.
31. Eldred, E., Lindsley, D., and Buchwald, J.: The effect of cooling on mammalian muscle spindles, Exp. Neurol. 2:144–157, 1960.
32. Evans, T., Ingersoll, C., and Knight, K.: Agility following the application of cold therapy, J. Athl. Train. 30(3):231–234, 1995.
33. Fischer, E., Soloman, S.: Physiologic responses to heat and cold. In Licht, S., editor. Therapeutic heat, New Haven, CT, 1965, Elizabeth Licht.
34. Gallant, S., Knight, K., and Ingersoll, C.: Cryotherapy effects on leg press and vertical jump force production, J. Athl. Train. 31(2):S18, 1996.
35. Golestani, S., Pyle, M., and Threlkeld, A.J.: Joint position sense in the knee following 30 min of cryotherapy, J. Athl. Train. 34(2):S–68, 1999.
36. Grant, A.: Massage with ice (cryokinetics) in the treatment of painful conditions of the musculoskeletal system, Arch. Phys. Med. Rehabil. 45:233–238, 1964.
37. Grecier, M., Kendrick, Z., and Kimura, I.: Immediate and delayed effects of cryotherapy on functional power and agility, J. Athl. Train. 31(Suppl.):S–32, 1996.
38. Griffin, J., Karselis, T.: Physical agents for physical therapists, ed. 2, Springfield, IL, 1988, Charles C Thomas.
39. Guyton, A.: Medical physiology, ed. 6, Philadelphia, 1991, W.B. Saunders.

40. Hatzel, B., Weidner, T., and Gehlsen, G.: Mechanical power and velocity following cryotherapy and ankle taping, J. Athl. Train. (Suppl.) 36(2S):S-89, 2001.

41. Hautkappe, M., Roizen, M., Toledano, A., et al.: Review of the effectiveness of capsaicin for painful cutaneous disorders and neural dysfunction, Clin. J. Pain 14(2):97–106, 1998.

42. Hayden, C.: Cryokinetics in an early treatment program, J. Am. Phys. Ther. Assoc. 44:11, 1964.

43. Haynes, S.C., Perrin, D.H.: Effects of a counterirritant on pain and restricted range of motion associated with delayed onset muscle soreness, J. Sport Rehabil. 1(1):13–18, 1992.

44. Hedenberg, L.: Functional improvement of the spastic hemiplegic arm after cooling, Scand. J. Rehabil. Med. 2:154–158, 1970.

45. Hill, J., Sumida, K.: Acute effect of 2 topical counterirritant creams on pain induced by delayed-onset muscle soreness, J. Sport Rehabil. 11(3):202, 2002.

46. Ho, S., Illgen, R., and Meyer, R.: Comparison of various icing times in decreasing bone metabolism and blood in the knee, Am. J. Sports Med. 23(1):74–76, 1995.

47. Hocutt, J., Jaffe, R., and Rylander, C.: Cryotherapy in ankle sprains, Am. J. Sports Med. 10(3):316–319, 1992.

48. Ichiyama, R.M., Ragan, B.G., Bell, G.W., and Iwamoto, G.A.: Effects of topical analgesics on the pressor response evoked by group III and IV muscle afferents, Med. Sci. Sports Exerc. 34(9):1440–1445, 2002.

49. Jameson, A., Kinzey, S., and Hallam, J.: Lower-extremity-joint cryotherapy does not affect vertical ground-reaction forces during landing, J. Sport Rehabil. 10(2):132, 2001.

50. Kimura, I.F., Gulick, D.T., and Thompson, G.T.: The effect of cryotherapy on eccentric plantar flexion peak torque and endurance, J. Athl. Train. 32(2):124–126, 1997.

51. Knight, C.A., Rutledge, C.R., Cox, M.E., et al.: Effect of superficial heat, deep heat, and active exercise warm-up on the extensibility of the plantar flexors, Phys. Ther. 81:1206–1214, 2001.

52. Knight, K.: Cryotherapy in sports injury management, Champaign, IL, 1995, Human Kinetics.

53. Knight, K.: Cryotherapy: theory, technique and physiology, Chattanooga, TN, 1985, Chattanooga Corporation.

54. Knight, K.: Effects of hypothermia on inflammation and swelling, Athl. Train. 11:7–10, 1976.

55. Knight, K.: Ice for immediate care of injuries, Phys. Sports Med. 10(2):137, 1982.

56. Knight, K., Aquino, J., and Johannes S.: A reexamination of Lewis' cold induced vasodilation in the finger and the ankle, Athl. Train. 15:248–250, 1980.

57. Knight, K., Ingersoll, C., and Trowbridge, C.: The effects of cooling the ankle, the triceps surae or both on functional agility, J. Athl. Train. 29(2):165, 1994.

58. Knight, K., Londeree, B.: Comparison of blood flow in the ankle of uninjured subjects during therapeutic applications of heat, cold, and exercise, Med. Sci. Sports Exerc. 12(1):76–80, 1980.

59. Knight, K.L., Rubley, M.D., and Ingersoll, C.D.: Pain perception is greater during ankle ice immersion than during ice pack application, J. Athl. Train. 35(2):S-45, 2000.

60. Knott, M., Barufaldi, D.: Treatment of whiplash injuries, Phys. Ther. 41:8, 1961.

61. Knutsson, E.: Topical cryotherapy in spasticity, Scand. J. Rehabil. Med. 2:159–163, 1970.

62. Knutsson, E., Mattson, E.: Effects of local cooling on monosynaptic reflexes in man, Scand. J. Rehabil. Med. 1:126–132, 1969.

63. Kolb, P., Denegar, C.: Traumatic edema and the lymphatic system, Athl. Train. 18:339–341, 1983.

64. Krause, B.A., Hopkins, J.T., and Ingersoll, C.D.: The relationship of ankle temperature during cooling and rewarming to the human soleus H reflex, J. Sport Rehabil. 9(3):253–262, 2000.

65. Kuligowski, L.A., Lephart, S.M., and Frank, P.: Effect of whirlpool therapy on the signs and symptoms of delayed-onset muscle soreness, J. Athl. Train. 33(3):222–228, 1998.

66. LaRiviere, J., Osternig, L.: The effect of ice immersion on joint position sense, J. Sport Rehabil. 3(1):58–67, 1994.

67. Lee, J.C., Lin, D.T., and Hong C.: The effectiveness of simultaneous thermotherapy with ultrasound and electrotherapy with combined AC and DC current on the immediate pain relief of myofascial trigger points, J. Musculoskeletal Pain 5(1):81–90, 1997.

68. Lehman, J.: Therapeutic heat and cold, ed. 3, Baltimore, MD, 1982, Williams & Wilkins.

69. Leonard, K., Horodyski, M.B., and Kaminski, T.: Changes in dynamic postural stability following cryotherapy to the ankle and knee, J. Athl. Train. 34(2):S-68, 1999.

70. Lewis, T.: Observations upon the reactions of the vessels of the human skin to cold, Heart 15:177–208, 1930.

71. Licht, S.: Therapeutic heat and cold, New Haven, CT, 1965, Elizabeth Licht.

72. Lippold, O., Nicholls, J., and Redfearn, J.: A study of the afferent discharge produced by cooling a mammalian muscle spindle, J. Physiol. 153:218–231, 1960.

73. Lowden, B., Moore, R.: Determinants and nature of intramuscular temperature changes during cold therapy, Am. J. Phys. Med. 54(5):223–233, 1975.

74. Mancuso, D., Knight, K.: Effects of prior skin surface temperature response of the ankle during and after a 30-minute ice pack application, J. Athl. Train. 27:242–249, 1992.

75. McKeon, P., Dolan, M., and Gandloph, J.: Effects of dependent positioning cool water immersion CWI and high-voltage electrical stimulation HVES on non-traumatized limb volumes, J. Athl. Train. (Suppl.) 38(2S): S-35, 2003.

76. McMaster, W.: A literary review on ice therapy in injuries, Am. J. Sports Med. 5(3):124–126, 1977.

77. Merrick, M.A., Jutte, L., and Smith, M.: Cold modalities with different thermodynamic properties produce different surface and intramuscular temperatures, J. Athl. Train. 38(1):28–33, 2003.

78. Merrick, M.A., Jutte, L.S., and Smith, M.E.: Intramuscular temperatures during cryotherapy with three different cold modalities, J. Athl. Train. 35(2):S-45, 2000.

79. Merrick, M.A., Knight, K., and Ingersoll C.: The effects of ice and compression wraps on intramuscular temperatures at various depths, J. Athl. Train. 28(3):236–245, 1993.

80. Merrick, M.A., Knight, K., and Ingersoll, C.: The effects of ice and elastic wraps on intratissue temperatures at various depths, J. Athl. Train. 28(2):156, 1993.

81. Mickey, C., Bernier, J., and Perrin, D.: Ice and ice with nonthermal ultrasound effects on delayed onset muscle soreness, J. Athl. Train. 31(2):S19, 1996.

82. Miglietta, O.: Electromyographic characteristics of clonus and influence of cold, Arch. Phys. Med. Rehabil. 45:508, 1964.

83. Misasi, S., Morin, G., and Kemler, D.: The effect of a toe cap and bias on perceived pain during cold water immersion, J. Athl. Train. 30(1):149–156, 1995.

84. Moore, R.: Uses of cold therapy in the rehabilitation of athletes: recent advances, Proceedings 19th American Medical Association National Conference on the medical aspects of sports, San Francisco, June 1977.

85. Moore, R., Nicolette, R., and Behnke, R.: The therapeutic use of cold (cryotherapy) in the care of athletic injuries, Athl. Train. 2:613, 1967.

86. Murphy, A.: The physiological effects of cold application, Phys. Ther. 40(2):112–115, 1960.

87. Myer, J.W., Draper, D., and Durrant, E.: The effect of contrast therapy on intramuscular temperature in the human lower leg, J. Athl. Train. 29(4):318–322, 1994.

88. Myer, J.W., Measom, G., Durrant, E., and Fellingham, G.W.: Cold- and hot-pack contrast therapy: subcutaneous and intramuscular temperature change, J. Athl. Train. 32(3): 238–241, 1997.

89. Myer, J.W., Measom, G., and Fellingham, G.W.: Temperature changes in the human leg during and after two methods of cryotherapy, J. Athl. Train. 33(1):25–29, 1998.

90. Myer, J.W., Myer, K., and Measom, G.: Muscle temperature is affected by overlying adipose when cryotherapy is administered, J. Athl. Train. 36(1):32–36, 2001.

91. Myer, K.A., Myer, J.W., and Measom, G.J.: Overlying adipose significantly effects intramuscular temperature change during crushed ice pack therapy, J. Athl. Train. 34(2):S–69, 1999.

92. Nelson, A.J., Ragan, B.G., Bell, G.W., and Iwamoto, G.A.: Capsaicin based analgesic balm decreases the pressor response evoked by muscle afferents, Med. Sci. Sports Exerc. 36(3): 444–450, 2004.

93. Nosaka, K., Sakamoto, K., and Newton, M.: Influence of pre-exercise muscle temperature on responses to eccentric exercise, J. Athl. Train. 39(2):132–137, 2004.

94. Olson, J., Stravino, V.: A review of cryotherapy, Phys. Ther. 62(8):840–853, 1972.

95. Otte, J., Merrick, M., and Ingersoll, C.: Subcutaneous adipose tissue thickness changes cooling time during cryotherapy, J. Athl. Train. (Suppl.) 36(2S):S-91, 2001.

96. Paduano, R., Crothers, J.: The effects of whirlpool treatments and age on a one-leg balance test, Phys. Ther. 74(5):S70, 1994.

97. Pincivero, D., Gieck, J., and Saliba, E.: Rehabilitation of a lateral ankle sprain with cryokinetic and functional progressive exercise, J. Sport Rehabil. 2(3):200–207, 1993.

98. Prentice, W: An electromyographic analysis of the effectiveness of heat or cold and stretching for inducing relaxation in injured muscle, J. Orthop. Sports Phys. Ther. 3(3):133–146, 1982.

99. Ragan, B.G., Marvar, P.J., and Dolan, M.G.: Effects of magnesium sulfate and warm baths on nontraumatized ankle volumes, J. Athl. Train. 35(2):S–43, 2000.

100. Ragan, B., Nelson, A., and Bell, G.: Menthol based analgesic balm attenuates the pressor response evoked by muscle afferents, J. Athl. Train. (Suppl.) 38(2S):S-34, 2003.

101. Rivers, D., Kimura, I., and Sitler, M.: The influence of cryotherapy and Aircast bracing on total body balance and proprioception, J. Athl. Train. 30(2):S15, 1995.

102. Rocks, A.: Intrinsic shoulder pain syndrome, Phys. Ther. 59(2):153–159, 1979.

103. Rogers, J., Knight, K., and Draper, D.: Increased pressure of application during ice massage results in an increase in calf skin numbing, J. Athl. Train. (Suppl.) 36(2S):S-90, 2001.

104. Rubley, M., Denegar, C., and Buckley, W.: Cryotherapy, sensation and isometric-force variability, J. Athl. Train. 38(2): 113–119, 2003.

105. Ruiz, D., Myrer, J., and Durrant, E.: Cryotherapy and sequential exercise bouts following cryotherapy on concentric and eccentric strength in the quadriceps, J. Athl. Train. 28(4): 320–323, 1993.

106. Sawyer, P., Uhl, T., and Yates, J.: Effects of muscle temperature on hamstring flexibility, J. Athl. Train. (Suppl.) 37(2S):S-103, 2002.

107. Schnatz, A., Kimura, I., and Sitler, M.: Influence of cryotherapy thermotherapy and neoprene ankle sleeve on total body balance and proprioception, J. Athl. Train. 31(2):S32, 1996.

108. Schuler, D., Ingersoll, C., and Knight, K.: Local cold application to foot and ankle, lower leg of both effects on a cutting drill, J. Athl. Train. 31(2):S35, 1996.

109. Serwa, J., Rancourt, L., and Merrick, M.: Effect of varying application pressures on skin surface and intramuscular temperatures during cryotherapy, J. Athl. Train. (Suppl.) 36(2S): S-90, 2001.

110. Smith, K., Draper, D., and Schulthies, S.: The effect of silicate gel hot packs on human muscle temperature, J. Athl. Train. 30(2):S33, 1995.

111. Smith, K., Newton, R.: The immediate effect of contrast baths on edema, temperature and pain in postsurgical hand injuries, Phys. Ther. 74(5):S157, 1994.

112. Sreniawski, S., Cordova, M., and Ingeroll, C.: A comparison of hot packs and light or moderate exercise on rectus femoris temperature, J. Athl. Train. (Suppl.) 37(2S):S-104, 2002.

113. Stillwell, K.: Therapeutic heat and cold. In Krusen F., Kootke F., and Ellwood P., editors. Handbook of physical medicine and rehabilitation, Philadelphia, PA, 1971, W.B. Saunders.

114. Sumida, K., Greenberg, M., and Hill, J.: Hot gel packs and reduction of delayed-onset muscle soreness 30 minutes after treatment, J. Sport Rehabil. 12(3):221–228, 2003.

115. Taylor, B., Waring, C., and Brasher, T.: The effects of therapeutic application of heat or cold followed by static stretch on hamstring muscle length, JOSPT 21(5):283–286, 1995.

116. Thieme, H., Ingersoll, C., and Knight, K.: Cooling does not affect knee proprioception, J. Athl. Train. 31(1):8–11, 1996.

117. Thieme, H., Ingersoll, C., and Knight, K.: The effect of cooling on proprioception of the knee, J. Athl. Train. 28(2):158, 1993.

118. Thompson, G., Kimura, I., and Sitler, M.: Effect of cryotherapy on eccentric and peak torque and endurance, J. Athl. Train. 29(2):180, 1994.

119. Travell, J.: Ethyl chloride spray for painful muscle spasm, Arch. Phys. Med. Rehabil. 32:291–298, 1952.

120. Travell, J.: Rapid relief of acute "stiff neck" by ethyl chloride spray, Am. Med. Wom. Assoc. 4(3):89–95, 1949.

121. Travell, J., Simons, D.: Myofascial pain and dysfunction: the trigger point manual, Baltimore, 1983, Williams & Wilkins.

122. Tremblay, F., Estaphan, L., and Legendre, M.: Influence of local cooling on proprioceptive acuity in the quadriceps muscle, J. Athl. Train. 36(2):119–123, 2001.

123. Trowbridge, C., Draper, D., and Jutte, L.: A comparison of the capsicum back plaster, the ABC back plaster and the Therma-Care Heatwrap on paraspinal muscle and skin temperature, J. Athl. Train. (Suppl.) 37(2S):S–102, 2002.

124. Tsang, K.K.W., Buxton, B.P., Guion, W.K., et al.: The effects of cryotherapy applied through various barriers, J. Sport Rehabil. 6(4):343–354, 1997.

125. Tsang, K.H., Hertel, J., and Denegar, C.: The effects of gravity dependent positioning following elevation on the volume of the uninjured ankle, J. Athl. Train. 35(2):S–50, 2000.

126. Weston, M., Taber, C., and Casagranda, L.: Changes in local blood volume during cold gel pack application to traumatized ankles, J. Orthop. Sports Phys. Ther. 19(4):197–199, 1994.

127. Whittaker, T., Lander, J., and Brubaker, D.: The effect of cryotherapy on selected balance parameters, J. Athl. Train. 29(2):180, 1994.

128. Zankel, H.: Effect of physical agents on motor conduction velocity of the ulnar nerve, Arch. Phys. Med. Rehabil. 47(12): 787–792, 1966.

129. Zemke, J.E., Andersen, J.C., and Guion, K.: Intramuscular temperature responses in the human leg to two forms of cryotherapy: ice massage and icebag, J. Orthop. Sports Phys. Ther. 27(4):301–307, 1998.

SUGGESTED READINGS

Abraham, E.: Whirlpool therapy for treatment of soft tissue wounds complicated by extremity fractures, J. Trauma 4:222, 1974.

Abraham, W.: Heat vs. cold therapy for the treatment of muscle injuries, Athl. Train. 9(4):177, 1974.

Abramson, D., Bell, B., and Tuck, S.: Changes in blood flow, oxygen uptake and tissue temperatures produced by therapeutic physical agents: effect of indirect or reflex vasodilation, Am. J. Phys. Med. 40:5–13, 1961.

Abramson, D., Mitchell, R., and Tuck, S.: Changes in blood flow, oxygen uptake and tissue temperatures produced by a topical application of wet heat, Arch. Phys. Med. Rehabil. 42:305, 1961.

Abramson, D., Tuck, S., and Zayas, A.: The effect of altering limb position on blood flow, oxygen uptake and skin temperature, J. Appl. Physiol. 17:191, 1962.

Abramson, D., Tuck, S., and Chu, L.: Effect of paraffin bath and hot fomentation on local tissue temperature, Arch. Phys. Med. Rehabil. 45:87, 1964.

Abramson, D., Tuck, S., Chu, L.: Indirect vasodilation in thermotherapy, Arch. Phys. Med. Rehabil. 46:412, 1965.

Abramson, D.: Physiologic basis for the use of physical agents in peripheral vascular disorders, Arch. Phys. Med. Rehabil. 46:216, 1965.

Abramson, D., Chu, L., and Tuck, S.: Effect of tissue temperatures and blood flow on motor nerve conduction velocity, JAMA 198:1082, 1966.

Abramson, D., Tuck, S., and Lee, S.: Comparison of wet and dry heat in raising temperature of tissues, Arch. Phys. Med. Rehabil. 48:654, 1967.

Airhihenbuwa, C., St. Pierre, R., and Winchell, D.: Cold vs. heat therapy: a physician's recommendations for first aid treatment of strain, Emergency 19(1):40–43, 1987.

Arnheim, D., Prentice, W.: Principles of athletic training, ed. 9, New York, 1997, McGraw-Hill.

Ascenzi, J.: The need for decontamination and disinfection of hydrotherapy equipment, vol. 1, Surgikos, 1980, Asepsis Monograph.

Austin, K.: Diseases of immediate type hypersensitivity. In Isselbacher, K., Adams, R., and Braumwald E., editors. Harrison's principles of internal medicine, ed. 9, New York, 1980, McGraw-Hill.

Barnes, L.: Cryotherapy: putting injury on ice, Phys. Sportsmed. 7(6):130–136, 1979.

Basur, R., Shephard, E., and Mouzos G.: A cooling method in the treatment of ankle sprains, Practitioner 216:708, 1976.

Beasley, R., Kester, N.: Principles of medical-surgical rehabilitation of the hand, Med. Clin. North Am. 53:645, 1969.

Belitsky, R., Odam, S., and Humbley-Kozey, C.: Evaluation of the effectiveness of wet ice, dry ice, and cryogen packs in reducing skin temperature, Phys. Ther. 67:1080, 1987.

Benoit, T., Martin, D., and Perrin, D.: Effect of clinical application of heat and cold on knee joint laxity, J. Athl. Train. 30(2):S31, 1995.

Benson, T., Copp, E.: The effects of therapeutic forms of heat and ice on the pain threshold of the normal shoulder, Rheumatol. Rehabil. 13:101, 1974.

Berne, R., Levy, M.: Cardiovascularphysiology, ed. 4, St. Louis, MO, 1981, C.V. Mosby.

Bickle, R.: Swimming pool management, Physiotherapy 57:475, 1971.

Bierman, W.: Therapeutic use of cold, JAMA 157:1189–1192, 1955.

Bocobo, C.: The effect of ice on intra-articular temperature in the knee of the dog, Am. J. Phys. Med. Rehabil. 70:181, 1991.

Boes, M.: Reduction of spasticity by cold, J. Am. Phys. Ther. Assoc. 42(1):29–32, 1962.

Boland, A.: Rehabilitation of the injured athlete. In Strauss, R.A., editor. Physiology, Philadelphia, PA, 1979, W.B. Saunders.

Borrell, R., Henley, E., and Purvis H.: Fluidotherapy: evaluation of a new heat modality, Arch. Phys. Med. Rehabil. 58:69, 1977.

Borrell, R., Parker, R., and Henley, E.: Comparison of in vivo temperatures produced by hydrotherapy, paraffin wax treatment, and fluidotherapy, Phys. Ther. 60(10):1273–1276, 1980.

Boyer, T., Fraser, R., and Doyle, A.: The haemodynamic effects of cold immersion, Clin. Sci. 19:539, 1980.

Boyle, R., Balisteri, F., and Osborne, F.: The value of the Hubbard tank as a diuretic agent, Arch. Phys. Med. Rehabil. 45:505, 1964.

Chastain, P.: The effect of deep heat on isometric strength, Phys. Ther. 58:543, 1978.

Clarke, K., editor: Fundamentals of athletic training: physical therapy procedures, Chicago, IL, 1971, AMA Press.

Claus-Walker, J.: Physiological responses to cold stress in healthy subjects and in subjects with cervical cord injuries, Arch. Phys. Med. Rehabil. 55:485, 1974.

Clements, J., Casa, D., and Knight, J.C.: Ice-water immersion and cold-water immersion provide similar cooling rates in runners with exercise-induced hyperthermia, J. Athl. Train. 37(2):146–150, 2002.

Clendenin, M., Szumski, A.: Influence of cutaneous ice application on single motor units in humans, Phys. Ther. 51(2):166–175, 1971.

Cobb, C., Devries, H., and Urban, R.: Electrical activity in muscle pain, Am. J. Phys. Med. 54:80, 1975.

Cobbold, A., Lewis, O.: Blood flow to the knee joint of the dog: effect of heating, cooling and adrenaline, J. Physiol. 132:379, 1956.

Cohen, A., Martin, G., and Waldin, K.: The effect of whirlpool bath with and without agitation on the circulation in normal and diseased extremities, Arch. Phys. Med. Rehabil. 30:212, 1949.

Conolly, W., Paltos, N., and Tooth, R.: Cold therapy: an improved method, Med. J. Aust. 2:424, 1972.

Cook, D., Georgouras K.: Complications of cutaneous cryotherapy, Med. J. Aust. 161(3):210–213, 1994.

Cordray, Y., Krusen, E.: Use of hydrocollator packs in the treatment of neck and shoulder pains, Arch. Phys. Med. Rehabil. 39:105, 1959.

Covington, D., Bassett, F.: When cryotherapy injures, Phys. Sportsmed. 21(3):78–79, 1993.

Crockford, G., Hellon, R.: Vascular responses of human skin to infrared radiation, J. Physiol. 149:424, 1959.

Crockford, G., Hellon, R., and Parkhouse, J.: Thermal vasomotor response in human skin mediated by local mechanism, J. Physiol. 161:10, 1962.

Culp, R., Taras, J.: The effect of ice application versus controlled cold therapy on skin temperature when used with postoperative bulky hand and wrist dressings: a preliminary study, J. Hand. Ther. 8(4):249–251, 1995.

Currier, D., Kramer, J.: Sensory nerve conduction: heating effects of ultrasound and infrared, Physiother. Can. 34:241, 1982.

Dawson, W., Kottke, P., and Kubicek, W.: Evaluation of cardiac output, cardiac work, and metabolic rate during hydrotherapy exercise in normal subjects, Arch. Phys. Med. Rehabil. 46:605, 1965.

Day, M.: Hypersensitive response to ice massage: report of a case, Phys. Ther. 54:592, 1974.

DeLateur, B., Lehmann, J.: Cryotherapy. In Lehmann, J., editor. Therapeutic heat and cold, ed. 3, Baltimore, MD, 1982, Williams & Wilkins.

Devries, H.: Quantitative electromyographic investigation of the spasm theory of muscle pain, Am. J. Phys. Med. 45:119, 1966.

Draper, D., Schulthies, S., and Sorvisto, P.: Temperature changes in deep muscles of humans during ice and ultrasound therapies: an in vivo study, J. Orthop. Sports Phys. Ther. 21(3):153–157, 1995.

Drez, D.: Therapeutic modalities for sports injuries, Chicago, IL, 1989, Yearbook.

Drez, D., Faust, D., and Evans, J.: Cryotherapy and nerve palsy, Am. J. Sports Med. 9:256, 1981.

Edwards, H., Harris, R., and Hultman, E.: Effect of temperature on muscle energy metabolism and endurance during successive isometric contractions, sustained to fatigue, of the quadriceps muscle in man, J. Physiol. 220:335, 1972.

Epstein, M.: Water immersion: modern researchers discover the secrets of an old folk remedy, Sciences 205:12, 1979.

Eyring, E., Murray, W.: The effect of joint position on the pressure of intraarticular effusion, J. Bone Joint Surg. 46[A](6):1235, 1964.

Farry, P., Prentice, N.: Ice treatment of injured ligaments: an experimental model, N.Z. Med. J. 9:12, 1950.

Folkow, B., Fox, R., and Krog, J.: Studies on the reactions of the cutaneous vessels to cold exposure, Acta Physiol. Scand. 58: 342, 1963.

Fountain, F., Gersten, J., and Senger, O.: Decrease in muscle spasm produced by ultrasound, hot packs and IR, Arch. Phys. Med. Rehabil. 41:293, 1960.

Fox, R.: Local cooling in man, Br. Ed. Bull. 17(1):14–18, 1961.

Fox, R., Wyatt, H.: Cold induced vasodilation in various areas of the body surface in man, J. Physiol. 162:259, 1962.

Gammon, G., Starr, I.: Studies on the relief of pain by counterirritation, J. Clin. Invest. 20:13, 1941.

Gerig, B.: The effects of cryotherapy upon ankle proprioception (abstract), Athl. Train. 25:119, 1990.

Gieck, J.: Precautions for hydrotherapeutic devices, Clin. Manage. 3:44, 1953.

Golland, A.: Basic hydrotherapy, Physiotherapy 67:258, 1951.

Green, G., Zachazewski, J., and Jordan, S.: A case conference: peroneal nerve palsy induced by cryotherapy, Phys. Sportsmed. 17:63, 1989.

Greenberg, R.: The effects of hot packs and exercise on local blood flow, Phys. Ther. 52:273, 1972.

Halkovich, I., Personius, W., and Clamann, H.: Effect of fluorimethane spray on passive hip flexion, Phys. Ther. 61:185, 1981.

Halvorson, G.: Therapeutic heat and cold for athletic injuries, Phys. Sportsmed. 18:87, 1990.

Harb, G.: The effect of paraffin bath submersion on digital blood flow in patients with Raynaud's syndrome, Phys. Ther. 73(6): S9, 1993.

Harrison, R.: Tolerance of pool therapy by ankylosing spondylitis patients with low vital capacity, Physiotherapy 67:296, 1981.

Hayes, K.: Heat and cold in the management of rheumatoid arthritis, Arth. Care Res. 6(3):156–166, 1993.

Head, M., Helms, P.: Paraffin and sustained stretching in the treatment of burn contractures, Burns 4:136, 1977.

Healy, W., Seidman, J., and Pfeifer B.: Cold compressive dressing after total knee arthroplasty, Clin. Orthop. Rel. Res. 299:143–146, 1994.

Hellerbrand, T., Holutz, S., and Eubarik, I.: Measurement of whirlpool temperature, pressure and turbulence, Arch. Phys. Med. Rehabil. 32:17, 1950.

Hendier, E., Crosbie, R., and Hardy, J.: Measurement of heating of the skin during exposure to infrared radiation, J. Appl. Physiol. 12:177, 1958.

Henricksen, A., Fredricksson, K., and Persson, I.: The effect of heat and stretching on the range of hip motion, J. Orthop. Sports Phys. Ther. 6:110, 1984.

Ho, S., Coel, M., and Kagawa, R.: The effects of ice on blood flow and bone metabolism in knees, Am. J. Sports Med. 22(4):537–540, 1994.

Hocutt, J., Jaffe, R., and Rylander, R.: Cryotherapy in ankle sprains, Am. J. Sports Med. 10:316, 1982.

Holcomb, W., Mangus, B., Tandy, R.: The effect of icing with the Pro-Stim Edema Management System on cutaneous cooling, J. Athl. Train. 31(2):126–129, 1996.

Holmes, G.: Hydrotherapy as a means of rehabilitation, Br. J. Phys. Med. 5:93, 1942.

Horton, B., Brown, G., and Roth, G.: Hypersensitiveness to cold with local and systemic manifestations of a histamine-like character: its amenability to treatment, JAMA 107:1263, 1936.

Horvath, S., Hollander, L.: Intra-articular temperature as a measure of joint reaction, J. Clin. Invest. 28:469, 1949.

Hunter, J., Mackin, E.: Edema and bandaging. In Hunter, J., editor. Rehabilitation of the hand, ed. 1, St. Louis, MO, 1978, C.V. Mosby.

Ingersoll, C., Mangus, B.: Sensations of cold reexamined: a study using the McGill pain questionnaire, Athl. Train. 26:240, 1991.

Ingersoll, C., Mangus, B., and Wolf, S.: Cold-induced pain: habituation to cold immersion (abstract), Athl. Train. 25:126, 1990.

Jamison, C., Merrick, M., and Ingersoll, C.: The effects of post cryotherapy exercise on surface and capsular temperature, J. Athl. Train. (Suppl.) 36(2S):S-91, 2001.

Jessup, G.: Muscle soreness: temporary distress of injury? Athl. Train. 15(4):260, 1950.

Jezdirisky, J., Marek, I., and Ochonsky, P.: Effects of local cold and heat therapy on traumatic oedema of the rat hind paw. 1. Effects of cooling on the course of traumatic oedema, Acta Universitatis Palackianae Olomucensis Facultatis Medicae 66:155, 1973.

Johnson, D.: Effect of cold submersion on intramuscular temperature of the gastrocnemius muscle, Phys. Ther. 59:1238, 1979.

Johnson, J., Leider, F.: Influence of cold bath on maximum handgrip strength, Percept. Mot. Skills 44:323, 1977.

Kaempffe, F.: Skin surface temperature after cryotherapy to a casted extremity, J. Orthop. Sports Phys. Ther. 10(11):448–450, 1989.

Kaul, M., Herring, S.: Superficial heat and cold: how to maximize the benefits, Phys. Sportsmed. 22(12):65–72, 74, 1994.

Kessler, R., Hertling, D.: Management of common musculoskeletal disorders, Philadelphia, PA, 1953, Harper & Row.

Knight, K.: Ankle rehabilitation with cryotherapy, Phys. Sportsmed. 7(11):133, 1979.

Knight, K., Han, K., and Rubley, M.: Comparison of tissue cooling and numbness during application of Cryo5 air cooling, crushed ice packs, ice massage, and ice water immersion, J. Athl. Train. (Suppl.) 37(2S):S-103, 2002.

Knight, K., Rubley, M., and Brucker, J.: Knee surface temperature changes on uninjured subjects during and following application of three post-operative cryotherapy devices, J. Athl. Train. (Suppl.) 36(2S):S-90, 2001.

Kowal, M.: Review of physiological effects of cryotherapy, J. Orthop. Sports Phys. Ther. 6(2):66–73, 1953.

Kramer, J., Mendryk, S.: Cold in the initial treatment of injuries sustained in physical activity programs, Can. Assoc. Health Phys. Ed. Rec. J. 45(4):27–29, 38–40, 1979.

Krause, B., Ingersoll, C., and Edwards, J.: Ankle joint and triceps surae muscle cooling produce similar changes in the soleus H:M Ratio, J. Athl. Train. (Suppl.) 36(2S):S-50, 2001.

Krause, B., Ingersoll, C., and Edwards, J.: Ankle ice immersion facilitates the soleus Hoffman Reflex and muscle response, J. Athl. Train. (Suppl.) 38(2S):S-48, 2003.

Krusen, E.: Effects of hot packs on peripheral circulation, Arch. Phys. Med. Rehabil. 31:145, 1950.

Landen, B.: Heat or cold for the relief of low back pain? Phys. Ther. 47:1126, 1967.

Lane, L.: Localized hypothermia for the relief of pain in musculoskeletal injuries, Phys. Ther. 51:182, 1971.

Lawrence, S., Cosgray, N., and Martin, S.: Using heat modalities for therapeutic hamstring flexibility: a comparison of pneumatherm moist heat pack and a control, J. Athl. Train. (Suppl.) 37(2S):S-101, 2002.

Lee, J., Warren, M., and Mason, S.: Effects of ice on nerve conduction velocity, Physiotherapy 64:2, 1978.

Lehmann, J.: Effect of therapeutic temperatures on tendon extensibility, Arch. Phys. Med. Rehabil. 51:481, 1970.

Lehmann, J., Brurmer, G., and Stow, R.: Pain threshold measurements after therapeutic application of ultrasound, microwaves and infrared, Arch. Phys. Med. Rehabil. 39:560, 1958.

Lehmann, J., Silverman, J., and Baum, B.: Temperature distributions in the human thigh produced by infrared, hot pack and microwave applications, Arch. Phys. Med. Rehabil. 41:291, 1966.

Levine, M., Kabat, H., and Knott, M.: Relaxation of spasticity by physiological techniques, Arch. Phys. Med. Rehabil. 35:214, 1954.

Levy, A., Marmar, E.: The role of cold compression dressings in the postoperative treatment of total knee arthroplasty, Clin. Orthop. Rel. Res. (297):174–178, 1993.

Lundgren, C., Muren, A., and Zederfeldt, B.: Effect of cold vasoconstriction on wound healing in the rabbit, Acta Chir. Scand. 118:1, 1959.

Magness, J., Garrett, T., and Erickson, D.: Swelling of the upper extremity during whirlpool baths, Arch. Phys. Med. Rehabil. 51:297, 1970.

Major, T., Schwingharner, J., and Winston, S.: Cutaneous and skeletal muscle vascular responses to hypothermia, Am. J. Physiol. 240 (Heart Circ. Physiol. 9):H868, 1981.

Marek, I., Jezdinsky, J., and Ochonsky, P.: Effects of local cold and heat therapy on traumatic oedema of the rat hind paw. II. Effects of various kinds of compresses on the course of traumatic oedema, Acta Univ. Palacki. Olomuc. Fa. Med. 66:203, 1973.

Matsen, F., Questad, K., and Matsen, A.: The effect of local cooling on post fracture swelling, Clin. Orthop. 109:201, 1975.

McDowell, J., McFarland, E., and Nalli, B.: Use of cryotherapy for orthopaedic patients, Orthop. Nurs. 13(5):21–30, 1994.

McGowen, H.: Effects of cold application on maximal isometric contraction, Phys. Ther. 47:185, 1967.

McGray, R., Patton, N.: Pain relief at trigger points: a comparison of moist heat and shortwave diathermy, J. Orthop. Sports Phys. Ther. 5:175, 1984.

McMaster, W.: Cryotherapy, Phys. Sportsmed. 10(11):112–119, 1982.

McMaster, W., Liddie, S.: Cryotherapy influence on posttraumatic limb edema, Clin. Orthop. 150:283–287, 1980.

McMaster, W., Liddie, S., and Waugh, T.: Laboratory evaluation of various cold therapy modalities, Am. J. Sports Med. 6(5): 291–294, 1978.

Mense, S.: Effects of temperature on the discharges of muscle spindles and tendon organs, Pflugers Arch. 374:159, 1978.

Mermel, J.: The therapeutic use of cold, J. Am. Osteopath. Assoc. 74:1146–1157, 1975.

Michalski, W., Sequin, J.: The effects of muscle cooling and stretch on muscle spindle secondary endings in the cat, J. Physiol. 253:341–356, 1975.

Michlovitz, S.: Thermal agents in rehabilitation, Philadelphia, PA, 1995, F.A. Davis.

Miglietta, O.: Action of cold on spasticity, Am. J. Phys. Med. 52(4):198–205, 1973.

Nelson, A., Ragan, B., and Bell, G.: Capsaicin based analgesic balm decreases the pressor response evoked by muscle afferents, J. Athl. Train. (Suppl.) 38(2S):S-34, 2003.

Newton, T., Lchnikuhi, D.: Muscle spindle response to body heating and localized muscle cooling: implications for relief of spasticity, J. Am. Phys. Ther. Assoc. 45(2):91, 105, 1965.

Noonan, T., Best, T., and Seaber, A.: Thermal effects on skeletal muscle tensile behavior, Am. J. Sports Med. 21(4):517–522, 1993.

Nylin, J.: The use of water in therapeutics, Arch. Phys. Med. Rehabil. 13:261, 1932.

Oliver, R., Johnson, D., and Wheelhouse, W.: Isometric muscle contraction response during recovery from reduced intramuscular temperature, Arch. Phys. Med. Rehabil. 60:126–129, 1979.

Panus, P., Carroll, J., and Gilbert, R.: Gender-dependent responses in humans to dry and wet cryotherapy, Phys. Ther. 74(5):S156, 1994.

Perkins, J., Mao-Chih, L., and Nicholas, C.: Cooling and contraction of smooth muscle, Am J. Physiol. 163:14, 1950.

Petajan, H., Watts, N.: Effects of cooling on the triceps surae reflex, Am. J. Phys. Med. 42:240–251, 1962.

Pope, C.: Physiologic action and therapeutic value of general and local whirlpool baths, Arch. Phys. Med. Rehabil. 10:498, 1929.

Preston, D., Irrgang, J., Bullock, A.: Effect of cold and compression on swelling following ACL reconstruction, J. Athl. Train. 28(2):166, 1993.

Price, R.: Influence of muscle cooling on the vasoelastic response of the human ankle to sinusoidal displacement, Arch. Phys. Med. Rehabil. 71(10):745–748, 1990.

Price, R., Lehmann, J., Boswell, S.: Influence of cryotherapy, on spasticity at the human ankle, Arch. Phys. Med. Rehabil. 74(3):300–304, 1993.

Randall, B., Imig, C., and Hines, H.: Effects of some physical therapies on blood flow, Arch. Phys. Med. Rehabil. 33:73, 1952.

Randt, G.: Hot tub folliculitis, Phys. Sports Med. 11:75, 1983.

Ritzmann, S., Levin, W.: Cryopathies: a review, Arch. Intern. Med. 107:186, 1961.

Roberts, P.: Hydrotherapy: its history, theory and practice, Occup. Health 235:5, 1981.

Schaubel, H.: Local use of ice after orthopedic procedures, Am. J. Surg. 72:711, 1946.

Schultz, K.: The effect of active exercise during whirlpool on the band, unpublished thesis, San Jose, CA, 1982, San Jose State University.

Shelley, W., Caro, W.: Cold erythema: a new hypersensitivity syndrome, JAMA 180:639, 1962.

Simonetti, A., Miller, R., and Gristina, J.: Efficacy of povidone-iodine in the disinfection of whirlpool baths and hubbard tanks, Phys. Ther. 52:450, 1972.

Steve, L., Goodhart, P., and Alexander, J.: Hydrotherapy burn treatment: use of chloramine-T against resistant microorganisms, Arch. Phys. Med. Rehabil. 60:301, 1979.

Stewart, B., Basmajian, J.: Exercises in water. In Basmaiian, J., editor. Therapeutic exercise, ed. 3, Baltimore, MD, 1978, Williams & Wilkins.

Streator, S., Ingersoll, C., and Knight, K.: The effects of sensory information on the perception of cold-induced pain, J. Athl. Train. 29(2):166, 1994.

Strandness, D.: Vascular diseases of the extremities. In Isselbacher, K., Adams, R., and Braunwald, E., editors. Harrison's principles of internal medicine, ed. 9, New York, 1980, McGraw-Hill.

Taber, C., Contryman, K., and Fahrenbach, J.: Measurement of reactive vasodilation during cold gel pack application to non-traumatized ankles, Phys. Ther. 72:294, 1992.

Travell, J., Simons, D.: Myofascial pain and dysfunction: the trigger point manual, Baltimore, MD, 1983, Williams & Wilkins.

Urbscheit, N., Johnston, R., and Bishop, B.: Effects of cooling on the ankle jerk and H-response in hemiplegic patients, Phys. Ther. 51:983, 1971.

Wakim, K., Porter, A., and Krusen, K.: Influence of physical agents and of certain drugs on intra-articular temperature, Arch. Phys. Med. Rehabil. 32:714, 1951.

Walsh, M.: Relationship of band edema to upper extremity position and water temperature during whirlpool treatments in normals, Unpublished thesis. Philadelphia, PA, 1983, Temple University.

Warren, G.: The use of heat and cold in the treatment of common musculoskeletal disorders. In Kessler, R., Hertling, D. Management of common musculoskeletal disorders, Philadelphia, PA, 1983, Harper & Row.

Warren, G., Lehmann, J., and Koblanski, N.: Heat and stretch procedures: an evaluation using rat tail tendon, Arch. Phys. Med. Rehabil. 57:122, 1976.

Watkins, A.: A manual of electrotherapy, ed. 3, Philadelphia, PA, 1972, Lea & Febiger.

Waylonis, G.: The physiological effect of ice massage, Arch. Phys. Med. Rehabil. 48:37–42, 1967.

Weinberger, A., Lev, A.: Temperature elevation of connective tissue by physical modalities, Crit. Rev. Phys. Rehabil. Med. 3:121, 1991.

Wessman, M., Kottke, F.: The effect of indirect heating on peripheral blood flow, pulse rate, blood pressure and temperature, Arch. Phys. Med. Rehabil. 48:567, 1967.

Whitelaw, G., DeMuth, K., and Demos H.: The use of the Cryo/Cuff versus ice and elastic wrap in the postoperative care of knee arthroscopy patients, Am. J. Knee Surg. 8(1):28–30, 1995.

Whitney, S.: Physical agents: heat and cold modalities. In Scully, R., Barnes, M., editors. Physical therapy, Philadelphia, PA, 1987, J.B. Lippincott.

Whyte, H., Reader, S.: Effectiveness of different forms of heating, Ann. Rheum. Dis. 10:449, 1951.

Wickstrom, R., Polk, C.: Effect of whirlpool on the strength endurance of the quadriceps muscle in trained male adolescents, Am. J. Phys. Med. 40:91, 1961.

Wilkerson, G.: Treatment of inversion ankle sprain through synchronous application of focal compression and cold, Athl. Train. 26:220, 1991.

Wolf, S., Basmajian, J.: Intramuscular temperature changes deep to localized cutaneous cold stimulation, Phys. Ther. 53(12): 1284–1288, 1973.

Wolf, S., Ledbetter, W.: Effect of skin cooling on spontaneous EMG activity in triceps surae of the decerebrate cat, Brain Res. 91:151–155, 1975.

Wright, V., Johns, R.: Physical factors concerned with the stiffness of normal and diseased joints, Bull. Johns Hopkins Hosp. 106:215, 1960.

Wyper, D., McNiven, D.: Effects of some physiotherapeutic agents on skeletal muscle blood flow, Physiotherapy 62:83, 1976.

Yackzan, L., Adams, C., and Francis, K.: The effects of ice massage in delayed muscle soreness, Am. J. Sports Med. 12(2):159–165, 1984.

Zankel, H.: Effect of physical agents on motor conduction velocity of the ulnar nerve, Arch. Phys. Med. Rehabil. 47:787, 1966.

Zeiter, V.: Clinical application of the paraffin bath, Arch. Phys. Ther. 20:469, 1939.

Zislis, J.: Hydrotherapy. In Krusen, F., editor. Handbook of physical medicine and rehabilitation, ed. 2, Philadelphia, PA, 1971, W.B. Saunders.

GLOSSARY

analgesia Loss of sensibility to pain.

anesthesia Loss of sensation.

conduction Heat loss or gain through direct contact.

congestion Presence of an abnormal amount of blood in the vessels resulting from an increase in blood flow or obstructed venous return.

consensual heat vasodilation Vasodilation and increased blood flow will spread to remote areas, causing increased metabolism in the unheated area.

contrast bath Hot (106°F) and cold (50°F) treatments in a combined sequence to stimulate superficial capillary vasodilation or vasoconstriction.

convection Heat loss or gain through the movement of water molecules across the skin.

conversion Changing from one energy form into another.

cryokinetics The use of cold and exercise in the treatment of pathology or disease.

cryotherapy The use of cold in the treatment of pathology or diseases.

edema Excessive fluid in cells.

erythema Redness of the skin.

fluidotherapy A modality of dry heat using a finely divided solid suspended in a stream with the properties of liquid.

hunting response A reflex vasodilation that occurs in response to cold approximately 15 minutes into the treatment. This has been demonstrated to be only an increase in temperature and not necessarily a change in blood flow.

hydrocollator A synthetic hot (170°F) or cold (0°F) gel used as an adjunctive modality to stimulate a rise or fall in tissue temperature.

hydrotherapy Cryotherapy and thermotherapy techniques that use water as the medium for heat transfer.

hyperemia Presence of an increased amount of blood in part of the body.

inflammation A redness of the skin caused by capillary dilation.

indication The reason to prescribe a remedy or procedure.

infrared That portion of the electromagnetic spectrum associated with thermal changes; located adjacent to the red portion of the visible light spectrum. That part of the electromagnetic spectrum dealing with infrared wavelengths.

metabolites Waste products of metabolism or catabolism.

myofascial pain A type of referred pain associated with trigger points.

PROCEDURE	EVALUATION		
	1	2	3
3. Position patient.			
a. Place patient in a well-supported, comfortable position.			
b. Expose body part to be treated.			
c. Drape patient to preserve patient's modesty, protect clothing, but allow access to body part.			
4. Inspect body part to be treated.			
a. Check light touch perception.			
b. Check circulatory status (pulses, capillary refill).			
c. Verify that there are no open wounds or rashes.			
d. Assess function of body part (e.g., ROM, irritability).			
5. Apply ice pack.			
a. Warn the patient that you are going to put the ice pack on the body part to be treated, then do so. Make sure the draping will catch any water that melts from the ice pack.			
b. Set a timer for the appropriate treatment time (generally about 20 minutes), and give the patient a signaling device. Make sure the patient understands how to use the signaling device.			
c. Check the patient's response verbally after the first 2 minutes, then about every 5 minutes. Perform a visual check of the area if the patient reports any unusual sensation. If wheals or welts appear, or if the skin color changes to absolute white within the first 4 minutes of treatment, stop the treatment.			
6. Complete the treatment.			
a. When the treatment time is over, remove the ice pack and dry the area with a towel.			
b. Remove material used for draping, assist the patient in dressing as needed.			
c. Dispose of the unmelted ice in a sink.			
d. Have the patient perform appropriate therapeutic exercise or apply tape or compression wrap as indicated.			
e. Clean the treatment area and equipment according to normal protocol.			
7. Assess treatment efficacy.			
a. Ask the patient how the treated area feels.			
b. Visually inspect the treated area for any adverse reactions (e.g., wheals, welts).			
c. Perform functional tests as indicated.			

LAB ACTIVITY

COLD WHIRLPOOL

DESCRIPTION

A whirlpool is a tank filled with water of a particular temperature, depending on the desired therapeutic effect. The tank also contains a turbine or pump that creates convection currents in the water. Although water that is any temperature below the temperature of the body surface could be considered "cold," generally water at 10–16°C is used. Because water from the tap is rarely this cold, ice must be added to the tank. Crushed ice results in the most rapid cooling of the water, and all ice must be melted before the turbine is turned on.

Using the turbine insures that a layer of warm water does not develop adjacent to the skin, thus providing a more effective cooling of the tissues. Because the limb is in a dependent position, any effect of the cooling on decreasing soft tissue swelling may be negated; using a compression bandage during the treatment may help in reducing the effects of dependency. As with a warm whirlpool, the patient should not be left unattended and should be warned against touching any part of the turbine.

PHYSIOLOGIC EFFECTS

Vasoconstriction
Superficial anesthesia
Decreased local metabolism
Decreased connective tissue elasticity

THERAPEUTIC EFFECTS

Decreased or prevented swelling
Decreased pain
Decreased inflammation
Decreased secondary tissue damage

INDICATIONS

The principal indication for a cold whirlpool is to provide therapeutic cooling of a larger area of the body than can be achieved readily with an ice or cold pack. Also, irregularly shaped areas of the body can be treated with total contact. In addition, the patient can perform active exercise during the application, or the therapist can perform joint mobilization on the injured limb while immersed in the water.

In addition, use of a cold whirlpool may minimize inflammation and swelling following a therapeutic exercise session. The advantage of a cold whirlpool over an ice or cold pack is the greater area that can be treated; a disadvantage is the possibility of increased swelling when the limb is in a dependent position.

CONTRAINDICATIONS

- Lack of normal temperature sensibility
- Cold hypersensitivity (urticaria or hemoglobinuria)
- Vasospastic disorders (e.g., Raynaud's disease)
- Coronary artery disease
- Hypertension

COLD WHIRPOOL

PROCEDURE	EVALUATION		
	1	2	3
1. Check supplies and equipment.			
a. Obtain towels for padding the edge of the whirlpool tank, as well as for drying the treated part.			
b. Check temperature of tank, ensure all ice is melted before applying treatment.			
c. Position chair of correct height next to whirlpool.			
2. Question patient.			
a. Verify identity of patient (if not already verified).			
b. Verify the absence of contraindications.			
c. Ask about previous cryotherapy or whirlpool treatments, check treatment notes.			
3. Position patient.			
a. Have patient sit on chair with body part out of water.			
b. Expose body part to be treated.			
c. Drape patient to preserve patient's modesty, protect clothing, but allow access to body part.			
4. Inspect body part to be treated.			
a. Check light touch perception.			
b. Check circulatory status (pulses, capillary refill).			
c. Verify that there are no open wounds or rashes.			
d. Assess function of body part (e.g., ROM, irritability).			
5. Administer cold whirlpool.			
a. Pad edge of tank with toweling, warn patient that the water is cold, then place body part in water.			
b. Instruct patient to keep away from all parts of the turbine.			
c. Turn on the turbine, adjust the aeration, agitation, and direction of the water being pumped.			
d. Check the patient's response verbally and visually about every 2 minutes. Remind the patient to tell you if the area starts hurting or if sensation is lost.			
6. Complete the treatment.			
a. Turn off the turbine at the completion of the treatment time.			
b. Remove the body part from the water and dry it off.			
c. Assist the patient in dressing as needed and instruct in therapeutic exercise as indicated.			
d. Clean the treatment area and equipment according to normal protocol.			
7. Assess treatment efficacy.			
a. Ask the patient how the treated area feels.			
b. Visually inspect the treated area for any adverse reactions (e.g., wheals, welts).			
c. Perform functional tests as indicated.			

VAPOCOOLANT COLD SPRAY

DESCRIPTION

Vapocoolant sprays, such as Fluori-Methane are liquids that are sprayed on the skin. Thermal energy from the body is absorbed by the liquids, which have low boiling points; therefore, the liquid almost immediately evaporates. As it evaporates, thermal energy is removed from the body, resulting in a superficial cooling.

Fluori-Methane, a mixture of 85 percent trichloromonofluoromethane and 15 percent dichlorodifluoromethane, is not flammable and is nontoxic. Ethyl chloride is flammable, and therefore is not recommended for use.

PHYSIOLOGIC EFFECTS

Superficial anesthesia

THERAPEUTIC EFFECTS

Inhibition of painful trigger points
Decrease in pain with stretching musculotendinous tissue

INDICATIONS

Vapocoolant sprays are used mostly for the treatment of trigger points and for stretching of tight musculotendinous tissue. Trigger points are a poorly understood phenomenon, but many pain syndromes are ascribed to active trigger points. Two relatively common treatments for trigger points are deep friction massage (similar to vigorous acupressure) and stretching of the muscle the trigger point is located within. Because direct pressure on and stretching of the trigger points is painful, the area can be sprayed with a vapocoolant to decrease the pain during the treatment.

In a similar manner, if a musculotendinous strain has resulted in a loss of range of motion, spraying the skin over the injured muscle may decrease the pain perception while the therapist stretches the body part. Care must be taken to not overstretch the tissue and produce further injury.

CONTRAINDICATIONS

- Lack of normal temperature sensibility
- Cold hypersensitivity (urticaria or hemoglobinuria)
- Vasospastic disorders (e.g., Raynaud's disease)

VAPOCOOLANT COLD SPRAY

PROCEDURE	EVALUATION		
	1	2	3
1. Check supplies.			
a. Obtain vapocoolant.			
b. Obtain toweling or other draping materials needed.			
2. Question patient.			
a. Verify identity of patient (if not already verified).			
b. Verify the absence of contraindications.			
c. Ask about previous cryotherapy treatments, check treatment notes.			

PROCEDURE	EVALUATION		
	1	2	3
3. Position patient.			
a. Place patient in a well-supported, comfortable position.			
b. Expose body part to be treated.			
c. Drape patient to preserve patient's modesty, protect clothing, but allow access to body part.			
4. Inspect body part to be treated.			
a. Check light touch perception.			
b. Check circulatory status (pulses, capillary refill).			
c. Verify that there are no open wounds or rashes.			
d. Assess function of body part (e.g., ROM, irritability).			
5. Apply vapocoolant.			
a. Position body part such that the area to be treated is on a stretch.			
b. Protect the patient's eyes and ensure the patient does not inhale fumes.			
c. Holding the vapocoolant upside down, with the nozzle at about a 30-degree angle from the perpendicular with the skin, and about 45 cm from the skin, spray the skin from distal to proximal.			
d. Spray in one direction only three to four times, then apply direct pressure or increased stretch as indicated and tolerated by the patient. Repeat the procedure as needed after the skin has rewarmed.			
e. Check the patient's response frequently during the treatment.			
6. Complete treatment.			
a. On attainment of the desired therapeutic effect (or up to four repetitions of spray-and-stretch or pressure or to patient tolerance), inspect the treated body part for adverse reactions.			
b. Remove draping materials, assist the patient in dressing as needed.			
c. If further therapeutic exercise is indicated, instruct the patient to perform it.			
d. Clean the treatment area and equipment according to normal protocol.			
7. Assess treatment efficacy.			
a. Ask the patient how the treated area feels.			
b. Visually inspect the treated area for any adverse reactions (e.g., wheals, welts).			
c. Perform functional tests as indicated.			

LAB ACTIVITY

CONTRAST BATH

DESCRIPTION

A contrast bath involves the alternating immersion of the involved body part in warm water and cold water. Usually, the wrist and hand or foot and ankle are treated, though the entire upper or lower member could be treated using two whirlpool tanks. The duration of immersion in each temperature water is variable, as is the number of times immersed during a single treatment session. A suggested sequence is to start with 3 minutes in warm, followed by 1 minute in cold, with the sequence repeated five times (e.g., 3W-1C-3W-1C-3W-1C-3W-1C-3W-1C); however, some therapists recommend starting and ending with warm water. The warm water should be 40–41°C and the cold water 10–16°C.

PHYSIOLOGIC EFFECTS

Alternating vasodilation and vasoconstriction

THERAPEUTIC EFFECTS

Variable effects on swelling
Decreased pain

INDICATIONS

Contrast baths are often used in the subacute and chronic stages of recovery. Most of the information regarding benefits of contrast baths is anecdotal; there is little research documenting the efficacy of this treatment.

CONTRAINDICATIONS

- Lack of normal temperature sensibility
- Cold hypersensitivity (urticaria or hemoglobinuria)
- Vasospastic disorders (e.g., Raynaud's disease)

CONTRAST BATH

PROCEDURE	EVALUATION		
	1	2	3
1. Check supplies and equipment.			
a. Obtain towels, containers, ice, timer, and so on.			
b. Check temperature of water in each container.			
2. Question patient.			
a. Verify identity of patient (if not already verified).			
b. Verify the absence of contraindications.			
c. Ask about previous cryotherapy or thermotherapy, treatments, check treatment notes.			
3. Position patient.			
a. Have patient sit in a comfortable position.			
b. Expose body part to be treated.			
c. Drape patient to preserve patient's modesty, protect clothing, but allow access to body part.			

PROCEDURE	EVALUATION		
	1	2	3
4. Inspect body part to be treated.			
a. Check light touch perception.			
b. Check circulatory status (pulses, capillary refill).			
c. Verify that there are no open wounds or rashes.			
d. Assess function of body part (e.g., ROM, irritability).			
5. Administer contrast bath.			
a. Set timer for appropriate interval, help patient immerse body part fully into warm water; start timer.			
b. After the timer goes off, set it for the next interval. Warn patient that the cold water will feel very cold; help patient immerse body part fully into cold water; start timer.			
c. Continue the cycles until the treatment is complete. Usually, the patients can time each immersion themselves.			
d. Check the patient's response verbally and visually about every 2 minutes. Remind the patient to tell you if the area starts hurting or if sensation is lost.			
6. Complete the treatment.			
a. Remove the body part from the water and dry it off.			
b. Assist the patient in dressing as needed and instruct in therapeutic exercise as indicated.			
c. Clean the treatment area and equipment according to normal protocol.			
7. Assess treatment efficacy.			
a. Ask the patient how the treated area feels.			
b. Visually inspect the treated area for any adverse reactions (e.g., wheals, welts).			
c. Perform functional tests as indicated.			

LAB ACTIVITY

CRYO-CUFF

DESCRIPTION

A Cryo-Cuff has three parts: a cuff that holds chilled water, a cooler that holds water and ice, and a connecting tube. Cuffs are fabricated for numerous body joints including ankle, knee, and shoulder. A major advantage of a Cryo-Cuff is that the cuff can conform to a joint's unique shape, providing both cold and compression simultaneously.

PHYSIOLOGIC EFFECTS

Superficial anesthesia
Decreased local metabolism

THERAPEUTIC EFFECTS

Decreased swelling
Decreased pain
Decreased inflammation

INDICATIONS

The primary indication for the use of a Cryo-Cuff is in the acute phase of a soft-tissue injury or immediately following surgery of a joint. The cooling and compression of the injured area will provide analgesia and help prevent the development of edema or effusion. The Cryo-Cuff may assist in the resolution of swelling by altering the Starling-Landis forces at the capillary bed.

A Cryo-Cuff is also useful in minimizing or preventing increased inflammation or pain following a session of therapeutic exercise. The depth of anesthesia achieved with a Cryo-Cuff is generally considerably less than with an ice massage.

CONTRAINDICATIONS

- Lack of normal temperature sensibility
- Cold hypersensitivity (urticaria or hemoglobinuria)
- Vasospastic disorders (e.g., Raynaud's disease)
- Coronary artery disease
- Hypertension

CRYO-CUFF

PROCEDURE	EVALUATION		
	1	2	3
1. Check supplies.			
a. Obtain wet towel to wrap joint in, an appropriate amount of ice to fill cooler, and a sheet or towels for draping.			
b. Add water and ice to cooler for appropriate mix.			
2. Question patient.			
a. Verify identity of patient (if not already verified).			
b. Verify the absence of contraindications.			
c. Ask about previous cryotherapy treatments, check treatment notes.			

PROCEDURE	EVALUATION		
	1	2	3
3. Position patient.			
a. Place patient in a well-supported, comfortable position.			
b. Expose the joint to be treated.			
c. Drape patient to preserve patient's modesty, protect clothing, but allow access to body part.			
4. Inspect joint to be treated.			
a. Check light touch perception.			
b. Check circulatory status (pulses, capillary refill).			
c. Verify that there are no open wounds or rashes.			
d. Assess function of body part (e.g., ROM, irritability).			
5. Apply empty Cryo-Cuff to joint as indicated, close Velcro straps, and connect tubing from cooler to cuff.			
a. Warn the patient that you are going to fill the Cryo-Cuff, and then do so by opening cooler air vent and raising the cooler above the cuff until the cuff is full. Close the cooler air vent. Elevate the joint as required.			
b. Set a timer for the appropriate treatment time (generally about 15 min), and give the patient a signaling device. Make sure the patient understands how to use the signaling device.			
c. Check the patient's response verbally after the first 2 minutes, then about every 5 minutes. Perform a visual check of the area if the patient reports any unusual sensation. If wheals or welts appear, or if the skin color changes to absolute white within the first 4 minutes of treatment, stop the treatment.			
d. Rechill cuff as needed. Reconnect tube to cuff, open air vent, lower cooler to floor and completely drain water from cuff. Allow water to rechill, then repeat filling cuff.			
6. Complete the treatment.			
a. When the treatment time is over, remove the Cryo-Cuff and dry the area with a towel.			
b. Remove material used for draping, assist the patient in dressing as needed.			
c. Have the patient perform appropriate therapeutic exercise as indicated.			
d. Clean the treatment area and equipment according to normal protocol.			
7. Assess treatment efficacy.			
a. Ask the patient how the treated area feels.			
b. Visually inspect the treated area for any adverse reactions.			
c. Perform functional tests as indicated.			

LAB ACTIVITY

WARM WHIRLPOOL

DESCRIPTION

A whirlpool is a tank filled with water of a particular temperature, depending on the desired therapeutic effect. The tank also contains a turbine or pump that creates convection currents in the water. Although water that is any temperature above the temperature of the body surface could be considered "warm," generally water at 35–43°C is used. If the entire body is to be immersed, temperatures above 38°C should not be used to avoid interference with thermoregulation. The use of the turbine avoids the development of a layer of cooler water adjacent to the body part, thus producing more uniform warming. Because of the dependent position of the body part in the whirlpool and the increased temperature of the body part, a warm whirlpool may increase soft tissue swelling; even in noninjured limbs, there may be a considerable increase in interstitial fluid following a warm whirlpool.

Because the turbine is powered by electricity, it is generally prudent to not let the patient touch any part of the turbine. Also, patients should not be left in the whirlpool unattended; this is true whether the entire body or only a limb is immersed.

PHYSIOLOGIC EFFECTS

Vasodilation
Decreased pain perception
Increased local metabolism
Increased connective tissue plasticity
Decreased isometric strength (transient)

THERAPEUTIC EFFECTS

Decreased pain
Increased soft tissue extensibility
Sedative

INDICATIONS

The principal indication for a warm whirlpool is to provide therapeutic warming of a larger area of the body than can be achieved readily with a hot pack. The effective depth of therapeutic heating is the same at approximately 1 cm. In addition, the patient can perform active exercise during the application, or the therapist can perform joint mobilization on the injured limb while immersed in the water. Some therapists use whirlpool for cleaning a limb after removal of a cast; equally effective and at less cost is a shower.

The primary therapeutic effect of superficial heating is to increase the ability of the collagen to remodel. Therefore, heating the tissue is beneficial following a period of reduced mobility if the soft tissue has shortened. In addition, the tissue viscosity is reduced, resulting in a greater ease of motion through the available range of motion.

CONTRAINDICATIONS

- Lack of normal temperature sensibility
- Peripheral vascular disease with compromised circulation
- Over tumors
- Coronary artery disease

WARM WHIRLPOOL

PROCEDURE	EVALUATION		
	1	2	3
1. Check supplies and equipment.			
a. Obtain towels for padding the edge of the whirlpool tank, as well as for drying the treated part.			
b. Check temperature of tank before applying treatment.			
c. Position chair of correct height next to whirlpool.			
2. Question patient.			
a. Verify identity of patient (if not already verified).			
b. Verify the absence of contraindications.			
c. Ask about previous thermotherapy or whirlpool treatments, check treatment notes.			
3. Position patient.			
a. Have patient sit on chair with body part out of water.			
b. Expose body part to be treated.			
c. Drape patient to preserve patient's modesty, protect clothing, but allow access to body part.			
4. Inspect body part to be treated.			
a. Check light touch perception.			
b. Check circulatory status (pulses, capillary refill).			
c. Verify that there are no open wounds or rashes.			
d. Assess function of body part (e.g., ROM, irritability).			
5. Administer warm whirlpool.			
a. Pad edge of tank with toweling; ask patient to tell you if the water is too hot, then place body part in water.			
b. Instruct patient to keep away from all parts of the turbine.			
c. Turn on the turbine, adjust the aeration, agitation, and direction of the water being pumped.			
d. Check the patient's response verbally and visually about every 2 minutes. Remind the patient to tell you if the area starts hurting or if sensation is lost.			
6. Complete the treatment.			
a. Turn off the turbine at the completion of the treatment time.			
b. Remove the body part from the water and dry it off.			
c. Assist the patient in dressing as needed and instruct in therapeutic exercise as indicated.			
d. Clean the treatment area and equipment according to normal protocol.			
7. Assess treatment efficacy.			
a. Ask the patient how the treated area feels.			
b. Visually inspect the treated area for any adverse reactions (e.g., wheals, welts).			
c. Perform functional tests as indicated.			

LAB ACTIVITY

HYDROCOLLATOR PACKS

DESCRIPTION

Commercially available hot packs (*hydrocollator packs*) are usually a canvas cover filled with a hydrophilic substance such as bentonite. Hot packs are kept in a commercial water-filled container that maintains a temperature of approximately 71°C. The packs are wrapped in six to eight layers of dry towels to protect the patient from burns; commercial hot pack covers provide approximately four thicknesses of toweling. After use, the hot pack should be returned to the cabinet for at least 30 minutes to insure reheating. Hot packs provide only superficial heating; the maximum depth of therapeutic heating is only about 1 cm, and occurs within 10 minutes of application.

PHYSIOLOGIC EFFECTS

Vasodilation
Decreased pain perception
Increased local metabolism
Increased connective tissue plasticity
Decreased isometric strength (transient)

THERAPEUTIC EFFECTS

Decreased pain
Increased soft tissue extensibility

INDICATIONS

The principal indication for a hot pack is to provide therapeutic warming of superficial tissues. Tissues that are deeper than 1 cm do not reach a therapeutic temperature range of 30–40°C. Therefore, if the target tissue is deeper than 1 cm (e.g., the spinal facet joints), a hot pack will not be effective. Other joints, such as the knee, wrist, and ankle, can be effectively heated with a hot pack.

The primary therapeutic effect of superficial heating is to increase the ability of the collagen to remodel. Therefore, heating the tissue is beneficial following a period of reduced mobility if the soft tissue has shortened. In addition, the tissue viscosity is reduced, resulting in a greater ease of motion through the available range of motion. Although generally not a problem, in case of extreme pressure sensitivity, the weight of a hot pack may be more than the patient can tolerate. In these cases, Fluidotherapy or a warm whirlpool may be helpful.

CONTRAINDICATIONS

- Lack of normal temperature sensibility
- Peripheral vascular disease with compromised circulation
- Over tumors

HYDROCOLLATOR PACKS

PROCEDURE	EVALUATION		
	1	2	3
1. Check supplies.			
a. Obtain dry towels to wrap hot pack in, sheet or towels for draping, timer, signaling device.			
b. Check cabinet for appropriate temperature.			
2. Question patient.			
a. Verify identity of patient (if not already verified).			
b. Verify the absence of contraindications.			
c. Ask about previous thermotherapy treatments, check treatment notes.			
3. Position patient.			
a. Place patient in a well-supported, comfortable position.			
b. Expose body part to be treated.			
c. Drape patient to preserve patient's modesty, protect clothing, but allow access to body part.			
4. Inspect body part to be treated.			
a. Check light touch perception.			
b. Check circulatory status (pulses, capillary refill).			
c. Verify that there are no open wounds or rashes.			
d. Assess function of body part (e.g., ROM, irritability).			
5. Apply hot pack.			
a. Wrap hot pack in towels to provide six to eight layers of towel between the hot pack and the patient. If using a commercial hot pack cover, use at least one layer of towel to keep the cover clean.			
b. Inform the patient that you are going to put the hot pack on the body part to be treated, then do so.			
c. Set a timer for the appropriate treatment time and give the patient a signaling device. Make sure the patient understands how to use the signaling device.			
d. Check the patient's response after the first 5 minutes by asking the patient how it feels as well as visually checking the area under the hot pack. If the area is blotchy, additional toweling may be needed. Recheck verbally about every 5 minutes. A visual inspection every 5 minutes is not inappropriate.			
6. Complete the treatment.			
a. When the treatment time is over, remove the hot pack and dry the area with a towel.			
b. Remove material used for draping, assist the patient in dressing as needed.			
c. Have the patient perform appropriate therapeutic exercise as indicated.			
d. Clean the treatment area and equipment according to normal protocol.			
7. Assess treatment efficacy.			
a. Ask the patient how the treated area feels.			
b. Visually inspect the treated area for any adverse reactions.			
c. Perform functional tests as indicated.			

LAB ACTIVITY

PARAFFIN BATH

DESCRIPTION

Paraffin baths consist of dipping and removing or immersing the body part in a mixture of wax and mineral oil. The ratio of wax and mineral oil is about 7:1, which results in a substance with a melting point of about 47.8°C, a specific heat of about 0.65 cal/g/°C, and a therapeutic temperature range of 48–54°C. Because of the low specific heat, much higher temperatures can be tolerated than if water is used. The paraffin is kept in a thermostatically controlled cabinet.

Paraffin provides a superficial heat, with a depth of therapeutic heating of about 1 cm. However, because paraffin is generally used only for the hands and feet, the depth of penetration is adequate to warm these joints to a therapeutic range.

The two basic techniques of application of paraffin involve repeated dipping of the body part in the mixture, then covering the body part with plastic and toweling. The advantage of this method is that the body part can then be elevated, reducing the potential for swelling. The second method involves dipping the body part in the paraffin once, letting it dry for a few seconds, then immersing the body part for the duration of the treatment. The advantage of this technique is that the source of heat is constant, so the therapeutic temperature can be maintained for a longer period.

PHYSIOLOGIC EFFECTS

Vasodilation
Decreased pain perception
Increased local metabolism
Increased connective tissue plasticity
Decreased isometric strength (transient)

THERAPEUTIC EFFECTS

Decreased pain
Increased soft tissue extensibility

INDICATIONS

The principal indication for a paraffin bath is to provide therapeutic warming of superficial tissues. This is particularly effective in the hands and feet following a period of immobilization. The increased connective tissue plasticity that occurs with warming will enhance the effectiveness of therapeutic exercise.

Paraffin baths are also helpful in alleviation of pain caused by arthritic changes in the hands and feet. Caution should be exercised in using paraffin (or any heating agent) during an acute phase of arthritic pain and swelling.

CONTRAINDICATIONS

- Lack of normal temperature sensibility
- Peripheral vascular disease with compromised circulation
- Over tumors

PARAFFIN BATH

PROCEDURE	EVALUATION		
	1	2	3
1. Check supplies.			
a. Obtain plastic bag and towels to wrap body part in, timer, signaling device.			
b. Check cabinet for appropriate temperature.			
2. Question patient.			
a. Verify identity of patient (if not already verified).			
b. Verify the absence of contraindications.			
c. Ask about previous thermotherapy treatments; check treatment notes.			
3. Prepare patient.			
a. Have patient remove all jewelry from body part, wash well and dry thoroughly.			
b. Explain to the patient that after dipping the body part into the paraffin, there should be no movement of the body part for the duration of the treatment.			
4. Inspect body part to be treated.			
a. Check light touch perception.			
b. Check circulatory status (pulses, capillary refill).			
c. Verify that there are no open wounds or rashes.			
d. Assess function of body part (e.g., ROM, irritability).			
5. Apply paraffin.			
a. Guide the body part into the paraffin, making sure the patient does not contact the bottom of the cabinet or the heating coils.			
b. After 2 or 3 seconds, remove the body part, and keep it above the paraffin so that none of the paraffin drips onto the floor. Reimmerse the body part, and repeat until the appropriate number of dips have been completed, or reimmerse for the duration of the treatment.			
c. Set a timer for the appropriate treatment time and give the patient a signaling device. Make sure the patient understands how to use the signaling device.			
d. Check the patient's response after the first 5 minutes by asking the patient how it feels. Recheck verbally about every 5 minutes.			
6. Complete the treatment.			
a. When the treatment time is over, remove the towel and plastic bag. Help the patient remove the paraffin, and either return the paraffin to the cabinet, or throw away according to local protocol.			
b. Have the patient thoroughly wash and dry the body part.			
c. Have the patient perform appropriate therapeutic exercise as indicated.			
d. Clean the treatment area and equipment according to normal protocol.			
7. Assess treatment efficacy.			
a. Ask the patient how the treated area feels.			
b. Visually inspect the treated area for any adverse reactions.			
c. Perform functional tests as indicated.			

LAB ACTIVITY

INFRARED LAMPS

DESCRIPTION

Infrared lamps provide superficial (1 mm or less) heating. Because of the extremely limited penetration, they are not capable of elevating connective tissue temperatures to a therapeutic level. Therefore, their primary effect is one of mild analgesia, and their use is very limited.

PHYSIOLOGIC EFFECTS

Cutaneous vasodilation
Decreased pain perception

THERAPEUTIC EFFECTS

Decreased pain

INDICATIONS

The principal indication for infrared lamp heating is localized pain. Elevation of skin temperature may decrease the perception of pain for a short time.

CONTRAINDICATIONS

- Lack of normal temperature sensibility
- Peripheral vascular disease with compromised circulation
- Over tumors

INFRARED LAMPS

PROCEDURE	EVALUATION		
	1	2	3
1. Check supplies.			
a. Obtain sheet or towels for draping, timer, signaling device.			
b. Check lamp for frayed power cords, integrity of lamp and shields, and so on.			
2. Question patient.			
a. Verify identity of patient (if not already verified).			
b. Verify the absence of contraindications.			
c. Ask about previous thermotherapy treatments, check treatment notes.			
3. Position patient.			
a. Place patient in a well-supported, comfortable position.			
b. Expose body part to be treated, have patient remove all jewelry from the area.			
c. Drape patient to preserve patient's modesty, protect clothing, but allow access to body part.			
4. Inspect body part to be treated.			
a. Check light touch perception.			
b. Check circulatory status (pulses, capillary refill).			
c. Verify that there are no open wounds or rashes.			
d. Assess function of body part (e.g., ROM, irritability).			

PROCEDURE	EVALUATION		
	1	2	3
5. Apply infrared light.			
a. Position lamp such that the bulb is parallel to the body part being treated (such that the energy will strike the body at a 90° angle), and is 45–60 cm away from the patient. Measure and record the distance from the lamp to the closest part of the body being treated.			
b. Inform the patient that they should feel only a mild warmth; if it is hot, they should inform you. Start the lamp.			
c. Set a timer for the appropriate treatment time and give the patient a signaling device. Make sure the patient understands how to use the signaling device.			
d. Check the patient's response after the first 5 minutes by asking the patient how it feels as well as visually checking the area being treated. Recheck visually and verbally about every 5 minutes.			
6. Complete the treatment.			
a. When the treatment time is over, move the lamp away from the patient; dry the area with a towel. Turn the intensity control to zero.			
b. Remove material used for draping, assist the patient in dressing as needed.			
c. Have the patient perform appropriate therapeutic exercise as indicated.			
d. Clean the treatment area and equipment according to normal protocol.			
7. Assess treatment efficacy.			
a. Ask the patient how the treated area feels.			
b. Visually inspect the treated area for any adverse reactions.			
c. Perform functional tests as indicated.			

LAB ACTIVITY

FLUIDOTHERAPY

DESCRIPTION

Fluidotherapy is a device manufactured by Henley International of Sugarland, TX. Heated air is forced through a container filled with cellulose particles; when heated, the cellulose takes on fluidlike characteristics. The body part to be treated is immersed in the cellulose particles, and the particles are circulated in the container, thus providing elevation of tissue temperature and a mechanical stimulation of the skin. The temperature of the unit is adjustable within a range of about 39–48°C.

There are several advantages to using Fluidotherapy to treat affected hands or feet. The source of heat is constant, so the tissue temperature can be maintained at a therapeutic level for the duration of the treatment. The body part can be exercised during the treatment, either actively or passively by the therapist. The mechanical stimulation of the skin with the cellulose particles may provide some analgesic effect and may help desensitize the injured area.

PHYSIOLOGIC EFFECTS

Vasodilation
Decreased pain perception
Increased local metabolism
Increased connective tissue plasticity
Decreased isometric strength (transient)

THERAPEUTIC EFFECTS

Decreased pain
Increased soft tissue extensibility

INDICATIONS

The principal indication for Fluidotherapy is to provide therapeutic warming of a larger area of the body than can be achieved readily with a hot pack. In addition, the patient can perform active exercise during the application, or the therapist can perform joint mobilization on the injured limb while in the unit.

The primary therapeutic effect of superficial heating is to increase the ability of the collagen to remodel. Therefore, heating the tissue is beneficial following a period of reduced mobility if the soft tissue has shortened. In addition, the tissue viscosity is reduced, resulting in a greater ease of motion through the available range of motion.

CONTRAINDICATIONS

- Lack of normal temperature sensibility
- Peripheral vascular disease with compromised circulation
- Over tumors
- Coronary artery disease

FLUIDOTHERAPY

PROCEDURE	EVALUATION		
	1	2	3
1. Check supplies and equipment.			
a. Obtain timer, signaling device, and so on.			
b. Check temperature of Fluidotherapy unit before applying treatment.			
c. Position chair of correct height next to unit.			

PROCEDURE	EVALUATION		
	1	2	3
2. Question patient.			
a. Verify identity of patient (if not already verified).			
b. Verify the absence of contraindications.			
c. Ask about previous thermotherapy treatments, check treatment notes.			
3. Position patient.			
a. Have patient remove jewelry from area to be treated and thoroughly wash and dry area.			
b. Have patient sit on chair next to unit.			
c. Expose body part to be treated.			
d. Drape patient to preserve patient's modesty, protect clothing, but allow access to body part.			
4. Inspect body part to be treated.			
a. Check light touch perception.			
b. Check circulatory status (pulses, capillary refill).			
c. Verify that there are no open wounds or rashes.			
d. Assess function of body part (e.g., ROM, irritability).			
5. Administer Fluidotherapy.			
a. With the agitation off, open the sleeved portion of the unit.			
b. Instruct patient to insert body part into cellulose particles, reminding them to tell you if the temperature is too hot.			
c. Fasten the sleeve around the body part to prevent the cellulose particles from being blown out of the unit, and start the agitation.			
d. Check the patient's response verbally after about 5 minutes. Remind the patient to tell you if the heating sensation becomes uncomfortable.			
e. Instruct the patient in any indicated therapeutic exercise to be performed during the treatment.			
6. Complete the treatment.			
a. Turn off the agitation at the completion of the treatment time.			
b. Remove the body part from the unit, having the patient brush or shake off as much of the cellulose as possible.			
c. Assist the patient in dressing as needed and instruct in therapeutic exercise as indicated.			
d. Clean the treatment area and equipment according to normal protocol.			
7. Assess treatment efficacy.			
a. Ask the patient how the treated area feels.			
b. Visually inspect the treated area for any adverse reactions (e.g., wheals, welts).			
c. Perform functional tests as indicated.			

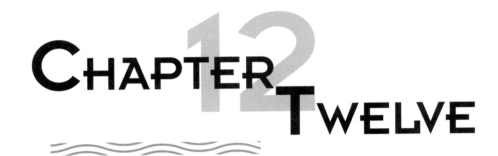

CHAPTER TWELVE

THERAPEUTIC ULTRASOUND

DAVID O. DRAPER and
WILLIAM E. PRENTICE

OBJECTIVES

Following completion of this chapter, the student therapist will be able to:

✓ Analyze the transmission of acoustic energy in biologic tissues relative to waveforms, frequency, velocity, and attenuation.

✓ Break down the basic physics involved in the production of a beam of therapeutic ultrasound.

✓ Compare both the thermal and nonthermal physiologic effects of therapeutic ultrasound.

✓ Evaluate specific techniques of application of therapeutic ultrasound and how they may be modified to achieve treatment goals.

✓ Choose the most appropriate and clinically effective uses for therapeutic ultrasound.

✓ Explain the technique and clinical application of phonophoresis.

✓ Identify the contraindications and precautions that should be observed with therapeutic ultrasound.

Ultrasound is one of the most widely used modalities in physical therapy

In the medical community, ultrasound is a modality that is used for a number of different purposes, including diagnosis, destruction of tissue, and as a therapeutic agent. Diagnostic ultrasound has been used for more than 30 years for the purpose of imaging internal structures. Most typically, diagnostic ultrasound is used to image the fetus during pregnancy. Ultrasound has also been used to produce extreme tissue hyperthermia that has been demonstrated to have tumoricidal effects in cancer patients.

In clinical practice, ultrasound is one of the most widely used therapeutic modalities in addition to superficial heat and cold and electrical stimulating currents.[26] It has been used for therapeutic purposes as a valuable tool in the rehabilitation of many different injuries primarily for the purpose of stimulating the repair of soft-tissue injuries and for relief of pain,[42] although some studies have questioned its efficency as a tretment modality.[5]

As discussed in Chapter 1, ultrasound is a form of acoustic rather than electromagnetic energy. Ultrasound is defined as inaudible, acoustic vibrations of high frequency that may produce either thermal or nonthermal physiologic effects.[57] The use of ultrasound as a therapeutic agent may be extremely effective if the therapist has an adequate understanding of its effects on biologic tissues and of the physical mechanisms by which these effects are produced.[42]

ULTRASOUND AS A THERMAL MODALITY

In Chapters 10 and 11, heat is discussed as a treatment modality. Warm whirlpools, paraffin baths, and hot packs, to name a few, all produce therapeutic heat. However, the depth of penetration of these modalities is superficial and at best only 1–2 cm.[106] Ultrasound, along with diathermy, has traditionally been classified as a "deep heating modality" and has been used primarily for the purpose of elevating tissue temperatures.

Suppose a patient is lacking dorsiflexion. It is determined through evaluation that a tight soleus is the problem, and as a therapist your desire is to use thermotherapy followed by stretching. Will superficial heat adequately prepare this muscle to be stretched? Since the soleus lies deep under the gastrocnemius muscle, it is beyond the reach of superficial heat.

One of the advantages of using ultrasound over other thermal modalities is that it can provide deep heating.[104] The heating effects of silicate gel hot packs and warm whirlpools have been compared with ultrasound. At an intramuscular depth of 3 cm, a 10-minute hot pack treatment yielded an increase of 0.8°C, whereas at this same depth, 1 MHz ultrasound has raised muscle temperature nearly 4°C in 10 minutes.[36,107] At 1 cm below the fat surface, a 4-minute warm whirlpool (40.6°C) raised the temperature 1.1°C; however, at this same depth, 3 MHz ultrasound raised the temperature 4°C in 4 minutes.[36,38,110]

Ultrasound and diathermy = deep heating modalities

Ultrasound = acoustic energy

TRANSMISSION OF ACOUSTIC ENERGY IN BIOLOGIC TISSUES

Unlike electromagnetic energy, which travels most effectively through a vacuum, acoustic energy relies on molecular collision for transmission. Molecules in a conducting medium will cause vibration and minimal displacement of other surrounding molecules when set into vibration, so that eventually this "wave" of vibration has propagated through the entire medium. Sound waves travel in a manner similar to waves created by a stone thrown into a pool of water. Ultrasound is a mechanical wave in which energy is transmitted by the vibrations of the molecules of the biologic medium through which the wave is traveling.[136]

longitudinal wave The primary waveform in which ultrasound energy travels in soft tissue with the molecular displacement along the direction in which the wave travels.

TRANSVERSE VERSUS LONGITUDINAL WAVES

There are two types of waves that can travel through a solid medium, **longitudinal** and **transverse waves**. In a longitudinal wave, the molecular displacement is along the direction in which the wave travels. Within this longitudinal wave pathway are regions of high molecular density referred to as **compressions** (the molecules are squeezed together) and regions of lower molecular density called **rarefactions** (the molecules spread out) (Fig. 12-1). This is much like the squeezing and spreading action when using a child's toy "slinky." In a transverse wave, the molecules are displaced in a direction perpendicular to the direction in which the wave is moving. Although longitudinal waves travel both in solids and liquids, transverse waves can travel only in solids. Because soft tissues are more like liquids, ultrasound travels primarily as a longitudinal wave; however, when it contacts bone a transverse wave results.[136]

transverse wave Occurring only in bone, the molecules are displaced in a direction perpendicular to the direction in which the ultrasound wave is moving.

rarefactions Regions of lower molecular density (i.e., a small amount of ultrasound energy) within a longitudinal wave.

FREQUENCY OF WAVE TRANSMISSION

The *frequency* of audible sound ranges between 16 and 20 KHz (kilohertz = 1000 cycles per second). Ultrasound has a frequency above 20 kHz. The frequency range for therapeutic ultrasound is between 0.75 and 3 MHz (megahertz = 1,000,000 cycles per second). The higher the frequency of the sound waves emitted from a sound source, the less the sound will diverge and thus a more focused beam of sound is produced.

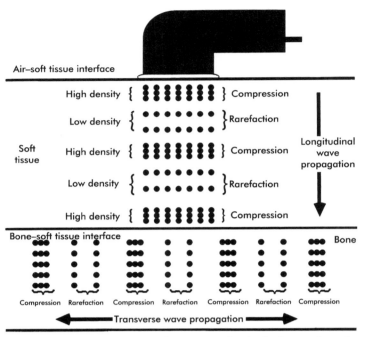

•**Figure 12-1** Ultrasound travels through soft tissue as a longitudinal wave alternating regions of high molecular density (compressions) and areas of low molecular density (rarefactions). Transverse waves are found primarily in bone.

In biologic tissues, the lower the frequency of the sound waves, the greater the depth of penetration. Higher frequency sound waves are absorbed in the more superficial tissues.

VELOCITY

The *velocity* at which this vibration or sound wave is propagated through the conducting medium is directly related to the density. Denser and more rigid materials will have a higher velocity of transmission. At a frequency of 1 MHz, sound travels through soft tissue at 1540 m/sec and through compact bone at 4000 m/sec.[148]

ATTENUATION

attenuation A decrease in energy intensity as the ultrasound wave is transmitted through various tissues owing to scattering and dispersion.

Penetration and absorption are inversely related.

As the ultrasound wave is transmitted through the various tissues, there will be **attenuation** or a decrease in energy intensity. This decrease is owing to either *absorption* of energy by the tissues or *dispersion* and *scattering* of the sound wave that results from reflection or refraction.[136]

Ultrasound penetrates through tissue high in water content and is absorbed in dense tissues high in protein where it will have its greatest heating potential.[63] The capability of acoustic energy to penetrate or be transmitted to deeper tissues is determined by the frequency of the ultrasound as well as the characteristics of the tissues through which ultrasound is traveling. Penetration and absorption are inversely related. Absorption increases as the frequency increases, thus less energy is transmitted to the deeper tissues.[87] Tissues that are high in water content have a low rate of absorption, whereas tissues high in protein have a high absorption rate.[43] Fat has a relatively low absorption rate, and muscle absorbs considerably more. Peripheral nerve absorbs at a rate twice that of muscle. Bone, which is relatively superficial, absorbs more ultrasonic energy than any of the other tissues (Table 12-1).

When a sound wave encounters a boundary or an interface between different tissues, some of the energy will scatter owing to reflection or refraction. The amount of energy reflected, and conversely the amount of energy that will be transmitted to

TABLE 12-1   Relationship Between Penetration and Absorption (1 MHz)

Medium	Absorption	Penetration
Water	1	1200
Blood plasma	23	52
Whole blood	60	20
Fat	390	4
Skeletal muscle	663	2
Peripheral nerve	1193	1

From Griffin, J.E.: J. Am. Phys. Ther. 46(1):18–26, 1966. Reprinted with permission of the American Physical Therapy Association.

deeper tissues, is determined by the relative magnitude of the **acoustic impedances** of the two materials on either side of the interface. Acoustic impedance may be determined by multiplying the density of the material by the speed at which sound travels inside it. If the acoustic impedance of the two materials forming the interface is the same, all of the sound will be transmitted and none will be reflected. The larger the difference between the two acoustic impedances, the more energy is reflected and the less that can enter a second medium (Table 12-2).[143]

Sound passing from the transducer to air will be almost completely reflected. Ultrasound is transmitted through fat. It is both reflected and refracted at the muscular interface. At the soft tissue-bone interface virtually all of the sound is reflected. As the ultrasound energy is reflected at tissue interfaces with different acoustic impedances, the intensity of the energy is increased as the reflected energy meets new energy being transmitted, creating what is referred to as a **standing wave** or a "**hot spot.**" This increased level of energy has the potential to produce tissue damage. Moving the sound transducer or using pulsed wave ultrasound can help to minimize the development of hot spots.[43]

BASIC PHYSICS OF THERAPEUTIC ULTRASOUND

COMPONENTS OF A THERAPEUTIC ULTRASOUND GENERATOR

An ultrasound generator consists of a high frequency electrical generator connected through an oscillator circuit and a transformer via a coaxial cable to a transducer housed in a type of insulated applicator (Fig. 12-2). The oscillator circuit produces a sound beam at a specific frequency that is adjusted by the manufacturer to the frequency requirements of the transducer. The control panel of an ultrasound unit usually has a timer that can be preset, a power meter, an intensity control, a duty cycle control switch, a selector for continuous or pulsed modes, and possibly output power in response to tissue loading, and automatic shut-off in case of overheating of the transducer. Recently dual soundheads and dual frequency choices have become standard equipment on ultrasound units (Fig. 12-3). Table 12-3 provides a list of the most desirable features in an ultrasound generator.

TABLE 12-2   The Percentage of the Incident Energy Reflected at Tissue Interfaces[98]

Interface	Percent Reflection
Soft tissue/air	99.9
Water/soft tissue	0.2
Soft tissue/fat	1.0
Soft tissue/bone	15–40

From Ward, A.R.: Electricity fields and waves in therapy, Maricksville, NSW, Australia, Science Press, 1986.

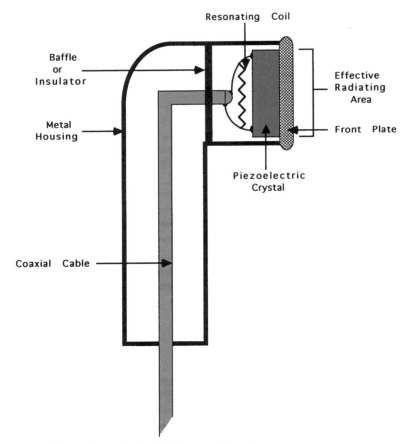

•Figure 12-2 The anatomy of a typical ultrasound transducer.

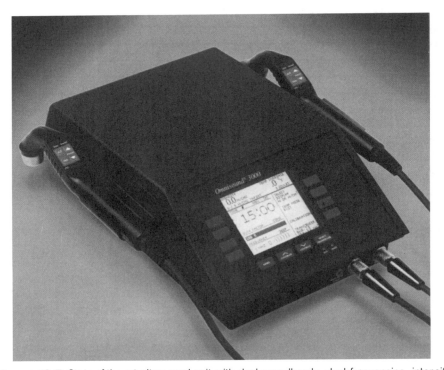

•Figure 12-3 State-of-the-art ultrasound unit with dual soundheads, dual frequencies, intensity, and frequency controls located on transducers, and preprogrammed temperature increase settings (manufactured by Physio Technology, Inc., Topeka, KS).

TABLE 12-3 The State-of-the-Art "Ultimate" Ultrasound Machine Would Contain the Following

---

Low BNR (4:1)
High ERA (nearly matches the size of the soundhead)
Multiple frequencies (1 and 3 MHz)
Multiple sized soundheads
Sensing device that shuts off the unit when overheating
Well insulated to be used underwater
Output jack for combination therapy
Several pulsed duty cycles
High quality synthetic crystal
Transducer handle that maintains the operator's wrist in a natural, relaxed
    position
Durable transducer face that will protect the crystal if dropped
Computer controlled timer that makes adjustments in treatment duration as
    the intensity is adjusted (much like iontophoresis where the treatment time
    adjusts according to the dose applied)

It must be added that several studies have demonstrated significant differences in the effectiviness of different ultrasound units produced by a variety of manufacturers in raising tissue temperatures.[72,73] It is also critical to make certain that ultrasound units are routinely tested and recalibrated to make certain that selected treatment parameters are actually being produced by the ultrasound unit.[2]

TRANSDUCER

The transducer, also referred to as an applicator or a soundhead, must be matched to particular units and are generally not interchangeable.[28] The transducer consists of some piezoelectric crystal, such as quartz, or synthetic ceramic crystals made of lead zirconate or titanate, barium titanate, or nickel-cobalt ferrite of approximately 2–3 mm in thickness. It is the crystal within the transducer that converts electrical energy to acoustic energy through mechanical deformation of the piezoelectric crystal.

Piezoelectric Effect

When an alternating electrical current generated at the same frequency as the crystal resonance is passed through the piezoelectric crystal, the crystal will expand and contract, creating what is referred to as the **piezoelectric effect**. There are two forms of this piezoelectric effect (Fig. 12-4). A *direct* piezoelectric effect is the generation of an electrical voltage across the crystal when it is compressed or expanded. An *indirect* or *reverse* piezoelectric effect is created when an alternating current moves through the crystal, producing compression or expansion. It is this change in voltage polarity that causes the crystal to expand and contract and thus vibrate at the frequency of the electrical oscillation. Thus, the reverse piezoelectric effect is used to generate ultrasound at a desired frequency.

piezoelectric effect When an alternating electrical current generated at the same frequency as the crystal resonance is passed through the piezoelectric crystal, the crystal will expand and contract or vibrate at the frequency of the electrical oscillation thus generating ultrasound at a desired frequency.

Effective Radiating Area (ERA)

That portion of the surface of the transducer that actually produces the sound wave is referred to as the **effective radiating area (ERA)**. ERA is dependent on the surface area of the crystal and ideally nearly matches the diameter of the transducer faceplate (Fig. 12-5).[42] The ERA is determined by scanning the transducer at a distance of 5 mm from the radiating surface and recording all areas in excess of 5 percent of the maximum power output found at any location on the surface of the transducer. The acoustic energy is contained with a focused cylindrical beam that is roughly the same diameter as the soundhead.[143]

Because the effective radiating area is always smaller than the transducer surface, the size of the transducer is not indicative of the actual radiating surface. A very common mistake

effective radiating area The total area of the surface of the transducer that actually produces the sound-wave.

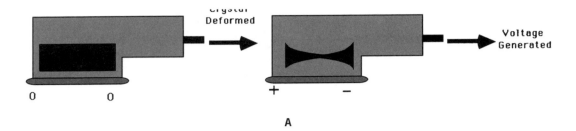

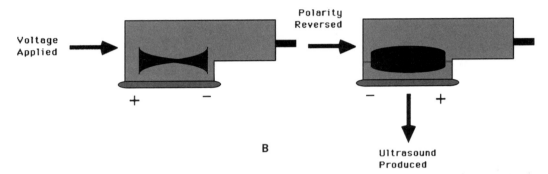

•**Figure 12-4** Piezoelectric effect. **A.** In a direct piezoelectric effect, a mechanical deformation of the crystal generates a voltage. **B.** In the reverse piezoelectric effect, as the alternating current reverses polarity, the crystal expands and contracts, producing ultrasound energy.

is to assume that because you have a large transducer surface the entire surface radiates ultrasound output. This is generally not true, particularly with larger 10-cm^2 transducers. There is really no point in having a large transducer with a small radiating surface as it only mechanically limits the coupling in smaller areas (see Fig. 12-5). The transducer ERA should match the total size of the soundhead as closely as possible for ease of application to various body surfaces, in order to maintain the most effective coupling.

The appropriate size of the area to be treated using ultrasound is two to three times the size of the ERA of the crystal.[17,126] To support this premise, peak temperature in human muscle was measured during 10 minutes of 1 MHz ultrasound delivered at 1.5 W/cm^2 (Fig. 12-6). The treatment size for 10 subjects was 2 ERA, and for the other 10 it was 6 ERA. The 2-ERA group's temperature increased 3.6°C (moderate to vigorous heating); whereas subjects' temperature in the 6-ERA group only increased

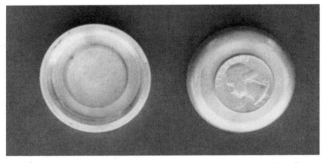

•**Figure 12-5** Left, photo of a quarter-sized crystal mounted to the inside of the transducer faceplate. A quarter (right) is placed on the transducer face to illustrate that this crystal is smaller than the faceplate. Ideally, they should be closer to the same size.

Temperature During 1-MHz Ultrasound Treatment
Comparing 2 & 6 ERA at 1.5 W/cm²

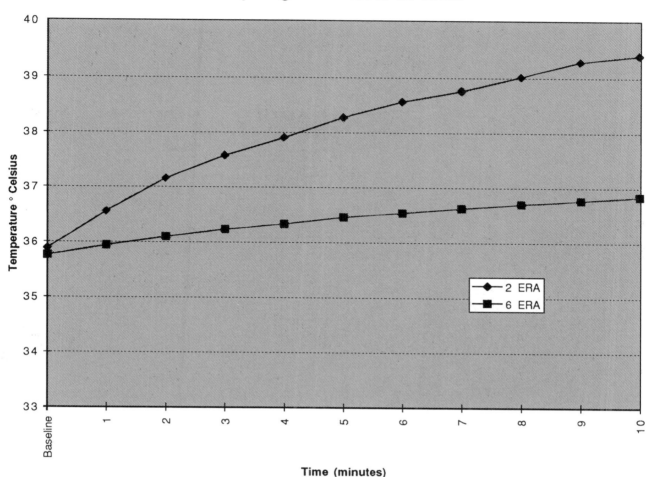

Time (minutes)

•**Figure 12-6** This graph illustrates that ultrasound is ineffective in heating areas much larger than twice the size of the transducer face. Mean temperature increase for 2 ERA was 3.4°C and only 1.1°C for an area six times the effective radiating area ERA. (From Chudliegh, D., Schulthies, S.S., Draper, D.O., and Myrer, J.W.: Muscle temperature rise with 1 MHz ultrasound in treatment sizes of 2 and 6 times the effective radiating area of the transducer, Master's thesis, Brigham Young University, July 1997.)

1.1°C (mild heating). A similar study showed that 3 MHz ultrasound at an intensity of 1 W/cm² significantly increased patellar tendon temperature at both two times and four times ERA. However, the 2-ERA size provided higher and longer heating than the 4-ERA size.[18] Thus, ultrasound is most effectively used for treating small areas.[34] Hot packs, whirlpools, and shortwave diathermy have an advantage over ultrasound in that they can be used to heat much larger areas.

FREQUENCY OF THERAPEUTIC ULTRASOUND

Therapeutic ultrasound produced by a piezoelectric transducer has a frequency range between 0.75 and 3.0 MHz. Frequency is the number of wave cycles completed each second. The majority of the older ultrasound generators are set at a frequency of 1 MHz (meaning the crystal is deforming 1 million times per sec), whereas some of the newer models also contain the 3 MHz frequency (the crystal is deforming 3 million times per sec). Certainly, a generator that can be set between 1 and 3 MHz affords the therapist the greatest treatment flexibility.

A common misconception is that intensity determines the depth of ultrasonic penetration, thus high intensities (1.5 or 2 W/cm^2) are used for deep heating, and low intensities (<1 W/cm^2) are used for superficial heating. However, depth of tissue penetration is determined by ultrasound frequency and not by intensity.[55] Ultrasound energy generated at 1 MHz is transmitted through the more superficial tissues and absorbed primarily in the deeper tissues at depths of 2–5 cm (Fig. 12-7).[36] A 1 MHz frequency is most useful in patients with high percent body fat cutaneously and whenever

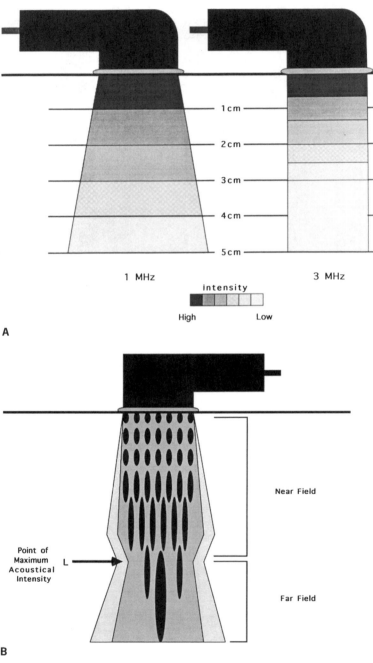

•**Figure 12-7 A.** The ultrasound energy attenuates as it travels through soft tissue. At 1 MHz, the energy can penetrate to the deeper tissues although the beam diverges slightly. At 3 MHz the effects are primarily in the superficial tissues and the beam is less divergent. **B.** In the near field the distribution of energy is nonuniform. In the far field energy distribution is more uniform but the beam is more divergent. L represents the point of highest acoustic intensity.

desired effects are in the deeper structures, such as the soleus or piriformis muscles.[57] At 3 MHz the energy is absorbed in the more superficial tissues with a depth of penetration between 1 and 2 cm, making it ideal for treating superficial conditions such as plantar fasciitis, patellar tendinitis, and epicondylitis.[148]

As previously mentioned, attenuation is the decrease in the energy of ultrasound as the distance it travels through tissue increases. The rate of absorption, and therefore attenuation, increases as the frequency of the ultrasound increases.[80] The 3 MHz frequency is not only absorbed more superficially, it is also absorbed three times faster than 1 MHz ultrasound. This faster rate of absorption results in faster peak heating in tissues. It has been demonstrated that 3 MHz ultrasound heats human muscle three times faster than 1 MHz ultrasound.[36]

THE ULTRASOUND BEAM

If the wavelength of the sound is larger than the source that produced it, then the sound will spread in all directions.[143] Such is the case with audible sound, thus explaining why it is possible for a person behind you to hear your voice almost as well as a person in front of you. In the case of therapeutic ultrasound, the sound is less divergent, thus concentrating energy in a limited area (1 MHz at a velocity 1540 m/sec in soft tissue and a wavelength of 1.5 mm, emitted from a transducer that is larger than the wavelength at approximately 25 mm in diameter).

The larger the diameter of the soundhead, the more focused or **collimated** the beam. Smaller soundheads produce a more divergent beam. Also, the beam from ultrasound generated at a frequency of 1 MHz is more divergent than ultrasound generated at 3 MHz (see Fig. 12-7).

Within this cylindrical beam the distribution of sound energy is highly nonuniform, particularly in an area close to the transducer referred to as the near field or near zone (Fig. 12-7B). The near field is a zone of spatially fluctuating ultrasound strength. The fluctuation occurs because of differences in pressure created by the waves emitted from the transducer. As the beam moves away from the transducer, the waves eventually become indistinguishable, arriving at a certain point simultaneously, creating a point of highest acoustic intensity.[143] The point of maximum acoustic intensity can be determined by calculating the distance (L) from the surface of the transducer:

$$L = \frac{D^2}{4W}$$

where D is the diameter of the transducer and W is the wavelength.[87] From this point the beam moves into the far field or far zone where the distribution of energy is much more uniform but the beam becomes more divergent.

Beam Nonuniformity Ratio

Ultrasound beams are not homogeneous along their longitudinal axis; some points are of higher intensity than others away from the transducer surface. The amount of variability of intensity within the ultrasound beam is indicated by the **beam nonuniformity ratio (BNR)**. This ratio is determined by using an underwater microphone (acoustic hydrophone) to measure the maximal point intensity of the transducer to the average intensity across the transducer surface. For example, a BNR of 2 to 1 means when the average output intensity is 1 W/cm^2, the peak or maximal point intensity of the beam is 2 W/cm^2. Optimally the BNR would be 1 to 1; however, because this is not possible, the BNR should fall between 2 and 6. Some ultrasound units have BNRs as high as 8 to 1. Peak intensities of 8 W/cm^2 have been shown to damage tissue; therefore, the patient runs a risk of tissue damage if intensities greater than 1 W/cm^2 are used on a machine with an 8 to 1 BNR. The lower the BNR, the more uniform the output and therefore the lower the chance of developing "hot spots" of concentrated energy. The Food and Drug Administration requires all ultrasound units to list the BNR, and the therapist should be aware of the BNR for that particular unit.[51]

Treatment Tip
The lower the frequency of ultrasound the less the energy is absorbed in the superficial tissues, and thus the deeper it penetrates. The majority of the sound waves generated from the 3 MHz treatment would be absorbed in the muscle or tendon. Also, when treating subcutaneous structures 3 MHz heats more rapidly, and is more comfortable than 1 MHz.

3 MHz = superficial heat
1 MHz = deep heat

collimated beam A focused, less divergent beam of ultrasound energy produced by a large diameter transducer.

Treatment area = 2–3 ERA

CASE STUDY 12-1
ULTRASOUND

Background: An 18-year-old college freshman sustained a fracture of the fifth metacarpal of the left hand during a prank in the dormitory. The fracture required gauntlet cast immobilization for 6 weeks. At the time of cast removal the patient noted significant restriction of motion and weakness in the left wrist. A referral was initiated. Physical examination revealed flexion 0–45 degrees, extension 0–30 degrees with radial and ulnar deviation unaffected. There was point tenderness at the callus site on the shaft of the fifth metacarpal. Finger motion was grossly within normal limits at all constituent joints.

Impression: Wrist capsule motion restriction secondary to immobilization, muscular weakness secondary to immobilization.

Treatment Plan: A course of therapeutic ultrasound was initiated to decrease joint stiffness through increased collagen-connective tissue extensibility. Given the small and irregular surface of the wrist joint, underwater coupling was chosen as the mode of ultrasound delivery. After checking the left wrist and hand for any rashes or open wounds and verifying that sensation and circulation were normal in the distal portion of the extremity the left forearm, wrist, and hand were immersed in a plastic basin filled with warm water. An ultrasound treatment of 1.5 W/cm2 for 6 minutes was applied to the dorsal aspect of the left wrist. Patient reported a mild sensation of warmth. At the conclusion of the treatment the patient was instructed in active and active-assistive wrist mobilization exercises.

Response: Following initial ultrasound treatment and exercise patient experienced a 10-degree improvement in both flexion and extension range of motion. At the completion of the sixth treatment wrist range of motion was within normal limits, and the patient was aggressively pursuing a wrist curl strengthening regimen. Ultrasound treatments were discontinued at that time with efforts focused on strengthening and functional use of the left upper extremity.

The rehabilitation professional employs therapeutic agent modalities to create an optimum environment for tissue healing while minimizing the symptoms associated with the trauma or condition.

Discussion Questions

- What tissues were injured or affected?
- What symptoms were present?
- What phase of the injury healing continuum did the patient present for care in?
- What are the therapeutic agent modality's biophysical effects (direct, indirect, depth, and tissue affinity)?
- What are the therapeutic agent modality's indications and contraindications?
- What are the parameters of the therapeutic agent modality's application, dosage, duration, and frequency in this case study?
- What other therapeutic agent modalities could be utilized to treat this injury or condition? Why? How?

Ultrasound may be continuous or pulsed.

The high peak intensities associated with high BNRs are responsible for much of the discomfort or periosteal pain often associated with ultrasound treatment.[68] Therefore, the higher the BNR the more important it is to move the transducer faster during treatment to avoid hot spots and areas of tissue damage or cavitation. Figure 12-8 shows the high beam homogeneity of a low BNR transducer and the typical beam profile of a high BNR transducer at 3 MHz output frequency.

Some researchers give little credence to BNR as a factor in good ultrasound equipment and say that it has little effect in treatment quality. Their rationale is that good treatment technique is much more important than the BNR.[58] However, most would agree that a continuous thermal ultrasound treatment is effective only if it is tolerated by the patient, and if it produces uniform heating through the tissues.[72] Some have speculated that a beam flowing from a poor-quality ultrasound crystal might be a reason patients experience pain and might cause uneven heating of tissue. Patient compliance should be better when thermal ultrasound is delivered via an ultrasound device with a low beam nonuniformity ratio. This will encourage patients to return for needed ultrasound treatments and allow the therapist to increase the intensity to the point where the patient feels local heat. When a heat modality is applied to tissue, it only makes sense that the patient should feel heat. If warmth is not felt, either the therapist is moving the soundhead too fast, or the intensity is too low.

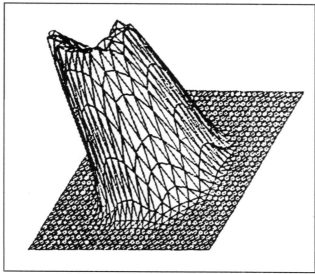

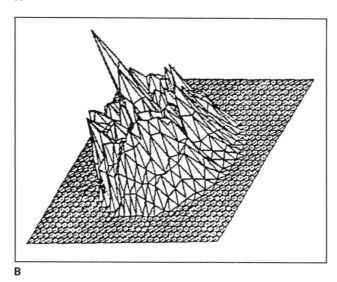

•**Figure 12-8 A.** Graphic representation of a low BNR of 2 to 1. **B.** Graphic representation of a high BNR of 6 to 1.

PULSED VERSUS CONTINUOUS WAVE ULTRASOUND

Virtually all therapeutic ultrasound generators can emit either continuous or pulsed ultrasound waves. If **continuous wave ultrasound** is used, the sound intensity remains constant throughout the treatment, and the ultrasound energy is being produced 100 percent of the time (Fig. 12-9).

With **pulsed ultrasound** the intensity is periodically interrupted, with no ultrasound energy being produced during the off period (Fig. 12-10). When using pulsed ultrasound, the average intensity of the output over time is reduced. The percentage of time that ultrasound is being generated (pulse duration) over one pulse period is referred to as the **duty cycle**.

$$\text{Duty cycle} = \frac{\text{duration of pulse (on time)} \times 100}{\text{pulse period (on time + off time)}}$$

Thus, if the pulse duration is 1 msec and the total pulse period is 5 msec, the duty cycle would be 20 percent. Therefore, the total amount of energy being delivered to the tissues would be only 20 percent of the energy delivered if a continuous wave was

continuous wave ultrasound The sound intensity remains constant throughout the treatment and the ultrasound energy is being produced 100 percent of the time.

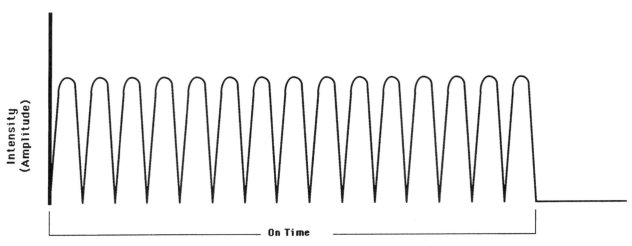

•Figure 12-9 In continuous ultrasound, energy is constantly being generated.

being used. The majority of ultrasound generators have duty cycles that are preset at either 20 or 50 percent; however, some provide several optional duty cycles. Occasionally the duty cycle is also referred to as the *mark:space* ratio.

Continuous ultrasound is most commonly used when thermal effects are desired. The use of pulsed ultrasound results in a reduced average heating of the tissues. Pulsed ultrasound or continuous ultrasound at a low intensity will produce nonthermal or mechanical effects that may be associated with soft tissue healing.

pulsed ultrasound The intensity is periodically interrupted with no ultrasound energy being produced during the off period. When using pulsed ultrasound, the average intensity of the output over time is reduced.

AMPLITUDE, POWER, AND INTENSITY

Amplitude is a term used to describe the magnitude of the vibration in a wave. It is the maximum distance from equilibrium that any particle reaches. Amplitude is used to describe either the movement of particles in the medium through which it travels in units of distance (centimeters or meters), or the variation in pressure found along the path of the wave in units of pressure (Newtons/meter^2).[28]

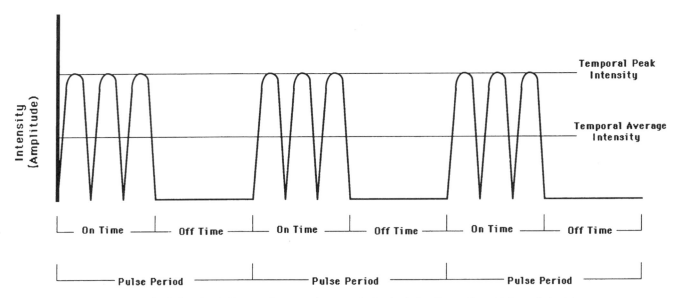

•Figure 12-10 In pulsed ultrasound, energy is generated only during the on time. Duty cycle is determined by the ratio of on time to pulse period.

Power is the total amount of ultrasound energy in the beam and is expressed in watts. **Intensity** is a measure of the rate at which energy is being delivered per unit area. Because power and intensity are unevenly distributed in the beam, several varying types of intensities must be defined.

Spatial-averaged intensity is the intensity of the ultrasound beam averaged over the area of the transducer. It may be calculated by dividing the power output in watts by the total effective radiating area of the soundhead in cm² and is indicated in watts per square centimeter (W/cm²). If ultrasound is being produced at a power of 6 W and the effective radiating area of the transducer is 4 cm², the spatial-averaged intensity would be 1.5 W/cm². On many ultrasound units, both the power in watts and the spatial-average intensity in W/cm² may be displayed. If the power output is constant, increasing the size of the transducer will decrease the spatial-averaged intensity.

Spatial peak intensity is the highest value occurring within the beam over time. With therapeutic ultrasound, maximum intensities can range between 0.25 and 3.0 W/cm².

Temporal peak intensity, sometimes also referred to as *pulse-averaged intensity*, is the maximum intensity during the on period with pulsed ultrasound, indicated in W/cm² (see Fig. 12-10).

Temporal-averaged intensity is important only with pulsed ultrasound and is calculated by averaging the power during both the on and off periods. For a pulsed sound beam with a duty cycle of 20 percent with a temporal peak intensity of 2.0 W/cm², temporal-averaged intensity would be 0.4 W/cm². It should be pointed out that on some machines, the intensity setting indicates the temporal peak intensity or on time, whereas on others it shows the temporal-averaged intensity or the mean of the on-off intensity (see Fig. 12-10).[106]

Spatial-averaged temporal peak (SATP) intensity is the maximum intensity occurring in time of the spatially averaged intensity. The SATP intensity is simply the spatial average during a single pulse.

There are no definitive rules that govern selection of specific ultrasound intensities during treatment, yet using too much may likely damage tissues and exacerbate the condition.[143] One recommendation is that the lowest intensity of ultrasound energy at the highest frequency that will transmit the energy to a specific tissue should be used to achieve a desired therapeutic effect.[106] Some guidance for selecting intensities has come from published reports from those who have obtained successful, yet subjective, clinical outcomes. Table 12-4 provides a summary of various studies from the literature that have made recommendations regarding intensities, frequencies, and treatment mode.[106]

It is important to remember that everyone's tolerance to heat is different, and thus ultrasound intensity should always be adjusted to patient tolerance.[68] At the beginning of the treatment, turn the intensity to the point where the patient feels deep warmth, and then back the intensity down slightly until gentle heating is felt.[33,34] During the treatment ask the patient for feedback, and make the necessary intensity adjustments. This idea only applies to continuous mode ultrasound because pulsed ultrasound generally does not produce heat. Regardless, the treatment should never produce reports of pain. If the patient reports that the transducer feels hot at the skin surface, it is likely that the coupling medium is inadequate, and possible that the piezoelectric crystal has been damaged and the transducer is overheating.

Ultrasound treatments should be temperature dependent, not time dependent. Thermal ultrasound is used in order to bring about certain desired effects, and tissues

amplitude Describes the magnitude of the vibration in a wave. It is the maximum distance from equilibrium that any particle reaches.

power The total amount of ultrasound energy in the beam and is expressed in watts.

intensity A measure of the rate at which energy is being delivered per unit area.

TABLE 12-4	Ultrasound Rate of Heating Per Minute[36]	
Intensity (W/cm²)	1 MHz (°C)	3 MHz (°C)
0.5	0.04	0.3
1.0	0.2	0.6
1.5	0.3	0.9
2.0	0.4	1.4

respond according to the amount of heat they receive.[91,92] Any significant adjustment in the intensity must be countered with an adjustment in the treatment time. It is possible that ultrasound treatments of the future will be like iontophoresis, where the treatment time is dependent on the dosage delivered. For this reason, it is likely that the new generation of ultrasound generators will have the capability of automatically decreasing treatment time as the intensity is increased and increasing treatment time as the intensity is decreased (see Fig. 12-3).

It should also be added that different ultrasound devices will in all likelihood produce different intensities and different outputs during treatments despite the fact that the selected treatment parameters may be identical. Therefore the therapeutic effects may be different from one therapeutic ultrasound device to the next.[102]

PHYSIOLOGIC EFFECTS OF ULTRASOUND

Therapeutic ultrasound may induce clinically significant responses in cells, tissues, and organs through both thermal effects and nonthermal biophysical effects.[12,42–44,55,80,115,136,143,148] Ultrasound will affect both normal and damaged biologic tissues. It has been suggested that damaged tissue may be more responsive to ultrasound than normal tissue.[46] When ultrasound is applied for its thermal effects, nonthermal biophysical effects will also occur that may damage normal tissues.[80] If appropriate, treatment parameters are selected; however, nonthermal effects can occur with minimal thermal effects.

THERMAL EFFECTS

The ultrasound wave attenuates as it travels through the tissue. Attenuation is caused primarily by the conversion of ultrasound energy into heat through absorption and to some extent by scattering and beam deflection. Traditionally, ultrasound has been used primarily to produce a tissue temperature increase.[9,54,94,97,129,141] The clinical effects of using ultrasound to heat tissues are similar to other forms of heat that may be applied, including the following:[91]

1. An increase in the extensibility of collagen fibers found in tendons and joint capsules
2. Decrease in joint stiffness
3. Reduction of muscle spasm
4. Modulation of pain
5. Increased blood flow
6. Mild inflammatory response that may help in the resolution of chronic inflammation

It has been suggested that for the majority of these effects to occur the tissues must be raised to a level of 40–45°C for a minimum of 5 minutes.[43] Others are of the opinion that absolute temperatures are not the key, but rather how much the temperature rises above baseline.[91–93] They report that tissue temperature increases of 1°C increase metabolism and healing, increases of 2–3°C decrease pain and muscle spasm, and increases of 4°C or greater increase extensibility of collagen and decrease joint stiffness.[16,17,91] It has been shown that temperatures above 45°C may be potentially damaging to tissues, yet patients usually experience pain prior to these extreme temperatures.[36]

Ultrasound at 1 MHz with an intensity of 1 W/cm^2 has been reported to raise soft tissue temperature by as much as 0.86°C/min in tissues with a poor vascular supply.[123] It has been shown that 3 MHz ultrasound at 1 W/cm^2 to raise human patellar tendon temperatures 2°C/min.[18] In muscle, which is quite vascular, 1 and 3 MHz ultrasound at 1 W/cm^2 increase the temperature 0.2 and 0.6°C/min, respectively.[36] It has also been demonstrated that tissue temperature increases were significantly increased by preheating the treatment area prior to initiating or ultrasound treatment.[70]

The primary advantage of ultrasound over other nonacoustic heating modalities is that tissues high in collagen, such as tendons, muscles, ligaments, joint capsules, joint menisci, intermuscular interfaces, nerve roots, periosteum, cortical bone, and other deep tissues may be selectively heated to the therapeutic range without causing a significant tissue temperature increase in skin or fat.[137] Ultrasound will penetrate skin and fat with little attenuation.[40]

The thermal effects of ultrasound are related to frequency. As indicated earlier, an inverse relationship exists between depth of penetration and frequency. Most of the energy in a sound wave at 3 MHz will be absorbed in the superficial tissues. At 1 MHz there will be less attenuation, and the energy will penetrate to the deeper tissues, selectively heating them. It has been suggested that 3 MHz ultrasound should be the recommended modality in the heating of tissue structures to a depth level of 2.5 cm. One MHz treatment will not produce the temperatures (>4°C change or 40°C absolute temperature) needed to heat the structures of the body effectively.[67]

Heating will occur with both continuous and pulsed ultrasound, depending on the intensity of the total current being delivered to the patient. Significant thermal effects will be induced whenever the upper end of the available intensity range is used. Regardless of whether ultrasound is pulsed or continuous, if the spatial-averaged temporal-averaged intensity is in the 0.1–0.2 W/cm^2 range, the intensity is too low to produce a tissue temperature increase and only nonthermal effects will occur.[43]

Unlike the other heating modalities discussed in this text, whenever ultrasound is used to produce thermal changes, nonthermal changes also simultaneously occur.[44] An understanding of these nonthermal changes, therefore, is essential.

NONTHERMAL EFFECTS

The nonthermal effects of therapeutic ultrasound include **cavitation** and **acoustic microstreaming** (Fig. 12-11). Cavitation is the formation of gas-filled bubbles that expand and compress owing to ultrasonically induced pressure changes in tissue fluids.[43,136] Cavitation may be classified as being either *stable* or *unstable*. In stable cavitation, the bubbles expand and contract in response to regularly repeated pressure changes over many acoustic cycles. In unstable or transient cavitation, there are violent large excursions in bubble volume before implosion and collapse occurs after only a few cycles. Therapeutic benefits are derived only from stable cavitation, whereas the collapse of bubbles is thought to create increased pressure and high temperatures that may cause local tissue damage. Unstable cavitation clearly should be avoided. It is likely that high intensity, low frequency ultrasound may produce unstable cavitation, particularly if standing waves develop at tissue interfaces.[43]

Cavitation results in an increased flow in the fluid around these vibrating bubbles. Microstreaming is the unidirectional movement of fluids along the boundaries of cell membranes resulting from the mechanical pressure wave in an ultrasonic field.[43,136] Microstreaming produces high viscous stresses, which can alter cell membrane structure and function due to changes in cell membrane permeability to sodium and calcium ions important in the healing process. As long as the cell membrane is not damaged, microstreaming can be of therapeutic value in accelerating the healing process.[43]

It has been well documented that the nonthermal effects of therapeutic ultrasound in the treatment of injured tissues may be as important, if not more important, than the thermal effects. Therapeutically significant nonthermal effects have been identified in soft tissue repair via stimulation of fibroblast activity, which produces an increase in protein synthesis, tissue regeneration, increased blood flow in chronically ischemic tissues, bone healing and repair of nonunion fractures, and in phonophoresis.[46,69,120] Treatment with therapeutic levels of ultrasound may alter the course of the immune response. Ultrasound effects a number of biologic processes associated with injury repair.

The literature provides a number of examples in which exposure of cells to therapeutic ultrasound under nonthermal conditions modified cellular functions. Nonthermal levels of ultrasound are reported to modulate membrane properties, alter cellular

acoustic microstreaming The unidirectional movement of fluids along the boundaries of cell membranes resulting from the mechanical pressure wave in an ultrasonic field.

cavitation The formation of gas-filled bubbles that expand and compress because of ultrasonically induced pressure changes in tissue fluids.

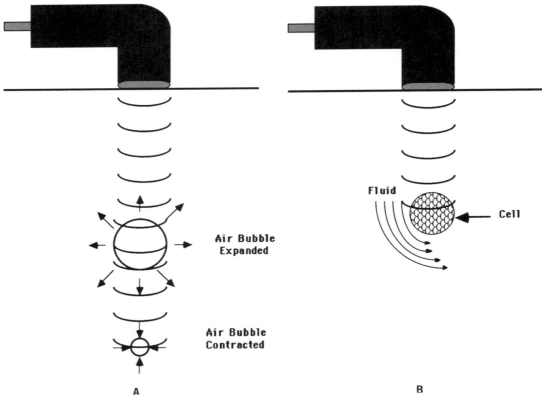

•Figure 12-11 Nonthermal effects of ultrasound. **A.** Cavitation is the formation of gas-filled bubbles that expand and compress owing to ultrasonically induced pressure changes in tissue fluids. **B.** Microstreaming is the unidirectional movement of fluids along the boundaries of cell membranes resulting from the mechanical pressure wave in an ultrasonic field.

Treatment Tip

The nonthermal effects of cavitation and microstreaming can be maximized while minimizing the thermal effects by using a spatial-averaged temporal-averaged intensity of 0.1 to 0.2 W/cm² with continuous ultrasound. This range may also be achieved using a low temporal-averaged intensity by pulsing a higher temporal-peak intensity of 1.0 W/cm² at a duty cycle of 20 percent, to give a temporal average intensity of 0.2 W/cm².

proliferation, and produce increases in proteins associated with inflammation and injury repair.[77] Combined, these data suggest that nonthermal effects of therapeutic ultrasound can modify the inflammatory response. The concept of the absorption of ultrasonic energy by enzymatic proteins leading to changes in the enzymes activity is not novel.[77] However, recent reports demonstrating that ultrasound affects enzyme activity and possibly gene regulation provide sufficient data to present a probable molecular mechanism of ultrasound's nonthermal therapeutic action. The frequency resonance hypothesis describes two possible biologic mechanisms that may alter protein function as a result of the absorption of ultrasonic energy. First, absorption of mechanical energy by a protein may produce a transient conformational shift (modifying the three-dimensional structure) and alter the protein's functional activity. Second, the resonance or shearing properties of the wave (or both) may dissociate a multimolecular complex, thereby disrupting the complex's function.[77]

The nonthermal effects of cavitation and microstreaming can be maximized while minimizing the thermal effects by using a spatial-averaged temporal-averaged intensity of 0.1–0.2 W/cm² with continuous ultrasound. This range may also be achieved using a low temporal-averaged intensity by pulsing a higher temporal-peak intensity of 1.0 W/cm² at a duty cycle of 20 percent, to give a temporal average intensity of 0.2 W/cm².

ULTRASOUND TREATMENT TECHNIQUES

The principles and theories of therapeutic ultrasound are well understood and documented. However, specific practical recommendations as to how ultrasound may best be applied to a patient therapeutically are quite controversial and are based primarily on the experience of the clinicians who have used it. Even though there are numerous laboratory and clinically based reports in the literature, treatment procedures and parameters are highly variable, and many contradictory results and conclusions have been presented in the literature.[106]

FREQUENCY OF TREATMENT

It is generally accepted that acute conditions require more frequent treatments over a shorter period of time, whereas more chronic conditions require fewer treatments over a longer period of time.[106] Ultrasound treatments should begin as soon as possible following injury, ideally within hours but definitely within 48 hours to maximize effects on the healing process.[56,114,116] Acute conditions may be treated using low intensity or pulsed ultrasound once or even twice daily for 6–8 days until acute symptoms such as pain and swelling subside. In chronic conditions, when acute symptoms have subsided, treatment may be done on alternating days.[134] Ultrasound treatment should continue as long as there is improvement. Assuming that appropriate treatment parameters are chosen and the ultrasound generator is functioning properly, if no improvement is noted following three or four treatments, ultrasound should be discontinued, or different parameters (i.e., duty cycle, frequency) employed.

The question is often asked, "How many ultrasound treatments can be given?" It must be pointed out that most of the research regarding treatment longevity has been performed on animals, and it takes quite a leap of logic to assume that the same negative effects would occur in humans. If the correct parameters are followed using a high-quality, recently calibrated ultrasound machine, treatments could occur daily for several weeks. In the past, it has been recommended that ultrasound be limited to 14 treatments in the majority of conditions, although this has not been documented scientifically. More than 14 treatments can reduce both red and white blood cell counts. After these 14 treatments some authors advise avoiding ultrasound use for 2 weeks.[57]

DURATION OF TREATMENT

In the past, modality textbooks have been quite vague with respect to treatment time, and generally the suggested duration has been too short.[68,132] Typically recommended treatment times have ranged between 5 and 10 minutes in length; however, these times may be insufficient. The length of the treatment is dependent on several factors: the size of the area to be treated; the intensity in W/cm^2; the frequency; and the desired temperature increase. As stated previously, specific temperature increases are required to achieve beneficial effects in tissue. The therapist must determine what the desired effects of the treatment are before a treatment duration is set (Fig. 12-12). There is little research defining the application duration needed to increase tissue temperature to the target range during ultrasound at varying application intensities. Likewise, there are few data describing the effect of ultrasound intensity on the final temperature reached.[95]

An accepted recommendation is that ultrasound be administered in an area two times the ERA (roughly twice the size of the soundhead). If thermal effects are desired in an area larger than this, obviously the treatment time needs to be increased.

The higher the intensity applied in W/cm^2, the shorter the treatment time, and vice versa. It just does not make clinical sense to treat one patient at 1 W/cm^2 and another at 2 W/cm^2 at identical treatment durations when both patients require vigorous heating. Based on this scenario, it could be hypothesized that patient two will produce tissue temperature increases of twice that of patient one. However, it has been shown that an ultrasound treatment using a 1 MHz frequency and an intensity level of 1.0 W/cm^2 increases intramuscular tissue to higher temperatures than a 2.0 W/cm^2 intensity at a depth of 4 cm[95]

Ultrasound frequency (MHz) not only determines the depth of penetration, it also determines the rate of heating. The energy produced with 3 MHz ultrasound is absorbed three times faster than that produced from 1 MHz ultrasound, the result of which is faster heating. Ultrasound at 3 MHz consistently heats tissues three

Ideal BNR = 1:1

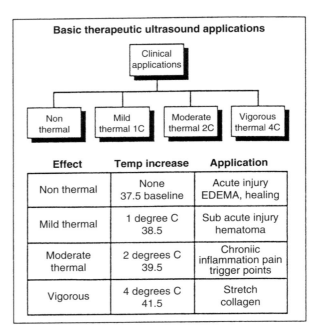

Basic therapeutic ultrasound applications

Effect	Temp increase	Application
Non thermal	None 37.5 baseline	Acute injury EDEMA, healing
Mild thermal	1 degree C 38.5	Sub acute injury hematoma
Moderate thermal	2 degrees C 39.5	Chroniic inflammation pain trigger points
Vigorous	4 degrees C 41.5	Stretch collagen

•**Figure 12-12** It is important to have a treatment goal and to adjust the ultrasound treatment time accordingly.

times faster than 1 MHz, thus reducing the required treatment duration by one-third.[32,36] The desired temperature increase is also a factor in determining the duration of an ultrasound treatment. Table 12-4 displays the rate of muscle temperature increase per minute, per W/cm^2, at various intensities and frequencies.[36] Based on this information, the therapist can determine the appropriate duration of an ultrasound treatment. For example, a patient has limited range of motion because of scar tissue buildup from a chronic hamstring strain at the musculotendinous junction. An appropriate goal would be to vigorously heat the muscle (an increase of 4°C) and immediately perform passive hamstring stretching. If 1 MHz ultrasound were used at an intensity of 2 W/cm^2, the 4°C increase would take about 10 minutes. At 2 minutes into the treatment, however, the patient complains that the treatment is too hot. Most of us would respond by decreasing the intensity, but we may forget to increase the treatment time. In this case if we decreased the intensity to 1.5 W/cm^2, we would need to add 2 minutes to the treatment time in order to ensure a 4°C increase in muscle temperature. It is important to note that this chart requires a treatment size of two to three ERA, and these temperatures were reported in muscle. It has also been suggested that tendon heats over three times faster than muscle.[18]

COUPLING METHODS

The greatest amount of reflection of ultrasonic energy occurs at the air-tissue interface. To ensure that maximal energy will be transmitted to the patient, the face of the transducer should be parallel with the surface of the skin so that the ultrasound will strike the surface at a 90 degree angle. If the angle between the transducer face and the skin is greater than 15 degree a large percentage of the energy will be reflected and the treatment effects will be minimal.[135]

Reflection at the air-tissue interface can be further reduced by applying the ultrasound via the use of some coupling agent. The purpose of the **coupling medium** is to exclude air from the region between the patient and the transducer so that ultrasound can get to the area to be treated.[143] The acoustical impedance of the coupling medium

coupling medium A substance used to decrease the acoustical impedance at the air-skin interface and thus facilitate the passage of ultrasound energy.

should match the impedance of the transducer and should be slightly higher than the skin. Also, the medium should have a low coefficient of absorption to minimize attenuation in the coupling medium. It is important that the medium remains free of air bubbles during treatment. The coupling agent should be viscous enough to act as a lubricant as the transducer is moved over the surface of the skin.[106]

The coupling medium should be applied to the skin surface and the ultrasound transducer should be in contact with the coupling medium before the power is turned on. If the transducer is not in contact with the skin via the coupling medium, or if for some reason the transducer is lifted away from the treatment area, the piezoelectric crystal may be damaged and the transducer can overheat.

A number of studies have looked at the efficacy of different coupling media in transmitting ultrasound.[4,40,43,126] Water, light oils, topical analgesics,[12,119] gel packs,[85,105] gel pads,[103] and various brands of ultrasonic gel have been recommended as coupling agents. The recommendations of these studies have proven to be somewhat contradictory. Essentially it appears that all of these agents have very similar acoustic properties and are effective as coupling agents.[29]

When using ultrasound in the treatment of patients with partial and full-thinkness wounds, treatments are performed over a hydrogel sheet (i.e., Nu-Gel, ClearSite, etc.) or semipermeable film dressing (i.e., J&J Bioclusive, Tegaderm). Transmissivity of wound care products used to deliver acoustic energy during ultrasound treatment of wounds varies greatly among dressing products.[84]

Water is an effective coupling medium, but its low viscosity reduces its suitability in surface application. To reach the temperature increase obtained with gel, higher intensities need to be used with water.[75] Light oils, such as mineral oil and glycerol, have relatively higher absorption coefficients and are somewhat difficult to clean up following treatment. Water-soluble gels seem to have the most desirable properties necessary for a good coupling medium.[29,40] Perhaps the only disadvantage is that the salts in the gel may damage the metal face of the transducer with improper cleaning. Out of convenience, some therapists have used massage lotion instead of ultrasound gel; however, experience has revealed that massage lotion is not an adequate ultrasound conducting medium. Table 12-5 describes a technique that can be used to check the relative transmission capability of a medium.

EXPOSURE TECHNIQUES

Direct Contact

Direct application of ultrasound involves actual contact between the applicator and the skin, with a sufficient amount of couplant between. A layer of gel should be applied to the treatment area in sufficient amounts to maintain good contact and lubrication between the transducer and the skin, but not so much that air pockets may form from movement of the transducer. A thin film of gel should also be applied directly to the transducer face before transmission begins (Fig. 12-13).[106] A direct technique of exposure may be used as long as the surface being treated is larger than the diameter of the transducer. If a smaller surface area is to be treated, a smaller transducer should be used so that direct application can still be performed.

TABLE 12-5	Technique That Can Be Used to Check the Relative Transmission Capability of a Medium

Encircle the transducer with tape while leaving about 2 cm of tape exposed (making a tape tube).
Fill the tape tube with 1 cm thickness of ultrasound gel medium.
Fill the tube to the top with water.
Adjust the intensity and watch the water bubble.
Repeat the procedure yet substitute the gel with the medium you are testing.
If the water has little or no bubbles, your desired medium is not a good couplant after all.

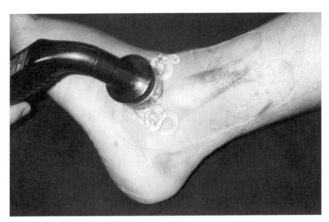

•**Figure 12-13** Ultrasound may be applied directly through some gel-like coupling medium.

Heating of the ultrasound gel prior to treatment has been recommended to improve the thermal effects of ultrasound in deeper tissues; however, this is not the case. Because ultrasound heats only through conversion of mechanical vibration to heat and not through conduction, heating of the gel will have no effect in the deeper tissues.[51] The only rationale for heating cold ultrasound gel is strictly for patient comfort and compliance.

Recently several manufacturers of analgesic creams have been promoting their use as ultrasound couplants (i.e., Biofreeze, T-prep).[112,119] Patients are treated with ultrasound via a conducting medium of gel mixed with their product.[111] One company recommended a mixture of two parts gel to one part analgesic cream (this has recently been changed to 80 percent gel to 20 percent cream), whereas another recommended a 50/50 ratio of ultrasound gel and their analgesic cream. Small mixtures of analgesic creams with 80 or 90 percent gel may produce significant heating, but as yet have not been tested. Some of these products have been shown to actually impede the transmission of ultrasound. Many of these over-the-counter medications presently used are only minimally effective as ultrasound couplants.[3] If a patient wants the added benefits of heat and analgesia, first massage the balm into the area, then apply 100 percent ultrasound gel followed by ultrasound. Perceptions of heat by the patient may not indicate actual temperature increases within the muscle when using analgesic creams.[111] Until further research is performed in this area, it is suggested that the practice of using analgesic creams mixed with ultrasound gel be discontinued when vigorous heating is desired. Figure 12-14 displays the results of research involving two such products and their effect on muscle temperature increase via ultrasound.

Water soluble gels = best coupling medium

FLEX-ALL VS. BIOFREEZE

Depth (cm)	50/50 Flex-all; gel (°C)	50/50 Biofreeze; gel (°C)	100% Gel (°C)
3	2.8	1.8	3.4
5	1.8	1.3	2.5

Muscle temperature increase from continuous 1-MHz ultrasound at 1.5 W/cm² for 10 minutes.

•**Figure 12-14** Two popular analgesic creams were mixed with ultrasound gel and used as coupling media. Only the treatments that used 100 percent ultrasound gel as the couplant yielded temperatures consistent with vigorous heating. We conclude that these creams, although they might decrease pain perception, actually impede ultrasound transmission. *Note:* These manufacturers are now recommending mixtures of 80 percent ultrasound gel with 20 percent of their product.

Immersion

Although direct application with gel has been shown to be the most effective application technique, there are some instances where water immersion is warranted. The immersion technique is recommended if the area to be treated is smaller than the diameter of the available transducer or if the treatment area is irregular with bony prominences (Fig. 12-15). A plastic, ceramic, or rubber basin should be used, because a metal basin or whirlpool will reflect some of the ultrasound, increasing the intensity near the basin walls. Tap water seems to be just as effective as degassed water as a coupling medium for the immersion technique and less likely to produce surface heating than mineral oil or glycerin.[56,126] The transducer should be moved parallel to the surface being treated at a distance of 0.5–1 cm.[148] If air bubbles accumulate on the transducer or over the treatment area, they may be wiped away quickly during the treatment. In order to ensure adequate heating, the intensity should be increased, possibly as much as 50 percent.[41]

Bladder Technique

If for some reason the treatment area cannot be immersed in water, a bladder technique can be used in which a balloon, surgical glove, or even a condom have been filled with water and the ultrasound energy is transmitted from the transducer to the treatment surface through this bladder (Fig. 12-16). Generally the use of the bladder technique is not recommended. Nevertheless it is occasionally used. Both sides of the balloon should be coated with gel to assure better contact. Recently, commercial gel packs have gained popularity and several studies have demonstrated their efficacy as a coupling medium.[8,85,105] Treatments using a bladder filled with either gel or silicone have also been used at higher ultrasound intensities[4] (Figure 12-16B).

MOVING THE TRANSDUCER

In the past, treatment techniques that involve both moving the transducer and holding the transducer stationary have been recommended. The stationary technique was most often used when the treatment area was small or when pulsed ultrasound was used at a

Treatment Tip
When using a large soundhead to treat over bony prominences the immersion technique done in a plastic or rubber tub can be effective. Also the bladder technique could be used to make certain that there is consistent contact between the soundhead and the coupling medium.

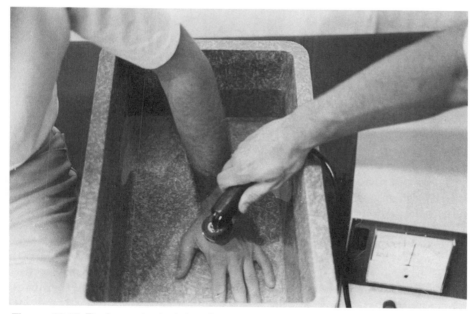

•**Figure 12-15** The immersion technique is recommended when using ultrasound over irregular surfaces.

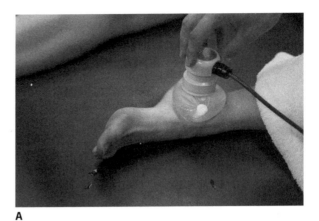

A

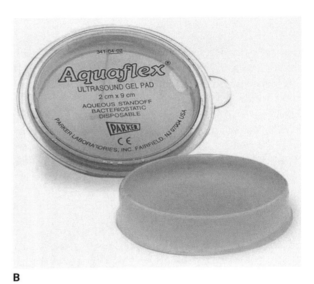

B

•Figure 12-16 Although not recommended, the bladder technique may also be used over irregular surfaces. Move the transducer at 4 cm/sec.

low temporal-averaged intensity. However, because of the nonuniformity of the ultrasound beam, the energy distribution in the tissue is uneven, thus creating potential tissue-damaging "hot spots."[148] If the ultrasound beam is stationary, the spatial-peak intensity determines the point of maximal temperature increase. With the moving technique, the spatial-averaged intensity gives the most reasonable measure of the average rate of heating within the treatment area.[136] This stationary technique has been demonstrated to produce disruption of blood flow, platelet aggregation, and damage to the venous system, therefore the stationary technique is no longer recommended.[147]

Moving the transducer during treatment leads to a more even distribution of energy within the treatment area, especially if the unit has a low BNR.[16] This can reduce the damaging effects of standing waves, particularly those which are most likely to occur at bone-tissue interfaces. Overlapping circular motions or a longitudinal stroking pattern can be used. The transducer should be moved slowly at approximately 4 cm/sec, covering a treatment area that is two to three times larger than the ERA of the transducer.[86,104] Movement speed of the transducer is BNR-dependent, and the higher the BNR the more important it is to move the transducer faster during treatment to avoid periosteal irritation and transient cavitation.[68,132] However, moving the transducer too rapidly decreases the total amount of energy absorbed per unit area. Rapid movement of the soundhead causes the therapist to slip into treating a larger area, thus the desired temperatures may not be attained.

Equipment with a low BNR usually allows for a slower stroking movement of the ultrasound transducer. Slow strokes are more controlled and can easily be contained to a small area (2 ERA). Slow movement of the applicator results in evenly distributed sound waves throughout the area, whereas a fast moving transducer will not allow for adequate absorption of the sound waves, and sufficient heating will not occur. If the patient complains of pain, decrease the output intensity, while making the appropriate adjustments in treatment duration. The transducer should be kept in maximum contact with the skin via some coupling agent.

During the administration of ultrasound, it is possible that the amount of pressure at the transducer may affect the physiologic response to and the outcome of the treatment.[83] It has been demonstrated that applying an excessive amount of pressure could decrease the acoustic transmissivity, damage the crystal in the transducer, or make the patient uncomfortable. It is recommended that the therapist apply firm, consistent pressure during treatment.[83]

RECORDING ULTRASOUND TREATMENTS

It is recommended that the therapist report or record the specific parameters used in an ultrasound treatment when completing treatment records or progress notes so that the treatment may be reproduced or altered. The parameters which should be recorded include frequency, spatial-averaged temporal peak intensity, whether the beam is pulsed or continuous, the duty factor (if pulsed), effective radiating surface area of the transducer, duration of the treatment, and the number of treatments per week.[106]

A typical treatment might be recorded as 3 MHz, at 1.0 W/cm², pulsed at 20 percent (0.2) duty factor, 5-cm transducer head, 5 minutes, four times per week.

CLINICAL APPLICATIONS FOR THERAPEUTIC ULTRASOUND

Ultrasound is generally recognized clinically as one of the most effective and widely used modalities in the treatment of many soft tissue and bony lesions. Considering the extensive use of ultrasound in treating soft tissue injuries, until the past decade there has been relatively little documented evidence from the medical community concerning the efficacy of this modality (however, research in this area is increasing). Many of the decisions as to how ultrasound should be used are empirically based on personal opinion and experience. This section summarizes the various clinical applications of therapeutic ultrasound used in a clinical setting.

SOFT-TISSUE HEALING AND REPAIR

Soft-tissue healing and repair may be accelerated by both thermal and nonthermal ultrasound.[42,47,53] Repair of soft tissues involves three phases of healing: inflammation, proliferation, and remodeling. Ultrasound does not seem to have any anti-inflammatory effects; rather, it is thought to accelerate the inflammatory phase of healing.

It has been shown that a single treatment with ultrasound can stimulate the release of histamine from mast cells.[66] The mechanism for this may be attributed primarily to nonthermal effects involving cavitation and streaming that increase the transport of calcium ions across the cell membrane, thus stimulating release of histamine by the mast cells.[43] Histamine attracts polymorphonuclear leukocytes that "clean up" debris from the injured area, along with monocytes whose primary function is to release chemotactic agents and growth factors that stimulate fibroblasts and endothelial cells to form a collagen-rich, well-vascularized tissue used for the development of new connective tissue that is essential for rapid repair. Thus, ultrasound can be effective in facilitating the process of inflammation, and therefore healing, if applied after bleeding has stopped but still within

Ultrasound accelerates the inflammatory process.

CASE STUDY 12-2
ULTRASOUND

Background: A 12-year-old junior high school student sustained a deep bruise of the left quadriceps muscle in a fall from his skateboard. The parents were advised by their pediatrician to apply cold initially and then moist heat until the problem resolved. At this time, 1 month postinjury, there remains significant restriction of left knee motion. A referral was initiated to physical therapy at the parent's request. Physical examination revealed active knee motion of only 10–65 degrees. There was point tenderness and a well-demarcated hematoma palpable in the middle third of the vastus lateralis.

Impression: Knee motion restriction secondary to soft-tissue contusion and hematoma formation.

Treatment Plan: A course of pulsed therapeutic ultrasound was initiated to decrease the hematoma formation through increased collagen-connective tissue extensibility and reabsorption of the extracellular debrise from the original contusion. The patient reported a mild sensation of warmth. At the conclusion of the treatment, the patient was instructed in active and active-assistive knee range-of-motion exercises.

Response: Following initial US treatment and exercise, patient experienced a 10-degree improvement in knee flexion and extension range of motion. At the completion of the tenth treatment session, knee range of motion was within normal limits, and the patient was aggressively pursuing a quadriceps-strengthening regimen. Ultrasound treatments were discontinued at that time with efforts focused on strengthening and functional use of the left lower extremity.

The rehabilitation professional employs physical agent modalities to create an optimum environment for tissue healing while minimizing the symptoms associated with the trauma or condition.

Discussion Questions

- What tissues were injured/affected?
- What symptoms were present?
- What phase of the injury-healing continuum did the patient present for care in?
- What are the physical agent modality's biophysical effects (direct/indirect/depth/tissue affinity)?
- What are the physical agent modality's indications/contraindications?
- What are the parameters of the physical agent modality's application/dosage/duration/frequency in this case study?
- What other physical agent modalities could be utilized to treat this injury or condition? Why? How?

Further Discussion Questions

- Which ultrasound frequency would be optimal for this patient's condition?
- Could you utilize continuous ultrasound output? Why? Why not?
- What would be your response to the patient's complaint of a "dull ache" during the treatment?
- Given the patient's age, are there any additional precautions you should take in utilizing ultrasound?

the first few hours after injury during the early stages of inflammation.[43] It has been suggested that this response occurs using pulsed ultrasound at 0.5 W/cm^2 with a duty cycle of 20 percent for 5 minutes or continuous ultrasound at 0.1 W/cm^2.[44]

These treatments have been described as being "proinflammatory" and are of value in accelerating repair in short-term or acute inflammation.[131] However, in chronic inflammatory conditions, the proinflammatory effects are of questionable value.[66] If an inflammatory stimulus such as overuse remains, the response to therapeutic ultrasound is of questionable value.[8]

Pitting edema is a condition that sometimes provides a challenge for therapists. Pitting edema may be treated with continuous 3 MHz ultrasound at intensities of 1–1.5 W/cm^2. The heat seems to liquefy the "gel-like" cellular debris. The limb is then elevated, massaged, or EMS used to pump the fluid and promote lymphatic drainage.

During the proliferative phase of healing, a connective tissue matrix is produced into which new blood vessels will grow. Fibroblasts are mainly responsible for producing this connective tissue. Fibroblasts exposed to therapeutic ultrasound are stimulated to produce more collagen that gives connective tissue most of its strength.[65] Again, cavitation and streaming alter cell membrane permeability to calcium ions that facilitate increases in collagen synthesis and in tensile strength. The intensity levels of therapeutic ultrasound that produce these changes during the proliferative phase are too low to be entirely thermal. It has been demonstrated that heating with continuous ultrasound may be more effective than stretching alone for increasing the extensibility of dense connective tissue.[125]

Ultrasound does not appear to be effective in enhancing postexercise muscle strength recovery or in diminishing delayed-onset muscle soreness.[121,138] Although treatment with pulsed ultrasound can promote the satellite cell proliferation phase of the myoregeneration, it does not seem to have significant effects on the overall morphologic manifestations of muscle regeneration.[124]

SCAR TISSUE AND JOINT CONTRACTURE

During remodeling, collagen fibers are realigned along lines of tensile stresses and strains, forming scar tissue. This process may continue for months or even years. In scar tissue, collagen never attains the same pattern and remains weaker and less elastic than normal tissue prior to injury. Scar tissue in tendons, ligaments, and capsules surrounding joints can produce joint contractures that limit range of motion. Increased tissue temperatures increase the elasticity and decrease the viscosity of collagen fibers. Because the deeper tissues surrounding joints that most often restrict range are rich in collagen, ultrasound is the treatment modality of choice.[90,148]

A number of studies have investigated the effects of ultrasound treatment on scar tissue and joint contracture. Ultrasound has been demonstrated to increase mobility in mature scar.[7] A greater residual increase in tissue length with less potential damage is produced through preheating with ultrasound prior to stretching, or by putting the joint on stretch while insonating.[38,89,128] Tissue extensibility increases when continuous ultrasound is applied at higher intensities causing vigorous heating of tissues.[59] Thigh, periarticular structures, and scar tissues become significantly more extensible following treatment with ultrasound involving thermal effects at intensities of 1.2–2.0 W/cm^2.[89] Scar tissue can be softened if treated with ultrasound at an early stage.[116] Dupuytren's contracture shows a beneficial effect on long-standing contracted bands of scar and a decrease in pain when treated early on with ultrasound.[99]

The majority of the earlier studies attributed the effectiveness of ultrasound to thermal effects and used continuous moderate intensities between 0.5 and 2.0 W/cm^2.

STRETCHING OF CONNECTIVE TISSUE

Collagenous tissue when stressed is fairly rigid, yet when heated it becomes much more yielding.[59,89] However, the combination of heat and stretching theoretically produces a residual lengthening of connective tissue, which increases according to the force applied.[101]

Preevent heating and stretching to improve range of motion are commonly recommended before exercise in an attempt to prevent musculotendinous injury. Active exercise appears to be more effective than ultrasound for increasing intramuscular temperature, however, the temperature increases do not appear to influence range of motion.[23]

The time period of vigorous heating when tissues will undergo the greatest extensibility and elongation is referred to as the **"stretching window."**[38,128] It should be added that the existence of this stretching window is theoretical and has not been conclusively demonstrated to exist.[10] To explain this concept, We refer to the analogy of the plastic spoon.[16] When a plastic spoon is dipped in hot water it softens, and by pulling on the ends, we are able to stretch it. As the plastic cools, however, it hardens and is no longer able to be stretched. Likewise, if we vigorously heat tissue it becomes more pliable and less resistant to stretch, yet as the tissue cools it withstands stretching, and can actually be damaged if too great of a force is applied.

Treatment Tip
To heat a large area in the low back, the best treatment choice is to use either hydrocollator packs or diathermy rather than ultrasound. If depth of penetration is a concern, then shortwave diathermy is the treatment modality of choice.

The rate of tissue cooling following continuous ultrasound at both 1 and 3 MHz frequencies has been determined (Fig. 12-17).[38,128] Thermistor probes were inserted 1.2 cm below the skin's surface and ultrasound was applied. The treatment raised the tissue temperature 5.3°C for the 3-MHz frequency. The average time it took for the temperature to drop each degree as expressed in minutes and seconds was: 1°C = 1:20; 2°C = 3:22; 3°C = 5:50; 4°C = 9:13; 5°C = 14:55. In this case, the temperature remained in the vigorous heating phase for only 3.3 minutes following an ultrasound treatment.

The same methods were used to determine the stretching window at 1 MHz. The temperature was recorded 4 cm deep in the muscle. It took 2 minutes for the temperature to drop 1°C, and a total of 5.5 minutes to drop 2°C. The deeper muscle cools at a slower rate than superficial muscle because the added tissue serves as a barrier to escaping heat. Regardless, tissue heated by ultrasound loses its heat at a fairly rapid rate; therefore, stretching, friction massage, or joint mobilization should be performed immediately postultrasound. To increase the duration of the stretching window, it is recommended that stretching be done during and immediately after ultrasound application.

Indications
- Acute and postacute conditions (ultrasound with nonthermal effects)
- Soft tissue healing and repair
- Scar tissue
- Joint contracture
- Chronic inflammation
- Increase extensibility of collagen
- Reduction of muscle spasm
- Pain modulation
- Increase blood flow
- Soft tissue repair
- Increase in protein synthesis
- Tissue regeneration
- Bone healing
- Repair of nonunion fractures
- Inflammation associated with myositis ossificans
- Plantar warts
- Myofascial trigger points

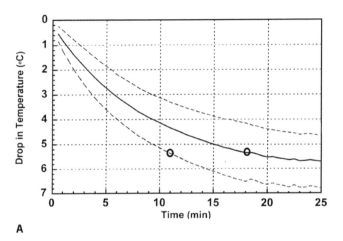

A

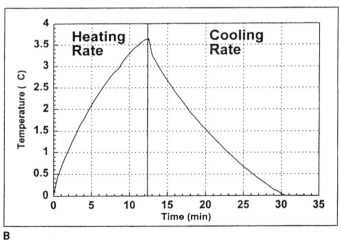

B

•**Figure 12-17 A.** Rate of temperature decay following 3-MHz ultrasound treatments. Solid line = mean temperature decay. Hatched lines = 1 standard deviation above and below the mean. Oval = time to preultrasound baseline. **B.** Rate of temperature increase during 1-MHz ultrasound applied at 1.5 W/cm², followed by the rate of temperature decay at termination of insonation. The thermistor was 4 cm deep in the triceps surae muscle.[34,108]

It appears that ultrasound and stretching increases range of motion more than stretching alone immediately following treatment. However, there is no significant difference between the two techniques over the long term.[35]

CHRONIC INFLAMMATION

There are few clinical or experimental studies that discuss the effects of therapeutic ultrasound on the chronic inflammations (tendinitis, bursitis, epicondylitis). Treatment of bicipital tendinitis with ultrasound decreases pain and tenderness, and increases range of motion.[48] Although earlier studies have shown ultrasound to be effective in treating pain and increasing range of motion in subacromial bursitis, a more recent study shows no improvement in the general condition of the shoulder when using continuous ultrasound at 1.0–2.0 W/cm^2.[30] Ultrasound applied at an intensity of 1.0–2.0 W/cm^2 at a 20-percent duty cycle significantly enhanced recovery in patients with epicondylitis.[8]

In these chronic inflammatory conditions, ultrasound seems to be effective in increasing blood flow for healing and for pain reduction through heating.[148]

BONE HEALING

Since bone is a type of connective tissue, damaged bone progresses through the same stages of healing as other soft tissues, the major difference being the deposition of bone salts.[146] Several researchers have observed acceleration of fracture repair following treatment with ultrasound.[22,120,133,142] It has been shown that the application of ultrasound within the first 2 weeks postfibular fracture during the inflammatory and proliferative stages increases the rate of healing. Treatment parameters were 0.5 W/cm^2 at a duty cycle of 20 percent for 5 minutes, four times per week.[45] Ultrasound was effectively used to stimulate bone repair following osteotomy and fixation of the tibia in rabbits.[13]

Treatment given during the first 2 weeks after injury is sufficient to accelerate bony union. However, ultrasound given to an unstable fracture during the phase of cartilage formation may cause proliferation of cartilage and consequent delayed bony union.[42] It appears that nonthermal mechanisms are most responsible for the accelerated bone healing.[106]

Several researchers have looked at the use of ultrasound over growing epiphyses.[26,62,139] Although results have been somewhat inconsistent, some form of damage was observed in each study, including premature closure of the epiphysis, epiphyseal displacement, widening of the epiphyseal, fractures, condyle erosion, and shortening of the bones. The degree of destruction appears to be unpredictable; therefore, it is not recommended that ultrasound be applied to growing bone.[57]

Ultrasonic Bone Growth Stimulators

Two types of bone growth stimulators currently exist: electrical and ultrasonic. An electrical bone growth stimulator (EBS) uses electric current to promote bone healing. The current may generate a direct, direct pulsating, or pulsating electromagnetic field (PEMF). An ultrasonic bone growth stimulator uses ultrasound for accelerated fracture healing.[22] It is a pulsed, low-intensity, ultrasound device that provides nonthermal, specifically programmed ultrasonic stimulation to accelerate bone repair. The device is characterized by a main operating unit, with an external power supply that is connected to a treatment head module, which is affixed to a mounting fixture that is centered over the fracture site. This nonthermal device is specifically programmed to promote accelerated fracture healing, but does not increase the temperature of the tissue and therefore can be administered by the patient at home in one daily 20-minute treatment. Healing times of fresh fractures appear to be significantly decreased among those receiving low intensity ultrasound stimulation.[22]

11. Phonophoresis is a technique in which ultrasound is used to drive molecules of a topically applied medication, usually either anti-inflammatories or analgesics, into the tissues.

12. In a clinical setting, ultrasound is frequently used in combination with other modalities, including hot packs, cold packs, and electrical stimulating currents, to produce specific treatment effects.

13. Although ultrasound is a relatively safe modality if used appropriately, the therapist must be aware of the various contraindications and precautions.

14. For ultrasound to be effective, the therapist must pay particular attention to correct parameters such as intensity, frequency, duration, and treatment size.

REVIEW QUESTIONS

1. What is therapeutic ultrasound, and what are its two primary physiologic effects?

2. How does an ultrasound wave travel through biologic tissues, and what happens to the acoustic energy within those tissues?

3. How does the transducer convert electrical energy into acoustic energy?

4. How does the frequency affect the ultrasound beam within the tissues?

5. What are the differences between continuous and pulsed ultrasound?

6. What are the potential thermal effects of ultrasound?

7. How can the nonthermal effects of ultrasound facilitate the healing process?

8. What is the relationship between treatment intensity and treatment duration in effecting a temperature increase in the tissues?

9. What are the various coupling agents and exposure techniques that may be used when treating a patient with ultrasound?

10. What are the various clinical applications for using ultrasound in treating injuries?

11. What is the purpose of using a phonophoresis treatment?

12. How should ultrasound be used in combination with other therapeutic modalities?

REFERENCES

1. Antich, T.J.: Phonophoresis: the principles of the ultrasonic driving force and efficacy in treatment of common orthopedic diagnosis, J. Orthop. Sport Phys. Ther. 4(2):99–103, 1982.

2. Artho, P.A., Thyne, J.G., Warring, B.P., et al.: A calibration study of therapeutic ultrasound units, Phys. Ther. 82:257–263, 2002.

3. Ashton, D.F., Draper, D.O., and Myrer, J.W.: Temperature rise in human muscle during ultrasound treatments using Flex-All as a coupling agent, J. Athl. Train. 33(2):136–140, 1998.

4. Balmaseda, M.T., Fatehi, M.T., and Koozekanani, S.H.: Ultrasound therapy: a comparative study of different coupling medium, Arch. Phys. Med. Rehabil. 67:147, 1986.

5. Baker, K.G., Robertson, V.J., and Duck, F.A.: A review of therapeutic ultrasound: biophysical effects, Phys. Ther. 81: 1351–1358, 2001.

6. Benson, H.A.E., McElnay, I.C.: Transmission of ultrasound energy through topical pharmaceutical products, Physiotherapy 74:587, 1988.

7. Bierman, W.: Ultrasound in the treatment of scars, Arch. Phys. Med. Rehabil. 35:209, 1954.

8. Bishop, S., Draper, D., and Knight, K.: Human tissue temperature rise during ultrasound treatments with the Aquaflex Gel Pad, J. Athl. Train. 39(2):126–131, 2004.

9. Black, K., Halverson, J.L., Maierus, K., and Soderbere, G.L.: Alterations in ankle dorsiflexion torque as a result of continuous ultrasound to the anterior tibial compartment, Phys. Ther. 64(6):910–913, 1984.

10. Bly, N.N.: The use of ultrasound as an enhancer for transcutaneous drug delivery: phonophoresis, Phys. Ther. 75(6):89–95, 1995.

11. Bly, N., McKenzie, A., West, J., and Whitney, J.: Low dose ultrasound effects on wound healing: a controlled study with Yucatan pigs, Arch. Phys. Med. Rehabil. 73:656–664, 1992.

12. Boone, L., Ingersol, C.D., and Cordova, M.L.: Passive hip flexion does not increase during or following ultrasound treatment of the hamstring musculature, J. Athl. Train. 34(2):S-70, 1999.

13. Brueton, R.N., Campbell, B.: The use of geliperm as a sterile coupling agent for therapeutic ultrasound, Physiotherapy 73:653, 1987.

14. Cagnie, B., Vinck, E., Rimbaut, S., and Vanderstraeten, G.: Phonophoresis versus topical application of ketoprofen: comparison between tissue and plasma levels, Phys. Ther. 83:707–712, 2003.

15. Cameron, M., Monroe, L.: Relative transmission of ultrasound by media customarily used for phonophoresis, Phys. Ther. 72(2):142–148, 1992.

16. Castel, J.C.: Electrotherapy application in clinical for neuromuscular stimulation and tissue repair. Presented at the 46th Annual Clinical Symposium of the National Athletic Trainer's Association; June 16, 1995, Indianapolis.

17. Castel, J.C.: Therapeutic ultrasound. Rehabil. Ther. Prod. Rev. Jan/Feb:22–32, 1993.

18. Chan, A.K., Myrer, J.W., Measom, G., and Draper, D.: Temperature changes in human patellar tendon in response to therapeutic ultrasound, J. Athl. Train. 33(2):130–135, 1998.

19. Ciccone, C., Leggin, B., and Callamaro, J.: Effects of ultrasound and trolamine salicylate phonophoresis on delayed-onset muscle soreness, Phys. Ther. 71(9):666–675, 1991.

20. Clarke, G.R., Stenner, L.: Use of therapeutic ultrasound, Physiotherapy 62(6):85–190, 1976.

21. Craig, J.A., Bradley, J., Walsh, D.M., et al.: Delayed onset muscle soreness: lack of effect of therapeutic ultrasound in humans, Arch. Phys. Med. Rehabil. 80(3):318–323, 1999.

22. Conner, C.: Use of an ultrasonic bone-growth stimulator to promote healing of a Jones fracture, Athl. Ther. Today 8(1):37–39, 2003.

23. Crumley, M., Nowak, P., and Merrick, M.: Do ultrasound, active warm-up and passive motion differ on their ability to cause temperature and range of motion changes? J. Athl. Train. (Suppl.) 36(2S):S-92, 2001.

24. Currier, D.P., Kramer, I.F.: Sensory nerve conduction: heating effects of ultrasound and infrared, Physiother. Can. 34:241, 1982.

25. Darrow, H., Schulthies, S., and Draper, D.: Serum dexamethasone levels after Decadron phonophoresis, J. Athl. Train. 34(4):338–341, 1999.

26. DeForest, R.E., Henick, J.F., and Janes, J.M.: Effects of ultrasound on growing bone: an experimental study, Arch. Phys. Med. Rehabil. 34:21, 1953.

27. Delacerda, F.G.: Ultrasonic techniques for treatment of plantar warts in patients, J. Orthop. Sports Phys. Ther. 1:100, 1979.

28. Docker, M.F.: A review of instrumentation available for therapeutic ultrasound, Physiotherapy 73(4):154, 1987.

29. Docker, M.F., Foulkes, D.J., and Patrick, M.K.: Ultrasound couplants for physiotherapy, Physiotherapy 68(4):124–125, 1982.

30. Downing, D.S., Weinstein, A.: Ultrasound therapy of subacromial bursitis (abstr), Phys. Ther. 66:194, 1986.

31. Draper, D.O.: Current research on therapeutic ultrasound and pulsed short-wave diathermy. Presented at Physio Therapy Research Seminars Japan, Nov. 17, 1996, Sendai, Japan.

32. Draper, D.O.: Guidelines to enhance therapeutic ultrasound treatment outcomes, Athl. Ther. Today 3(6):7, 1998.

33. Draper, D.O.: Ten mistakes commonly made with ultrasound use: Current research sheds light on myths, Athl. Train. Sports Health Care Perspect. 2:95–107, 1996.

34. Draper, D.O.: The latest research on therapeutic ultrasound: clinical habits may need to be changed. Presented at the 46th Annual Meeting and Clinical Symposium of the National Athletic Trainer's Association; June 16, 1995, Indianapolis, IN.

35. Draper, D.O., Anderson, C., and Schulthies, S.S.: Immediate and residual changes in dorsiflexion range of motion using an ultrasound heat and stretch routine, J. Athl. Train. 33(2):141–144, 1998.

36. Draper, D.O., Castel, J.C., and Castel, D.: Rate of temperature increase in human muscle during 1 MHz and 3 MHz continuous ultrasound, J. Orthop. Sports Phys. Ther. 22:142–150, 1995.

37. Draper, D.O., Harris, S.T., and Schulthies, S.: Hot pack and 1-MHz ultrasound treatments have an additive effect on muscle temperature increase, J. Athl. Train. 33(1):21–24, 1998.

38. Draper, D.O., Ricard, M.D.: Rate of temperature decay in human muscle following 3 MHz ultrasound: the stretching window revealed, J. Athl. Train. 30:304–307, 1995.

39. Draper, D.O., Schulthies, S., Sorvisto, P., and Hautala, A.: Temperature changes in deep muscles of humans during ice and ultrasound therapies: an in-vivo study, J. Orthop. Sports Phys. Ther. 21:153–157, 1995.

40. Draper, D.O., Sunderland, S.: Examination of the law of Grotthus-Draper: does ultrasound penetrate subcutaneous fat in humans? J. Athl. Train. 28:246–250, 1993.

41. Draper, D.O., Sunderland, S., Kirkendall, D.T., and Ricard, M.D.: A comparison of temperature rise in the human calf muscles following applications of underwater and topical gel ultrasound, J. Orthop. Sports Phys. Ther. 17:247–251, 1993.

42. Dyson, M.: The use of ultrasound in sports physiotherapy. In Grisogono, V., editor. Sports injuries (international perspectives in physiotherapy), Edinburgh, 1989, Churchill Livingstone.

43. Dyson, M.: Mechanisms involved in therapeutic ultrasound, Physiotherapy 73(3):116–120, 1987.

44. Dyson, M.: Therapeutic application of ultrasound. In Nyborg, W.L., Ziskin, M.C., editors. Biological effects of ultrasound, Edinburgh, 1985, Churchill-Livingstone.

45. Dyson, M., Brookes, M.: Stimulation of bone repair by ultrasound (abstr.), Ultrasound Med. Biol. 8(Suppl. 50):50, 1982.

46. Dyson, M., Luke, D.A.: Induction of mast cell degranulation in skin by ultrasound, IEEE Trans. Ultrasonics. Ferroelectrics Freq. Control UFFC-33:194, 1986.

47. Dyson, M., Pond, J.B.: The effect of pulsed ultrasound on tissue regeneration, J. Physiother. 105–108, 1970.

48. Echternach, J.L.: Ultrasound: an adjunct treatment for shoulder disability, Phys. Ther. 45:565, 1965.

49. El Hag, M., Coghlan, K., and Christmas, P.: The anti-inflammatory effects of dexamethasone and therapeutic ultrasound in oral surgery, Br. J. Oral Maxillofac. Surg. 23:17, 1985.

50. Fahey, S., Smith, M., and Merrick, M.: Intramuscular temperature does not differ among hydrocortisone preparations during exercise, J. Athl. Train. 35(2):S-47, 2000.

51. Ferguson, B.A.: A practitioner's guide to ultrasonic therapy equipment standard, U.S. Dept. of Health and Human Services, Public Health Service, Food and Drug Administration, Rockville, MD, 1985.

52. Ferguson, H.N.: Ultrasound in the treatment of surgical wounds, Physiotherapy 67:12, 1981.

53. Finucane, S., Sparrow, K., and Owen, J.: Low-intensity ultrasound enhances MCL healing at 3 and 6 weeks post injury, J. Athl. Train. (Suppl.) 38(2S):S-23, 2003.

54. Frizell, L.A., Dunn, F.: Biophysics of ultrasound; bioeffects of ultrasound. In Lehmann, J.F., editor. Therapeutic heat and cold, ed. 3, Baltimore, MD, 1982, Williams & Wilkins.

55. Fyfe, M.C., Bullock, M.: Therapeutic ultrasound: some historical background and development in knowledge of its effects on healing, Aust. J. Physiother. 31(6):220–224, 1985.

56. Fyfe, M.C., Chahl, L.A.: The effect of single or repeated applications of "therapeutic" ultrasound on plasma extravasation during silver nitrate induced inflammation of the rat hindpaw ankle joint, Ultrasound Med. Biol. 11:273, 1985.

57. Gann, N.: Ultrasound: current concepts, Clin. Manage. 11(4):64–69, 1991.

58. Gatto, J., Kimura, I.F., and Gulick, D.: Effect of beam nonuniformity ratio of three ultrasound machines on tissue phantom temperature, J. Athl. Train. 34(2):S-69, 1999.

59. Gersten, J.W.: Effect of ultrasound on tendon extensibility, Am. J. Phys. Med. 34:662, 1955.

60. Girardi, C.Q., Seaborne, D., and Savard-Goulet, F.: The analgesic effect of high voltage galvanic stimulation combined with ultrasound in the treatment of low back pain: a one group pretest/posttest study, Physiother. Can. 36(6):327–333, 1984.

61. Gorkiewicz, R.: Ultrasound for subacromial bursitis, Phys. Ther. 64:46, 1984.

62. Griffin, J.E., Echternach, J.L., and Price, R.E.: Patients treated with ultrasonic-driven hydrocortisone and ultrasound alone, Phys. Ther. 47:594–601, 1967.

63. Griffin, J.E., Karsalis, T.C.: Physical agents for physical therapists, Springfield, IL, 1978, Charles C Thomas.

64. Gum, S.L., Reddy, G.K., Stehno-Bittel, L., and Enwemeka, C.S.: Combined ultrasound, electrical stimulation, and laser promote collagen synthesis with moderate changes in tendon biomechanics, Am. J. Phys. Med. Rehabil. 76(4):288–296, 1997.

65. Harvey, W., Dyson, M., and Pond, J.B.: The simulation of protein synthesis in human fibroblasts by therapeutic ultrasound, Rheumat. Rehabil. 14:237, 1975.

66. Hashish, I., Harvey, W., and Harris, M.: Antiinflammatory effects of ultrasound therapy: evidence for a major placebo effect, Br. J. Rheumatol. 25:77, 1986.

67. Hayes, B., Sandrey, M., and Merrick, M.: The differences between 1 MHz and 3 MHz ultrasound in the heating of subcutaneous tissue, J. Athl. Train. (Suppl.) 36(2S):S-92, 2001.

68. Hecox, B., Mehreteab, T.A., and Weisbergm, J.: Physical agents: a comprehensive text for physical therapists, Norwalk, CT, 1994, Appleton & Lange.

69. Hogan, R.D., Burke, K.M., and Franklin, T.D.: The effect of ultrasound on microvascular hemodynamics in skeletal muscle: effects during ischemia, Microvasc. Res. 23:370, 1982.

70. Holcomb, W., Blank, C.: The effects of superficial heating before 1-MHz ultrasound on tissue temperature, J. Sport Rehabil. 12(2):95–103, 2003.

71. Holcomb, W.R., Blank, C., and Davis, C.: The effect of superficial pre-heating on the magnitude and duration of temperature elevation with 1 MHz ultrasound, J. Athl. Train. 35(2):S-48, 2000.

72. Holcomb, W., Joyce, C.: A comparison of the effectiveness of two commonly used ultrasound units, J. Athl. Train. (Suppl.), 36(2S):S-89, 2001.

73. Holcomb, W., Joyce, C.: A comparison of temperature increases produced by 2 commonly used ultrasound units, J. Athl. Train. 38(1):24–27, 2003.

74. Holdsworth, L.K., Anderson, D.M.: Effectiveness of ultrasound used with hydrocortisone coupling medium or epicondylitis clasp to treat lateral epicondylitis: pilot study, Physiotherapy 79(1):19–25, 1993.

75. Jennings, Y., Biggs, M., and Ingersoll, C.: The effect of ultrasound intensity and coupling medium on gastrocnemius tissue temperature, J. Athl. Train. (Suppl.) 37(2S):S-42, 2002.

76. Johns, L., Colloton, P.: Effects of ultrasound on spleenocyte proliferation and lymphokine production, J. Athl. Train. (Suppl.) 37(2S):S-42, 2002.

77. Johns, L.: Nonthermal effects of therapeutic ultrasound, J. Athl. Train. 37(3):293–299, 2002.

78. Kahn, J.: Iontophoresis and ultrasound for post-surgical temporomandibular trismus and paresthesia, Phys. Ther. 60(3):307–308, 1980.

79. Kent, H.: Plantar wart treatment with ultrasound, Arch. Phys. Med. Rehabil. 40:15, 1959.

80. Kitchen, S., Partridge, C.: A review of therapeutic ultrasound: Part 1, background and physiological effects, Physiotherapy 76(10):593–595, 1990.

81. Kitchen, S., Partridge, C.: A review of therapeutic ultrasound: Part 2, the efficacy of ultrasound, Physiotherapy 76(10):595–599, 1990.

82. Kleinkort, I.A., Wood, F.: Phonophoresis with 1 percent versus 10 percent hydrocortisone, Phys. Ther. 55:1320, 1975.

83. Klucinec, B., Denegar, C., and Mahmood, R.: The transducer pressure variable: its influence on acoustic energy transmission, J. Sport Rehabil. 6(1):47–53, 1997.

84. Klucinec, B., Scheidler, M., Denegar, C., et al.: Effectiveness of wound care products in the transmission of acoustic energy, Phys. Ther. 80:469–476, 2000.

85. Klucinec, B., Scheidler, M., and Denegar, C.: Transmission of coupling agents used to deliver acoustic energy over irregular surfaces, J. Orthop. Sports Phys. Ther. 30(5):263–269, 2000.

86. Kramer, J.F.: Ultrasound: evaluation of its mechanical and thermal effects, Arch. Phys. Med. Rehabil. 65:223, 1984.

87. Kremkau, F.: Physical conditioning. In Nyborg, W.L., Ziskin, M.C., editors. Biological effects of ultrasound, Edinburgh, 1985, Churchill Livingstone.

88. Lee, J.C., Lin, D.T., and Hong, C.: The effectiveness of simultaneous thermotherapy with ultrasound and electrotherapy with combined AC and DC current on the immediate pain relief of myofascial trigger points, J. Musculoskeletal Pain 5(1):81–90, 1997.

89. Lehmann, J.F.: Clinical evaluation of a new approach in the treatment of contracture associated with hip fracture after internal fixation, Arch. Phys. Med. Rehabil. 42:95, 1961.

90. Lehmann, J.F.: Effect of therapeutic temperatures on tendon extensibility, Arch. Phys. Med. Rehabil. 51:481, 1970.

91. Lehmann, J.F., de Lateur, B.J.: Therapeutic heat. In Lehmann, J.F., editor. Therapeutic heat and cold, ed. 4, Baltimore, MD, 1990, Williams & Wilkins.

92. Lehmann, J.F., de Lateur, B.J., and Silverman, D.R.: Selective heating effects of ultrasound in human beings, Arch. Phys. Med. Rehabil. 46:331, 1966.

93. Lehman, J.F., de Lateur, B.J., Stonebridge, J.B., and Warren, G.: Therapeutic temperature distribution produced by ultrasound as modified by dosage and volume of tissue exposed, Arch. Phys. Med. Rehabil. 48:662–666, 1967.

94. Lowden, A.: Application of ultrasound to assess stress fractures, Physiotherapy 72(3):160–161, 1986.

95. Leonard, J., Merrick, M., and Ingersoll, C.: A comparison of ultrasound intensities on a 10 minute 1.0 MHz ultrasound treatment, J. Athl. Train. (Suppl.) 36(2S):S-91, 2001.

96. Lundeberg, T., Abrahamsson, P., and Haker, E.: A comparative study of continuous ultrasound, placebo ultrasound and rest in epicondylalgia, Scand. Rehabil. Med. 20:99, 1988.

97. MacDonald, B.L., Shipster, S.B.: Temperature changes induced by continuous ultrasound, S. Afr. J. Physiother. 37(1):13–15, 1981.

98. Makuloluwe, R.T., Mouzas, G.L.: Ultrasound in the treatment of sprained ankles, Practitioner 218:586–588, 1977.

99. Markham, D. E., and Wood, M.R.: Ultrasound for Dupytren's contracture, Physiotherapy 66(2):55–58, 1980.

100. Merrick, M.A.: Does 1-MHz ultrasound really work? Athl. Ther. Today 6(6):48–54, 2001.

101. Merrick, M.A.: Ultrasound and range of motion examined, Athl. Ther. Today 5(3):48–49, 2000.

102. Merrick, M.A., Bernard, K.D., and Devor, S.T.: Identical 3-MHz ultrasound treatments with different devices produce different intramuscular temperatures, J. Orthop. Sports Phys. Ther. 33(7):379–385, 2003.

103. Merrick, M.A., Mihalyov, M.R., and Roethemeier, J.L.: A comparison of intramuscular temperatures during ultrasound treatments with coupling gel or gel pads, J. Orthop. Sports Phys Ther. 32(5):216–220, 2002.

104. Michlovitz, S.: Thermal agents in rehabilitation, Philadelphia, PA, 1996, F.A. Davis.

105. Mihaloyvov, M.R., Roethmeier, J.L., and Merrick, M.A.: Intramuscular temperature does not differ between direct ultrasound application and application with commercial gel packs, J. Athl. Train. 35(2):S-47, 2000.

106. McDiarmid, T., Burns, P.N.: Clinical applications of therapeutic ultrasound, Physiotherapy 73:155, 1987.

107. Middlemast, S., Chatterjee, D.S.: Comparison of ultrasound and thermotherapy for soft tissue injuries, Physiotherapy 64:331, 1978.

108. Moll, M.J.: A new approach to pain: lidocaine and decadron with ultrasound, USAF Medical Service Digest, May–June 8, 1977.

109. Munting, E.: Ultrasonic therapy for painful shoulders, Physiotherapy 64:180, 1978.

110. Myrer, J.W., Draper, D.O., and Durrant, E.: Contrast therapy and intramuscular temperature in the human leg, J. Athl. Train. 29:318–322, 1994.

111. Myrer, J.: Measom, G., and Fellingham, G.: Intramuscular temperature rises with topical analgesics used as coupling agents during therapeutic ultrasound, J. Athl. Train. 36(1):20–26, 2001.

112. Myrer, J.W., Measom, G., and Fellingham, G.W.: Significant intramuscular temperature rise obtained when topical analgesics Nature's Chemist and Biofreeze were used as coupling agents during ultrasound treatment, J. Athl. Train. 35(2):S-48, 2000.

113. Nwuga, V.C.B.: Ultrasound in treatment of back pain resulting from prolapsed intervertebral disc, Arch. Phys. Med. Rehabil. 64:88, 1983.

114. Oakley, E.M.: Application of continuous beam ultrasound at therapeutic levels, Physiotherapy 64(4):103–104, 1978.

115. Partridge, C.J.: Evaluation of the efficacy of ultrasound, Physiotherapy 73(4):166–168, 1987.

116. Patrick, M.K.: Applications of pulsed therapeutic ultrasound, Physiotherapy 64(4):3–104, 1978.

117. Penderghest, C., Kimura, I., and Gulick, D.: Double blind clinical efficacy study of pulsed phonophoresis on perceived pain associated with symptomatic tendinitis, J. Sport Rehabil. (7):9–19, 1998.

118. Performance Standards for Sonic, Infrasonic, and Ultrasonic Radiation Emitting Products: 21 CFR 1050:10 Federal Register 43:7166, 1978.

119. Pesek, J., Kane, E., and Perrin, D.: T-Prep ultrasound gel and ultrasound does not effect local anesthesia, J. Athl. Train. (Suppl.) 36(2S):S-89, 2001.

120. Pilla, A.A., Figueiredo, M., Nasser, P., et al.: Non-invasive low intensity pulsed ultrasound: a potent accelerator of bone repair, Proceedings of the 36th Annual Meeting, Orthopaedic Research Society, New Orleans, 1990.

121. Plaskett, C., Tiidus, P.M., and Livingston, L.: Ultrasound treatment does not affect post exercise muscle strength recovery or soreness, J. Sport Rehabil. 8(1):1–9, 1999.

122. Portwood, M.M., Lieberman, S.S., and Taylor, R.G.: Ultrasound treatment of reflex sympathetic dystrophy, Arch. Phys. Med. Rehabil. 68:116, 1987.

123. Quade, A.G., Radzyminski, S.F.: Ultrasound in verruca plantaris, J. Am. Podiatric Assoc. 56:503, 1966.

124. Rantanen, J., Thorsson, O., Wollmer, P., et al.: Effects of therapeutic ultrasound on the regeneration of skeletal myofibers after experimental muscle injury, Am. J. Sports Med. 27(1):54–59, 1999.

125. Reed, B., Ashikaga, T., and Flemming, B.C.: Effects of ultrasound and stretch on knee ligament extensibility, J. Orthop. Sports Phys. Ther. 30(6):341–347, 2000.

126. Reid, D.C., Cummings, G.E.: Factors in selecting the dosage of ultrasound with particular reference to the use of various coupling agents, Physiother. Can. 63:255, 1973.

127. Rimington, S., Draper, D.O., Durrant, E., and Fellingham, G.W.: Temperature changes during therapeutic ultrasound in the precooled human gastrocnemius muscle, J. Athl. Train. 29:325–327, 1994.

128. Rose, S., Draper, D.O., Schulthies, S.S., and Durrant, E.: The stretching window part two: rate of thermal decay in deep muscle following 1 MHz ultrasound, J. Athl. Train. 31:139–143, 1996.

129. Sandler, V., Feingold, P.: The thermal effect of pulsed ultrasound, S. Afr. J. Physiother. 37(1):10–12, 1951.

130. Smith, K., Draper, D.O., Schulthies, S.S., and Durrant, E.: The effect of silicate gel hot packs on human muscle temperature. Presented at the 46th Annual Meeting and Clinical Symposium of the National Athletic Trainer's Association; June 15, 1995; Indianapolis, IN. Abstract published in J. Athl. Train. 30:S-33, 1995.

131. Snow, C.J., Johnson, K.A.: Effect of therapeutic ultrasound on acute inflammation, Physiother. Can. 40:162, 1988.

132. Starkey, C.: Therapeutic modalities for athletic trainers, Philadelphia, PA, 1999, F.A. Davis.

133. Stein, T.: Ultrasound: exploring benefits on bone repair, growth and healing, Sports Med. Update 13(1):22–23, 1998.

134. Strapp, E., Guskiewicz, K., and Hackney, A.: The cumulative effects of multiple phonophoresis treatments on dexamethasone and cortisol concentrations in the blood, J. Athl. Train. 35(2):S-47, 2000.

135. Summer, W., Patrick, M.K.: Ultrasonic therapy, New York, 1964, American Elsevier.

136. Ter Haar, C.: Basic physics of therapeutic ultrasound, Physiotherapy 73(3):110–113, 1987.

137. Ter Haar, G., Hopewell, J.W.: Ultrasonic heating of mammalian tissue in vivo, Br. J. Cancer 45(Suppl. V):65–67, 1982.

138. Tiidus, P., Cort, J., and Woodruf, S., Ultrasound treatment and recovery from eccentric-exercise-induced muscle damage, J. Sport Rehabil. 11(4):305–314, 2002.

139. Vaughen, I.L., Bender, L.F.: Effect of ultrasound on growing bone, Arch. Phys. Med. Rehabil. 40:158, 1959.

140. Vaughn, D.T.: Direct method versus underwater method in treatment of plantar warts with ultrasound, Phys. Ther. 53:396, 1973.

141. Ward, A.R.: Electricity fields and waves in therapy, Marrickville, NSW, Australia, 1986, Science Press.

142. Werden, S.J., Bennell, K.K., and McMeeken, J.M.: Can conventional therapeutic ultrasound units be used to accelerate fracture repair? Phys. Ther. Rev. 4(2):117–126, 1999.

143. Williams, R.: Production and transmission of ultrasound, Physiotherapy 73(3):113–116, 1987.

144. Williams, A.R., McHale, I., and Bowditchm, M.: Effects of MHz ultrasound on electrical pain threshold perception in humans, Ultrasound Med. Biol. 13:249, 1987.

145. Wing, M.: Phonophoresis with hydrocortisone in the treatment of temporomandibular joint dysfunction, Phys. Ther. 62:32–33, 1982.

146. Woolf, N.: Cell, Tissue and disease, ed. 2, London, 1986, Bailliere Tindall.

147. Zarod, A.P., Williams, A.R.: Platelet aggregation in vivo by therapeutic ultrasound, Lancet 1:1266, 1977.

148. Ziskin, M., McDiarmid, T., and Michlovitz, S.: Therapeutic ultrasound. In Michlovitz, S., editor. Thermal agents in rehabilitation, Philadelphia, PA, 1996, F.A. Davis.

SUGGESTED READINGS

Abramson, D.I.: Changes in blood flow, oxygen uptake and tissue temperatures produced by therapeutic physical agents. I. Effect of ultrasound, Am. J. Phys. Med. 39:51, 1960.

Aldes, I.H., Grabin, S.: Ultrasound in the treatment of intervertebral disc syndrome, Am. J. Phys. Med. 37:199, 1958.

Allen, K.G.R., Battye, C.K.: Performance of ultrasonic therapy instruments, Physiotherapy 64(6):174–179, 1978.

Antich, T.J.: Physical therapy treatment of knee extensor mechanism disorders: comparison of four treatment modalities, J. Orthop. Sports Phys. Ther. 8:255, 1986.

Aspelin, P., Ekberg, O., Thorsson, O., and Wilhelmsson, M.: Ultrasound examination of soft tissue injury in the lower limb in patients, Am. J. Sports. Med. 20(5):601–603, 1992.

Banties, A., Klomp, R.: Transmission of ultrasound energy through coupling agents, Physiother. Sport 3:9–13, 1979.

Bare, A., McAnaw, M., and Pritchard, A.: Phonophoretic delivery of 10% hydrocortisone through the epidermis of humans as determined by serum cortisol concentration, Phys. Ther. 76(7): 738–749, 1996.

Bearzy, H.J.: Clinical applications of ultrasonic energy in the treatment of acute and chronic subacromial bursitis, Arch. Phys. Med. Rehabil. 34:228, 1953.

Behrens, B.J., Michlovitz, S.L.: Physical agents: theory and practice for the physical therapist assistant, Philadelphia, PA, 1996, F.A. Davis.

Benson, H.A., McElnay, J.C., and Harland, R.L.: Use of ultrasound to enhance percutaneous absorption of benzydamine, Phys. Ther. 69(2): 113–118, 1989.

Bickford, R.H., Duff, R.S.: Influence of ultrasonic irradiation on temperature and blood flow in human skeletal muscle, Circ. Res. 1:534, 1953.

Billings, C., Draper, D., and Schulthies, S.: Ability of the Omnisound 3000 Delta T to reproduce predictable temperature increases in human muscle, J. Athl. Train. 31(Suppl.):S-47, 1996.

Bondolo, W.: Phenylbutazone with ultrasonics in some cases of anhrosynovitis of the knee, Arch. Orthopaed. 73:532–540, 1960.

Borrell, R.M., Parker, R., and Henley, E.J.: Comparison of in vitro temperatures produced by hydrotherapy paraffin wax treatment and fluidotherapy, Phys. Ther. 60:1273–1276, 1984.

Brueton, R.N., Blookes, M., and Heatley, F.W.: The effect of ultrasound on the repair of a rabbit's tibial osteotomy held in rigid external fixation, J. Bone Joint Surg. 69B:494, 1987.

Buchan, J.F.: Heat therapy and ultrasonics, Practitioner, 208:130–131, 1972.

Buchtala, V.: The present state of ultrasonic therapy, Br. J. Phys. Med. 15:3, 1952.

Bundt, F.B.: Ultrasound therapy in supraspinatus bursitis, Phys. Ther. Rev. 38:826, 1958.

Burns, P.N., Pitcher, E.M.: Calibration of physiotherapy ultrasound generators, Clin. Phys. Physiol. Measure 5:37(abstr.), 1984.

Byl, N.: The use of ultrasound as an enhancer for transcutaneous drug delivery: phonophoresis, Phys. Ther. 75(6):539–553, 1995.

Callam, M.J., Harper, D.R., Dale, J.J., et al.: A controlled trial of weekly ultrasound therapy in chronic leg ulceration, Lancet 2(8552):204, 1987.

Cerino, LE., Ackerman, E., and Janes, J.M.: Effects of ultrasound on experimental bone tumor, Surg. For. 16:466, 1965.

Cherup, N., Urben, J., and Bender, L.F.: The treatment of plantar warts with ultrasound, Arch. Phys. Med. Rehabil. 44:602, 1963.

Chan, A.K., Siealmann, R.A., and Guy, A.W.: Calculations of therapeutic heat generated by ultrasound in fat-muscle-bone layers, Inst. Electric. Electron. Eng. Trans. Biomed. Eng. BME-2t. 280–284, 1973.

Cline, P.D.: Radiographic follow-up of ultrasound therapy in calcific bursitis, Phys. Ther. 43:16, 1963.

Coakley, W.T.: Biophysical effects of ultrasound at therapeutic intensities, Physiotherapy 94(6):168–169, 1978.

Conger, A.D., Ziskin, M.C., and Wittels, H.: Ultrasonic effects on mammalian multicellular tumor spheroids, Clin. Ultrasound 9:167, 1981.

Conner-Kerr, T., Franklin, M., and Smith, S.: Efficacy of using phonophoresis for the delivery of dexamethasone to human transdermal tissues, JOSPT 23(1):79, 1996.

Costentino, A.B., Cross, D.L., Harrington, R.J., and Sodarberg, G.L.: Ultrasound effects on electroneuromyographic measures in sensory fibres of the median nerve, Phys. Ther. 63(11):1788–1792, 1983.

Creates, V.: A study of ultrasound treatment to the painful perineum after childbirth, Physiotherapy 73:162, 1987.

Currier, D.F., Greathouse, D., and Swift, T.: Sensory nerve conduction: effect of ultrasound, Arch. Phys. Med. Rehabil. 59:181, 1978.

DeDeyne, P., Kirsh-Volders, M.: In vitro effects of therapeutic ultrasound on the nucleus of human fibroblasts, Phys. Ther. 75(7):629–634, 1995.

DiIorio, A., Frommelt, T., and Svendsen, L.: Therapeutic ultrasound effect on regional temperature and blood flow, J. Athl. Train. 31(Suppl.):S-14, 1996.

Duarte, L.R.: The stimulation of bone growth by ultrasound, Arch. Orthop. Trauma Surg. 101:153–159, 1983.

Dyson, M.: The production of blood cell stasis and endothelial damage in the blood vessels of chick embryos treated with ultrasound in a stationary wave field, Ultrasound Med. Biol. 11:133, 1974.

Dyson, M.: The stimulation of tissue regeneration by means of ultrasound, Clin. Sci. 35:273, 1968.

Dyson, M., Pond, J.B.: The effect of pulsed ultrasound on tissue regeneration, Physiotherapy 56(6):134–142, 1970.

Dyson, M., Suckling, J.: Stimulation of tissue repair by ultrasound: a survey of mechanisms involved, Physiotherapy 64:105, 1978.

Dyson, M., ter Haar, G.R.: The response of smooth muscle to ultrasound (abstr.). In Proceedings from an International Symposium on Therapeutic Ultrasound, Winnipeg, Manitoba, September 10, 1981.

Dyson, M., Woodward, B., and Pond, J.B.: Flow of red blood cells stopped by ultrasound, Nature 232:572–573, 1971.

Edwards, M.I.: Congenital defects in guinea pigs: prenatal retardation of brain growth of guinea pigs following hyperthermia during gestation, Teratology 2:329, 1969.

Enwemeka, C.S.: The effects of therapeutic ultrasound on tendon healing, Am. J. Phys. Med. Rehabil. 68(6):283–287, 1989.

Falconer, J., Hayes, K.W., and Ghang, R.W.: Therapeutic ultrasound in the treatment of musculoskeletal conditions, Arthritis Care Res. 3(2):85–91, 1990.

Farmer, W.C.: Effect of intensity of ultrasound on conduction of motor axons, Phys. Ther. 48:1233–1237, 1968.

Faul, E.D., Imig, C.J.: Temperature and blood flow studies after ultrasonic irradiation, Am. J. Phys. Med. 34:370, 1955.

Fieldhouse, C.: Ultrasound for relief of painful episiotomy scars, Physiotherapy 65:217, 1979.

Forrest, G., Rosen, K.: Ultrasound: effectiveness of treatments given under water, Arch. Phys. Med. Rehabil. 70:28, 1989.

Fountain, F.P., Gersten, J.W., and Sengu, O.: Decrease in muscle spasm produced by ultrasound, hot packs and IR, Arch. Phys. Med. Rehabil. 41:293, 1960.

Franklin, M., Smith, S., and Chenier, T.: Effect of phonophoresis with dexamethasone on adrenal function, JOSPT 22(3):103–107, 1995.

Friedar, S.: A pilot study: the therapeutic effect of ultrasound following partial rupture of achilles tendons in male rats, J. Orthop. Sports Phys. Ther. 10:39, 1988.

Fyfe, M.C.: A study of the effects of different ultrasonic frequencies on experimental oedema, Aust. J. Physiother. 25(5):205–207, 1979.

Fyfe, M.C., Bullock, M.: Acoustic output from therapeutic ultrasound units, Aust. J. Physiother. 32(1):13–16, 1986.

Fyfe, M.C., Chahl, L.A.: The effect of ultrasound on experimental oedema in rats, Ultrasound. Med. Biol. 6:l07, 1980.

Gantz, S.: Increased radicular pain due to therapeutic ultrasound applied to the back, Arch. Phys. Med. Rehabil. 70:493–494, 1989.

Garrett, A.S., Garrett, M.: Letters: ultrasound for herpes zoster pain, J. Roy. College Gen. Practice. Nov., 709, 1982.

Gersten, J.W.: Effect of metallic objects on temperature rises produced in tissues by ultrasound, Am. J. Phys. Med. 37:75, 1958.

Goddard, D.H., Revell, P.A., and Cason, J.: Ultrasound has no anti-inflammatory effect, Ann. Rheum. Dis. 42:582–584, 1983.

Gracewski, S.M., Wagg, R.C., and Schenk, E.A.: High-frequency attenuation measurements using an acoustic microscope, J. Acoustic Soc. Am. 83(6):2405–2409, 1988.

Grant, A., Sleep, J., Mclntosh, J., and Ashurst, H.: Ultrasound and pulsed electromagnetic energy treatment for peroneal trauma. A randomized placebo-controlled trial, Br. J. Obstet. Gynecol. 96:434–439, 1989.

Grieder, A., Vinton P., Cinott W., et al.: An evaluation of ultrasonic therapy for temperomandibular joint dysfunction, Oral Surg. 31:25, 1971.

Griffin, J.E.: Transmissiveness of ultrasound through tap water, glycerin, and mineral oil, Phys. Ther. 60:1010, 1980.

Griffin, J.E.: Patients treated with ultrasonic driven cortisone and with ultrasound alone, Phys. Ther. 47:594, 1967.

Griffin, J.E., Touchstone, J.C.: Low intensity phonophoresis of cortisol in swine, Phys. Ther. 48(10):1336–1344, 1968.

Griffin, J.E., Touchstone, J.C.: Ultrasonic movement of cortisol into pig tissue: 1. movement into skeletal muscle, Am. J. Phys. Med. 42:77–85, 1962.

Griffin, J.E., Touchstone, J.C., and Liu, A.: Ultrasonic movement of cortisol into pig tissues; II. peripheral nerve, Am. J. Phys. Med. 4:20, 1965.

Halle, J.S., Franklin, R.J., and Karalfa, B.L.: Comparison of four treatment approaches for lateral epicondylitis of the elbow, J. Orthop. Sports Phys. Ther. 8:62, 1986.

Halle, J.S., Scoville, C.R., and Greathouse, D.G.: Ultrasound's effect on the conduction latency of superficial radial nerve in man, Phys. Ther. 61:345, 1981.

Hamer, J., Kirk, J.A.: Physiotherapy and the frozen shoulder: a comparative trial of ice and ultrasound therapy, N.Z. Med. 83(3):191, 1976.

Hansen, T.I., Kristensen, J.H.: Effects of massage: shortwave and ultrasound upon 133Xe disappearance rate from muscle and subcutaneous tissue in the human calf, Scand. J. Rehabil. Med. 5:197, 1973.

Harris, S., Draper, D., and Schulthies, S.: The effect of ultrasound on temperature rise in preheated human muscle, J. Athl. Train. 30(Suppl.):S-42, 1995.

Hashish, I., Hai, H.K., Harvey, W., et al.: Reduction of post-operative pain and swelling by ultrasound treatment, a placebo effect, Pain 33:303–311, 1988.

Hekkenberg, R.T., Oosterbaan, W.A., and van Beekum, W.T.: Evaluation of ultrasound therapy devices, Physiotherapy 72:390, 1986.

Hill, C.R., ter Haar, G.: Ultrasound and non-ionizing radiation protection. In Suess, M.J., editor. WHO Regional Publication, European Series No. 10. World Health Organization, Copenhagen, 1981.

Hogan, R.D., Burke, K.M., and Franklin, T.D.: The effect of ultrasound on microvascular hemodynamics in skeletal muscle: effects during ischemia, Microvasc. Res. 23:370, 1982.

Hone, C-Z., Liu, H.H., and Yu, J.: Ultrasound thermotherapy effect on the recovery of nerve conduction in experimental compression neuropathy, Arch. Phys. Med. Rehabil. 69:410–414, 1988.

Hustler, J.E., Zarod, A.P., and Williams, A.R.: Ultrasonic modification of experimental bruising in the guinea-pig pinna, Ultrasound 16:223–228, 1978.

Imig, C.J., Randall, B.F., and Hines, H.M.: Effect of ultra-sonic energy on blood flow, Am. J. Phys. Med. 53:100–102, 1954.

Inaba, M.K., Piorkowski, M.: Ultrasound in treatment of painful shoulder in patients with hemiplegia, Phys. Ther. 52:737, 1972.

Jones, R.I.: Treatment of acute herpes zoster using ultrasonic therapy, Physiotherapy 70:94, 1984.

Klemp, P., Staberg, B., Korsgard, J., et al.: Reduced blood flow in fibromyotic muscles during ultrasound therapy, Scand. J. Rehabil. Med. 15:21–23, 1982.

Kramer, J.F.: Sensory and motor nerve conduction velocities following therapeutic ultrasound, Aust. J. Physiother. 33(4):235–243, 1987.

Kramer, J.F.: Effect of ultrasound intensity on sensory nerve conduction velocity, Physiother. Can. 37:5–10, 1985.

Kramer, J.F.: Effects of therapeutic ultrasound intensity on subcutaneous tissue temperature and ulnar nerve conduction velocity, Am. J. Phys. Med. 64:9, 1985.

Kuitert, J.H.: Ultrasonic energy as an adjunct in the management of radiculitis and similar referred pain, Am. J. Phys. Med. 33:61, 1954.

Kuitert, J.H., Harr, E.T.: Introduction to clinical application of ultrasound, Phys. Ther. Rev. 35:19, 1955.

LaBan, M.M.: Collagen tissue: implications of its response to stress in vitro, Arch. Phys. Med. Rehabil. 43:461, 1962.

Lehmann, J.F.: Heating of joint structures by ultrasound, Arch. Phys. Med. Rehabil. 49:28, 1968.

Lehmann, J.F.: Heating produced by ultrasound in bone and soft tissue, Arch. Phys. Med. Rehabil. 48:397, 1967.

Lehmann, J.F.: Therapeutic temperature distribution produced by ultrasound as modified by dosage and volume of tissue exposed, Arch. Phys. Med. Rehabil. 48:662, 1967.

Lehmann, J.F.: Ultrasound effects as demonstrated in live pigs with surgical metallic implants, Arch. Phys. Med. Rehabil. 40:483, 1959.

Lehmann, J.F., Biegler, R.: Changes of potentials and temperature gradients in membranes caused by ultrasound, Arch. Phys. Med. Rehabil. 35:287, 1954.

Lehmann, J.F., Brunner, G.D., and Stow, R.W.: Pain threshold measurements after therapeutic application of ultrasound. microwaves and infrared, Arch. Phys. Med. Rehabil. 39:560, 1958.

Lehmann, J.F., Erickson, D.J., and Martin, G.M.: Comparative study of the efficiency of shortwave, microwave and ultrasonic diathermy in heating the hip joint, Arch. Phys. Med. Rehabil. 40:510, 1959.

Lehmann, J.R., Henrick, J.F.: Biologic reactions to cavitation: a consideration for ultrasonic therapy, Arch. Phys. Med. Rehabil. 34:86, 1953.

Lehmann, J.F., Stonebridge, J.B., de Lateur, B.J., et al.: Temperatures in human thighs after hot pack treatment followed by ultrasound, Arch. Phys. Med. Rehabil. 59:472–475, 1978.

Lehmann, J.F., Warren, C.C., and Scham, S.M.: Therapeutic heat and cold, Clin. Orthop. 99:207–245, 1974.

Levenson, J.L., Weissberg, M.P.: Ultrasound abuse: a case report, Arch. Phys. Med. Rehabil. 64: 90–91, 1983.

Lloyd, J.J., Evans, J.A.: A calibration survey of physiotherapy equipment in North Wales, Physiotherapy 74(2):56–61, 1988.

Lota, M.I., Darling, R.C.: Change in permeability of the red blood cell membrane in a homogeneous ultrasonic field, Arch. Phys. Med. Rehabil. 36:282, 1955.

Lyons, M.E., Parker, K.J.: Absorption and attenuation in soft tissues II: experimental results, Inst. Electric. Electron. Eng. Trans. Ultrason. Ferroelect. Freq. Contr. 35:4, 1988.

Madsen, P.W., Gersten, J.W.: Effect of ultrasound on conduction velocity of peripheral nerves, Arch. Phys. Med. Rehabil. 42:645–649, 1963.

Massoth, A., Draper, D., and Kirkendall, D.: A measure of superficial tissue temperature during 1 MHz ultrasound treatments delivered at three different intensity settings, J. Athl. Train. 28(2):166, 1993.

Maxwell, L.: Therapeutic ultrasound and the metastasis of a solid tumor, J. Sport Rehabil. 4(4):273–281, 1995.

Maxwell, L.: Therapeutic ultrasound: its effects on the cellular and molecular mechanisms of inflammation and repair, Physiotherapy 78(6):421–425, 1992.

McDiarmid, T., Burns, P.N., and Lewith, G.T.: Ultrasound and the treatment of pressure sores, Physiotherapy 71:661, 1985.

McLaren, J.: Randomized controlled trial of ultrasound therapy for the damaged perineum (abstr.), Clin. Phys. Physiol. Measure 5:40, 1984.

Michlovitz, S.L., Lynch, P.R., and Tuma, R.F.: Therapeutic ultrasound: its effects on vascular permeability (abstr.), Fed. Proc. 41:1761, 1982.

Mickey, D., Bernier, J., and Perrin, D.: Ice and ice with nonthermal ultrasound effects on delayed onset muscle soreness, J. Athl. Train. 31(Suppl.):S-19, 1996.

Miller, D.L.: A review of the ultrasonic bioeffects of microsonation, gas body activation and related cavitation-like phenomena, Ultrasound Med. Biol. 13(8):443–470, 1987.

Mortimer, A.J., Dyson, M.: The effect of therapeutic ultrasound on calcium uptake in fibroblasts, Ultrasound Med. Biol. 14:499–508, 1988.

Mummery, C.L.: The effect of ultrasound on fibroblasts in vitro, PhD thesis, London University, 1978.

National Council on Radiation Protection and Measurements (NCRP) Report No 74 (BioloSica) effects of ultrasound, mechanisms and clinical applications, NCRP, Bethesda, MD, p. 197, 1983.

Newman, M.K., Kill, M., and Frampton, G.: Effects of ultrasound alone and combined with hydrocortisone injections by needle or hydrospray, Am. J. Phys. Med. 37:206, 1958.

Novak, E.J.: Experimental transmission of lidocaine through intact skin by ultrasound, Arch. Phys. Med. Rehabil. 45:231, 1964.

Oakley, E.M.: Evidence for effectiveness of ultrasound treatment in physical medicine, Br. J. Cancer 45(Suppl. V):233–237, 1982.

Olson, S., Bowman, J., and Condrey, K.: Transdermal delivery of hydrocortisone, lidocaine, and menthol in subjects with delayed onset muscle soreness, J. Orthop. Sports Phys. Ther. 19(1):69, 1994.

Paaske, W.P., Hovind, H., and Seyerson, P.: Influence of therapeutic ultrasonic irradiation on blood flow in human cutaneous, subcutaneous and muscular tissues, Scand. J. Clin. Lab. Invest. 31:389, 1973.

Paul, B.: Use of ultrasound in the treatment of pressure sores in patients with spinal cord injury, Arch. Phys. Med. Rehabil. 41:438, 1960.

Payne, C.: Ultrasound for post-herpetic neuralgia, Physiotherapy 70:96, 1984.

Penderghest, C., Kimura, I., and Sitler, M.: Double blind clinical efficacy study of dexamethasone-lidocaine pulsed phonophoresis on perceived pain associated with symptomatic tendinitis, J. Athl. Train. 31(Suppl.):S-47, 1996.

Popspisilova, L., Rottova, A.: Ultrasonic effect on collagen synthesis and deposition in differently localised experimental granulomas, Acta Chirurgica Plastica 19:148–157, 1977.

Reid, D.C.: Possible contraindications and precautions associated with ultrasound therapy. In Mortimer, A., Lee, N., editors. Proceedings of the International Symposium on Therapeutic Ultrasound, Canadian Physiotherapy Association, Winnipeg, 1981.

Reynolds, N.L.: Reliable ultrasound transmission (letter), Phys. Ther. 72(8):611, 1992.

Roberts, M., Rutherford, J.H., and Harris, D.: The effect of ultrasound on flexor tendon repairs in the rabbit, Hand 14:17, 1982.

Robinson, S., Buono, M.: Effect of continuous-wave ultrasound on blood flow in skeletal muscle, Phys. Ther. 75(2):145–150, 1995.

Roche, C., West, J.: A controlled trial investigating the effects of ultrasound on venous ulcers referred from general practitioners, Physiotherapy 70(12):475–477, 1984.

Rowe, R.J., Gray, I.M.: Ultrasound treatment of plantar warts, Arch. Phys. Med. Rehabil. 46:273, 1965.

Shambereer, R.C., Talbot, T.L., Tipton, H.W., et al.: The effect of ultrasonic and thermal treatment of wounds, Plast. Reconstruct. Surg. 68(6):880–870, 1981.

Sicard-Rosenbaum, L., Lord, D., and Danoff, J.: Effects of continuous therapeutic ultrasound on growth and metastasis of subcutaneous murine tumors, Phys. Ther. 75(1):3–12, 1995.

Smith, W., Winn, F., and Farette, R.: Comparative study using four modalities in shinsplint treatments, J. Orthop. Sports Phys. Ther. 8:77, 1986.

Sokoliu, A.: Destructive effect of ultrasound on ocular tissues. In Reid, J.M., Sikov, M.R., editors. Interaction of ultrasound and biological tissues, DHEW Pub (FDA) 73-8008, 1972.

Soren, A.: Evaluation of ultrasound treatment in musculoskeletal disorders, Physiotherapy 61:214–217, 1965.

Soren, A.: Nature and biophysical effects of ultrasound, J. Occup. Med. 7:375, 1965.

Stevenson, J.H.: Functional, mechanical, and biochemical assessment of ultrasound therapy on tendon healing in chicken toe, Plast. Reconstruct. Surg. 77:965, 1986.

Stewart, H.F.: Survey of use and performance of ultrasonic therapy equipment in Pinelles County, Phys. Ther. 54:707, 1974.

Stewart, H.F., Abzug, J.L., and Harris, G.F.: Considerations in ultrasound therapy and equipment performance, Phys. Ther. 80(4):424–428, 1980.

Stoller, D.W., Markholf, K.L., Zager, S.A., and Shoemaker, S.C.: The effects of exercise ice and ultrasonography on torsional laxity of the knee joint, Clin. Orthop. Rel. Res. 174:172–150, 1983.

Stratford, P.W., Cevy, D.R., Gauldie, S., et al.: The evaluation of phonophoresis and friction massage as treatments for extensor carpi radialis tendinitis: a randomized controlled trial, Physiother. Can. 41:93, 1989.

Stratton, S.A., Heckmann. R., and Francis, R.S.: Therapeutic ultrasound: its effect on the integrity of a nonpenetrating wound, J. Orthop. Sports Phys. Ther. 5:278, 1984.

Talaat, A.M., El-Dibany, M.M., and El-Garf, A.: Physical therapy in the management of myofascial pain dysfunction syndrome, Am. Otol. Rhinol. Laryngol. 95:225, 1986.

Taylor, E., Humphry, R.: Survey of therapeutic agent modality use, Am. J. Occup. Ther. 46(10):924–931, 1991.

Ter Haar, G.: Basic physics of therapeutic ultrasound, Physiotherapy 64(4):100–103, 1978.

Ter Haar, C., Dyson, M., and Oakley, E.M.: The use of ultrasound by physiotherapists in Britain, 1985, Ultrasound Med. Biol. 13:659, 1987.

Ter Haar, G., Wyard, S.J.: Blood cell banding in ultrasonic standing waves: a physical analysis, Ultrasound Med. Biol. 4:111–123, 1978.

Van Levieveld, D.W.: Evaluation of ultrasonics and electrical stimulation in the treatment of sprained ankles. A controlled study, Ugesrk-Laeger 141(16):1077–1080, 1979.

Ward, A., Robertson, V.: Comparison of heating of nonliving soft tissue produced by 45 KHz and 1 MHz frequency ultrasound machines, JOSPT 23(4):258–266, 1996.

Warren, C.G., Koblanski, I.N., and Sigelmann, R.A.: Ultrasound coupling media: their relative transmissivity, Arch. Phys. Med. Rehabil. 57:218, 1976.

Warren, C.G., Lehmann, J.F., and Koblanski, N.: Heat and stretch procedures: an evaluation using rat tail tendon, Arch. Phys. Med. Rehabil. 57:122, 1976.

Wells, P.E., Frampton, V., and Bowsher, D., editors: Pain: management and control in physiotherapy, London, 1988, Heinemann.

Wells, P.N.: Biomedical ultrasonics, London, 1977, Academic Press.

Williams, A.R., McHale, I., and Bowditch, M.: Effects of MHz ultrasound on electrical pain threshold perception in humans, Ultrasound Med. Biol. 13:249, 1987.

Williamson, J.B., George, T.K., Simpson, D.C., et al.: Ultrasound in the treatment of ankle sprains, Injury 17:76–178, 1986.

Wilson, A.G., Jamieson, S., and Saunders, R.: The physical behaviour of ultrasound, N.Z. J. Physiotherapy. 12(1):30–31, 1984.

Wood, R.W., Loomis, A.L.: The physical and biological effects of high frequency waves of great intensity, Philosoph. Mag. 4:417, 1927.

Wright, E.T., Haase, K.H.: Keloid and ultrasound, Arch. Phys. Med. Rehabil. 52:280, 1971.

Wyper, D.J., McNiven, D.R., and Donnelly, T.J.: Therapeutic ultrasound and muscle blood flow, Physiotherapy 64:321, 1978.

Zankei, H.T.: Effects of physical agents on motor conduction velocity of the ulnar nerve, Arch. Phys. Med. Rehabil. 47:787–792, 1966.

GLOSSARY

acoustic impedance Determines the amount of ultrasound energy reflected at tissue interfaces.

acoustic microstreaming The unidirectional movement of fluids along the boundaries of cell membranes resulting from the mechanical pressure wave in an ultrasonic field.

amplitude Describes the magnitude of the vibration in a wave. It is the maximum distance from equilibrium that any particle reaches.

attenuation A decrease in energy intensity as the ultrasound wave is transmitted through various tissues owing to scattering and dispersion.

beam nonuniformity ratio (BNR) Indicates the amount of variability of intensity within the ultrasound beam and is determined by the maximal point intensity of the transducer to the average intensity across the transducer surface.

cavitation The formation of gas-filled bubbles that expand and compress owing to ultrasonically induced pressure changes in tissue fluids.

collimated beam A focused, less divergent beam of ultrasound energy produced by a large diameter transducer.

compressions Regions of high molecular density (i.e., a great amount of ultrasound energy) within the longitudinal wave.

continuous wave ultrasound The sound intensity remains constant throughout the treatment, and the ultrasound energy is being produced 100 percent of the time.

coupling medium A substance used to decrease the acoustical impedance at the air-skin interface and thus facilitates the passage of ultrasound energy.

duty cycle The percentage of time that ultrasound is being generated (pulse duration) over one pulse period, which is also referred to as the mark to space ratio.

effective radiating area The total area of the surface of the transducer that actually produces the sound wave.

hot spots Areas at tissue interfaces that may become overheated.

intensity A measure of the rate at which energy is being delivered per unit area.

longitudinal wave The primary waveform in which ultrasound energy travels in soft tissue, with the molecular displacement along the direction in which the wave travels.

phonophoresis A technique in which ultrasound is used to drive a topical application of a selected medication into the tissues.

piezoelectric effect When an alternating electrical current generated at the same frequency as the crystal resonance is passed through the piezoelectric crystal, the crystal will expand and contract or vibrate at the frequency of the electrical oscillation, thus generating ultrasound at a desired frequency.

power The total amount of ultrasound energy in the beam and is expressed in watts.

pulsed ultrasound The intensity is periodically interrupted with no ultrasound energy being produced during the off period. When using pulsed ultrasound, the average intensity of the output over time is reduced.

rarefactions Regions of lower molecular density (i.e., a small amount of ultrasound energy) within a longitudinal wave.

standing wave As the ultrasound energy is reflected at tissue interfaces with different acoustic impedances, the intensity of the energy is increased as the reflected energy meets new energy being transmitted, forming waves of high energy that can potentially damage surrounding tissues.

stretching window The time period of vigorous heating when tissues will undergo their greatest extensibility and elongation.

transverse wave Occurring only in bone, the molecules are displaced in a direction perpendicular to the direction in which the ultrasound wave is moving.

LAB ACTIVITY

ULTRASOUND

DESCRIPTION

Therapeutic ultrasound is a physical agent modality utilized in sports medicine for the purpose of elevating tissue temperature, stimulating the repair of musculoskeletal soft tissues, modulating pain, and in the case of phonophoresis, driving medicinal molecules into a local tissue. Ultrasound is a high frequency, inaudible acoustic sound wave that may produce either thermal or nonthermal physiologic effects within the body. When applied to biologic tissues ultrasound may induce significant responses in cells, tissues, and organs. Ultrasound is one of the most widely utilized physical agent modalities in addition to the thermotherapies and electrotherapies.

PHYSIOLOGIC EFFECTS

Thermal effects
    Elevated tissue temperature
    Increased blood flow
    Increased tissue extensibility
    Increased local metabolism
    Altered nerve conduction velocity

Nonthermal effects
    Cavitation
    Fluid movement
    Increased cellular membrane permeability
    Acoustic microstreaming
    Stimulation of fibroblast activity

THERAPEUTIC EFFECTS

    Increased collagen tissue extensibility
    Decreased joint stiffness
    Reduction of muscle spasm
    Modulation of pain
    Increased blood flow
    Mild inflammatory response
    Stimulation of tissue regeneration

INDICATIONS

The primary indication for the use of therapeutic ultrasound by the therapist is in the acute and chronic treatment of soft tissue dysfunction, that is, strains, sprains, contusions with associated symptoms of pain, and muscular spasm. Ultrasound has also been successfully employed to enhance soft tissue and bone healing. Ultrasound can also be employed to percutaneously deliver selected medications to areas of inflammation.

CONTRAINDICATIONS

- Areas of impaired pain or temperature sensation
- Areas of impaired circulation
- Epiphyseal areas in children
- Not over reproductive organs
- Not over eyes, heart, spinal cord, or cervical/stellate ganglia
- Not over cemented joint prostheses
- Not over malignancies

ULTRASOUND

PROCEDURE	EVALUATION		
	1	2	3
1. Check supplies and equipment.			
a. Obtain appropriate ultrasound unit (1 or 3 MHz), towels, and coupling gel.			
2. Question patient.			
a. Verify identity of patient.			
b. Verify the absence of contraindications.			
c. Ask about previous ultrasound treatments and check previous treatment notes.			
3. Position patient.			
a. Place patient in a well-supported, comfortable position.			
b. Expose body part to be treated.			
c. Drape patient to preserve patient's modesty, protect clothing, but allow access to body part.			
4. Inspect body part to be treated.			
a. Check sensation.			
b. Check circulatory status.			
c. Verify that there are no rashes or open wounds.			
d. Assess function of body part (e.g., ROM, strength, irritability).			
5. Apply indicated technique: Select continuous or pulsed output and verify output intensity is at 0 before turning unit power on.			
a. Direct coupling.			
i. Apply layer of coupling gel to treatment surface.			
ii. Establish treatment duration dependent on size of area to be treated (i.e., 5 min for each 16-square-in area).			
iii. Maintain contact between soundhead and treatment surface, moving soundhead in circular or linear overlapping strokes at a rate of 2–4 in/sec; observe for air bubble formation.			
iv. Adjust treatment intensity: 0.5–1.0 W/cm^2 for superficial tissues and 1.0–2.0 W/cm^2 for deeper tissues.			
v. Monitor patient response during treatment; if patient reports warmth or ache, reduce intensity by 10 percent and continue treatment.			
b. Bladder coupling.			
i. Fill a balloon or condom with tepid, degassed water.			
ii. Apply layer of coupling gel to bladder.			
iii. Apply layer of coupling gel to treatment surface.			
iv. Place bladder over treatment surface.			
v. Establish treatment duration dependent on size of area to be treated (i.e., 5 min for each 16-square-in area).			
vi. Maintain contact between soundhead and treatment surface, moving soundhead in circular or linear overlapping strokes at a rate of 2–4 in/sec; observe for air bubble formation.			
vii. Adjust treatment intensity: 0.5–1.0 W/cm^2 for superficial tissues and 1.0–2.0 W/cm^2 for deeper tissues, intensity may need to be increased.			
viii. Monitor patient response during treatment; if patient reports warmth or ache, reduce intensity by 10 percent and continue treatment.			

PROCEDURE	EVALUATION		
	1	2	3
c. Underwater coupling.			
i. Fill a plastic or ceramic nonconductive basin with tepid degassed water of sufficient depth to cover treatment surface.			
ii. Immerse the body part into the basin.			
iii. Establish treatment duration dependent on size of area to be treated (i.e., 5 min for each 16-square-in area).			
iv. Maintain soundhead parallel to treatment surface at a distance of 0.5–3 cm, moving soundhead in circular or linear overlapping strokes at a rate of 2–4 in/sec; observe for air bubble formation on soundhead and wipe away.			
v. Adjust treatment intensity: 0.5–1.0 W/cm^2 for superficial tissues and 1.0–2.0 W/cm^2 for deeper tissues, intensity may need to be increased.			
vi. Monitor patient response during treatment; if patient reports warmth or ache, reduce intensity by 10 percent and continue treatment.			
d. Phonophoresis.			
i. Cleanse treatment surface with alcohol or soap and water.			
ii. Apply medication in glycerol cream, oil, or other vehicle in lieu of coupling gel.			
iii. Establish treatment duration dependent upon size of area to be treated (i.e., 5 min for each 16-square-in area).			
iv. Maintain contact between soundhead and treatment surface, moving soundhead in circular or linear overlapping strokes at a rate of 2–4 in/sec; observe for air bubble formation.			
v. Adjust treatment intensity: 0.5–1.0 W/cm^2 for superficial tissues and 1.0–2.0 W/cm^2 for deeper tissues. Intensity may need to be decreased.			
vi. Monitor patient response during treatment; if patient reports warmth or ache, reduce intensity by 10 percent and continue treatment.			
6. Terminate treatment.			
a. Zero out ultrasound unit control before removing soundhead.			
b. Clean soundhead of excess gel or medication in vehicle.			
c. Clean treatment surface of excess gel or medication in vehicle.			
d. Visually inspect the treated area.			
e. Remove draping material and have patient dress.			
7. Assess treatment efficacy.			
a. Ask the patient how the treated area feels.			
b. Record treatment parameters.			
8. Instruct the patient in any indicated exercise.			
9. Return equipment to storage after cleaning.			

PART 4 FOUR

LIGHT THERAPY

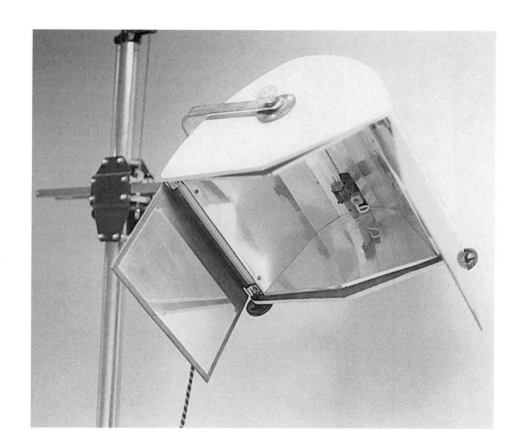

CHAPTER THIRTEEN

LOW-LEVEL LASER THERAPY

ETHAN SALIBA

SUSAN FOREMAN-SALIBA

OBJECTIVES

Following completion of this chapter, the student therapist will be able to:

- ✓ Identify the different types of lasers.
- ✓ Explain the physical principles used to produce laser light.
- ✓ Contrast the characteristics of the helium neon and gallium arsenide low-power lasers.
- ✓ Analyze the therapeutic applications of lasers in wound and soft-tissue healing, edema reduction, inflammation, and pain.
- ✓ Demonstrate the application techniques of low-power lasers.
- ✓ Describe the classifications of lasers.
- ✓ Incorporate the safety considerations in the use of lasers.
- ✓ Be aware of the precautions and contraindications for low-power lasers.

L ASER is an acronym that stands for light amplification of stimulated emissions of radiation. Despite the image presented in science-fiction movies, lasers offer valuable applications in the industrial, military, scientific, and medical environments. Einstein in 1916 was the first to postulate the theorems that conceptualized the development of lasers. The first work with amplified electromagnetic radiation dealt with MASERs (microwave amplification of stimulated emission of radiation). In 1955, Townes and Schawlow showed it was possible to produce stimulated emission of microwaves beyond the optical region of the electromagnetic spectrum. This work with stimulated emission soon extended into the optical region of the electromagnetic spectrum, resulting in the development of devices called optical masers. The first working optical maser was constructed in 1960 by Theodore Maiman when he developed the synthetic ruby laser. Other types of lasers were devised shortly afterward. It was not until 1965 that the term LASER was substituted for optical masers.[34]

Although lasers are relatively new, they have gone through extensive advances and refinements in a very short time. Lasers have been incorporated into numerous everyday applications that range from audio discs and supermarket scanning to communication and medical applications. This chapter provides an overview of lasers, but deals principally with the application of low-level lasers as they are used in conservative management of medical conditions.

LASER = Light Amplification for the Stimulated Emission of Radiation

laser A device that concentrates high energies into a narrow beam of coherent, monochromatic light; Light Amplification of the Stimulated Emission of Radiation.

PHYSICS

Light is a form of electromagnetic energy that has **wavelengths** between 100 and 10,000 nanometers (nm = 10^{-9}) within the electromagnetic spectrum.[34] Visible light ranges from 400 (violet) to 700 nm (red). Beyond the red portion of the visual range is the **infrared** and microwave region, and below the violet end are the ultraviolet, x-ray, gamma, and cosmic ray regions (Fig. 13-1). Light energy is transmitted through space as waves that contain tiny "energy packets" called **photons.** Each photon contains a definite amount of energy, depending on its wavelength (color).

Basics of the atomic theory are used to explain the principles of laser generation. The atom is the smallest particle of an element that retains all the properties of that element. The atom is divisible into fundamental particles called neutrons, protons, and electrons. Neutrons and positively charged protons are contained in the nucleus of the atom. **Electrons**, which are negatively charged, are equal in number to the protons and orbit the nucleus at distinct energy levels.

If an atom gains or loses an electron, it will become a negatively or positively charged ion, respectively. The polarity difference between the positively charged nucleus and negatively charged electrons keeps the electrons orbiting the nucleus at these distinct energy levels. Electrons neither absorb nor radiate energy as long as they are maintained in their distinct orbit. An electron will stay in its lowest energy level **(ground state)** unless it absorbs an adequate amount of energy to move it to one of its higher orbital levels. (Fig. 13-2). If an electron changes orbit, it will either gain or lose a distinct amount (quanta) of energy; it cannot exist between orbits.

If a photon of adequate energy level collides with an electron of an atom, it will cause the electron to change levels. When this occurs, the atom is said to be in an **excited state**. The atom stays in this excited state only momentarily and releases an identical photon (energy level) to the one it absorbed, which returns it to a ground state. This process is called **spontaneous emission** (Fig. 13-1). Energy levels are particular to the type of atom; therefore, an electron accepts only the precise amount of energy that will move it from one energy level to another. Another means of exciting atoms other than with photon collision is with an electrical discharge. The energy is generated by collision of electrons that are accelerated in an electrical field.[23]

STIMULATED EMISSIONS

The concept of **stimulated emission** was postulated by Einstein and is essential to the working principle of lasers.[28] It states that a photon released from an excited atom would stimulate another similarly excited atom to de-excite itself by releasing an identical photon.[34] The triggering photon would continue on its way unchanged, and the

stimulated emission When a photon interacts with an atom already in a high energy state and decay of the atomic system occurs, releasing two photons.

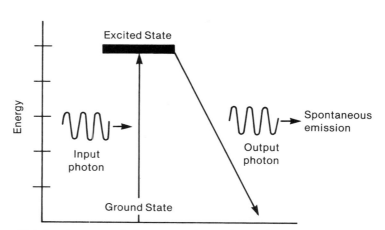

•**Figure 13-1** Spontaneous emission occurs when a photon changes energy level.

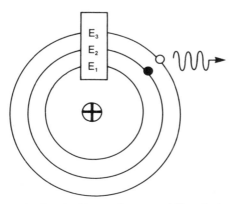

•Figure 13-2 When energy is absorbed by an atom, an orbiting electron can become excited to a higher orbit. As the electron drops back to its original level, energy (photon) is released.

subsequent photon released would be identical in frequency, direction, and phase. These two photons would promote the release of additional identical photons as long as other excited atoms were present. A critical factor for this occurrence is having an environment with unlimited excited atoms, which is termed **population inversion**. Population inversion occurs when there are more atoms in an excited state than in a ground state. It is caused by applying an external power source to the lasing medium. The released photons are identical in phase, direction, and **frequency**. To contain them, and to generate more photons, mirrors are placed at both ends of the chamber. One mirror is totally reflective, whereas the other is semipermeable. The photons are reflected within the chamber, which amplifies the light and stimulates the emission of other photons from excited atoms. Eventually, so many photons are stimulated that the chamber cannot contain the energy. When a specific level of energy is attained, photons of a particular wavelength are ejected through the semipermeable mirror.[28] Thus, amplified light through stimulated emissions (LASER) is produced (Fig. 13-3).

The laser light is emitted in an organized manner rather than in a random pattern as from a light bulb. Three properties distinguish the laser from incandescent and fluorescent light sources: **coherence**, **monochromaticity**, and **collimation**.[34]

Coherence means all photons of light emitted from individual gas molecules are the same wavelength and that the individual light waves are in phase with one another.

coherence Property of identical phase and time relationship. All photons of laser light are the same wavelength.

Three Properties of LASER
• Coherence
• Monochromaticity
• Collimation

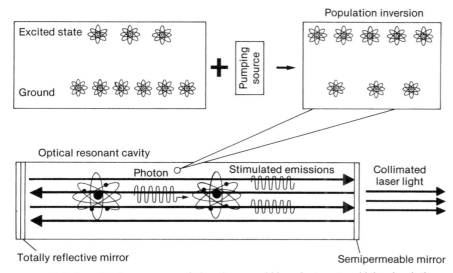

•Figure 13-3 Pumping is a process of elevating an orbiting electron to a higher level, thus creating population inversion, which is essential for laser operation.

Most Commonly Used LASERS
- Helium neon (HeNe)
- Gallium arsenide (GaAs)

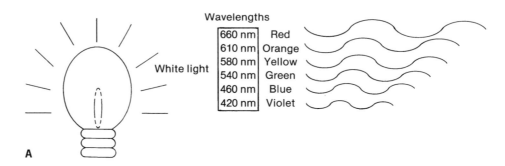

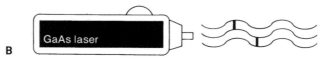

•**Figure 13-4 A.** White light contains electromagnetic energy of all wavelengths (colors) that are superimposed on each other. **B.** Laser light is monochromatic (single wavelength), coherent (in phase), and collimated (minimal divergence).

Normal light, on the other hand, is composed of many wavelengths that superimpose their phases on one another.

Monochromaticity refers to the specificity of light in a single, defined wavelength; if the specificity is in the visible light spectrum, it is only one color. The laser is one of the few light sources that produces a specific wavelength.

divergence The bending of light rays away from each other; the spreading of light.

The laser beam is well collimated, that is, there is minimal divergence of the photons.[1] That means the photons move in a parallel fashion, thus concentrating a beam of light (Fig. 13-4).

TYPES OF LASERS

Lasers are classified according to the nature of the material placed between two reflecting surfaces. There are potentially thousands of different types of lasers, each with specific wavelengths and unique characteristics, depending on the lasing medium utilized. The lasing mediums used to create lasers include the following categories: crystal and glass (solid-state), gas and excimer, semiconductor, liquid dye, and chemical.

Crystal lasers include the synthetic ruby (aluminum oxide and chromium) and the neodymium, yttrium, aluminum, garnet (Nd:YAG) lasers, among others. Synthetic, rather than natural materials are used to ensure purity of the medium, which is necessary for the physical characteristics of lasers to occur.[16]

Gas lasers were developed in 1961, shortly after the first ruby laser. The gas lasers developed include the helium neon (HeNe), argon, and carbon dioxide (CO_2) along with numerous others. The HeNe laser is one type of low-power device under investigation in the United States for application in physical medicine.

Semiconductor or **diode lasers** were developed in 1962 after the production of gas (HeNe) lasers. The gallium arsenide (GaAs) was the first diode laser developed and is another low-power laser under investigation in the United States for application in physical medicine.

Liquid lasers are also known as dye lasers because they use organic dyes as the lasing medium. By varying the mixture of the dyes, the wavelengths of the laser can be varied.

Chemical lasers are usually extremely high powered and frequently used for military purposes.[23]

Lasers can be categorized as either high or low power, depending on the intensity of energy they deliver. High-power lasers are also known as "hot" lasers because of the thermal responses they generate. These are used in the medical realms in numerous areas, including surgical cutting and coagulation, ophthalmologic, dermatologic, oncologic, and vascular specialties. The use of low-level lasers for wound healing and pain management is a relatively new area of application in medicine. These lasers produce a maximal output of less than 1 milliwatt (1 mW = 1/1000 W) in the United States and work by causing photochemical, rather than thermal, effects. No tissue warming occurs. The exact distinction of the power output that delineates a low- versus high-power laser varies. Low-level devices are considered any laser that does not generate an appreciable thermal response. This category can include lasers capable of producing up to 500 W of power (up to a class IV laser).[7] Low Level Laser Therapy (LLLT) is the dominant term in use today. In the literature Low Power Laser Therapy (LPLT) is also frequently used. "Therapeutic laser," "low-level laser," "low-power laser," or "low-energy laser" are also used for laser therapy. The term "soft laser" was originally used to differentiate therapeutic lasers from "hard lasers," i.e., surgical lasers. Several different designations then emerged, such as "MID laser" and "medical laser." "Biostimulating laser" is another term, with the disadvantage that one can also give inhibiting doses. The term "bioregulating laser" has thus been proposed. Other suggested names are "low-reactive-level laser," "low-intensity-level laser," "photobiostimulation laser," and "photobiomodulation laser."

Low-level lasers, which have been studied and used in Europe for the past 20 to 25 years, have been investigated in the United States for the past decade. The potential applications for low-power lasers include treatment of tendon and ligament injury, arthritis, edema reduction, soft-tissue injury, ulcer and burn care, scar tissue inhibition, and acutherapy.

LASER GENERATORS

Lasers require the following components to be operational.[23]

1. **Power supply:** Lasers use an electrical power supply that can potentially deliver up to 10,000 V and hundreds of amperes.
2. **Lasing medium:** This is the material that generates the laser light. It can include any type of matter: gas, solid, or liquid.
3. **Pumping device:** "Pumping" is the term used to describe the process of elevating an orbiting electron to a higher, "excited" energy level (see Fig. 13-3). This creates the population inversion that is essential for laser operation. The pumping device may be high voltage, photoflash lamps, radio-frequency oscillators, or other lasers. The pumping device is very specific to the type of lasing medium being used.
4. **Optical resonant cavity:** This contains the lasing medium. Once population inversion has occurred, this cavity, which contains the reflecting surfaces, directs the beam propagation.

The helium neon (HeNe) and gallium arsenide (GaAs) lasers are the two principal lasers currently under investigation in the United States for conservative management of medical conditions. The following discussion will concentrate on these two laser types.

HELIUM NEON LASERS

The HeNe gas laser uses a gas mixture of primarily helium with neon in a pressurized tube. This creates a laser in the red portion of the electromagnetic spectrum with a wavelength of 632.8 nm. The power output of the HeNe can vary, but typically runs from 1.0 to 10.0 mW, depending on the gas density used. Larger tubes are necessary for higher-power outputs, and each requires a precise power drive to operate.[6] Laser output can decrease, depending on the care of the equipment, on the number of operating hours, and whether **fiberoptics** are used. For example, rough handling can jar the reflecting surfaces, and a high number of hours in operation or poor fiberoptic quality can diminish the laser output.

CASE STUDY 13-1
LOW-LEVEL LASERS

Background: A 44-year-old man who has had Type I diabetes mellitus for 30 years presents for treatment of a non- or slow-healing lesion on his left foot. He has a mild peripheral sensory neuropathy, and developed a blister after going for a long run with new running shoes. The initial injury occurred 3 months ago, and there has been no change in the size of the lesion for the past month. The lesion is on the plantar surface of the foot, under the first metatarsal head. It is a full-thickness lesion, and is approximately 3 cm in diameter. The patient's medical condition is stable, and there are no other complaints.

Impression: Chronic dermal lesion on the left foot.

Treatment Plan: Daily treatment with a helium-neon laser was initiated. After cleansing the wound under aseptic conditions, the entire lesion was exposed to the HeNe light at 632.8 nm wavelength. The scanning technique was used to prevent contamination of the wound and equipment. The entire lesion was treated with an energy density of 4.0 J/cm^2.

Response: Photographs were taken on a weekly basis to document the effects of the treatment. After 3 weeks of daily treatment, the frequency was decreased to three sessions per week. After a total of 21 sessions (5 weeks), the lesion was healed. The patient was taught self-care, and techniques to prevent further injuries.

Discussion Questions

- What tissues were injured/affected?
- What symptoms were present?
- What phase of the injury-healing continuum did the patient present for care in?
- What are the physical agent modality's biophysical effects (direct/indirect/depth/tissue affinity)?
- What are the physical agent modality's indications/contraindications?
- What are the parameters of the physical agent modality's application/dosage/duration/frequency in this case study?
- What other physical agent modalities could be utilized to treat this injury or condition? Why? How?
- What is the mechanism of action of the laser energy?
- Why are patients with diabetes mellitus susceptible to cutaneous lesions?
- What precautions must be taken before treating a patient with a low-powered laser?
- What alternative treatment techniques would you consider? What are their advantages and disadvantages as compared to using a laser?

The rehabilitation professional employs physical agent modalities to create an optimum environment for tissue healing while minimizing the symptoms associated with the trauma or condition.

The HeNe laser in the United States delivers a power output of 1 mW through a fiber-optic tube in a continuous mode. Although the HeNe laser light is well collimated, the utilization of fiber-optics causes a divergence of the beam from 18–21 degrees.[7] Fiber-optics can decrease the output delivery 50 percent or more as the light travels from the lasing medium to the tip of the applicator. Fiber-optics are used to make the delivery more convenient because the size of the gas tube would make direct application difficult. HeNe lasers up to 6 mW have been manufactured for clinical use in Canada, which has fewer governmental restrictions than the United States. These higher-output lasers, although still considered low power, allow delivery of desired dosages in reduced time.[8]

GALLIUM ARSENIDE LASERS

The GaAs lasers utilize a diode to produce an infrared (invisible) laser at a wavelength of 904 nm.[3] Diode lasers are composed of semiconductor silicone materials that are precisely cut and layered. An electrical source is applied to each side, and lasing action is produced at the junction of the two materials. The cleaved surfaces function as partially reflecting surfaces that will ultimately produce coherent light (Fig. 13-5).[16]

Diode lasers produce a beam that is elliptically shaped so the lasers have a 10- to 35-degree divergence despite the fact that no fiber-optics are used.[23] The 904-nm laser

diode laser A solid-state semiconductor used as a lasing medium.

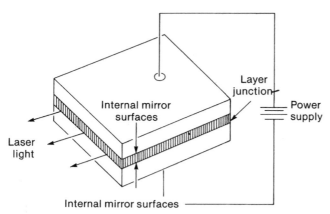

•**Figure 13-5** A diode is composed of silicone material that is cleaved and layered. The lasing action occurs at the junction of the layers when an electrical source is applied.

is delivered in a pulsed mode because of the heat produced at the junction of the diode chips. The GaAs laser manufactured in the United States has a peak power of 2 W but is delivered in a pulsed mode that decreases the average power to 0.4 mW output if delivered at 1000 Hz (see calculations in the Dosage section).

The application of additional layers of materials to other types of diodes allows their operation in a continuous mode at room temperature.[23] The continuous mode results in higher average power outputs from the lasers. Higher output diode lasers are manufactured for clinical applications in Canada and include the following:

780 nm wavelength with a 5 mW output, continuous mode delivery
810 nm wavelength with a 20 mW output, continuous mode delivery
830 nm wavelength with a 30 mW output, continuous mode delivery

These diodes are interchangeable in a single base unit.[8]

The laser units available in the United States have the ability to deliver both HeNe and GaAs lasers. The same device can both measure electrical impedance and deliver electrical point stimulation. The impedance detector allows hypersensitive or acupuncture points to be located. The point stimulator can be combined with laser application when treating pain. The electrical stimulation is believed to provide spontaneous pain relief, whereas the laser provides more latent tissue responses.[9]

LASER TREATMENT TECHNIQUES

The method of application of laser therapy is relatively simple, but certain principles of dosimetry should be discussed so the clinician can accurately determine the amount of laser energy delivered to the tissues. For general application, only the treatment time and the pulse rate vary. For research purposes, the investigator should measure the exact energy density emitted from the applicator before the treatments. Dosage is the most important variable in laser therapy and may be difficult to determine because of the variables mentioned previously (e.g., hours of operation or condition of the unit).

The laser energy is emitted from a handheld remote applicator. The GaAs laser houses the semiconductor elements in the tip of the applicator, whereas the HeNe lasers contain their componentry inside the unit and deliver the laser light to the target area via a fiber-optic tube. The fiber-optic assembly is fragile and should not be crimped or twisted excessively. The fiber-optics used with the HeNe and the elliptical shape of the GaAs laser create beam **divergence** with both devices. This divergence causes the beam's energy to spread out over a given area so that as the distance from the source increases, the intensity of the beam lessens.

Lasing Techniques
• Gridding
• Scanning
• Wanding

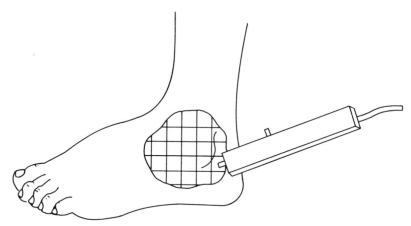

•**Figure 13-6** Grid application of laser. Laser aperture should be perpendicular to the surface. Lase each square centimeter of the injured area for the specified time. The aperture should be in light contact with the skin.

LASING TECHNIQUES

To administer a laser treatment, the tip should be in light contact with the skin and directed perpendicularly to the target tissue while the laser is engaged for the designated time. Commonly, a treatment area is divided into a grid of square centimeters, with each square centimeter stimulated for the specified time. This *gridding technique* is the most frequently utilized method of application and should be used whenever possible. Lines and points should not be drawn on the patient's skin, because this may absorb some of the light energy (Fig. 13-6). If open areas are to be treated, a sterilized clear plastic sheet can be placed over the wound to allow surface contact.

An alternative is a *scanning technique* in which there is no contact between the laser tip and the skin. With this technique, the applicator tip should be held 5–10 mm from the wound. Because beam divergence occurs, there is a decrease in the amount of energy as the distance from the target increases. The amount of energy lost becomes difficult to quantify accurately if the distance from the target is variable. Therefore, it is not recommended to treat at distances greater than 1 cm. When using a laser tip of 1 mm with 30 degrees of divergence, the red laser beam of the HeNe should fill an area the size of 1 cm^2 (Fig. 13-7). Although the infrared laser is invisible, the same consideration should be given when using the scanning technique. If the laser tip comes into contact

Treatment Tip

In treating myofascial trigger points, the therapist should use a gridding laser technique with the probe held perpendicular to the skin with light contact. The energy density should be set at 3 J/cm^2. The laser treatment can be combined with electrical stimulation using low-frequency (1–5 Hz) high-intensity current to produce pain modulation via the release of β-endorphin.

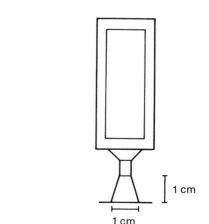

1 cm

1 cm

•**Figure 13-7** Scanning technique. When skin contact cannot be maintained, the remote should be held still in the center of the square centimeter grid at a distance of less than 1 cm. If using the HeNe laser, the red beam should fill a 1-cm^2 grid.

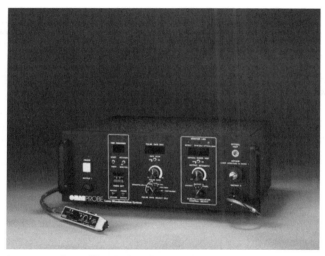

•**Figure 13-8** Low-power laser (Physio Technology, Ltd., Topeka, KS).

with an open wound, the tip should be cleaned thoroughly with a small amount of bleach or other antiseptic agents to prevent cross-contamination.

The scanning technique should be differentiated from the *wanding* technique, in which a grid area is bathed with the laser in an oscillating fashion for the designated time. As in the scanning technique, the dosimetry is difficult to calculate if a distance of less than 1 cm cannot be maintained. The wanding technique is not recommended because of irregularities in the dosages.

DOSAGE

The HeNe laser has a 1.0-mW average power output at the fiber tip and is delivered in the **continuous wave** mode. The GaAs laser has an output of 2 W but has only a 0.4-mW average power when pulsed at its maximum rate of 1000 Hz. The frequency of the GaAs is variable, and the clinician may choose a pulse rate of 1–1000 Hz, each with a pulse width of 200 nsec (nsec = 10^{-9}) (Figs. 13-8 and 13-9). Table 13-1 describes the contrasting specifications of these lasers.

The pulsed modes drastically reduce the amount of energy emitted from the laser. For example, a 2-W laser is pulsed at 100 Hz:

$$\textbf{Average power} = \textbf{pulse rate} \times \textbf{peak power} \times \textbf{pulse width}$$
$$= 100\,\text{Hz} \times 2\,\text{W} \times (2 \times 10^{-7}\,\text{sec})$$
$$= 0.04\,\text{mW}$$

This contrasts with the power output of 0.4-mW with the 1000 Hz rate. Therefore, it can be seen that adjustment of the pulse rate alters the average power, which significantly

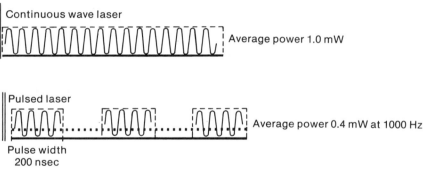

•**Figure 13-9** Continuous wave versus pulsed energies.

amplitudes than preinjury. The controls followed an expected course of recovery and did not reach normal levels even after 1 year.

The effect of HeNe irradiation on peripheral sensory nerve latency has been investigated on humans by Snyder-Mackler and Bork.[30] This double-blind study showed that exposure of the superficial radial nerve to low dosages of laser resulted in a significantly decreased sensory nerve conduction velocity, which may provide information about the pain-relieving mechanism of lasers. Other explanations for pain relief may be the result of hastened healing, anti-inflammatory action, autonomic nerve influence, and neurohumoral responses (serotonin, norepinephrine) from descending tract inhibition.[8,9]

Chronic pain has been treated with GaAs and HeNe lasers, and positive results have been observed empirically and through clinical research. Walker conducted a double-blind study to document analgesia after exposure to HeNe irradiation in chronic pain patients compared with sham treatments.[35] When the superficial sites of the radial, median, and saphenous nerves as well as painful areas were exposed to laser irradiation, there were significant decreases in pain and less reliance on medication for pain control. These preliminary studies suggest positive results, although pain modulation is difficult to measure objectively.

BONE RESPONSE

Future uses of laser irradiation include the treatment of other connective tissue structures, such as bone and articular cartilage. Schultz and colleagues studied various intensities of Nd:YAG laser on the healing of partial-thickness articular cartilage lesions in guinea pigs.[29] During the surgical procedure, the lesions were irradiated for 5 seconds, with intensities ranging from 25 to 125 J. After 4 weeks, the low-dosage group (25 J) had chondral proliferation, and by 6 weeks the defect had reconstituted to the level of the surface cartilage. Normal basophilia cells were present with staining, indicating normal cellular structures. The higher dosage groups and controls had little or no evidence of restoration of the lesion with cartilage. Bone healing and fracture consolidation have been investigated by Trelles and Mayayo.[33] An adapter was attached to an intramuscular needle so that the laser energy could be directed deeper to the periosteum. Rabbit tibial fractures showed faster consolidation with HeNe treatment of 2.4 J/cm^2 on alternate days. Histologic examination indicated more mature Haversian canals with detached osteocytes in the laser treated bone. There was also a remodeling of the articular line, which is impossible with traditional therapy.[32,33] The use of lasers for the treatment of nonunion fractures has begun in Europe.

SUGGESTED TREATMENT PROTOCOLS

Research suggests some laser densities for treating several clinical models. These average from 0.05 to 0.5 J/cm^2 for acute conditions and range from 0.5 to 3 J/cm^2 for more chronic conditions.[7] The responses of the tissues depend on the dosage delivered, although the type of laser used can also influence the effect. The response obtained with different dosages and with different lasers varies considerably among studies, leaving treatment parameters to be determined largely empirically. In the literature, there seems to be little differentiation when comparing the dosages of HeNe and GaAs lasers, although their depths of penetration differ significantly. The laser units produced in the United States have relatively little average power, so the tendency is to administer dosages in millijoules rather than Joules. Three to six treatments may be required before the effectiveness of laser therapy can be determined.

Although higher laser output is recommended to reduce treatment times, overstimulation should be avoided. The Arndt-Schultz principle that states more is not necessarily better is applicable with laser therapy. For this reason, laser should be administered at a maximum of once daily per treatment area. When using large dosages, treatment is recommended on alternate days. If the effects of laser plateau, the frequency of treatments should be reduced or the treatments discontinued for 1 week, at which time the treatment can be reinstated if needed.[32]

PAIN

The use of low-power lasers in the treatment of acute and chronic pain can be implemented in various manners. After proper diagnosis of the pain's etiology, the pathology site can be gridded. The entire area of injury should be lased as described previously. Table 13-3 lists some suggested treatment protocols for various clinical conditions. When trigger points are being treated, the probe should be held perpendicular to the skin with light contact. If a specific structure, such as a ligament, is the target tissue, the laser probe should be held in contact with the skin and perpendicular to that structure. When treating a joint, the patient should be positioned so that the joint is open to allow penetration of the energy to the intra-articular areas.

The treatment of acupuncture and trigger points with laser can be augmented with electrical stimulation for pain management. Reference to charts should be made to determine appropriate acupuncture points. The impedance detector in the laser remote enhances the ability to locate these sites. Points should be treated from distal to proximal for best results.

Occasionally patients may experience an increase in pain after a laser treatment. This phenomenon is believed to be the initiation of the body's normal responses to pain that have become dormant.[7] Laser has been found to help resolve the condition by enhancing normal physiologic processes needed to resolve the injury. As stated previously, several treatments should be administered before deeming the modality ineffective in pain management.

WOUND HEALING

Although ulcerations and open wounds are not common in an athletic training environment, contusions, abrasions, and lacerations can be treated with laser to hasten healing time and decrease infection[17] (see Chapter 3). The wound should be cleaned appropriately

Treatment Tip
In treating a new abrasion with a laser, the wound should first be cleaned appropriately and debrided as necessary. A scanning lasing technique with no direct contact should be done around the periphery of the abrasion. It is recommended that a HeNe laser be used at an energy density of 0.5-1 J/cm^2.

TABLE 13-3	Suggested Treatment Applications	
Application	**Laser Type**	**Energy Density**
Trigger point		
Superficial	HeNe	1-3 J/cm^2
Deep	GaAs	1-2 J/cm^2
Edema reduction		
Acute	GaAs	0.1-0.2 J/cm^2
Subacute	GaAs	0.2-0.5 J/cm^2
Wound healing (superficial tissues)		
Acute	HeNe	0.5-1 J/cm^2
Chronic	HeNe	4 J/cm^2
Wound healing (deep tissues)		
Acute	GaAs	0.05-0.1 J/cm^2
Chronic	GaAs	0.5-1 J/cm^2
Scar tissue	GaAs	0.5-1 J/cm^2

Copied with permission from Physio Technology.

and all debris and eschar removed. Heavy exudate that covers the wound will diminish the laser's penetration; therefore, lasing around the periphery of the wound is recommended. The scanning technique should be utilized over open wounds unless a clear plastic sheet is placed over the wound to allow direct contact. Opaque materials can absorb some of the laser energy and are not recommended. Facial lacerations can be treated with the laser, although care should be taken not to direct the beam into the patient's eyes. Risk of retinal damage from the low-power lasers used in the United States is low.

SCAR TISSUE

The laser energy affects only what is metabolically diminished and does not change normal tissue. Hypertrophic scars can be treated with lasers because of the bioinhibitive effects. Bioinhibition requires prolonged treatment times and may be clinically impractical because of the low power output of the lasers used in the United States. Pain and edema associated with pathologic scars have been effectively treated with low power lasers. Thick scars have varied vascularity, which makes laser transmission irregular; therefore, it is often recommended to treat the periphery of the scar rather than directly over it.

EDEMA AND INFLAMMATION

The primary action of laser application for control of edema and inflammation is through the interruption of the formation of intermediate substrates necessary for the production of inflammatory chemical mediators: kinins, histamines, and prostaglandins. Without these chemical mediators, the disruption of the body's homeostatic state is minimized and the extent of pain and edema is diminished. It is also believed that laser energy can optimize cell membrane permeability, which regulates interstitial osmotic hydrostatic pressures. Therefore, during tissue trauma, the flux of fluid into the intercellular spaces would be reduced. Laser treatment is usually applied by gridding over the involved areas or by treating related acupuncture points if the area of involvement is generalized.

SAFETY

Few safety considerations are necessary with the low-level laser. However, as the variety of lasers evolved and their uses increased in the United States, it became necessary to develop national guidelines not only for safety but also for therapeutic efficacy. The U.S. Food and Drug Administration's Center for Devices and Radiological Health now regulates the manufacture and sale of lasers in the United States.

Laser equipment commonly is grouped into four FDA classes, with simplified and well-differentiated safety procedures for each.[29]

Class I, or "exempt," lasers are considered nonhazardous to the body. All invisible lasers with average power outputs of 1 mW or less are class I devices. These include the GaAs lasers with wavelengths from 820 to 910 nm.[23] The invisible, infrared lasers should contain an indicator light to identify when the laser is engaged.

Class II, or "low-power," lasers are hazardous only if a viewer stares continuously into the source. This class includes visible lasers that emit up to 1 mW average power, such as the HeNe laser.

Class III, or moderate-risk, lasers can cause retinal injury within the natural reaction time. The operator and patient are required to wear protective eyewear. However, these lasers cannot cause serious skin injury or produce hazardous diffuse reflections from metals or other surfaces under normal use.[29]

Class IV, or high-power, lasers present a high risk of injury and can cause combustion of flammable materials. Other dangers are diffuse reflections that may harm the eyes and cause serious skin injury from direct exposure. These high-power lasers seldom are used outside research laboratories and restricted industrial environments.[29]

The low-level lasers used in treating sports injuries are categorized as classes I and II laser devices and class III medical devices. Class III medical devices include new or modified devices not equivalent to any marketed before May 28, 1976.[12] The U.S. Food and Drug Administration (FDA) has so far had a very strict policy on laser therapy. To use laser therapy on humans, it has been necessary to obtain approval by an institutional Review Board (IRB), established through a university, a manufacturer, or a hospital. Now, in accordance with a new policy established in 1999, the FDA has started to issue so-called Premarket Notifications, labeled 510(k). The FDA does not regulate physical therapists in the use of any laser product. They regulate the companies that manufacture and sell the laser products. A company must be approved by the FDA to market their device, and these companies are allowed to promote the medical use of their laser products ONLY for the specifically approved applications. Such an approval means that the specific laser approved can be sold, but the only claim the manufacturer can make is the indication described in the 510(k). To date the low-level laser is indicated for adjuncted use in the temporary relief of hand and wrist pain associated with carpal tunnel syndrome.[19] By requiring documentation of the results and side effects of lasers, the FDA regulations serve to generate scientific data to determine safety and efficacy of the device in question.

PRECAUTIONS AND CONTRAINDICATIONS

Contraindications
Cancerous tumors
Directly over eyes
Pregnancy

Lasers deliver nonionizing radiation, therefore, no mutagenic effects on DNA and no damage to the cells or cell membranes have been found.[8] No deleterious effects have been reported after low-power laser exposure, including carcinogenic responses, unless applied to already cancerous cells. Tumorous cells may proliferate when stimulated.[14] The following are some suggestions for laser use.

Laser should not be used over cancerous growths.

It is better to underexpose than to overexpose. If clinical results plateau, a reduction in dosage or treatment frequency may facilitate results.

Avoid direct exposure into the eyes because of possible retinal burns. If lasing for extended periods, as with wound healing, safety glasses are recommended to avoid exposure from reflection.

Although no adverse reactions have been documented, the use of laser during the first trimester of pregnancy is not recommended.

A small percentage of patients, especially those with chronic pain, may experience a syncope episode during the laser treatment. Symptoms usually subside within minutes. If symptoms exceed 5 minutes, no further treatments should be given.

CONCLUSION

The use of low-level lasers appears to have nothing but positive effects: This in itself should create a state of professional caution in deeming it a panacea modality. Currently, with these power outputs, lasers are recognized as nonsignificant risk devices. However, low-power lasers have not been granted recognition by the Food and Drug Administration as being a safe or effective modality. Although many empirical and clinical findings show promising results, more controlled studies are essential to determine the types of lasers and dosages that are required to attain reproducible results.

SUMMARY

1. The first working laser was the ruby laser developed in 1960 and was initially called an optical maser.
2. Visible light wavelengths range from 400 to 700 nm. Light is transmitted through space in waves and is comprised of photons emitted at distinct energy levels.

3. An atom is excited when energy is applied and raises an orbiting electron to a higher orbit. When the electron returns to its original orbit, it releases energy in the form of a photon, a process called spontaneous emission.

4. Stimulated emission occurs when the photon is released from an excited atom and promotes the release of an identical photon to be released from a similarly excited atom.

5. For lasers to operate, a medium of excited atoms must be generated. This is termed population inversion and results when an external energy source (pumping device) is applied to the medium.

6. Characteristics of laser light vary from conventional light sources in three manners: laser light is monochromatic (single color or wavelength), coherent (in phase), and collimated (minimal divergence).

7. Laser can be thermal (hot) or nonthermal (low power, soft, or cold). The categories of lasers include solid-state (crystal or glass), gas, semiconductor, dye, or chemical lasers.

8. Helium neon (HeNe; gas) and gallium arsenide (GaAs; semiconductor) lasers are two low-level lasers being investigated by the FDA for application in physical medicine. These low-level lasers are currently being used in the United States and other countries for wound and soft-tissue healing and pain relief.

9. HeNe lasers deliver a characteristic red beam with a wavelength of 632.8 nm. The laser is delivered in a continuous wave and has a direct penetration of 2–5 mm and an indirect penetration of 10–15 mm.

10. GaAs lasers are invisible and have a wavelength of 904 nm. They are delivered in a pulse mode and have an average power output of 0.4 mW. This laser has a direct penetration of 1–2 cm and an indirect penetration to 5 cm.

11. The proposed therapeutic applications of lasers in physical medicine include acceleration of collagen synthesis, decrease in microorganisms, increase in vascularization, and reduction of pain and inflammation.

12. The technique of laser application ideally is done with gentle contact with the skin surface and should be perpendicular to the target surface. Dosage appears to be the critical factor in eliciting the desired response, but exact dosimetry has not been determined. Dosage fluctuates by varying the pulse frequency and the treatment times.

13. The laser is applied by developing an imaginary grid over the target area. The grid is comprised of 1-cm squares and the laser is applied to each square for a predetermined time. Trigger or acupuncture points are also treated for painful conditions.

14. The FDA considers low-level lasers as low-risk investigational devices. For use in the United States, they require an IRB approval and informed consent prior to their use.

15. Although no deleterious effects have been reported, certain precautions and contraindications exist. Contraindications include lasing over cancerous tissue, directly into the eyes, and during the first trimester of pregnancy. Occasionally pain may initially increase when laser treatments begin but does not indicate cessation of treatment. A low percentage of patients have experienced a syncope episode during laser treatment, but this is usually self-resolving. If symptoms persist for longer than 5 minutes, future laser treatments are not advised.

16. Future research for determining efficacy and treatment parameters is critically needed to substantiate the application of low-power lasers in physical medicine.

REVIEW QUESTIONS

1. What does the acronym LASER stand for?
2. How does the laser use the concept of stimulate emission to produce a laser beam?
3. What are the characteristics of the helium neon and gallium arsenide low-power lasers?

4. What are the various therapeutic applications of lasers in wound and soft-tissue healing, edema reduction, inflammation, and pain reduction?

5. What are the scanning and gridding techniques of application of the laser?

6. What seems to be the most critical treatment parameter in eliciting a desired response?

7. What are the treatment precautions and contraindications for low-power lasers?

8. Where does the low-power laser stand in terms of FDA approval as a therapeutic modality?

REFERENCES

1. Abergel, R.: Biochemical mechanisms of wound and tissue healing with lasers, Second Canadian Low Power Medical Laser Conference, March, 1987.

2. Abergel, R., Lyons, R., and Castel, J.: Biostimulation of wound healing by lasers: experimental approaches in animal models and in fibroblast cultures, J. Dermatol. Surg. Oncol. 13:127–133, 1987.

3. Bartlett, W. Quillen, W., and Creer, R.: Effect of gallium-aluminum-arsenide triple-diode laser irradiationon evoked motor and sensory action potentials of the median nerve, J. Sport Rehabil. 11(1):12, 2002.

4. Bartlett, W.P., Quillen, W.S., and Gonzalez, J.L.: Effect of gallium aluminum arsenide triple-diode laser on median nerve latency in human subjects, J. Sport Rehabil. 8(2):99–108, 1999.

5. Bostara, M., Jucca, A., and Olliaro, P.: In vitro fibroblast and dermis fibroblast activation by laser irradiation at low energy, Dermatologica 168:157–162, 1984.

6. Castel, J.: Laser biophysics, Second Canadian Low Power Medical Laser Conference, Ontario, Canada, March, 1987.

7. Castel, M.: Personal communication, Downsview, Ontario, March, 1989, MEDELCO.

8. Castel, M.: A clinical guide to low power laser therapy, Downsview, Ontario, 1985, PhysioTechnology Ltd.

9. Cheng, R.: Combination laser/electrotherapy in pain management, Second Canadian Low Power Laser Conference, Ontario, Canada, March, 1987.

10. De Bie, R.A., De Vet, H.C.W., Lenssen, T.F., et al.: Low-level laser therapy in ankle sprains: a randomized clinical trial, Arch. Phys. Med. Rehabil. 79(11):1415–1420, 1998.

11. DeSimone, N.A., Christiansen, C., and Dore, D.: Bactericidal effect of .95 m W helium-neon and indium-gallium-aluminum-phosphate laser irradiation at exposure times of 30, 60, and 120 secs on photosensitized *Staphylococcus aureus* and *Pseudomonas aeruginosa* in vitro, Phys. Ther. 79(9):839–846, 1999.

12. Enwemeka, C.: Laser biostimulation of healing wounds: specific effects and mechanisms of action, J. Orthop. Sports Phys. Ther. 9:333–338, 1988.

13. Fact Sheet: Laser biostimulation, Rockville, MD, 1984, Center of Devices and Radiological Health, FDA.

14. Farnham, J.: Personal communication, Rockville, MD, March, 1989, Center of Devices and Radiological Health, FDA.

15. Gogia, P., Hurt, B., and Zirn, T.: Wound management with whirlpool and infrared cold laser treatment, Phys. Ther. 68: 1239–1242, 1988.

16. Hallmark, C., Horn, D.: Lasers: the light fantastic, ed. 2, Blue Ridge Summit, PA, 1987, TAB Books.

17. Hopkins, J., McCloda, T., and Seegmiller, J.: Effects of low-level laser on wound healing, J. Athl. Train. (Suppl.) 38(2S):S-33, 2003.

18. Hunter, J., Leonard, L., and Wilson, R.: Effects of low energy laser on wound healing in a porcine model, Lasers Surg. Med. 3:285–290, 1984.

19. Johnson, D.S.: Low-level laser therapy in the treatment of carpal tunnel syndrome, Athl. Ther. Today 8(2):30–31, 2003.

20. Kana, J., Hutschenreiter, G., and Haina, D.: Effect of low power density laser radiation on healing of open skin wounds in rats, Arch. Surg. 116:293–296, 1981.

21. Longo, L., Evangelista, S., and Tinacci, G.: Effect of diode-laser silver-arsenide-aluminum (Ag-As-Al) 904 nm on healing of experimental wounds, Lasers Surg. Med. 7:444–447, 1987.

22. Lyons, R., Abergel, R., and White, R.: Biostimulation of wound healing in vivo by a helium neon laser, Ann. Plast. Surg. 18: 47–77, 1987.

23. McComb, G.: The laser cookbook: 88 practical projects, Blue Ridge Summit, PA, 1988, TAB Books.

24. Mester, E., Mester, A., and Mester, A.: Biomedical effects of laser application, Laser Surg. Med. 5:31–39, 1985.

25. Mester, E., Spiry, T., and Szende, B.: Effect of laser rays on wound healing, Am. J. Surg. 122:532–535, 1971.

26. Rochkind, S., Nissan, M., and Barr-Nea, L.: Response of peripheral nerve to HeNe laser: experimental studies, Lasers Surg. Med. 7:441–443, 1987.

27. Schultz, R., Krishnamurthy, S., and Thelmo, W.: Effects of varying intensities of laser energy on articular cartilage: a preliminary study, Lasers Surg. Med. 5:577–588, 1985.

28. Shaffer, B.: Scientific basis of laser energy, Clin. Sports Med. 2(4):585–598, 2002.

29. Sliney, D., Wolkarsht, M.: Safety with lasers and other optical sources: a comprehensive handbook, New York, 1980, Plenum Press.

30. Snyder-Mackler, L., Bork, C.: Effect of helium neon laser irradiation on peripheral nerve sensory latency, Phys. Ther. 68:223–225, 1988.

31. Surinchak, J., Alago, M., and Bellamy, R.: Effects of low-level energy lasers on the healing of full-thickness skin defects, Lasers Surg. Med. 2:267–274, 1983.

32. Trelles, M.: Medical applications of laser biostimulation, Second Canadian Low Power Medical Laser Conference, Ontario, Canada, March, 1987.

33. Trelles, M., and Mayayo, E.: Bone fracture consolidates faster with low power laser, Lasers Surg. Med. 7:36–45, 1987.

34. Van Pelt, W., Stewart, H., and Peterson, R.: Laser fundamentals and experiments, Rockville, MD, 1970, U.S. Dept. HEW.

35. Walker, J.: Relief from chronic pain by low power laser irradiation, Neurosci. Lett. 43:339–344, 1983.

SUGGESTED READINGS

Abergel, R.: Biostimulation of procollagen production by low energy lasers in human skin fibroblast cultures, J. Invest. Dermatol. 82:395, 1984.

Baxter, G.: Therapeutic lasers theory and practice, New York, 1994, Churchill Livingstone.

Baxter, G., Bell, A., and Allen, J.: Low level laser therapy: current clinical practice in Northern Ireland, Physiotherapy 77:171–178, 1991.

Beckerman, H., de Bie, R., and Bouter L.: The efficacy of laser therapy for musculoskeletal and skin disorders: a criteria-based meta-analysis of randomized clinical trials, Phys. Ther. 72(7):483–491, 1992.

Bolton, P., Young, S., and Dyson, M.: Macrophage responsiveness to laser therapy with varying power and energy densities, Laser Ther. 3:105–112, 1991.

Bolton, P., Young, S., and Dyson, M.: Macrophage response to laser therapy: a dose response study, Laser Ther. 2:101–106, 1990.

Braverman, B., McCarthy, R., and Ivankovich, A.: Effect on helium neon and infrared laser irradiation on wound healing in rabbits, Lasers Surg. Med. 9:50–58, 1989.

Crous, L., Malherbe, C.: Laser and ultraviolet light irradiation in the treatment of chronic ulcers, Physiotherapy 44:73–77, 1988.

Cummings J.: The effect of low energy (HeNe) laser irradiation on healing dermal wounds in an animal model, Phys. Ther. 65:737, 1985.

Dreyfuss, P., Stratton, S.: The low-energy laser, electro-acuscope, and neuroprobe: treatment options remain controversial, Phys. Sportsmed. 21(8):47–50, 55–57, 1993.

Dyson, M., Young, S.: Effects of laser therapy on wound contraction and cellularity in mice, Laser Surg. Med. 1:125, 1986.

Fisher, B.: The effects of low power laser therapy on muscle healing following acute blunt trauma. Journal of Physical Therapy Science, 12(1): 49–55, 2000.

Flemming, L.A., Cullum, N.A., and Nelson, E.A.: A systematic review of laser therapy for venous leg ulcers, J. Wound Care 8(3):111–114, 1999.

Gogia, P., Marquez, R.: Effects of helium-neon laser on wound healing, Ostomy Wound Manage. 38(6):33, 36, 38–41, 1992.

Hayashi, K., Markel, M., and Thabit, G.: The effect of nonablative laser energy on joint capsular properties: an in vitro mechanical study using a rabbit model, Am. J. Sports Med. 23(4):482–487, 1995.

Herbert, K., Bhusate, L., and Scott, D.: Effect of laser light at 820 nm on adenosine nucleotide levels in human lymphocytes, Lasers Life Sci. 3:37–45, 1989.

Karu, T., Tiphlova, S., and Samokhina, M.: Effects of near infrared laser and superluminous diode irradiation on Escherichia coli division rate, IEEE J. Quant. Electron. 26:2162–2165, 1990.

Kramer, J., Sandrin, M.: Effect of low-power laser and white light on sensory conduction rate of the superficial radial nerve, Physiother. Can. 45(3):165–170, 1993.

Laakso, L., Richardson, C., and Cramond, T.: Factors affecting low level laser therapy, Aust. J. Physiother. 39(2):95–99, 1993.

Lam T., Abergerl R., and Meeker C.: Biostimulation of human skin fibroblasts: low energy lasers selectively enhance collagen synthesis, Laser Surg. Med. 3:328, 1984.

Lundeberg T., Haker E., and Thomas M.: Effect of laser versus placebo in tennis elbow, Scand. J. Rehabil. Med. 19:135–138, 1987.

Lyons, R., Abergel, R., and White, R.: Biostimulation of wound healing in vivo by a helium neon laser, Ann. Plast. Surg. 18:47–50, 1987.

Malm, M., Lundeberg, T.: Effect of low power gallium arsenide laser on healing of venous ulcers, Scand. J. Reconstruct. Hand Surg. 25:249–251, 1991.

Martin, D.: An investigation into the effects of low level therapy on arterial blood flow in skeletal muscle, Physiotherapy 81(9):562, 1995.

McMeeken, J., Stillman, B.: Perceptions of the clinical efficacy of laser therapy, Aust. J. Physiother. 39(2):101–106, 1993.

Mester, E., Jaszsagi-Nagy, E.: The effects of laser radiation on wound healing and collagen synthesis, Studia Biophysica 35(3):227, 1973.

Nussbaum, E., Biemann, I., and Mustard, B.: Comparison of ultrasound/ultraviolet-C and laser for treatment of pressure ulcers in patients with spinal cord injury, Phys. Ther. 74(9): 812–823, 1994.

Palmgren, N., Dahlin, J., and Beck, H.: Low level laser therapy of infected abdominal wounds after surgery, Lasers Surg. Med. 3(Suppl.):11, 1991.

Rockhind, S., Russo, M., and Nissan, M.: Systemic effect of low power laser on the peripheral and central nervous system, cutaneous wounds, and burns, Lasers Surg. Med. 9:174–182, 1989.

Saunders, L.: Laser versus ultrasound in the treatment of supraspinatus tendinosis: randomized controlled trial. PHYSIOTHERAPY, 89(6): 365–73, 2003.

Saperia, D., Glassberg, E., and Lyons, R.: Stimulation of collagen synthesis in human fibroblast cultures, Laser Life Sci. 1:61–77, 1986.

Swenson, R.S.: Therapeutic modalities in the management of nonspecific neck pain. Physical Therapy and Rehabilitation Clinics of North America, 14(3): 605–27, 2003.

Turner, J., Hode, L.: Laser therapy: clinical practice and scientific background, Grängesberg, Sweden, 2002, Prima Books.

Vasseljen, O.: Low-level laser versus traditional physiotherapy in the treatment of tennis elbow, Physiotherapy 78(5):329–334, 1992.

Waylonis, G., Wilke, S., and O'Toole, D.: Chronic myofascial pain: management by low-output helium-neon laser therapy, Arch. Phys. Med. Rehabil. 69(12):1017–1020, 1988.

Young, S.: Macrophage responsivity to light therapy, Lasers Surg. Med. 9:497–505, 1989.

Young, S., Dyson, M., and Bolton, P.: Effect of light on calcium uptake by macrophages. Presented at the Fourth International Biotherapy Association Seminar on Laser Biostimulation, Guy's Hospital, 1991, London.

Witt, J.D.: Interstitial laser photocoagulation for the treatment of osteoid osteoma, J. Bone Joint Surg. 82B(8): 1125–1128, 2000.

GLOSSARY

coherence Property of identical phase and time relationship. All photons of laser light are the same wavelength.

collimate To make parallel.

continuous wave An uninterrupted opposed to pulsed beam of laser light.

diode laser A solid-state semiconductor used as a lasing medium.

direct effect The tissue response that occurs from energy absorption.

divergence The bending of light rays away from each other; the spreading of light.

electron Fundamental particle of matter possessing a negative electrical charge and small mass.

excited state State of an atom that occurs when outside energy causes the atom to contain more energy than normal.

fiber-optic A solid glass or plastic tube that conducts light along its length.

frequency The number of cycles or pulses per second.

ground state The normal, unexcited state of an atom.

indirect effect A decreased response that occurs in deeper tissues.

infrared A portion of the electromagnetic spectrum between the visible and microwave regions. Wavelengths range from 780 to 100,000 nm.

laser A device that concentrates high energies into a narrow beam of coherent, monochromatic light (Light Amplification by the Stimulated Emission of Radiation).

monochromaticity The condition that occurs when a light source produces a single color or wavelength.

photon The basic unit of light; a packet or quanta of light energy.

population inversion A condition where more atoms exist in a high energy, excited state than those atoms that are in a normal ground state. This is required for lasing to occur.

spontaneous emission This occurs when an atom in a high energy state emits a photon and drops to a more stable ground state.

stimulated emission This occurs when a photon interacts with an atom already in a high energy state and decay of the atomic system occurs, releasing two photons.

wavelength The distance from peak to the same point on the next peak of an electromagnetic or acoustic wave.

LAB ACTIVITY

LOW-POWER LASER

DESCRIPTION

Low-power lasers produce a coherent, monochromatic, collimated light beam. They are used in the United States principally for pain modulation and wound healing. The two principal wavelengths used are 632.8 nm, produced by the helium neon (HeNe) laser, and 94 nm, produced by the gallium arsenide (GaAs) laser. Low-power (cold) lasers are distinguished from high-power (hot) lasers by the lack of thermal effects by the low-power lasers.

The mechanism of action of low-power laser energy is not clear. Whether the absorbed photons stimulating protein synthesis, thus promoting tissue healing, have a bactericidal effect on the wound or increase angiogenesis has not been established. The potential mechanisms for pain modulation are even less clear.

Although it has been suggested that laser energy may have indirect effects on tissue up to 5 cm deep, there is no convincing evidence of penetration this deep. How light energy absorbed by the superficial cells is conducted to underlying cells when the energy is nonionizing and nonthermal has not been explained.

It must be made crystal clear that the use of low power lasers for these purposes has not been approved by the U.S. Food and Drug Administration, the regulating body for medical devices. Individuals using low power lasers for these purposes must have an Investigational Device Exemption and should obtain informed consent from each patient before using the laser.

The physiologic and therapeutic effects of low power laser stimulation are not well established. Therefore, the indications, which are derived from the physiologic effects, are somewhat speculative.

PHYSIOLOGIC EFFECTS

Increased collagen synthesis by fibroblasts
Decreased nerve conduction velocity

THERAPEUTIC EFFECTS

Increased rate of wound closure
Increased tensile strength of wounds
Decreased perception of pain

INDICATIONS

Low-power laser stimulation may be helpful to optimize the rate of wound closure, modulate musculoskeletal pain, and remodel established scar tissue.

CONTRAINDICATIONS

There are no established contraindications to low-power laser application, but the light should not be directed at the eyes.

LOW-POWER LASER

PROCEDURE	EVALUATION		
	1	2	3
1. Check supplies.			
a. Obtain towels or sheets for draping.			
b. Check laser equipment for charged battery, broken or frayed cables, and so on.			
2. Question patient.			
a. Verify identity of patient (if not already verified).			
b. Verify the absence of contraindications.			
c. Ask about previous exposure to laser therapy; check treatment notes.			

PROCEDURE	EVALUATION		
	1	2	3
3. Position patient.			
a. Place patient in a well-supported, comfortable position.			
b. Expose body part to be treated.			
c. Drape patient to preserve patient's modesty, protect clothing, but allow access to body part.			
4. Inspect body part to be treated.			
a. Check light touch perception.			
b. Assess function of body part (e.g., ROM, irritability).			
5. Apply laser stimulation.			
a. Determine the area to be treated and visualize a grid overlying the treatment area. The grid should be divided into 1-cm squares.			
b. If the gridding technique is to be used, place the tip of the probe in light contact with the skin and administer the light to each square centimeter of area for the appropriate time to obtain the desired dosage.			
c. If the scanning technique is to be used, hold the tip of the probe within 1 cm of the skin and make sure the aperture of the probe is positioned such that the laser beam will be perpendicular to the skin. Administer the light to each square centimeter of area for the appropriate time to obtain the desired dosage.			
d. Ensure that the laser energy will not be directed at the patient's eyes.			
e. If the patient reports anything unusual, such as discomfort at the treatment site, nausea, and so on, discontinue treatment.			
f. Continue to monitor the patient during the duration of the treatment.			
6. Complete treatment.			
a. When the treatment time is over, discontinue application of the laser energy.			
b. Remove material used for draping, assist the patient in dressing as needed.			
c. Have the patient perform appropriate therapeutic exercise as indicated.			
d. Clean the treatment area and equipment according to normal protocol.			
7. Assess treatment efficacy.			
a. Ask the patient how the treated area feels.			
b. Visually inspect the treated area for any adverse reactions.			
c. Perform functional tests as indicated.			

CHAPTER FOURTEEN

ULTRAVIOLET THERAPY

J. MARC DAVIS

OBJECTIVES

Following completion of this chapter, the student therapist will be able to:

✓ Describe the position of ultraviolet radiation (UVR) in the electromagnetic spectrum and the relationship of UVR to other forms of electromagnetic energy.
✓ Explain how UVR raises energy levels within irradiated objects.
✓ Understand the effect of UVR on individual cells and human tissue and explain the tanning process.
✓ Recognize the effect of long-term exposure to UVR and the effect of UVR on the eyes.
✓ Demonstrate the physical setup and procedures for operating a UVR device, including safety precautions, the skin test, the inverse square law, and the cosine law.
✓ Articulate various clinical uses of UVR.

Ultraviolet radiation (UVR) is one of the oldest medical modalities. The physicians of ancient Egypt and Greece attributed many healing powers to sunlight, and in fact life itself would not be possible without the interaction of solar UVR and plant photosynthesis. Before this century the sun was the only satisfactory source of UVR, but now a wide selection of UVR generators is available.

This chapter serves to familiarize the student therapist with the properties of UVR, explain how UVR affects human tissue, and explore different UVR treatment apparatus and techniques. Subsequently, the therapist should be able to understand why UVR therapy can be effective in treating certain maladies, and therefore be able to correctly choose UVR therapy when it is the appropriate treatment for a given problem.

ULTRAVIOLET RADIATION

Ultraviolet radiation is the portion of the electromagnetic spectrum that ranges from 2000 to 4000 Å and is bordered below 2000 Å by x-ray and above 4000 Å by visible light (see Fig. 1-2). The UVR portion of the electromagnetic spectrum is further divided into three sections: UV-A, UV-B, and UV-C. Shortwave UV (UV-C, also called extreme UV, and far UV) ranges from 2000 to 2900 Å and is bactericidal.[28,34] UV-B (called middle UV and the sunburn spectrum) ranges from 2900 to 3200 Å and is associated with sunburn and age-related skin changes.[27-33] UV-A (near UV) ranges from 3200 to 4000 Å. Until recently little or no physiologic effect was attributed to UV-A, but recent research and clinical use of UV-A are showing possible benefits and hazards for UV-A exposure. The UVR apparatus most likely to be encountered in a clinical setting would generate UVR in the UV-B or UV-C range or in both ranges.[13]

The beneficial effects of UVR as a treatment modality are mediated by its limited absorption. Ultraviolet radiation is absorbed within the first 1–2 mm of human skin and most of the physiologic effects are superficial.[8] Therefore, the most effective use of UVR therapy is in the treatment of various skin disorders such as acne and psoriasis.[5,12,16]

EFFECT ON CELLS

Ultraviolet radiation is a form of energy. As such, when it contacts any surface, skin included, it must be either reflected or absorbed and transmitted. If UVR strikes the skin at a 90-degree angle, 90–95 percent of the energy will be absorbed. Most will be absorbed within the epidermis of the skin (80–90%), whereas the rest will reach the dermis.[8] As the UVR is absorbed within the tissue it causes the energy level of exposed atoms to increase. These atoms will quickly return to their normal energy state; however, the presence of excess energy causes chemical excitation within the cells of the exposed tissue. This chemical excitation is the cause of the various effects of UVR on living cells and tissue. Even a single exposure to UVR will cause chemical excitation within exposed cells, which leads to physiologic changes within these cells.

These physiologic changes are the result of a photochemical event that is the end product of the UVR-induced chemical excitation. This photochemical event results in an alteration of cell biochemistry and cellular metabolism. The synthesis of **DNA** and **RNA** is affected, leading to alterations in protein and enzyme production. As a consequence, cell protein structure can be altered, and this alteration of cellular protein and DNA may leave the cell inactive or dead.[28-33]

keratin The fibrous protein that forms the chemical basis of the epidermis.

Fortunately, defenses have evolved that protect microorganisms and cells that are exposed to a constant barrage of UVR from the sun. The damaged cells may be restored by enzymatic action or by simple deterioration of the damaged portion; the damaged segment may be replaced by normal material, or it may be bypassed when the cell reproduces.[28] DNA synthesis within cells of the human epidermis is suppressed for 24–48 hours following exposure to UVR in the range of 2500–2700 Å and is then followed by a period of increased DNA synthesis.[28,33]

EFFECT ON NORMAL HUMAN TISSUE

SHORT-TERM EFFECT ON SKIN

keratinocyte A cell that produces keratin.

Normal human skin consists of two layers, the superficial epidermis and the underlying dermis (Fig. 14-1). The epidermis is avascular and composed mostly of well-organized layers of **keratinocytes**. These produce **keratin**, the fibrous protective protein of the skin. The keratinocytes are produced from cells of the basal layer of the epidermis and then move upward through the epidermis. The dermis is divided into two layers, the papillary layer that contains a rich blood supply, and the reticular layer that is composed of heavy connective tissue and contains fibroblasts, histiocytes, and mast cells.

Erythema

When human skin is exposed to UVR, the individual cells react as previously described. However, the skin is a protective organ, covering the entire human exterior, and it will respond in a generalized manner over the entire area that is irradiated. This generalized response culminates in the development of an acute inflammatory reaction. The end results

CROSS SECTION OF SKIN

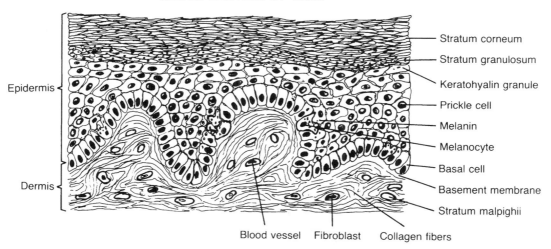

•**Figure 14-1** A cross section of the skin showing the dermis and epidermis layers.

of an active inflammation within the skin are **erythema** (the reddening of the skin associated with sunburn), **pigmentation** (tanning), and increased epidermal thickness.[8,17,28,33]

pigmentation Tanning of the skin from sun exposure.

Inflammation

Inflammation is the response of any human tissue, skin included, to an irritating or injurious substance or event. In the case of UVR exposure, the irritating substances are the end products of the previously described photochemical event and may include damaged DNA, RNA, and cell proteins. The inflammatory process removes these injurious and irritating substances from the skin. Because the appearance of these irritating substances does not occur immediately following UVR exposure, the inflammatory response is delayed. Normally it begins several hours after irradiation and peaks 8–24 hours following exposure.[28]

This inflammatory response is characterized by local vasodilation and increased capillary permeability. Theoretically this is caused by (1) the absorption of UVR by keratinocytes, leading to the release of substances that diffuse to the papillary dermis and cause vasodilation; or (2) the absorption of UVR by mast cells in the dermis that in turn release histamine, resulting in vasodilation.[8,17,28] Erythema is caused by this vasodilation and the subsequent increase of blood within the dermis. The increased capillary permeability permits certain proteins to move from the capillaries into the dermis. This results in a change in osmotic pressure; consequently, water is drawn into the area and edema occurs. Leukocytes, lymphocytes, and monocytes pass into the dermis and to a small degree into the epidermis. These cells phagocytize (consume or engulf) dead cells and other debris. At 24 hours the inflammatory process is completed, and at 30 hours the rebuilding begins. The reparative process is characterized by increased activity of the keratinocytes and results in a thickening of the epidermis **(hyperplasia)**.[28] This is protective; areas covered with a thick epidermis, such as the soles of the feet, do not sunburn.

hyperplasia An increase in the size of a tissue; in the skin, an increased thickness of the epidermis.

The acute effects of UVR exposure can be exacerbated if certain chemicals or medications are present on the skin or in the body. **Photosensitization** is a process in which a person becomes overly sensitive to UVR as a result of the excitation of a chemical by UVR exposure.[8] Any person taking a photosensitizing medication is very susceptible to the effects of UVR and should be treated accordingly. It should be noted that such an adverse reaction can occur even after limited exposure to natural sunlight. A list of common photosensitizing agents follows.

> Antibacterial and microbial agents
> > Tetracyclines: a group of broad-spectrum antibiotics
> > Sulfonamides: a group of synthetic antimicrobial drugs

CASE STUDY 14-1
ULTRAVIOLET THERAPY

Background: A 25-year-old man developed a psoriatic plaque over the region of the posterior aspect of his left elbow. After an unsuccessful regimen of oral medications and topical ointments, his dermatologist referred him for a regimen of ultraviolet therapy. The lesion measured 3 × 5 cm extending over the olecranon region. The patient was otherwise in a normal state of health and exhibited full active ROM and strength of the left upper extremity.

Impression: Active psoriasis.

Treatment Plan: After establishing the patient's MED (minimal erythemal dosage) as 30 seconds during an initial treatment session; a progressive program of exposure was begun to the posterior left elbow. Exposure began at 1 MED and increased by 1/2 MED each treatment session conducted on alternate days. When the patient reached 6 MED exposure, treatment was suspended pending physician reassessment.

Response: There was an increase in erythema noted around the margins of the lesion subsequent to initial UV exposure. Subsequent sessions did not produce any notable change from this initial response. A gradual reduction in plaque size was noted over the course of exposures, having decreased by 30 percent at the time treatment was suspended.

The rehabilitation professional employs therapeutic agent modalities to create an optimum environment for tissue healing while minimizing the symptoms associated with the trauma or condition.

Discussion Questions

- What tissues were injured or affected?
- What symptoms were present?
- What phase of the injury healing continuum did the patient present for care in?
- What are the therapeutic agent modality's biophysical effects (direct, indirect, depth, and tissue affinity)?
- What are the therapeutic agent modality's indications and contraindications?
- What are the parameters of the therapeutic agent modality's application, dosage, duration, and frequency in this case study?
- What other therapeutic agent modalities could be utilized to treat this injury or condition? Why? How?

Griseofulvin (Fulvicin, Grifulvin, Grisactin): an antibiotic with an additional antifungal action

Thiazide diuretics: A group of drugs that act on the kidney to increase sodium and water in the urine
    Chlorothiazide (Diuril)
    Hydrochlorothiazide (Hydrodiuril, Oretic, Esidrix)
    Methychlorothiazide (Enduron)

Other medications
    Phenothiazines (Thorazine): widely used tranquilizers
    Psoralens: a group of dermal pigmenting agents
    Sulfonylureas (Dymelor, Diabinese)
    Diphenhydramine (Benadryl): an antihistamine

Miscellaneous
    Sunscreens
    Tar
    Oral contraceptives
    Certain cosmetics[8,27,28]

TANNING

Tanning is the increase of pigmentation within the skin and is a protective mechanism activated by UVR exposure. An increase of **melanin,** the pigment responsible for darkening, within the skin causes the tan (see Fig. 14-1). The melanin functions as a biologic filter of UVR by scattering the radiation, absorbing the UVR, and dissipating the absorbed energy as heat.[33] The process of tanning is divided into two phases: immediate and delayed tanning.

Immediate tanning appears most often in darkly pigmented individuals and occurs immediately following UVR exposure. Immediate tanning represents the darkening of melanosomes already present in the skin. It begins to fade 1 hour after exposure and is hardly noticeable 3–8 hours later.[28,33] Delayed tanning is the result of the formation of new pigment (melanin) through the process of melanogenesis. The process is initiated by production of erythema (sunburn) within the skin. Melanogenesis occurs within the melanocytes of the basal layer of the epidermis (see Fig. 14-1), and the end products of this process are melanosomes, new pigment granules. These melanosomes are transferred from the melanocytes via nerve cells to nearby keratinocytes. As the keratinocytes gradually move outward to the skin's surface, the new pigment also migrates to the periphery. Delayed tanning usually becomes apparent 72 hours after UVR exposure.

erythema A redness of the skin caused by capillary dilation.

Human skin color is a baseline that is influenced by various environmental factors (exposure to solar radiation, occupation, leisure activities) and the genetically determined level of melanin within the skin.[8,34] Individuals of all races have the same number of melanocytes per unit area, but darker individuals are able to produce greater amounts of melanin.[7]

melanin A group of dark brown or black pigments that occur naturally in the eye, skin, hair, and other animal tissues.

LONG-TERM EFFECT ON SKIN

The most serious effects of long-term UVR exposure are premature aging of the skin and skin cancer.[20,30,31] Lightly pigmented individuals are more susceptible to these maladies. Premature aging of the skin is characterized by dryness, cracking, and a decrease in the elasticity of the skin, and it results from a change in the epidermis called solar elastosis. An alteration in the skin's elastic fibers causes solar elastosis and has been tentatively linked to UVR-induced DNA damage.[28]

Skin cancer is the most common malignant tumor found in humans and has been epidemiologically and clinically associated with solar UVR.[1,28,30,34] Damage to DNA is suspected as the cause of skin cancer, but the exact cause is yet unknown. The major types of skin cancer are basal cell carcinoma, which rarely metastasizes (spreads to other areas); squamous cell carcinoma, which metastasizes in 5 percent of all cases; and malignant melanoma, which metastasizes in a majority of cases.[28,30] Fortunately, the rate of cure exceeds 95 percent with early detection and treatment.

EFFECT ON EYES

For centuries it has been known that sunlight can have an adverse effect on vision. Snow blindness, the result of solar UVR being reflected from the snow to the unprotected eyes of winter outdoor enthusiasts, was first described in 375 BC.[33] Ultraviolet radiation exposure of the eyes causes an acute inflammation called **photokeratitis.** It is a delayed reaction occurring from 6 to 24 hours after exposure, but occasionally develops within 30 minutes. Conjunctivitis (inflammation of the mucous membrane that lines the inside of the eyelid) develops, accompanied by erythema of adjacent facial skin, and the injured person reports the sensation of a foreign body on the eye. Photophobia, increased tear production, and spasm of the ocular muscles may occur.[28,34] The acute reaction lasts from 6–24 hours, and all symptoms will generally clear by 48 hours with few residual effects. The eye, unlike the skin, does not develop a tolerance to UVR. The development of cataracts has been attributed to UVR, especially in wavelengths of greater than 2900 Å.[32,34]

photokeratitis An inflammation of the eyes caused by exposure to UVR.

CASE STUDY 14-2
ULTRAVIOLET THERAPY

Background: A 32-year-old woman developed psoriatic plaques over the region of the posterior aspect of both of her elbows. After an unsuccessful regimen of oral medications and topical ointments, her dermatologist referred her for a regimen of ultraviolet therapy. The lesions measured approximately 6 × 8 cm extending over the olecranon region. The patient was otherwise in a normal state of health and exhibited full active ROM and strength of her upper extremities.

Impression: Active psoriasis.

Treatment Plan: After establishing the patient's MED (minimal erythemal dosage) as 30 seconds during an initial treatment session; a progressive program of exposure was begun to the posterior aspect of the elbows. Exposure began at 1 MED and increased by ¹/₂ MED each treatment session conducted on alternate days. When the patient reached 6-MED exposure, treatment was suspended pending physician reassessment.

Response: There was an increase in erythema noted around the margins of the lesion subsequent to initial UV exposure. Subsequent sessions did not produce any notable change from this initial response. A gradual reduction in plaque size was noted over the course of exposures, having decreased by 30 percent at the time that treatment was suspended.

Discussion Questions

- What tissues were injured/affected?
- What symptoms were present?
- What phase of the injury-healing continuum did the patient present for care in?
- What are the physical agent modality's biophysical effects (direct/indirect/depth/tissue affinity)?
- What are the physical agent modality's indications/contraindications?
- What are the parameters of the physical agent modality's application/dosage/duration/frequency in this case study?
- What other physical agent modalities could be utilized to treat this injury or condition? Why? How?

The rehabilitation professional employs physical agent modalities to create an optimum environment for tissue healing while minimizing the symptoms associated with the trauma or condition.

SYSTEMIC EFFECTS

Systemic effect is photosynthesis of vitamin D.

The only systemic effect that can be objectively attributed to UVR is the photosynthesis of vitamin D following irradiation of the skin by UVR in the UV-B range.[19,32] The process is activated when the skin is irradiated by UVR at approximately 300 Å wavelength. This activates a complicated biochemical pathway that travels from the skin to the liver and kidneys and results in vitamin D being delivered to bones, intestines, various organs, and muscles. Vitamin D is responsible for regulating calcium and phosphorus, and after UVR exposure the absorption of these elements increases within the intestines and results in increased amounts of calcium and phosphorus within the blood. Consequently, UVR can be used as a treatment for disorders of calcium and phosphorus metabolism, such as rickets and tetany. Presently, the treatment of choice for such problems is dietary supplementation; however, if this is not effective, UVR is an acceptable alternative.

ULTRAVIOLET GENERATORS

Since the beginning of this century, many types of UVR generators have been developed, including the carbon arc lamp, fluorescent lamp, xenon compact arc lamp, and mercury arc lamps. Of these, the mercury arc lamps are the most common, and they have been found to be safe, effective, and easy to operate.

The **carbon arc lamp** is composed of two carbon electrodes that consist of carbon and certain inorganic salts and metals. Initially the two electrodes are in contact when the current is applied and then are moved slightly apart, causing the current to arc across this small gap. As the salts and metals within the electrodes become heated, UVR is emitted, the majority between 3500 and 4000 Å. The electrode gradually burns, and so the lamp will deteriorate and the electrodes must be replaced. This burning is noisy and causes an unpleasant odor, and the device requires a high electrical input.

The **xenon compact arc lamp** is composed of xenon gas enclosed in a vessel in which it is compressed to 20 times atmospheric pressure. An electric arc is passed through the gas, causing increased temperature. When the gas is heated to 6000°C (10,832°F), the atoms become incandescent and emit infrared, visible, and ultraviolet light waves. Most of the UVR is in the range of 3200–4000 Å. Caution must be exercised when using a device with gas under such high pressure, because rupture of the containing vessel could endanger the patient and operator.

The **mercury arc lamps** are divided into two categories, low-pressure and high-pressure mercury arcs. Both consist of mercury (a heavy metal in a liquid state) contained in a quartz envelope. When an electric arc is passed through the envelope, the mercury becomes vaporized and at 8000°C (14,432°F) the atoms become incandescent and emit ultraviolet, infrared, and visible light. In the low-pressure lamp, also called the cold quartz lamp, the temperature of the mercury electrons is greater than the mercury vapor, and the temperature of the quartz envelope is about 60°C—hot, but not dangerous. The UVR spectrum produced by low pressure lamps is limited to 1849 and 2537 Å. The 1849 Å wavelength is blocked by the quartz envelope, or it would combine with oxygen and produce ozone; 95 percent of the UVR produced by these lamps is the 2537 Å wavelength, which is highly germicidal. The low pressure mercury arc lamp does not require a warm up or cool down period, and it is used mainly where the bactericidal effect of UVR is desired.

A high-pressure mercury arc occurs when the mercury vapor temperature equals the mercury electron temperature and the pressure within the envelope reaches 1 atmosphere or more.[31] The quartz envelopes of these lamps become quite hot and may be cooled by a water jacket or circulating air; subsequently these are called hot quartz lamps. The UVR spectrum produced peaks at 2537, 2800, 2967, 3025, 3130, and 3660 Å.[8,17,32,33] The 2537 Å wavelength is absorbed by the increased density of the mercury vapor and does not pass from the lamp. Most of the UVR produced falls within the UV-B range. These lamps require a warm-up period before reaching peak efficiency and a cool down period after the current is stopped before the lamp can be restarted. The high pressure mercury arc lamps are mainly used to produce erythema and the accompanying photochemical reactions.

The **fluorescent ultraviolet lamp**, or "blacklight," is actually a low pressure mercury lamp. It consists of a tube of UV-transmitting glass that is coated with phosphors. The phosphors are fluorescing substances that absorb the UVR and then reemit it at a longer wavelength. Most of the UVR emitted ranges from 3000 to 4000 A, within the high UV-B and entire UV-A range.[32] These lamps are low powered and generally used in multiples. These lamps are used where exposure of several people simultaneously is desired.

The **mercury arc lamps** are the most likely kind of UVR lamp to be used in a clinical setting, and generally the lamps will be either a standing model or a hand-held model. The standing model consists of a mercury arc lamp surrounded by a reflector. The opening below the lamp and reflector can be closed by the use of shutters. The lamp, reflector, and shutters are supported by a column, and the height of the column is adjustable. At the base of the column is a housing that contains the electrical controls contained within the configuration of the unit (Fig. 14-2). The handheld unit is used for very local treatments and produces the bactericidal spectral bond of 2536 Å. It is very effective for treating local skin infections and, with the addition of a special lens, is used for diagnostic purposes.

UVR Generators
- Carbon arc lamp
- Xenon compact arc lamp
- Fluorescent ultraviolet lamp (blacklight)
- Mercury arc lamp

Mercury arc lamp most commonly used.

ULTRAVIOLET

PROCEDURE	EVALUATION		
	1	2	3
1. Check supplies.			
a. Obtain sheet or towels for draping, stopwatch, UV protection goggles for patient and therapist.			
b. Check lamp for frayed power cords, integrity of lamp and shields, and so on.			
c. Verify that the intensity control is at zero.			
2. Question patient.			
a. Verify identity of patient (if not already verified).			
b. Verify the absence of contraindications.			
c. Ask about previous ultraviolet treatments, check treatment notes.			
3. Position patient.			
a. Place patient in a well-supported, comfortable position.			
b. Expose body part to be treated; have patient remove all jewelry from the area.			
c. Drape patient to preserve patient's modesty and protect clothing, but allow access to body part. Insure that only the area you want to expose to UV is exposed; draping is crucial.			
4. Inspect body part to be treated.			
a. Check for precancerous skin lesions (e.g., keratoses).			
b. If treating for acne, attempt to quantify the number of lesions; if treating a wound, measure the size of the wound.			
5. Determine minimal erythemal dose (MED) of ultraviolet light on initial treatment day.			
a. Cut six 1-cm^2 holes of different shapes in a piece of cloth (e.g., stockinette) or stiff paper (e.g., file folder).			
b. Cover an area of the body away from the treatment area that has not been exposed to ultraviolet in the past few weeks (e.g., the abdomen or anterior forearm) with the paper or cloth.			
c. Position lamp such that the bulb is parallel to the body part being treated (such that the energy will strike the body at a 90° angle) and is about 75 cm away from the patient.			
d. Inform the patient that he or she should feel only a mild warmth; if it is hot, he or she should inform you. Start the lamp.			
e. Expose the first window for 30 seconds, then uncover the second window for an additional 30 seconds; continue exposing remaining windows every 15 seconds. If six windows are used, the first window will have been exposed for 120 seconds, the last for only 15 seconds.			
f. The MED is the duration of exposure that produces redness within 8 hours and disappears within 24 hours. Inform the patient to inspect the test area over the next 24-hour period and report the results on the next visit.			

PROCEDURE	EVALUATION		
	1	2	3
6. Apply ultraviolet light.			
a. Position lamp such that the bulb is parallel to the body part being treated (such that the energy will strike the body at a 90° angle) and is about 75 cm away from the patient.			
b. Inform the patient that he or she should feel only a mild warmth; if it is hot, he or she should inform you. Start the lamp.			
c. Expose the treatment area for the appropriate time (i.e., one MED for the first treatment, with an increase of 35% per treatment; if 1 day's treatment is missed, exposure should be the same as the last treatment).			
7. Complete the treatment.			
a. When the treatment time is over, move the lamp away from the patient and turn the output control to zero; dry the area with a towel.			
b. Remove material used for draping, assist the patient in dressing as needed.			
c. Clean the treatment area and equipment according to normal protocol.			
8. Assess treatment efficacy.			
a. Ask the patient how the treated area feels.			
b. Visually inspect the treated area for any adverse reactions.			
c. Perform functional tests as indicated.			

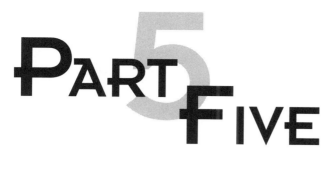

PART 5 FIVE

MECHANICAL MODALITIES

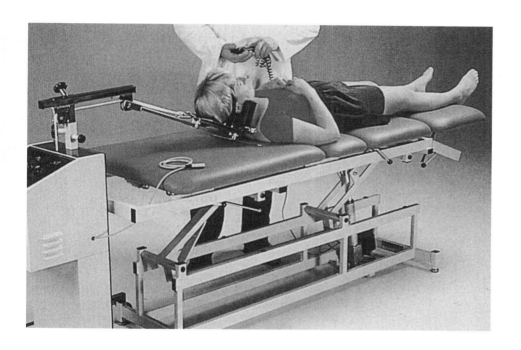

Chapter Fifteen

Spinal Traction

Daniel N. Hooker

OBJECTIVES

Following completion of this chapter, the student therapist will be able to:

✓ Analyze the physical effects and therapeutic value of traction on bone, muscle, ligaments, joint structures, nerve, blood vessels, and intervertebral disk.

✓ Evaluate the clinical advantages of using positional lumbar traction and inversion traction.

✓ Describe the clinical applications for using manual lumbar traction techniques including level specific manual traction and unilateral leg pull manual traction.

✓ Explain the setup procedures and treatment parameter considerations for using mechanical lumbar traction.

✓ Articulate the advantages of using a manual traction technique of the cervical spine.

✓ Demonstrate the setup procedure for mechanical traction techniques for the cervical spine.

Traction has been used since ancient times in the treatment of painful spinal conditions. Traction can be defined as a drawing tension applied to a body segment.[4]

In the clinical setting, traction may be performed *mechanically,* using a traction machine or ropes and pulleys to apply a traction force, or it may be performed *manually* by a therapist who understands the appropriate positions and intensities of the force being applied to the joints of the spine or the extremities. Some of the concepts of traction discussed in this chapter are generalizable to the treatment of the extremities; however, this discussion has been aimed specifically at cervical and lumbar spinal traction.

THE PHYSICAL EFFECTS OF TRACTION

EFFECTS ON SPINAL MOVEMENT

Traction encourages movement of the spine both overall and between each individual spinal segment.[2] Changes in overall spinal length and the amount of separation or space between each vertebra have been shown in studies of both the lumbar and the cervical spine (Fig. 15-1).[1,6,20,29,30,31,37,38]

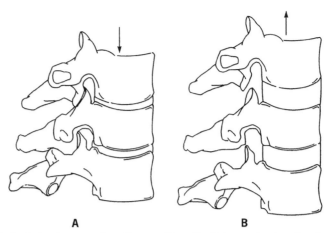

•**Figure 15-1 A.** Spine in normal resting position. **B.** Spine under traction load with overall increase in length and overall increased separation between vertebrae.

The amount of movement varies according to the position of the spine, the amount of force, and the length of time the force is applied. Separations of 1–2 mm per intervertebral space have been reported. This change is very transient, and the spine quickly returns to the previous intervertebral space relationships when traction is released and the erect posture is assumed.[10,18,25,31] Decreases in pain, paresthesia, or tingling while traction is applied may be caused by the physical separation of the vertebral segments and the resultant decrease in pressure on sensitive structures. If these changes occur while the patient is being treated with traction, the prognosis for the patient is good and traction should be continued as part of the treatment plan.[2,5,30] Any lasting therapeutic changes must be assumed to occur from adjustments or adaptations of the structures around the vertebrae in response to the traction.

EFFECTS ON BONE

Wolff's law Bone remodels itself and provides increased strength along the lines of the mechanical forces placed on it.

Bone changes, according to **Wolff's law,** usually occur in response to compressive or distractive loads. Traction places a distractive load on each of the vertebrae affected by the traction load. Although bone tissue adapts relatively quickly, bony changes do not occur fast enough to cause the symptom changes that occur with traction application. An intermittent traction with a rhythmic on and off load cycle not only provides distraction load but also promotes movement. The major effect of traction on the bone may come from the increase in spinal movement that reverses any immobilization-related bone weakness by increasing or maintaining bone density.

EFFECTS ON LIGAMENTS

The ligamentous structures of the spinal column are stretched by traction. Structural changes of the ligaments occur relatively slowly in response to mechanical stresses because ligaments have **viscoelastic properties** that allow them to resist shear forces and return to their original form following the removal of a deforming load.[2,5,29]

viscoelastic properties The property of a material to show sensitivity to rate of loading.

With rapid loading, the ligaments become stiffer or resistant to changes in length and are able to absorb a high load or force before failure occurs. With this type of loading, overstress could produce a significant injury.[5]

Slow loading rates allow the ligament to lengthen as it absorbs the force of the load. Overstress can still produce injury, but it is not as severe as in the high loading rates. The amount of **ligament deformation** accompanying a low rate of loading is higher than in rapid loading situations. Loading should be applied slowly and comfortably.[5] The ligament deformation allows the spinal vertebrae to move apart.

In ligaments shortened or contracted by an injury or a long-term postural problem, traction is important in restoring normal length. The traction force provides the stress that encourages the ligament to make adaptive changes in length and strength. The traction force in this instance would have to be heavy enough to stimulate adaptive changes but not heavy enough to overwhelm the ligament. In acute severely sprained ligaments, a traction force may overwhelm the ligament and have a negative effect on the healing process. Traction treatment should be a part of an overall treatment program that includes strengthening and flexibility exercises.[2]

When they are stretched, the ligaments put pressure on or move other structures within the ligamentous structure (**proprioceptive nerves**) and external to the ligament structure (**disk material, synovial fringes,** vascular structures, nerve roots). This pressure or movement can have a tremendous impact on painful problems if pressure on a sensitive structure (nerve, vascular) is reduced. Activation of the proprioceptive system also relieves pain by providing a gating effect similar to a transcutaneous electrical nerve stimulation treatment.[2,8]

proprioceptive nervous system System of nerves that provide information on joint movement, pressure, and muscle tension.

EFFECTS ON THE DISK

The mechanical tension created by the traction has an excellent effect on **disk protrusions** and disk-related pain. Normally, the disk helps to dissipate compressive forces while the spine is in an erect posture (Fig. 15-2A).

In the normal disk, internal pressure increases but the nucleus pulposus (fluid-like center of the fibrocartilaginous vertebral disk) does not move with changes in the weight-bearing forces as the spine moves from flexion to extension.[31] When an injury occurs to the disk structures and the disk loses its normal fullness, the vertebrae can move closer together. The annular fibers bulge just as an underinflated car tire bulges when compared with a normally inflated one (Fig. 15-2B).[31]

If the disk is damaged and movement occurs in a weight-bearing position, the disk nucleus will shift according to fluid-dynamic principles. Pressure on one side squeezes the nucleus in the opposite direction (Fig. 15-2C). If tears develop in the annular fibers, the nucleus will tend to take the path of least resistance and move in this direction (Fig. 15-2D).

disk protrusion The abnormal projection of the disk nucleus through some or all of the annular rings.

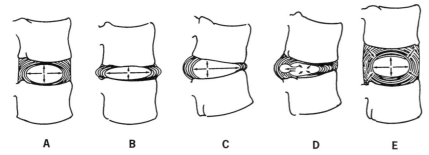

•**Figure 15-2** Fluid dynamics of the intervertebral disk. **A.** Normal disk in noncompressed position; internal pressure, indicated by arrows, is exerted relatively equally in all directions. The internal annular fibers contain the nuclear materials. **B.** Sitting or standing with compression of an injured disk causes the nucleus to become flatter. Pressure in this instance still remains relatively equal in all directions. **C.** In an injured disk, movement in the weight-bearing position causes a horizontal shift in the nuclear material. If this was forward bending, the bulge to the left would take place at the posterior annular fibers, whereas the anterior annular fibers would be slackened and narrow. **D.** Weakness of the annular wall would allow the nuclear material to create a herniation and possibly put pressure on sensitive structures in the area. **E.** When placed under traction, the intervertebral space expands, lowering the disk pressure. The taut annulus creates a centripetally directed force. Both these factors encourage the nuclear material to move and decrease the herniation and its effects.

annulus fibrosus The interlacing cross fibers of fibroelastic tissue that are attached to adjacent vertebral bodies that contain the nucleus pulposus.

Traction that increases the separation of the vertebral bodies decreases the central pressure in the disk space and encourages the **disk nucleus** to return to a central position. The mechanical tension of the **annulus fibrosus** and ligaments surrounding the disk also tends to force the nuclear material and cartilage fragments toward the center.[2,8,12,18,24,29,31]

Movement of these materials relieves pain and symptoms if they are compressing nervous or vascular structures. Decreasing the compressive forces also allows for better fluid interchange within the disk and spinal canal.[2,8] The reduction in **disk herniation** is unstable and the herniation tends to return when compressive forces return (Fig. 15-2D and E).[24,25]

The positive effect of traction in this instance may be destroyed by allowing the patient to sit after treatment. Minimizing compressive forces after treatment may be equally as important to the treatment's success as the traction.[2] The sitting posture increases the disk pressure, causing the nucleus to follow the path of least resistance and a return of the disk herniation.

EFFECTS ON ARTICULAR FACET JOINTS

facet joints Articular joints of the spine.

meniscoid structures A cartilage tip found on the synovial fringes of some facet joints.

The articular joints of the spine (**facet joints**) can be affected by traction, primarily through increased separation of the joint surfaces. **Meniscoid structures**, synovial fringes, or osteochondral fragments (calcified bone chips) impinged between joint surfaces are released and a dramatic reduction in symptoms is noticed when joint surfaces are separated. Increased joint separation decompresses the articular cartilage, allowing the synovial fluid exchange to nourish the cartilage. The separation may also decrease the rate of degenerative changes from osteoarthritis. Increased proprioceptive discharge from the facet joint structures provides some decrease in pain perception.[2,5,10,24]

EFFECTS ON THE MUSCULAR SYSTEM

Ligaments may be progressively stretched with traction.

The vertebral muscles can be effectively stretched by traction provided that the positions of the spine during traction are selected to optimize the stretch of particular muscle groups. The initial stretch should come from body positioning, and the addition of traction then provides some additional stretch. **Electromyographic recordings** of the spinal erector muscles during traction showed some decrease in EMG activity in most patients, indicating a muscular relaxation.[11,28] This effect can be enhanced by palpating the erector muscles and focusing the patient's attention on relaxing them. The muscular stretch lengthens tight muscle structures, or creates relaxation of contraction, allowing better muscular blood flow, and also activates muscle proprioceptors, providing even more of a gating influence on the pain. All these properties lead to a decrease in muscular irritation.[2,10,11,14,23,27]

EFFECTS ON THE NERVES

nerve root impingement Abnormal encroachment of some body tissue into the space occupied by the nerve root.

The nerve is the structure at which traction's effects are most often directed. Pressure on nerves or roots from bulging disk material, irritated facet joints, bony spurs, or narrowed foramen size causes the neurologic malfunctioning often associated with spinal pain. Tingling is usually the first clinical sign indicating that there is pressure on a nerve structure. If the pressure is not relieved or if damage of the nerve as a result of trauma or anoxia has resulted in an inflammation, the tingling may not respond to traction.[10,12,20,30,31,36,38]

Unrelieved pressure on a nerve causes slowing and eventual loss of impulse conduction. The signs of motor weakness, numbness, and loss of reflex become progressively more apparent and are indicative of nerve degeneration. Pain, tenderness, and muscular spasm are also associated with continued pressure on the nerve.

CASE STUDY 15-1
MECHANICAL TRACTION

Background: A 49-year-old man developed lower cervical pain 4 days ago after trimming trees in his yard for several hours. He has been referred for symptomatic treatment of his mechanical neck pain; there are no neural deficits, and no signs of a disk lesion. The patient is experiencing pain in the midline of the lower cervical area, and across the upper trapezius area bilaterally. His active range of motion is normal, but is painful at the end of range in all planes, and overpressure increases the symptoms. Extension (back bending) is the most painful motion.

Impression: Soft-tissue injury of the lower cervical spine.

Treatment Plan: To assist in pain relief, a 3-day per week course of intermittent mechanical cervical traction was initiated. The patient was positioned supine on the traction table, and the traction unit was adjusted to produce approximately 20 degrees of cervical flexion during traction. For the initial session, 20 lb of traction was applied, with four progressive steps up, and four regressive steps down. Each traction cycle consisted of 15 seconds of tension, followed by 20 seconds of rest. Total treatment time was 20 minutes. The target traction force was increased by 10 percent each session, to a maximum of 40 lb. In addition to the traction, active exercise was prescribed.

Response: The patient reported a transient increase in symptoms following the first two sessions, then a gradual resolution of the symptoms. There was a marked reduction in symptoms immediately following the third session; the relief persisted for approximately 2 hours. Cervical traction was discontinued after a total of six sessions, and the patient was instructed in a home exercise program. Two weeks later, the patient was asymptomatic.

Discussion Questions

- What tissues were injured/affected?
- What symptoms were present?
- What phase of the injury-healing continuum did the patient present for care in?
- What are the physical agent modality's biophysical effects (direct/indirect/depth/tissue affinity)?
- What are the physical agent modality's indications/contraindications?
- What are the parameters of the physical agent modality's application/dosage/duration/frequency in this case study?
- What other physical agent modalities could be utilized to treat this injury or condition? Why? How?
- What was the mechanism of injury to the cervical spine?
- What were the physiological effects of the cervical traction?
- Why was the supine position used for the treatment?
- What additional physical agents may have been helpful for this patient?
- What are the contraindications to cervical traction?
- Why were the symptoms initially increased?

The rehabilitation professional employs physical agent modalities to create an optimum environment for tissue healing while minimizing the symptoms associated with the trauma or condition.

Anything that decreases the pressure on the nerve increases the blood's circulation to the nerve, decreasing edema and allowing the nerve to return to normal functioning. Some degenerative changes are reversible, depending on the amount of degeneration and the amount of fibrosis that occur during the repair process.[2,10,36,38]

EFFECTS ON THE ENTIRE BODY PART

The previous discussion outlined the effect of traction on the major systems involved in spine-related pain and dysfunction. The complexity and interrelationships among these systems make determining specific causes of pain and dysfunction very difficult. Traction is not specific to one system but has an effect on each system, and collectively the effect can be very satisfactory. Traction can affect the pathologic process in any of the systems, and then all the structures involved can begin to normalize. Traction should not stand alone as a treatment but should be considered as part of an overall treatment plan, and each component of any spine-related dysfunction should be treated with other appropriate modalities.[1,2,5,8,23,30–32,38]

TRACTION TREATMENT TECHNIQUES

The literature on traction and its clinical effectiveness is somewhat limited.[6,8,12,24,31,37,39,45] Most of the clinical studies go into great depth about the pathology being treated, but unfortunately they provide only a cursory description of the traction setup, making duplication of the traction method difficult.[39]

The following discussion of specific traction setups is organized according to lumbar and cervical traction. Each of these areas will contain discussions of postural, manual, and machine-assisted traction. The traction setups mentioned in this chapter should be used as starting points in a treatment plan. The parameters of time, position, and traction force should be adapted to the patient, rather than forcing the patient to adapt to a predetermined traction setup.

The treatment plan should include the clinical criteria for judging the success and continued use of traction. Positive changes should occur within 5–8 treatment days if traction is going to be successful, for example, if a patient has a positive straight leg raise sign (i.e., pain in the back with a passive straight leg raise). This is a measurable clinical criterion that can be used to judge the treatment's success. If the straight leg raise test is positive at 20 degrees of hip flexion before and after traction, and after successive treatments the straight leg raise test is positive at increasing degrees of hip flexion, then the treatment can be considered successful.[26]

LUMBAR POSITIONAL TRACTION

> Traction is most often used to treat nerve root impingement.

Spinal nerve root impingement, from a variety of causes ranging from disk herniation or prolapse to spondylolisthesis, is the leading diagnosis for which traction is prescribed. Traction has also been used to treat joint hypomobility, arthritic conditions of the facet joints, mechanically produced muscle spasm, and joint pain.[2,11,12,30,31,36,40,45]

Normal spinal mechanics allow movements to occur that narrow or enlarge the intervertebral foramina. If the patient is placed in the supine position with hips and knees flexed, the lumbar spine bends forward and the spinous processes separate. This movement increases the size of the **intervertebral foramen** bilaterally (Fig. 15-3). The flexed postures used to treat low-back pain are examples of this positional traction.

> **unilateral foramen opening** Enlargement of the foramen on one side of a vertebral segment.

The greatest **unilateral foramen opening** occurs by positioning the patient sidelying with a pillow or blanket roll between the iliac crest and the lower border of the rib cage. The side on which increased foramen opening is desired should be superior. The roll should be close to the level of the spine where the traction separation is desired. The spine side bends around the roll (Fig. 15-4). The patient's hips and knees are then flexed until the lumbar spine is in a forward-bent position (Fig. 15-5A). This accentuates the opening of a foramen. Maximal opening can be achieved by adding trunk rotation toward the side of the superior shoulder (Fig. 15-5B).[31,36–38]

Positional traction is normally used when the patient is on a very restricted activity program because of low-back pain. The positions are used on a trial-and-error basis to determine maximum comfort and to attempt to relieve pressure on nerve roots.

The results of the patient evaluation should be used to determine whether the painful side should be up or down when using the sidelying positional traction technique. Protective scoliosis is the most obvious sign that will help determine patient position. If the patient leans away from the painful side, the painful side should be up (Fig. 15-6A). If the patient leans toward the painful side, the painful side should be down (Fig. 15-6B).

It should be added that the patient should be evaluated following the first treatment to determine changes in symptoms. Hopefully the patient will describe excellent results, but it is not uncommon to complain of increased pain.

The location of the pressure from the disk herniation was previously believed to cause these signs. Further research suggests that hand dominance may be more of a

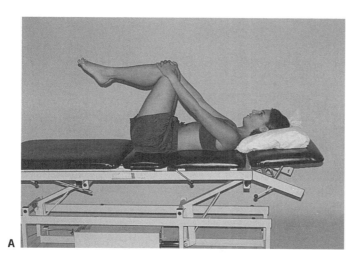

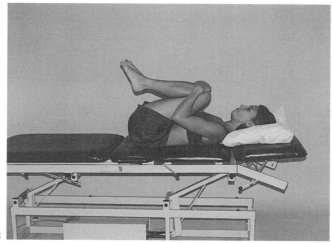

•**Figure 15-3 A.** Positional traction; **B.** Knees-to-chest posture can be used to increase the size of the lumbar intervertebral foramen bilaterally.

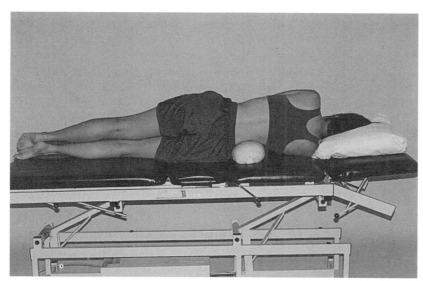

•**Figure 15-4** Positional traction; patient positioned sidelying with a blanket roll between iliac crest and rib cage. This increases the intervertebral foramen size of the left side of the lumbar spine.

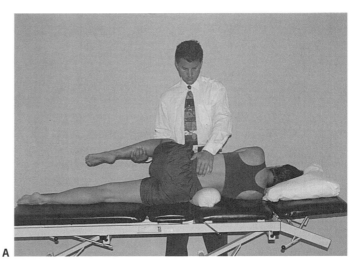

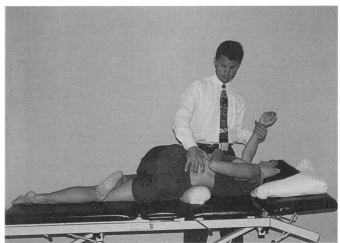

•**Figure 15-5** Positional traction; maximum opening of the intervertebral foramen of the left side of the patient's lumbar spine is achieved by flexing the upper hip and knee and rotating the patient's shoulders so he or she is looking over the left shoulder (left rotation).

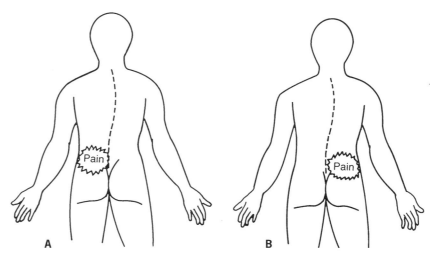

•**Figure 15-6 A.** Patient leaning away from the painful side. The patient's left side should be placed up while sidelying over a blanket roll to open up the upper foramen or the nerve roots away from the lateral herniation or both. **B.** Patient leaning toward the painful side. The patient's left side should be placed up while sidelying over a blanket roll to pull the nerve roots away from a medial herniation.

factor than herniation location in producing this scoliosis. However, the patient may be more compliant with the treatment regime if simple mechanical explanations such as pushing the herniation back into place are used.[33]

Patients with these symptoms may also be good candidates for unilateral traction.[2,5,30,31,35,38] Facet irritation is capable of causing similar scoliotic curves; in most instances the scoliosis is convex toward the painful side.

INVERSION TRACTION

Inversion traction, another positional traction, is used for prevention and treatment of back problems.[13] Specialized equipment or simply hanging upside down from a chinning bar places a person in the inverted position.[13] The spinal column is lengthened because of the stretch provided by the weight of the trunk. The force of the trunk in this position is usually calculated to be approximately 40 percent of body weight (Fig. 15-7).[19]

When the person is comfortable and able to relax, the length of the spinal column increases. These length changes coincide with decreases in spinal muscle activity.[1,2,6,7,17,21,22,28]

No research-supported protocols exist for this method of traction, although a slow progression of time in the inverted position seems to be best. One study suggests the electromyographic activity decreases after 70 seconds in the inverted position. If the patient is comfortable completely inverted, 70 seconds may be used as a minimum treatment time. The inverted position may be repeated two or three times at a treatment session, with a 2- to 3-minute rest between bouts. Longer treatment times also may enhance results. Maximum treatment times range from 10–30 minutes. Setup procedures are equipment-dependent and the manufacturer's protocols should be followed and modified as necessary to meet the needs of the patient.[1,2,3,9,28]

Blood pressure should be monitored while the patient is in the inverted position. If a rise of 20 mm of mercury above the resting diastolic pressure is found, the therapist should stop the treatment for that session.[2,3,28]

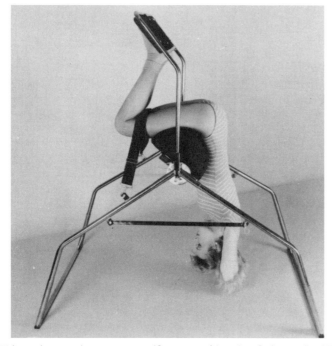

•**Figure 15-7** Inversion traction apparatus. (Courtesy of Lossing Orthopaedic, Minneapolis, MN 55404.)

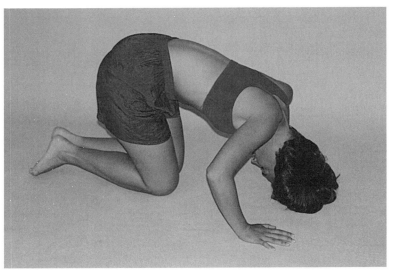

•**Figure 15-8** Inversion tolerance test position. Any vertigo, dizziness, or nausea may indicate that this patient is a poor candidate for inversion treatment.

Contraindications include hypertensive (140/90) individuals and anyone with heart disease or glaucoma. Patients with sinus problems, diabetes, thyroid conditions, asthma, migraine headaches, detached retinas, or hiatal hernias should consult their physicians before treatment is initiated.

Recent surgery or musculoskeletal problems to the lower limb may require modification of the inversion apparatus. In addition, meals or snacks should not be eaten during the hour before treatment to keep the patient comfortable.

One method of testing the patient's tolerance to the inverted position is to have the patient assume the hand-knee position and put his or her head on the floor, holding that position for 60 seconds. Any vertigo, dizziness, or nausea may indicate that this patient is a poor candidate for inversion and that the treatment progression should be very slow (Fig. 15-8).[1–3,6,7,9,17,21,22,28]

MANUAL LUMBAR TRACTION

Manual lumbar traction is used for lumbar spine problems to test the patient's tolerance to traction, to arrive at the most comfortable treatment setup, to make the traction as specific to one vertebral level as possible, and to provide the specificity needed for a traction mobilization of the spine. If the patient's back pain is diminished by having the therapist flex the patient's hips and knees to 90 degrees each and apply enough pressure under the calves to lift the buttocks off the table, then the patient is a good candidate for spine 90-90-degree traction. The disadvantage is that maintaining the large forces necessary for separation of the lumbar vertebrae for a period of time is difficult and energy-consuming for the therapist.[2,35,38]

Having a split table will eliminate most of the friction between the patient's body segments and the treatment table and is essential for effective delivery of manual lumbar traction (Fig. 15-9).[2,5,25,36,38] The therapist's effort does not cause separation of the vertebral segments unless the frictional forces are overcome first.

LEVEL-SPECIFIC MANUAL TRACTION

To make the traction specific to a vertebral level, the patient is positioned sidelying on the split table. For traction specific to L3-4, L4-5, and L5-S1 levels, the patient's

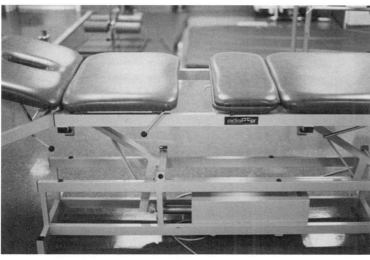

•**Figure 15-9** Split table with movable section to decrease frictional forces.

lumbar spine is flexed, using the patient's upper leg as a lever. The therapist palpates the interspinous area between two spinous processes. The upper spinous process is the one at which maximum effect is desired. When the lumbar spine flexes and the therapist feels the motion of the lower spinous process with the palpating hand, the foot is placed against the opposite leg so that further flexion is not allowed (see Fig. 15-5A). The patient's trunk is rotated by the therapist until motion of the upper spinous process is felt by the therapist. Trunk rotation should be passively produced by the therapist, positioning the patient's upper arm with hand on the rib cage, and pulling on the patient's lower arm, creating trunk rotation toward the upper arm. In this case it is rotation to the left (see Fig. 15-5B).

If lumbar levels T12, L1, L1-2, and L2-3 are to be given specific traction, the patient is again positioned sidelying. These levels require positioning in reverse order from the lower levels. First the trunk is rotated, then the lumbar spine is flexed.[2,5]

In both instances the rotation and flexion tighten and lock joint structures in which these motions have taken place, leaving the desired segment with more movement available than the upper or lower levels. When traction is applied, greater movement of the desired level occurs, whereas movement at other levels is minimized because of the joint locking created by the preliminary positioning.

The split table is then released and the therapist palpates the spinous processes of the selected intervertebral level, places his or her chest against the anterior superior iliac spine of the patient's upper hip, and leans toward the patient's feet. Enough force is used to cause a palpable separation of the spinous processes (Fig. 15-10). Intermittent movement is most easily accomplished, whereas sustained traction becomes physically more difficult.[2,5]

UNILATERAL LEG PULL MANUAL TRACTION

Unilateral leg pull traction has been used in the treatment of hip joint problems or difficult lateral shift corrections. A thoracic countertraction harness is used to secure the patient to the table. The therapist grabs the patient's ankle and brings the patient's hip into 30-degree flexion, 30-degree abduction, and full external rotation. A steady pull is applied until a noticeable distraction is felt (Fig. 15-11).[5]

In suspected sacroiliac joint problems, a similar setup can be used. A banana strap is placed through the groin on the side to be stretched. This strap will secure the patient in position. The therapist grabs the patient's ankle, brings his or her hip into 30-degree

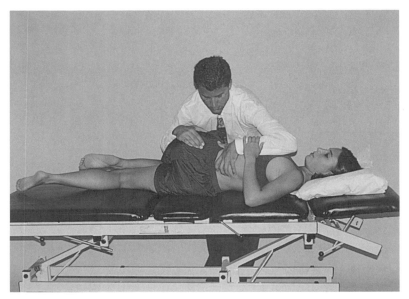

•Figure 15-10 Manual lumbar traction with maximum effect at a specific level. The therapist has positioned the patient for maximum effect and is palpating the interspinous area between the two spinous processes where maximum traction effect is desired. The therapist then places his or her chest against the anterior superior iliac spine and the patient's upper hip. The split table is released and the therapist leans toward the patient's feet, using enough force to cause a palpable separation of the spinous processes at the desired level.

flexion and 15-degree abduction, and then applies a sustained or intermittent pull to create a mobilizing effect on the sacroiliac joint (Fig. 15-12).[5]

As a preliminary to mechanical traction, manual traction is helpful in determining what degree of lumbar flexion, extension, or sidebending is most comfortable and will also give an indication of the treatment's success. The most comfortable position is usually the best therapeutic position.[5,35,37]

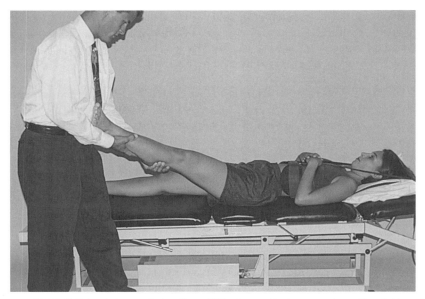

•Figure 15-11 Unilateral leg pull traction. With the patient secured to the table with a thoracic countertraction harness, the therapist brings the patient's hip into 30-degree flexion, 30-degree abduction, and maximum external rotation. A steady pull is then applied.

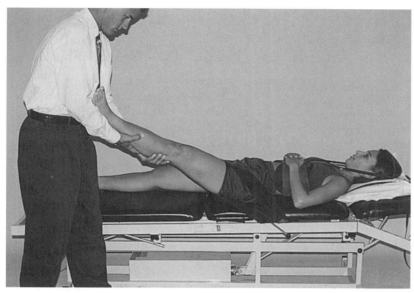

•Figure 15-12 Unilateral leg pull traction for sacroiliac joint problems. A strap is placed through the groin and secured to the table. The therapist brings the patient's hip into 30-degree flexion and 15-degree abduction, and then applies a traction force to the leg.

Patient comfort may have a bigger impact on the traction's results than the angle of pull, the force used, the mode, or the duration of the treatment. The inability of the patient to relax in any traction setup affects the traction's ability to cause a separation of the vertebrae. The lack of vertebral separation minimizes some of the traction's therapeutic benefits.[5,35,38]

MECHANICAL LUMBAR TRACTION

When using mechanical traction, the therapist will have to select and adjust the following seven parameters of the traction equipment and patient position.

Traction will return disk nucleus to a central position.

1. Body position: prone, supine, hip position, bilateral, or unilateral direction of pull
2. Force used
3. Intermittent traction: traction time and rest time
4. Sustained traction
5. Duration of treatment
6. Progressive steps
7. Regressive steps

The research on mechanical lumbar traction gives us a strong protocol for using traction to decrease disk protrusion and nerve root symptoms. The protocols for use in other pathologies are not supported by research, but clinical empiricism and inference from some of the research give a good working protocol. The therapist will need to match the traction treatment to the patient's symptoms and make adjustments based on the clinical results.[5,12,29,35,42]

Traction can relieve pressure on a nerve root.

PATIENT SETUP AND EQUIPMENT

A split table or other mechanism to eliminate friction between body segments and the table surface is a prerequisite to effective lumbar traction. Otherwise, most of the force applied would be spent overcoming the coefficient of friction (see Fig. 15-9).[1,2,5,17,25,36,38,42]

CASE STUDY 15-2
SPINAL TRACTION: LUMBAR

Background: A 58-year-old pharmacist has an 11-year history of recurrent low back pain. The onset was insidious, and he has developed episodes of moderately severe low back pain three or four times per year since the initial episode. This episode started 9 days ago after playing 18 holes of golf and is the most severe episode ever. He has constant pain in the right lumbo-sacral area, with radiation of the pain into the right buttock, and down the posterio-lateral aspect of the thigh and leg into the foot, with paresthesia in the lateral foot. He demonstrates weakness in the S1 myotome, a loss of the right ankle jerk, and positive tests for adverse neural tension on the right. He was referred to a neurosurgeon, who obtained an MRI. The MRI revealed a moderately large right posterio-lateral bulge of the intervertebral disc at L5S1, with a loss of disc height. The neurosurgeon recommended surgery, but the patient opted for a trial of conservative treatment. The patient was referred for lumbar traction and therapeutic exercise.

Impression: S1 nerve root compression due to L5S1 disc lesion.

Treatment Plan: Motorized static lumbar traction with the patient prone on the traction table was initiated. For the initial treatment session, the traction device was set to apply 14 kg (31 lb) of distractive force, which was equal to one-sixth of the patient's body weight. The force was increased in three steps over a 3-minute period, then the force was maintained at 14 kg for 4 minutes, then removed in two steps over a 2-minute period. Because this initial session did not exacerbate the patient's symptoms, therapeutic traction was administered on a daily basis starting the next day, with a distraction force of 41 kg (90 lb), or one-half of the patient's body weight. The traction increased to the therapeutic dose in three steps over a 3-minute period, the maximal force was maintained for 10 minutes, then decreased to 0 in two steps over a 2-minute period. The patient then performed therapeutic exercise to maintain a lordosis of the lumbar spine before getting off the table.

Response: Following each treatment session, the patient noted diminished peripheral and central symptoms for approximately 1 hour. There was no sustained improvement after 10 sessions, and the patient elected to return to the neurosurgeon for surgical treatment.

Discussion Questions

- What tissues were injured or affected?
- What symptoms were present?
- What phase of the injury-healing continuum did the patient present for care in?
- What are the physical agent modality's biophysical effects (direct, indirect, depth, and tissue affinity)?
- What are the physical agent modality's indications and contraindications?
- What are the parameters of the physical agent modality's application, dosage, duration, and frequency in this case study?
- What other physical agent modalities could be used to treat this injury or condition? Why? How?
- Why was the initial treatment applied with such a low force? If the patient had noted an increase in the symptoms following this initial session, how would the therapist have proceeded?
- How much force is needed to achieve distraction of the vertebrae? How much is required to damage the vertebral motion segment?
- Why was the therapeutic distraction force applied for only 10 minutes? What are the advantages and disadvantages of a shorter session? A longer session?
- What is the most likely reason the traction was not successful in this patient? Would the treatment have been more or less likely to be successful if it had been initiated immediately after the onset of the symptoms?

The rehabilitation professional employs physical agent modalities to create an optimum environment for tissue healing while minimizing the symptoms associated with the trauma or condition.

A nonslip traction harness is needed to transfer the traction force comfortably to the patient and to stabilize the trunk while the lumbar spine is placed under traction. A harness lined with a vinyl material is best because it adheres to the patient's skin and does not slip like the cotton-lined harness. Clothing between the harness and the skin will also promote slipping. The vinyl-sided harness does not have to be as constricting as the cotton-backed harness to prevent slippage, thus increasing the patient's comfort (Fig. 15-13).[5,36,38]

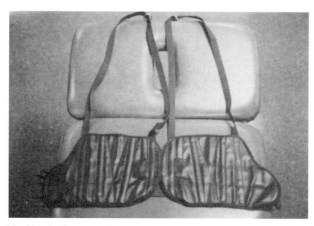

•**Figure 15-13** Vinyl-backed traction harness.

The harness can be applied when the patient is standing next to the traction table prior to treatment. The pelvic harness is applied so the contact pads and upper belt are at or just above the level of the iliac crest (Fig. 15-14).

Shirts should never be tucked under the pelvic harness because some of the tractive force would be dissipated pulling on the shirt material. The contact pads should be adjusted so that the harness loops provide a posteriorly directed pull, encouraging lumbar flexion (Fig. 15-15). The harness firmly adheres to the patient's hips.[5,36,38]

The rib belt is then applied in a similar manner with the rib pads positioned over the lower rib cage in a comfortable manner. The rib belt is then snugged up and the patient is positioned on the table (Fig. 15-16).[5,36,38]

The standing application of the traction harness is easier and more effective if the patient is to be placed in prone position for treatment (Fig. 15-17).[5,33,36] The traction harness can also be applied by laying it out on the traction table and having the patient lie down on top of it. The pads are then adjusted and the belts snugged with the patient lying down.

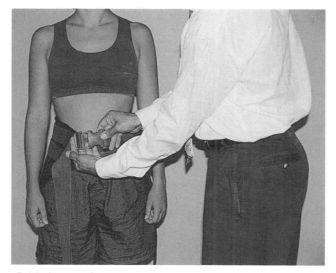

•**Figure 15-14** Pelvic harness for mechanical lumbar traction. The contact pads are applied so that the upper belt is at or just above the level of the iliac crest.

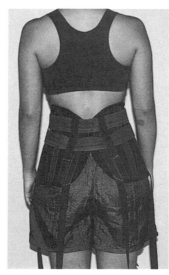

•**Figure 15-15** The traction straps from the pelvic harness should bracket the patient's buttocks if a lumbar flexion pull is desired. If a straight pull is desired, the pelvic harness should be adjusted so that the straps bracket the patient's lateral hip area.

BODY POSITION

Body position has been reported to have a substantial impact on traction results, but this has been empirically derived rather than research supported. The therapist needs a satisfactory understanding of the mechanics of the lumbar spine to make decisions about position that will best affect a patient's symptoms.[2,5,24,31,36,38,42]

Generally, the neutral spinal position allows for the largest intervertebral foramen opening, and it is usually the position of choice whether the patient is prone or supine. Extension beyond neutral lumbar spine causes the bony elements of the foramen to create a narrower opening. Lumbar spinal flexion beyond neutral causes the ligamentum flavum and other soft tissues to constrict the foramen's opening (Fig. 15-18).[35,37]

Saunders recommends the prone position with a normal to slightly flattened lumbar lordosis (an abnormal anterior curve) as the position of choice in disk protrusions.[36,38] The amount of lordosis may be controlled by using pillows under the

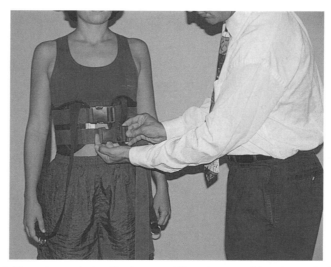

•**Figure 15-16** Thoracic countertraction harness. Rib pads are positioned over the lower rib cage.

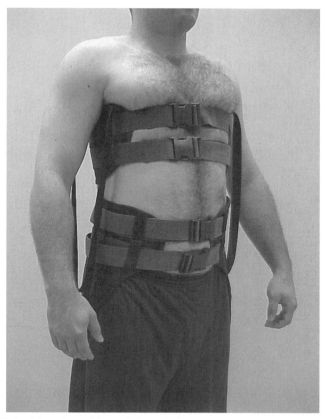

•**Figure 15-17** Applying the pelvic and thoracic harnesses may be easier if done while the patient is standing.

abdomen. The prone position also allows the easy application of other modalities to the pain area and an easier assessment of the amount of spinous process separation (Fig. 15-19).[5,36,38]

In traction applied to a patient in the supine position, hip position was found to affect vertebral separation. As hip flexion increased from 0 to 90 degrees, traction produced a greater posterior intervertebral space separation (Fig. 15-20).[34]

Unilateral pelvic traction also has been recommended when a stronger force is desired on one side of the spine. Patients with protective scoliosis, unilateral joint dysfunction, or unilateral lumbar muscle spasm with scoliosis may do quite well with this approach. Only one side of the pelvic harness is hooked to the traction device to accomplish this technique (Fig. 15-21).[38]

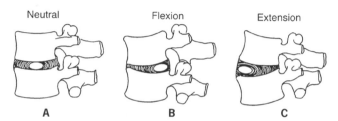

•**Figure 15-18 A.** Neutral lumbar spine position allows for the largest intervertebral foramen opening before traction is applied. **B.** Flexion puts pressure on the disk nucleus to move posterior, although it may tend to increase the posterior opening. Other soft tissue may also close the foramen opening. **C.** Extension beyond neutral tends to close the foramen down as the bony arches come closer together.

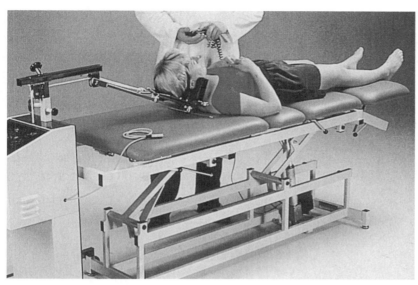

•**Figure 15-29** Mechanical cervical traction; patient in the supine position with traction harness placed so that maximum pull is exerted on the occiput and the patient is in a position of approximately 20–30 degrees of neck flexion.

A traction force above 20 lb, applied intermittently for a minimum of 7 seconds' traction time and with adequate rest time for recovery, is recommended (Fig. 15-30). This traction should be continued over 20–25 minutes. Higher forces up to 50 lb may produce increased separation, but the other parameters should remain the same. The average separation at the posterior vertebral area is 1–1.5 mm per space, while the anterior vertebral area separates approximately 0.4 mm per space. Greater separations are expected in the younger population than in the older population. Within 20–25 minutes from the time traction is stopped and normal sitting or standing postures are resumed, the vertebral separation returns to its previous heights. The upper cervical segments do not separate as easily as lower cervical segments.[8,10,24] The addition of pain-reducing and heating modalities will add to the benefits gained by the traction.[1,2,5,10,24]

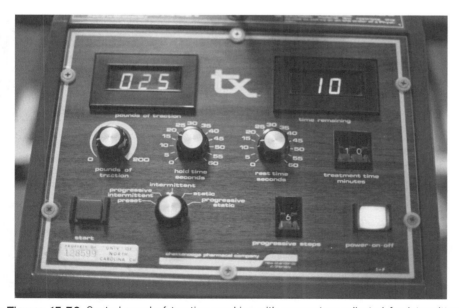

•**Figure 15-30** Control panel of traction machine with parameters adjusted for intermittent cervical traction.

CASE STUDY 15-3
SPINAL TRACTION: CERVICAL

Background: A 47-year-old woman noted an ache in the right midcervical area upon awakening this morning. While driving to work, she turned her head to the right before changing lanes, and noted an audible click with severe pain in the right midcervical area. After arriving at work, she continued to experience localized pain that gradually worsened over the next hour. She presented to the emergency room, where an examination (including radiographic) revealed no neurologic or bony injury. She was referred for treatment of an acute neck sprain. She does not have radiating pain, and the neurologic examination is negative. She holds her head tilted and rotated to the left, and any attempt at side bend or rotation to the right produces severe, localized right midcervical pain. She is very tender over the right articular pillar at C4-5, and passive mobility testing reveals a markedly restricted joint play at C4-5.

Impression: Acute locking of the cervical spine (C4-5).

Treatment Plan: Manual cervical traction. With the patient supine on a treatment table, the therapist placed one hand under the patient's head, with the palm over the occiput, thumb over one mastoid process, and the fingertips over the opposite mastoid process. The therapist's other hand was placed over the patient's forehead to avoid compressive forces on the temporo-mandibular joint. A gentle distraction force was applied (approximately 5 kg), with the line of force parallel to the long axis of the spine. The force was held for 3 seconds, then released for 10 seconds. This was repeated 10 times, with the distraction force gradually increased to a maximum of approximately 15 kilograms.

Response: A reassessment was performed after the 10th force application, and the patient was able to hold her neck in a neutral position. The cycle was repeated four more times, with a gradual improvement in cervical range of motion and a reduction in pain each time. After the fifth cycle, she was able to attain rotation and side bending to the right equal to approximately 80 percent that of the motion to the left. She was treated the following day with the same approach, and attained full, pain-free range of motion.

Discussion Questions

- What tissues were injured or affected?
- What symptoms were present?
- What phase of the injury-healing continuum did the patient present for care in?
- What are the physical agent modality's biophysical effects (direct, indirect, depth, and tissue affinity)?
- What are the physical agent modality's indications and contraindications?
- What are the parameters of the physical agent modality's application, dosage, duration, and frequency in this case study?
- What other physical agent modalities could be used to treat this injury or condition? Why? How?
- What is the mechanism for acute locking of the cervical spine?
- What are the advantages of manual traction over mechanical (motorized) traction for this patient? Disadvantages?
- Why was the distraction force applied parallel to the long axis of the spine? What advantages or disadvantages would there be to applying the force along an oblique axis?

The rehabilitation professional employs physical agent modalities to create an optimum environment for tissue healing while minimizing the symptoms associated with the trauma or condition.

INDICATIONS AND CONTRAINDICATIONS

As discussed throughout this chapter, there are a number of conditions for which spinal traction may be useful, including cases where there is impingement on a nerve root resulting from disk herniation, spondylolisthesis, narrowing within the intervertebral foramen, or osteophyte formation; degenerative joint diseases, subacute pain; joint hypomobility; discogenic pain; and muscle spasm.

Traction, except as a light mobilization, is contraindicated in acute sprains or strains (first 3–5 days), acute inflammation, or in any conditions in which movement is either undesirable or exacerbates the existing problem. In cases of vertebral joint instability, traction may perpetuate the instability or cause further strain. Certainly, the serious problems associated with tumors, bone diseases, osteoporosis, and infections in bones or joints are also contraindications. Patients who can potentially experience problems relating to the fitting of a harness, such as those with vascular conditions, pregnant females, or those with cardiac or pulmonary problems, should also avoid traction.

SUMMARY

1. Traction has been used to treat a variety of cervical and lumbar spine problems. The effect of traction on each system involved in the complex anatomic makeup of the spine needs to be considered when selecting traction as a part of a therapeutic treatment plan.

2. The traction protocol should be set up to manage a particular problem rather than applied in the same manner regardless of the patient or pathology. Traction is a flexible modality with an infinite number of variations available. This flexibility allows the therapist to adjust protocols to match the patient's symptoms and diagnosis.

3. Traction is capable of producing a separation of vertebral bodies; a centripetal force on the soft tissues surrounding the vertebrae; a mobilization of vertebral joints; a change in proprioceptive discharge of the spinal complex; a stretch of connective tissue; a stretch of muscle tissue; an improvement in arterial, venous, and lymphatic flow; and a lessening of the compressive effects of posture. Any of these effects can change the symptoms of the patient under treatment and help to normalize the patient's lumbar or cervical spine.

REVIEW QUESTIONS

1. What is traction and how may it be performed by the therapist?

2. What are the physical effects and therapeutic value of spinal traction on bone, muscle, ligaments, facet joints, nerve, blood vessels, and intervertebral disks?

3. What are the clinical advantages of using positional lumbar traction and inversion traction?

4. What are the clinical applications for using manual lumbar traction techniques, including level specific manual traction, and unilateral leg pull manual traction?

5. What are the setup procedures and treatment parameter considerations for using mechanical lumbar traction?

6. What are the advantages of using a manual traction technique of the cervical spine?

7. What is the setup procedure for mechanical and wall-mounted traction techniques for the cervical spine?

Indications and Contraindications for Spinal Traction

Indications
Impingement on a nerve root
Disk herniation
Spondylolisthesis
Narrowing within the intervertebral foramen
Osteophyte formation
Degenerative joint diseases
Subacute pain
Joint hypomobility
Discogenic pain
Muscle spasm or guarding
Muscle strain
Spinal ligament or connective tissues contractures
Improvement in arterial, venous, and lymphatic flow

Contraindications
Acute sprains or strains
Acute inflammation
Fractures
Vertebral joint instability
Any condition in which movement exacerbates the existing problem
Tumors
Bone diseases
Osteoporosis
Infections in bones or joints
Vascular conditions
Pregnancy
Cardiac or pulmonary problems

REFERENCES

1. Bridger, R.: Effect of lumbar traction on stature, Spine 15:522–524, 1990.
2. Burkhardt, S.: Course notes, cervical and lumbar traction seminar, Morgantown, WV, 1983.
3. Cooperman, J., Scheid, D.: Guidelines for the use of inversion, Clin. Manage. 4(1):6, 1984.
4. Dorland's illustrated medical dictionary, ed. 24, Philadelphia, PA, 1965, W.B. Saunders.
5. Erhard, R.: Course notes, cervical and lumbar traction seminar, Morgantown, WV, 1983.
6. Gianakopoulos, G.: Inversion devices: their role in producing lumbar distraction, Arch. Phys. Med. Rehabil. 68:100–102, 1985.
7. Goldman, R.: The effects of oscillating inversion on systemic blood pressure pulse, intraocular pressure and central retinal arterial pressure, Phys. Sports Med. 13(3):93–96, 1985.
8. Grieve, G.: Neck traction, Physiotherapy 6:260–265, 1982.
9. Gudenhoven, R.: Gravitational lumbar traction, Arch. Phys. Med. Rehabil. 59:510–512, 1978.
10. Harris, P.: Cervical traction: review of the literature and treatment guidelines, Phys. Ther. 57:910–914, 1977.

11. Hood, C.: Comparison of EMG activity in normal lumbar sacrospinalis musculature during continuous and intermittent pelvic traction, JOSPT 2:137–141, 1981.

12. Hood, L., Chrisman, D.: Intermittent pelvic traction in the treatment of the ruptured intervertebral disk, Phys. Ther. 48:21–30, 1968.

13. Houlding, M.: Clinical perspective. Inversion traction: a clinical appraisal, N.Z.J. Physiother. 26(2):23–24, 1998.

14. Jett, D.: Effect of intermittent, supine cervical traction on the myoelectric activity of the upper trapezius muscle in subjects with neck pain, Phys. Ther. 65:1173–1176, 1985.

15. Katavich, L.: Neural mechanisms underlying manual cervical traction, J. Manual Manipulative Ther. 7(1):20–25, 1999.

16. KeKosz, U.: Cervical and lumbopelvic traction, Post Grad. Med. 80(8):187–194, 1986.

17. Kent, B.: Anatomy of the trunk, Part I, Phys. Ther. 54: 722–744, 1974.

18. Kent, B.: Anatomy of the trunk, Part II, Phys. Ther. 54: 850–859, 1974.

19. Klatz, R.: Effects of gravity inversion on hypertensive subjects, Phys. Sports Med. 13(3):85–89, 1985.

20. Krause, M., Refshauge, K.M., Dessen, M., and Boland, R.: Lumbar spine traction: evaluation of effects and recommended application for treatment, Manual Ther. 5(2), 2000.

21. LaBan, M.: Intermittent traction: a progenitor of lumbar radicular pain, Arch. Phys. Med. Rehabil. 73:295–296, 1992.

22. LeMarr, J.: Cardiorespiratory responses to inversion, Phys. Sports Med. 11(11):51–57, 1983.

23. Letchuman, R., Deusinger, R.: Comparsion of sacrospinalis myoelectric activity and pain levels in patients undergoing static and intermittent lumbar traction, Spine 18:1261–1365, 1993.

24. Mathews, J.: The effects of spinal traction, Physiotherapy 58:64–66, 1972.

25. Mathews, J.: Dynamic discography: a study of lumbar traction, Ann. Phys. Med. 9:275–279, 1968.

26. Meszaros, T.F., Olson, R., and Kulig, K.: Effect of 10%, 30%, and 60% body weight traction on the straight leg raise test of symptomatic patients with low back pain, J. Orthop. Sports Phys. Ther. 30(10):595–601, 2000.

27. Murphy, M.: Effects of cervical traction on muscle activity, JOSPT 13:220–225, 1991.

28. Nosse, L.: Inverted spinal traction, Arch. Phys. Med. Rehabil. 59:367–370, 1978.

29. O'Donoghue, D.: Treatment of injuries to patients, ed. 3, Philadelphia, PA, 1978, W.B. Saunders.

30. Onel, D.: Computed tomographic investigation of the effects of traction on lumbar disc herniations, Spine 14:82–90, 1989.

31. Paris, S.: Course notes, basic course in spinal mobilization, Atlanta, GA, 1977.

32. Petulla, L.: Clinical observations with respect to progressive/regressive traction, JOSPT 7:261–263, 1986.

33. Porter, R., Miller, C.: Back pain and trunk list, Spine 11: 596–600, 1986.

34. Reilly, J.: Pelvic femoral position on vertebral separation produced by lumbar traction, Phys. Ther. 59:282–286, 1979.

35. Roaf, R.: A study of the mechanics of spinal injuries, J. Bone Joint Surg. 42B:810–819, 1960.

36. Saunders, D.: Use of spinal traction in the treatment of neck and back conditions, Clin. Orthop. 179:31–38, 1983.

37. Saunders, D.: Unilateral lumbar traction, Phys. Ther. 61: 221–225, 1981.

38. Saunders, D.: Lumbar traction, JOSPT 1:36–45, 1979.

39. Saunders, H.D.: The controversy over traction for neck and low back pain, Physiotherapy 84(6):285–288, 1998.

40. Sood, N.: Prone cervical traction, Clin. Manage. Phys. Ther. 7(6):37, 1987.

41. Stoddard, A: Traction for cervical nerve root irritation, Physiotherapy 40:48–49, 1954.

42. Strapp, E.J.: Lumbar traction: suggestions for treatment parameters, Sports Med. Update 13(4):9–11, 1998.

43. Varma, S.: The role of traction in cervical spondylosis, Physiotherapy 59:248–249, 1973.

44. Walker, G.: Goodley polyaxial cervical traction: a new approach to a traditional treatment, Phys. Ther. 66:1255–1259, 1986.

45. Weinert, A., Rizzo, T.: Non-operative management of multilevel lumbar disk herniations in an adolescent patient, Mayo Clin. Proc. 67:137–141, 1992.

SUGGESTED READINGS

Alice, M., Wong, M., and Chaupeng, I.: The traction angle and cervical intervertebral separation, Spine 17(2):136, 1992.

Beurskens, A., de Vet, H., and Koke, A.: Efficacy of traction for non-specific low back pain: a randomised clinical trial, Lancet 346(8990):1596–1600, 1995.

Beurskens, A., van der Heijden, G., and de Vet, H.: The efficacy of traction for lumbar back pain: design of a randomized clinical trial, J. Man. Physiol. Ther. 18(3):141–147, 1995.

Constantoyannis, C.: Intermittent cervical traction for cervical radiculopathy caused by large-volume herniated disks, J. Manipulative Physiol. Ther. 25(3):188–192, 2002.

Corkery, M.J.: The use of lumbar harness traction to treat a patient with lumbar radicular pain: a case report, Man. Manipulative Ther. 9(4):191–197, 2001.

Creighton, D.: Positional distraction, a radiological confirmation, J. Manual Man. Ther. 1(3):83–86, 1993.

Donkin, R.D.: Possible effect of chiropractic manipulation and combined manual traction and manipulation on tension-type headache: a pilot study, J. Neuromusc. Syst. 10(3):89–97, 2002.

Gilworth, G.: Cervical traction with active rotation, Physiotherapy 77(11):782–784, 1991.

Güvenol, K.: A comparison of inverted spinal traction and conventional traction in the treatment of lumbar disc herniations, Physiother. Theory Pract. 16(3):151–160, 2000.

Hariman, D.: The efficacy of cervical extension-compression traction combined with diversified manipulation and drop table adjustments in the rehabilitation of cervical lordosis: a pilot study, J. Man. Physiol. Ther. 18(5):323–325, 1995.

Harrison, D.E.: A new 3-point bending traction method for restoring cervical lordosis and cervical manipulation: a nonrandomized clinical controlled trial, Arch. Phys. Med. Rehabil. 83(4):447–453, 2002.

Harrison, D., Jackson, B., and Troyanovich, S.: The efficacy of cervical extension-compression traction combined with diversified manipulation and drop table adjustments in the rehabilitation of cervical lordosis: a pilot study, J. Man. Physiol. Ther. 18(5): 590–596, 1995.

Krause, M.: Lumbar spine traction: evaluation of effects and recommended application for treatment, Man. Ther. 5(2):72–81, 2000.

Lee, R.Y.: Loads in the lumbar spine during traction therapy, Aust. J. Physiother. 47(2):102–108, 2001.

Letchuman, R., Deusinger, R.: Comparison of sacrospinalis myoelectric activity and pain levels in patients undergoing static and intermittent lumbar traction, Spine 18(10):1361–1365, 1993.

Ljunggren, A., Walker, L., and Weber, H.: Manual traction vs. isometric exercise in patients with herniated intervertebral lumbar disks, Physiother. Theory Pract. 8:207, 1992.

Meszaros, T.F.: Effect of 10%, 30%, and 60% body weight traction on the straight leg raise test of symptomatic patients with low back pain, J. Orthop. Sports Phys. Ther. 30(10):595–601, 2000.

Nanno, M.: Effects of intermittent cervical traction on muscle pain. Flowmetric and electromyographic studies of the cervical paraspinal muscles, J. Nippon Med. School 61(2):137–147, 1994.

Pal, B., Magnion, P., and Hossian, M.: A controlled trial of continuous lumbar traction in the treatment of back pain and sciatica, Br. J. Rheumatol. 25:181, 1989.

Pellecchia, G.: Lumbar traction: a review of the literature, [review] JOSPT 20(5):262–267, 1994.

Pio, A., Rendina, M., and Benazzo, F.: The statics of cervical traction, J. Spinal Disord. 7(4):337–342, 1994.

Terahata, N., Ishihara, H., and Ohshima, H.: Effects of axial traction stress on solute transport and proteoglycan synthesis in the porcine intervertebral disc in vitro, Eur. Spine J. 3(6): 325–330, 1994.

Tesio, L., Merlo, A.: Autotraction versus passive traction: an open controlled study in lumbar disc herniation, Arch. Phys. Med. Rehabil. 74(8):871–876, 1993.

Trudel, G.: Autotraction, Arch. Phys. Med. Rehabil. 75(2): 234–235, 1994.

van der Heijden, G., Beurskens, A., and Koes, B.: The efficacy of traction for back and neck pain: a systematic, blinded review of randomized clinical trial methods, Phys. Ther. 75(2):93–104, 1995.

Wong, A., Leong, C., and Chen, C.: The traction angle and cervical intervertebral separation, Spine 17(2):136–138, 1992.

GLOSSARY

annulus fibrosus The interlacing cross-fibers of fibroelastic tissue that are attached to adjacent vertebral bodies that contain the nucleus pulposus.

anoxia Reduction of oxygen in body tissues below physiologic levels.

disk herniation The protrusion of the nucleus pulposus through a defect in the annulus fibrosus.

disk material Cartilaginous material from vertebral body surfaces, disk nucleus, or annulus fibrosus.

disk nucleus The protein polysaccharide gel that is contained between the cartilaginous endplates of the vertebrae and the annulus fibrosus.

disk protrusion The abnormal projection of the disk nucleus through some or all of the annular rings.

facet joints Articular joints of the spine.

fibrosis The formation of fibrous tissue in the injury repair process.

ligament deformation Lengthening distortion of ligament caused by traction loading.

meniscoid structures A cartilage tip found on the synovial fringes of some facet joints.

nerve root impingement Abnormal encroachment of some body tissue into the space occupied by the nerve root.

proprioceptive nervous system System of nerves that provides information on joint movement, pressure, and muscle tension.

spondylolisthesis Forward displacement of one vertebra over another.

synovial fringes Folds of synovial tissue that move in and out of the joint space.

traction Drawing tension applied to a body segment.

unilateral foramen opening Enlargement of the foramen on one side of a vertebral segment.

viscoelastic properties The property of a material to show sensitivity to rate of loading.

Wolff's law Bone remodels itself and provides increased strength along the lines of the mechanical forces placed on it.

LAB ACTIVITY

MECHANICAL TRACTION

DESCRIPTION

Mechanical traction has been used since ancient times in the treatment of painful spinal conditions. Simply, traction is applying tension to a body segment though a rope attached to various straps, halters, or devices. The therapeutic effect of traction is a function of the position of the spine, amount of traction force, and length of time the force is applied. Mechanical traction results in longitudinal separation of cervical or lumbar spinal segments with associated ligament, discal, neural, and muscular structures.

THERAPEUTIC EFFECTS

Separation of spinal segments
Elongation of muscle, ligament, and capsular tissue
Reduced intradiscal pressure

INDICATIONS

Mechanical traction is indicated to reduce the signs and symptoms of spinal compression. Appropriately applied mechanical traction can stretch facet joint capsules, increase the dimension of the intervertebral foramen thus increasing space for nerve roots, and alter intradiscal pressure. Paraspinal muscle tissues can also be elongated contributing to a reduction in the pain-spasm cycle, which frequently accompanies spinal dysfunction.

CONTRAINDICATIONS

- Spinal infection or malignancy
- Rheumatoid arthritis
- Osteoporosis
- Spinal hypermobility
- Acute stage injury
- Cardiac or respiratory insufficiency
- Pregnancy

MECHANICAL TRACTION

PROCEDURE	EVALUATION		
	1	2	3
1. Check supplies and equipment.			
a. Assemble towels, halters, harnesses, and belts.			
2. Question patient.			
a. Verify identity of patient.			
b. Verify the absence of contraindications.			
c. Ask about previous traction treatments and review treatment record.			
3. Apply and adjust appropriate halters, harnesses, and belts for indicated traction treatment.			
a. Cervical: Apply head halter beneath the occiput and mandible, attach to spreader bar.			
b. Lumbar: Attach pelvic harness snugly about the waist, beginning just above the iliac crests, thoracic rib belt snugly about the lower rib cage.			
c. Attach traction apparatus to unit: Take up and adjust for slack in the line.			

PROCEDURE	EVALUATION		
	1	2	3
4. Position patient for indicated traction treatment.			
a. Cervical: Supine lying with neck flexed 20–30 degrees.			
b. Lumbar: Supine hooklying with hips flexed and legs supported by pillows or stools.			
c. Lumbar: Prone lying in neutral.			
d. Ensure proper body alignment and pull off traction apparatus.			
4. Apply indicated traction poundage.			
a. Cervical: Adjust traction poundage beginning with 20 lb or as tolerated by the patient, (range 20–50 lb).			
b. Lumbar: Adjust traction poundage beginning with 65 lb or as tolerated by the patient (range 65–200 lb).			
5. Adjust traction duty cycle and treatment duration.			
a. Sustained: Less than 10 minutes.			
b. Intermittent: 3–10 seconds, on/off for 20–30 minutes			
6. Complete the treatment.			
a. Zero out equipment, turn power off.			
b. Slacken traction line.			
c. Remove the traction harness, halter, or belt.			
d. Have patient sit up slowly.			
e. Assess treatment efficacy.			
f. Record treatment parameters.			
7. Instruct the patient in any indicated exercise.			
8. Return equipment to storage after cleaning.			

CHAPTER 16 SIXTEEN

INTERMITTENT COMPRESSION DEVICES

DANIEL N. HOOKER

OBJECTIVES

Following completion of this chapter, the student therapist will be able to:

✓ Appraise the effectiveness of external compression on the accumulation and the reabsorption of edema following an athletic injury.
✓ Outline the setup procedure for intermittent external compression.
✓ Recognize the effects that changing a parameter might have on edema reduction.
✓ Review the clinical applications for using intermittent compression devices.

Edema accumulation following trauma is one of the clinical signs at which considerable attention is directed in first aid and therapeutic rehabilitation programs. **Edema** is defined as the presence of abnormal amounts of fluid in the extracellular tissue spaces of the body. Intermittent compression is one of the clinical modalities used to help reduce the accumulation of edema.

There are two distinct kinds of tissue swelling that are usually associated with injury. **Joint swelling,** marked by the presence of blood and joint fluid accumulated within the joint capsule, is one kind. This type of swelling occurs immediately following injury to a joint. Joint swelling is usually contained by the joint capsule and has the appearance and feel of a water balloon. If pressure is placed on the swelling, the fluid moves but it immediately returns when the pressure is released.

Lymphedema is the other variety of swelling encountered in athletic injuries. This type of swelling in the subcutaneous tissues results from an excessive accumulation of **lymph** and usually occurs over several hours following the injury. Intermittent compression can be used with both varieties, but it is usually more successful with **pitting edema.** The lymphatic system is the primary body system that deals with these injury induced changes.

THE LYMPHATIC SYSTEM

PURPOSES OF THE LYMPHATIC SYSTEM

The lymphatic system has four major purposes.

1. The fluid in the interstitial spaces is continuously circulating. As plasma and plasma proteins escape from the small blood vessels, they are picked up by the lymphatic system and returned to the blood circulation.

2. The lymphatic system acts as a safety valve for fluid overload and helps keep edema from forming. As the interstitial fluid increases, the interstitial fluid pressure increases, which causes an increase in the local lymph flow. The local lymphatic system can be overwhelmed by sudden local increases in the interstitial fluid and pitting edema will be the result.[35]

3. The homeostasis of the extracellular environment is maintained by the lymphatic system. The lymphatic system removes excess protein molecules and waste from the interstitial fluid. The large protein molecules and fluids that cannot reenter the circulatory vessels gain entry back into the blood circulation through the terminal lymphatics.

4. The lymphatic system also cleanses the interstitial fluid and provides a blockade to the spread of infection or malignant cells in the lymph nodes. The lymph nodes' ability is not clearly understood and is highly variable.[16]

STRUCTURE OF THE LYMPHATIC SYSTEM

The lymphatic system is a closed vascular system of **endothelial cell-lined** tubes that parallel the arterial and nervous system. The lymphatic capillaries are made of single-layered endothelial cells with **fibrils** radiating from the junctions of the endothelial cells (Fig. 16-1). These fibrils support the lymphatic capillaries and anchor them to the surrounding connective tissue. The capillary is surrounded by the interstitial fluid and tissues. These lymphatic capillaries are called the terminal lymphatics and they provide the entry way into the lymphatic system for the excess interstitial fluid and plasma proteins.

These lymphatic capillaries join together in a network of lymphatic vessels that eventually lead to larger collecting vessels in the extremities. The collecting vessels connect with the thoracic duct or the right lymphatic duct, which join the venous system in the left and right cervical area. As the lymph flows centrally up the system, the lymph moves through one or more lymph nodes. These nodes remove the foreign substances and are the primary area of lymphocyte activity.[16]

endothelial cell Cells that line the cavities of vessels.

lymph A transparent, slightly yellow liquid found in the lymphatic vessels.

fibrils Connective tissue fibers supporting the lymphatic capillaries.

PERIPHERAL LYMPHATIC STRUCTURE AND FUNCTION

Deep and superficial lymphatic collecting systems are found in the extremities. The terminal lymphatics in the skin and subcutaneous tissue drain into the superficial branches. Lymph channels in the fascial and bony layers drain into the deep branches.

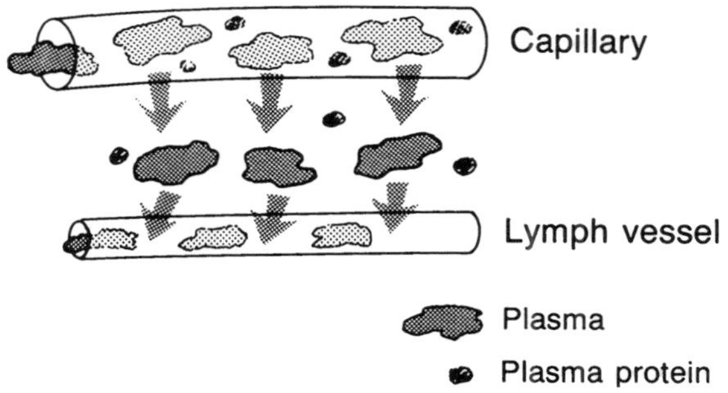

•**Figure 16-1** Plasma proteins outside the capillaries attract fluid to the intercellular space, leading to an abnormal "wet state" in the intercellular spaces. Plasma is absorbed back into the lymphatic spaces and away from the injured area.

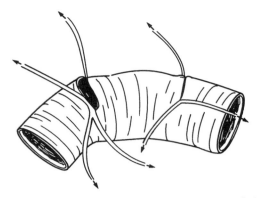

•**Figure 16-2** Lymphatic capillary with pore open to allow movement of plasma protein out of the intercellular space. As the intercellular fluid accumulates, the fibrils radiating from the seams in the lymphatic capillary pull the seam open to create a pore large enough for plasma proteins to enter.

In the superficial branches, the dermis is packed with two types of lymphatic channels. The channels closer to the surface have no valves, whereas those lying under the dermis and in the subcutaneous tissue do have valves. The valves are located approximately 1 cm apart and are similar in construction to the valves in veins. These structures prevent the back flow of lymph when pressure is applied. As with the blood vessels, the lymph system is concentrated on the medial side of the limbs.[16]

As the lymphatic system changes from the entry channels to the collecting channels, the lymphatic vessel changes to look similar to venous tissue. These vessels have smooth muscle and appear to have innervation from the sympathetic nervous system.

As the fluid or tissues move in the interstitial spaces, they push or pull on the fibrils supporting the terminal lymphatics (Fig. 16-2). This activity forces the endothelial cells to gap apart at their junctions, creating an opening in the terminal lymphatics for the entry of interstitial fluid, cellular waste, large protein molecules, plasma proteins, extracellular particles, and cells into the lymphatic channels. These junctions are constantly being pushed and pulled open and are then allowed to close, depending on the local activity. Once the interstitial fluid and proteins enter these channels, they become lymph. Terminal lymphatics in inflamed areas are dilated and an increased number of gaps in the capillary are present (Fig. 16-2).[11,16, 20,44,45]

If no tissue activity or interstitial volume increase takes place, these endothelial junctions remain closed. The interstitial fluid, however, can still enter the terminal lymphatics by moving across the endothelial cell, or by being transported across in a vesicle or cell organelle. This permeability is similar to the small blood vessels or capillaries (see Fig. 16-1).

Muscle activity, active and passive movements, elevated positions, respiration, and blood vessel pulsation, all aid in the movement of lymph by compressing the lymphatic vessels and allowing gravity to pull the lymph down the channels. The valves help by maintaining a unidirectional flow of lymph in response to pressure. The collecting lymph channels all have smooth muscle in their walls. These muscles can provide contractible activity that promotes lymph flow. These muscles have a natural firing frequency that simulates a rhythmic pumping action. There are also studies that indicate increased lymph flow during heating of animal limbs.[1–7,9,10,12,13,19,38,39,42–47]

INJURY EDEMA

Following a closed injury, changes in and around the site of the injury occur that have an impact on the accumulation of extracellular fluid and proteins in the local interstitial spaces. The direct effects of the injury include cell death, bleeding, the release of chemical

---

Movement of lymph occurs because of
- Muscle activity
- Active and passive motion
- Elevation
- Respiration
- Contraction of vessels

edema The presence of abnormal amounts of fluid in the extracellular tissue spaces of the body.

mediators to initiate and guide the healing process, and changes in local tissue electric currents. The first stage of the healing process is inflammation, which is characterized by local redness, heat, swelling, and pain. In addition, loss of function frequently occurs.

FORMATION OF PITTING EDEMA

These changes are brought about by changes in the local circulation. Local edema is formed by the plasma, plasma proteins, and cell debris from the damaged cells all moving into the interstitial spaces. This sudden volume change is compounded by the intact local circulatory responses to the chemical mediators of the inflammatory process. The hormones released by the injured cells stimulate the small arterioles, capillaries, and venules to vasodilate, enlarging the size of the vascular pool. This causes the local blood flow to slow down and the pressure within the blood vessels to increase. The endothelial cells in the blood vessel walls then separate or become more loosely bound to their neighboring cell. The permeability of the vessel increases, allowing more plasma, plasma proteins, and leucocytes to escape into the local area. The increase in the plasma proteins in the interstitial spaces causes the osmotic pressure to push more plasma into the area, forming an inflammatory exudate. This exudate forms too quickly for the lymphatic system to maintain the local equilibrium and pitting edema is formed (Fig. 16-3). This small increase in the plasma protein in the intercellular spaces causes an increase in the intercellular fluid volume by several hundred percent.[1,2,3,7,15,21,45,46]

This fluid in the form of a gel is trapped by both collagen fibers and proteoglycan molecules. The gel prevents the free flow of fluid, as seen in the joint fluid example. Clinically, this state is recognized as pitting edema. After finger pressure on the swollen part is released, a slight pit is left at the finger's previous location. Fluid is squeezed out of the intercellular space and time is needed for the fluid to move slowly back into that space (Fig. 16-3).

pitting edema A type of swelling that leaves a pitlike depression when the skin is compressed.

FORMATION OF LYMPHEDEMA

As the intercellular fluid becomes greater, the lymph begins to flow. If the edema causes an overdistention of the lymph capillaries, the entry pores become ineffective and lymphedema results. Constriction of lymph capillaries or larger lymphatic vessels from increased pressure also discourage lymph flow and cause intercellular fluid to increase.[1,2,3,7,15,21,45,46]

Using computerized tomography cross-sectional images, Airaksinen reported a 23 percent increase in the subcutaneous tissue, thickened skin, and muscular atrophy

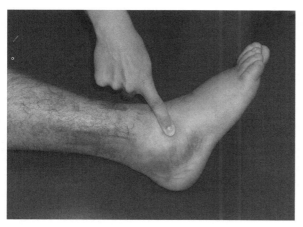

•**Figure 16-3** Ankle with pitting edema. Finger pressure squeezes fluid out of the intercellular space; an indentation is left when the pressure is removed.

CASE STUDY 16-1
INTERMITTENT COMPRESSION

Background: A 48-year-old male developed pain and edema in his right foot and ankle subsequent to stepping in a hole in his yard while mowing his lawn. He was treated at his local hospital's emergency room. He failed to comply with their instructions to elevate and ice the injured extremity and reported to his family physician 48 hours later with a moderately swollen and ecchymotic right ankle. The patient reported the obvious swelling, localized tenderness over the lateral aspect of the ankle, and difficulty with weight-bearing during ambulation. Physical examination revealed point tenderness at the ATF (anterior talofibular ligament), 2+ effusion—figure 8 girth increased by $3/4$ inch versus uninvolved side, and reduced ROM of dorsiflexion to 0 degrees/plantarflexion to 35 degrees. The ankle was stable to anterior drawer and talar tilt tests.

Impression: Subacute grade I inversion sprain right ankle.

Treatment Plan: In addition to reinstruction in home care principles; a course of intermittent compression was initiated to the right foot/ankle to mobilize the residual effusion/edema. The right lower extremity was elevated, pretreatment circumferential measurements taken, and stockingnette placed over the extremity. Treatment consisted of 60 mmHg pressure applied intermittently for 30 seconds on/10 seconds off cycles for 30 minutes duration. Posttreatment circumferential measures were taken and the patient was encouraged to attempt active and active-assisted ankle pumping exercise. Patient was fitted with a compression stocking and thermoplastic ankle stirrup for ambulation weight-bearing as tolerated.

Response: Postinitial treatment, patient's circumferential measures were reduced by $1/4$ inch. Dorsiflexion range of motion increased by 5 degrees. Over the course of five treatment sessions, effusion was resolved and active range of motion approached normal limits. Strengthening exercises were implemented and the patient continued to ambulate with the aid of the ankle stirrup. At the time of discharge the patient was essentially symptom free, independent in performing his strengthening regimen, and had returned to his yard work.

The rehabilitation professional employs therapeutic agent modalities to create an optimum environment for tissue healing while minimizing the symptoms associated with the trauma or condition.

Discussion Questions

- What tissues were injured or affected?
- What symptoms were present?
- What phase of the injury-healing continuum did the patient present for care in?
- What are the therapeutic agent modality's biophysical effects (direct, indirect, depth, and tissue affinity)?
- What are the therapeutic agent modality's indications and contraindications?
- What are the parameters of the therapeutic agent modality's application, dosage, duration, and frequency in this case study?
- What other therapeutic agent modalities could be utilized to treat this injury or condition? Why? How?

in patients following lower leg fracture and casting. They reported an 8 percent edema decrease in the subcutaneous compartment after intermittent compression. The mean area of the subfascial compartment remained the same, but the density of the muscle tissue increased after treatment. This study indicates that injury edema follows the path of least resistance and that tissues that have the least natural pressure exerted on them demonstrate the greatest accumulation of extra fluid. The skin and subcutaneous tissue appear to be the major site for pitting edema; the deep muscle and connective tissue have enough pressure to inhibit major accumulations in the deeper tissues.[3]

Clinical measurement of edema is reasonably accurate and correlates extremely well with both CT scan and volumetric measures. The standard clinical circumferential measurement of limb and joint are adequate to determine the treatment effects.[3,5]

THE NEGATIVE EFFECTS OF EDEMA ACCUMULATION

Edema compounds the extent of an injury by causing secondary hypoxic cellular death in the tissues surrounding the injured area. The edema increases the distance nutrients and oxygen must travel to nourish the remaining cells. This in turn adds to the injury debris in the damaged area and causes further edema to accumulate, thus perpetuating the cycle.[9]

Other ill effects of edema include the physical separation of torn tissue ends, pain, and restricted joint range of motion. Recovery times become more prolonged. If the edema persists, further problems with extremity function can occur, including infection, muscle atrophy, joint contractures, interstitial fibrosis, and reflex sympathetic dystrophy.[7,11,13]

TREATMENT OF EDEMA

Good first aid can minimize edema (Fig. 16-4). The use of ice, compression, electricity, elevation, and early gentle motion retards the accumulation of fluid and keeps the lymphatic system operating at an optimum level. Any treatment that encourages the lymph flow will decrease plasma protein content in the intercellular spaces and therefore decrease edema. The standard methods of treatment in most clinical settings include elevation, compression, and muscular contraction.

The force of gravity can be used to augment normal lymph flow. The swollen part can be elevated so that gravity does not resist the flow of lymph but encourages its movement. Elevation of the injured swollen part above heart level is all that is necessary. The higher the elevation, the greater the effect on the lymph flow.[32,36]

In an uninjured population, placing the legs in an elevated position significantly decreased ankle volume after 20 minutes, although the dependent position significantly increased ankle volumes. These findings could be expected to be the same in injured subjects, but the dependent position may markedly increase volume, whereas the elevated position may decrease volumes less well because of the injury to the tissue. In the majority of studies using postacute ankle sprain edema, elevation alone provided a significant posttreatment reduction in ankle volume,[3,5,25,32,36] although a more recent study has shown no effect.[40]

Rhythmic internal compression provided by muscle contraction also squeezes the lymph through the lymph vessels, improving its flow back to the vascular system. This

---

Edema is best treated with
- Elevation
- Compression
- Weight-bearing exercise
- Cryotherapy

Treatment Tip
When using intermittent compression following an acute ankle sprain, the compression boot should be applied with the inflation pressure set at about 60 mm, the on-off time at 30 sec on 30 sec off, and a total treatment time of 20 minutes initially. The on-off times and total treatment time can be increased over the next several days as tolerated.

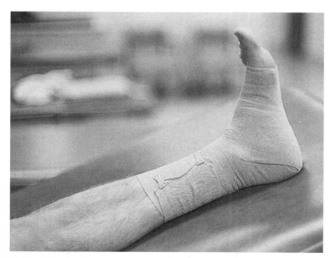

•**Figure 16-4** Ankle with elastic wrap compression in an elevated position.

muscle contraction can be accomplished through isometric or active exercise or through electrically induced muscle contraction. Several authors also advocate the use of noncontractable electric current for edema control and reduction. (See Chapter 6 for a discussion of electrical therapy for edema control.) When elevation is combined with muscle contraction, lymph flow benefits.[4,6,12]

External pressure also can be used to increase lymph flow. Massage, elastic compression, and intermittent pressure devices are the most often used external pressure devices. This external compression not only moves the lymph along but also may spread the intercellular edema over a larger area, enabling more lymph capillaries to become involved in removing the plasma proteins and water. External pressure from horseshoe, pads, and elastic wraps are also helpful in minimizing the accumulation or reaccumulation of edema in the injured area.[9,44,45,46]

Gardner has proposed that weight-bearing activities activate a powerful venous pump.[15] The pump consists of the venae comitantes of the lateral plantar artery. It is emptied immediately on weight-bearing and flattening of the plantar arch. Because this emptying occurs so rapidly, they believe that this process is mediated by the release of an **endothelial-derived relaxing factor** (EDRF) and is not related to muscular activity of the limb. The EDRF is liberated by sudden pressure changes, and it diffuses locally. Its major action is to relax the smooth muscle and stimulate blood flow rates in the veins.[18]

This phenomenon may explain the rapid decrease in edema that occurs when patients switch from a non-weight-bearing gait to a weight-bearing gait. Using this venous pump on lower leg edema is a reason to include early weight-bearing in a variety of injury treatment protocols.

Using an intermittent compression device to decrease postacute injury edema has recently been shown to have a good effect. The addition of cryotherapy to the intermittent compression has shown the best results in the reduction of postacute injury edema.[1,2,3,5,19,20,25,30,37,38,47]

INTERMITTENT COMPRESSION TREATMENT TECHNIQUES

Treatment Parameters
• Inflation pressure
• On-off times
• Total treatment time

There are three parameters available for adjustment when using most intermittent pressure devices: (1) inflation pressure; (2) on-off time sequence; and (3) total treatment time (Fig. 16-5). There are also intermittent pressure devices with multiple

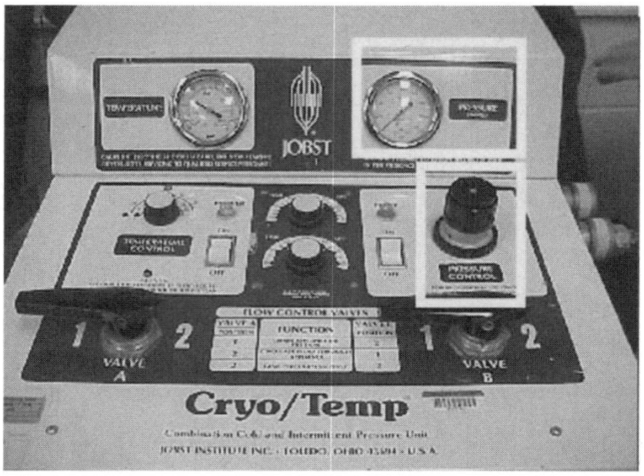

•**Figure 16-5** Pressure gauge and pressure control knob on an intermittent compression unit.

compartments that inflate distal to proximal with gradual reduced pressure in each compartment. These devices try to mimic the massage strokes used in edema removal.[19,20,25,42] Reduction in postacute injury edema does not require this graded sequential action, nor is postinjury edema reduction significantly enhanced by these devices.[25,42] All intermittent compression devices seem to have similar influences on edema.

Little research has been done comparing adjustments of these parameters with volumetric results. Empiricism and clinical trials have been used to design the established protocols.

INFLATION PRESSURES

Pressure settings have been loosely correlated with blood pressure and patient comfort to arrive at the therapeutic pressure. A pressure approximating the patient's diastolic blood pressure has been used in most treatment protocols. The arterial capillary pressures are approximately 30 mmHg, and any pressure that exceeds this should encourage reabsorption of the edema and movement of the lymph. Maximum pressure should correspond to the systolic blood pressure. Higher pressure would shut off arterial blood flow and create a potentially uncomfortable tissue response as a result of low blood flow.[1,2,3,11,13,21,23]

More may not necessarily be better. Enough pressure is needed to squeeze the lymphatic vessels and force the lymph to move. This should be accomplished with relatively low pressures, for example, 30–40 mmHg. The other mechanism in operation is the force of the hydrostatic pressure and pressure in the range of 40–50 mmHg should suffice to raise the interstitial fluid pressure higher than the blood vessel pressures.[13,21,23] Recommended inflation pressures for intermittent compression are 30–60 mm for the upper extremity and 40–80 mm for the lower extremity.

ON-OFF SEQUENCE

On and off time sequences are even more variable, with some protocols calling for a sequence of 30 seconds on, 30 seconds off; 1 minute on, 2 minutes off; whereas others reverse this to 2 minutes on, 1 minute off. Others use a 4 minutes on to 1 minute off ratio. One study has recommended using continuous compression for treating delayed onset muscle soreness.[22] If lymphatic massage is the primary vehicle used in this therapy, shorter on-off time sequences may have an advantage. The hydrostatic pressure vehicles require the longer on times. These time periods are not research-based, and the therapist is left to his or her own empirical judgment as to the optimum time sequence for each patient. Patient comfort should be the primary deciding factor here.

TOTAL TREATMENT TIME

Total treatment times have some basis in research, but again this is convenience or empirically based in many instances. Most of the protocols for primary lymphedema call for 3- to 4-hour treatments. This time frame has been effective for many patients.[1–3,5,12,13,19,20,22–25,29–33,35–39,42,44,47]

Researchers have shown a marked increase in lymph flow on initiation of massage; this flow decreases over a 10-minute period and stops when the massage is discontinued.[28,34] Clinical studies show significant gains in limb volume reduction after 30 minutes of compression.[1–3,5,12,24,25,29,30,35–37,38,44,47] In most situations, a 10- to 30-minute treatment seems adequate unless the edema is overwhelming in volume or is resistant to treatment. More treatment times per day may also be an advantage in controlling and reducing edema from various musculoskeletal injuries.

Treatment Tip
Joint swelling is usually contained in the joint capsule and feels very much like a water balloon. The fluid is easily moved around by simply applying pressure on one side of the joint. Lymphedema occurs in the subcutaneous tissues, has more of a gel-like feeling to it and leaves an indentation after finger pressure is removed.

It has also been suggested that the pressures indicated on the control panel may be substantially less than actual pressures in the cuff. Thus it is recommended that cuff target pressures be set at much lower levels than indicated above.[34]

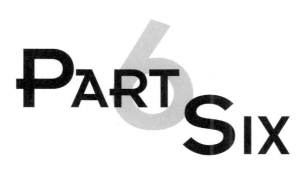

PART SIX

OTHER MODALITIES

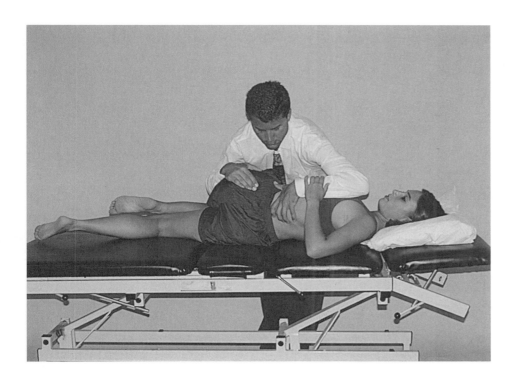

CHAPTER 17 SEVENTEEN

THERAPEUTIC MASSAGE

WILLIAM E. PRENTICE
CLAIRBETH LEHN

OBJECTIVES

Following completion of this chapter, the student therapist will be able to:

✓ Discuss the physiologic effects of massage differentiating between reflexive and mechanical effects.
✓ Apply specific treatment guidelines and considerations when administering massage.
✓ Demonstrate the various strokes involved with classic Hoffa massage.
✓ Describe connective tissue massage.
✓ Explain how acupressure massage is most effectively used and identify the relationship between acupuncture and trigger points.
✓ Explain how myofascial release can be used to restore normal functional movement patterns.
✓ Contrast special massage techniques, including Rolfing and Tragering.

THE VALUE OF MANUAL THERAPY TECHNIQUES

Manual therapy techniques, including massage, joint mobilization, and traction, as well as proprioceptive neuromuscular facilitation techniques, are being used more frequently in rehabilitation by the therapist. In recent years, therapists have tended to get caught up in some of the technologic advances that have been made available in rehabilitation equipment. These "high-tech" devices to a great extent have taken the place of what many consider to be the greatest tool available in the rehabilitation repertoire, our hands. It seems, however, that the pendulum is beginning to swing back in the other direction, and more therapists are incorporating manual therapy techniques into their rehabilitation regimens.

THE EVOLUTION OF MASSAGE AS A TREATMENT MODALITY

The earliest available medical records seem to indicate that massage played an important role in the treatment of sick and injured people.[30] A natural reaction when a part of the body hurts is to rub the injured area with a hand.

massage The act of rubbing, kneading, or stroking the superficial parts of the body with the hand or with an instrument.

In early writings pertaining to medical treatments little difference is shown between massage, as we know it, and general exercise of the body. In fact, although there are very detailed descriptions of techniques, one has a great deal of difficulty in making a determination as to exactly what is meant because the terminology is unfamiliar. Language changes with time.

In Europe during the Middle Ages, the influence of the Church of Rome and its religious teachings discouraged the use of massage as a healing practice. This brought the art to somewhat of a halt until enlightened individuals strove to bring medical knowledge into the forefront and scholars in the medical fields started to again delve into how and why the body functions as it does.

The word massage is derived from two sources. One is the Arabic verb *mass*, to touch, and the other is the Greek word massein, to knead. However, history shows that this was not an art exclusive to the Greeks and Arabs. The general knowledge of massage was also known and practiced by the Egyptians, Romans, Japanese, Persians, and Chinese.

In Sweden in the early part of the nineteenth century, Peter H. Ling (1776–1839), the acknowledged founder of curative gymnastics, used massage as a branch of gymnastics. He appears to be the founder of modern-day massage techniques with some incorporation of French massage techniques into his system.[15]

Massage techniques have changed dramatically in the past 50 years. They are based on the research and teachings of Albert Hoffa (1859–1907), James B. Mennell (1880–1957), and Gertrude Beard (1887–1971). Medical practitioners of the twentieth century have added a scientific basis to massage along with additional techniques and terms.[10] In modern-day preventative and rehabilitative therapy, massage is a widely used therapeutic modality that seems to be gaining renewed interest.[10,41]

PHYSIOLOGIC EFFECTS OF MASSAGE

Physiologic Effects of Massage
• Reflexive
• Mechanical

Massage is a mechanical stimulation of the tissues by means of rhythmically applied pressure and stretching.[75] Over the years many claims have been made relative to the therapeutic benefits of massage in the patient population, although few are based on well-controlled and designed studies.[2,3,6,8,65,66,73] Patients have used massage to increase flexibility and coordination as well as increase pain threshold; decrease neuromuscular excitability in the muscle being massaged; stimulate circulation, thus improving energy transport to the muscle; facilitate healing and restore joint mobility; and remove lactic acid, thus alleviating muscle cramps.[3,36,42,43,57,68] Conclusive evidence of the efficacy of massage as an ergogenic aid in the physically active population is lacking.[29]

How these effects may be accomplished is determined by the specific approaches used with massage techniques and how they are applied. Generally, the effects of massage may be either reflexive or mechanical.[14] The effect of massage on the nervous system differs greatly according to the method employed, pressure exerted, and duration of applications. Through the reflex mechanism, sedation is induced. Slow, gentle, rhythmical, and superficial effleurage may relieve tension and soothe, rendering the muscles more relaxed. This indicates an effect on sensory and motor nerves locally and some central nervous system response. The mechanical approach seeks to make mechanical or histologic changes in myofascial structures through direct force applied superficially.[14]

REFLEXIVE EFFECTS

Reflexive Effects
• Pain
• Circulation
• Metabolism

The first approach in massage therapy involves a reflexive mechanism. The reflexive approach attempts to exert effects through the skin and superficial connective tissues. Mobilization of soft tissue stimulates sensory receptors in the skin and superficial fascia.[14] If hands are passed lightly over the skin, a series of responses occur as a result of the sensory stimulus of cutaneous receptors. This reflex mechanism is believed to be an autonomic nervous system phenomenon.[5] The reflex stimulus can occur alone (i.e., unaccompanied by the mechanical mechanism). Mennell calls this the "reflex effect."[55] In itself, it is not an effect but the cause of an effect (i.e., causes sedation, relieves tension, increases blood flow).

Effects on Pain

The effect of massage on pain is probably regulated by both the gate control theory and through the release of endogenous opiates (see Chapter 4). In gate control, cutaneous stimulation of large diameter afferent nerve fibers effectively block transmission of pain information carried in small diameter nerve fibers. Stimulation of painful areas in the skin or myofascia can facilitate the release of β-endorphins and enkephalin, which essentially effect the transmission of pain-associated information in descending spinal tracts.

Effects on Circulation

The effect of massage on the circulation of the blood, according to Pemberton, takes place through a reflex influence on blood vessels from a sympathetic division in the nervous system.[59] He believes that vessels in the muscular system are emptied during massage, not only by being squeezed but also by this reflex action. Very light massage (effleurage) produces an almost instantaneous reaction through transient dilation of lymphatics and small capillaries. Heavier pressure brings about a more lasting dilation. If capillary dilation occurs, blood volume and blood flow increase, producing an increase in temperature in the area being massaged.[23]

Massage increases lymphatic flow.[25] In the lymphatic system, movement of fluid depends on forces outside of the system. Such factors as gravity, muscle contraction, movement, and massage can affect the flow of lymph. Increased lymphatic flow assists in the removal of edema.[13] When administering massage to an edematous part, elevation also helps to increase lymph flow.

It has been proposed that massage can promote lactate clearance following exercise. However, evidence suggests that increases in blood flow that occur from massage have little or no effect on lactate metabolism and its subsequent clearance from blood and tissues.[32,53]

Effects on Metabolism

Massage does not alter general metabolism appreciably.[59] There is no change in acid-base equilibrium of blood. Massage does not appear to have any significant effects on the cardiovascular system.[9] Massage metabolically augments a chemical balance. The increased circulation means increased dispersion of waste products and an increase of fresh blood and oxygen. The mechanical movements assist in the removal and hastens the resynthesis of lactic acid.

MECHANICAL EFFECTS

The second approach to massage is mechanical in nature. Techniques that stretch a muscle, elongate fascia, or mobilize soft-tissue adhesions or restrictions are all mechanical techniques. The mechanical effects are always accompanied by some reflex effects. As the mechanical stimulus becomes more effective, the reflex stimulus becomes less effective. Mechanical techniques should be performed after reflexive techniques. This is not to imply that mechanical techniques are more aggressive forms of massage. However, mechanical techniques are most often directed at deeper tissues, such as adhesions or restrictions in muscle, tendons, and fascia.

Effects on Muscle

The basic goal of massage on muscle tissue is to "maintain the muscle in the best possible state of nutrition, flexibility, and vitality so that after recovery from trauma or disease the muscle can function at its maximum."[75] Muscle massage is done either for mechanical stretching of the intramuscular connective tissue or to relieve pain and

CASE STUDY 17-1
Massage

Background: A 30-year-old stockbroker complains of chronic cervical myalgia ("My neck hurts."). There was no prior history of trauma and his family physician reported that his x-rays were within normal limits without evidence of degenerative changes or loss of disk space height. The patient reports no radiation of pain into the shoulders or upper extremities, but did complain of restriction in rotating his head to the left. The patient stated that he spends many hours each day at work cradling a telephone with his right side.

Impression: "Occupational Neck": Right Upper Trapezius and Sternocleidomastoid Muscle Spasm.

Treatment Plan: The patient was placed in a forward seated position with the head and neck supported by pillows on the treatment plinth. The arms were likewise supported by a pillow in the lap. A small amount of pre-warmed massage lotion was applied to the right upper quarter region and a Hoffa massage commenced with light effleurage stroking begun to the SCM and upper trapezius muscles. The light effleurage stroking was followed by several minutes of deep effleurage strokes, which identified several "trigger point" areas in each muscle. Petrissage was directed at each trigger point area for approximately 30 seconds, then the massage concluded with several more minutes of deep, then superficial effleurage strokes. At the completion of the massage, excess lotion was removed, then the patient was instructed in cervical and upper quarter active range-of-motion exercise. The patient was encouraged to perform his home range of motion exercises each a.m. and p.m.

Response: The patient reported immediate relief of his symptoms following the initial session of massage. He reported the ability to fully turn and bend his head and neck. The patient returned for two additional sessions of massage treatment and was educated as to postural habits that triggered his condition. He continued his range of motion exercises twice a day, added isometric strengthening exercises to his daily regimen, and monitored his postural habits at work. His employer subsequently added once weekly visits by a massage therapist as an employee benefit.

The rehabilitation professional employs therapeutic agent modalities to create an optimum environment for tissue healing while minimizing the symptoms associated with the trauma or condition.

Discussion Questions

- What tissues were injured or affected?
- What symptoms were present?
- What phase of the injury-healing continuum did the patient present for care in?
- What are the therapeutic agent modality's biophysical effects (direct, indirect, depth, and tissue affinity)?
- What are the therapeutic agent modality's indications and contraindications?
- What are the parameters of the therapeutic agent modality's application, dosage, duration, and frequency in this case study?
- What other therapeutic agent modalities could be utilized to treat this injury or condition? Why? How?

---

discomfort associated with myofascial trigger points. Massage has been shown to increase blood flow to skeletal muscle, and thus to increase venous return.[22,76] It has also been shown to retard muscle atrophy following injury.[68] Massage has also been shown to increase the range of motion in hamstring muscles owing to the combined decrease in neuromuscular excitability and stretching of muscle and scar tissue.[19] Massage does not increase strength or bulk of muscle, nor does it increase muscle tone.

Effect on Skin

Effects of massage on the skin include an increase in skin temperature, possibly as a result of direct mechanical effects, and indirect vasomotor action. It has also been found that increased sweating and decreased skin resistance to galvanic current result from massage.

If skin becomes adherent to underlying tissues and scar tissue is formed, friction massage usually can be used to mechanically loosen the adhesions and soften the scar. Massage toughens yet softens the skin. It acts directly on the surface of the skin to remove dead cells that result from prolonged casting of 6–8 weeks.

The effect of massage on scar tissue is that it stretches and breaks down the fibrous tissue. It can break down adhesions between skin and subcutaneous tissue and stretch contracted or adhered tissue.[58]

PSYCHOLOGIC EFFECTS OF MASSAGE

The psychologic effects of massage can be as beneficial to some patients as the physiologic effects. The "hands-on" effect helps patients feel as if someone is helping them. A general sedative effect can be most beneficial for the patient. Massage has been shown to lower psychoemotional and somatic arousal such as tension and anxiety.[48] The therapist's approach should inspire a feeling of confidence in the patient, and the patient should respond with a feeling of well-being—a feeling of being helped.

MASSAGE TREATMENT CONSIDERATIONS AND GUIDELINES

The therapist must have the basic essential knowledge of anatomy and of the particular area being treated. The physiology of the area to be treated and the total function of the patient must be considered. There should be an understanding of the existing pathology so that the process by which repair occurs is known. The therapist needs a thorough knowledge of massage principles and skillful techniques, as well as manual dexterity, coordination, and concentration in the use of massage techniques. The therapist also needs to exhibit such traits as patience, a sense of caring for the patient's welfare, and courteousness both in speech and manner.

Perhaps the most important tools in massage therapy are the hands of the clinician. They must be clean, warm, dry, and soft. The nails must be short and smooth. Washing of the hands before and after treatment must take place for sanitary reasons. If the therapist's hands are cold, they should be placed in warm water for a short period. Rubbing them together briskly helps to warm them, too.

Positioning is also important for the clinician. Correct positioning will allow relaxation, prevent fatigue, and permit free movement of arms, hands, and the body. Good posture will also help prevent fatigue and backache. The weight should rest evenly on both feet with the body in good postural alignment. When massaging a large area, the weight should shift from one foot to the other. You must be able to fit your hands to the contour of the area being treated. A good position is required to allow the correct application of pressure and rhythmic strokes during the procedure (Fig. 17-1).

The following points are important to consider when administering massage.

1. Pressure regulation should be determined by the type and amount of tissue present. It must also be governed by the patient's condition and which tissues are to be affected. The pressure must be delivered from the body, through the soft parts of the hands, and it is adjusted to contours of the patient's body parts.

2. Rhythm must be steady and even. The time for each stroke and time between successive strokes should be equal.

3. Duration depends on the pathology, size of the area being treated, speed of motion, age, size, and condition of the patient. One also should observe the response of the patient to determine duration of the procedure. Massage of the back or the neck area might take 15–30 minutes. Massage of a large joint (such as a hip or shoulder) may require less than 10 minutes.

4. If swelling is present in an extremity, treatment should begin with the proximal part. The purpose of this is to help facilitate the lymphatic flow proximally. The subsequent effects of distal massage in removing fluid or edema will be more efficient since the proximal resistance to lymphatic flow will be reduced. This technique has been referred to as the "uncorking effect."

5. Massage should never be painful, except possibly for friction massage, nor should it be given with such force that it causes ecchymosis (discoloration of the skin resulting from contusion).

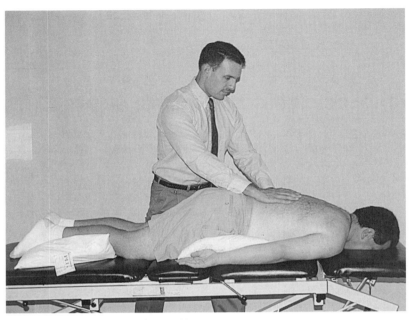

•**Figure 17-1** Position of therapist for stroking.

6. In general, the direction of forces should be applied in the direction of the muscle fibers (Fig. 17-2).

7. During a session, one should begin and end with effleurage. The maneuvers should increase progressively to the greatest energy possible and end by decreasing energy maneuvers.

8. The therapist must consider the position in which massage can best be given and be sure the patient is warm and in a comfortable, relaxed position.

9. The body part may be elevated if this is necessary and possible (Fig. 17-3).

10. The therapist should be in a position in which the whole body, as well as hands and arms, can be relaxed and the procedure accomplished without strain (see Fig. 17-1).

11. Sufficient lubricant should be used so that the therapist's hands will move smoothly along the skin surface (except in friction). The use of too much lubricant should be guarded against.

12. Massage should begin with superficial stroking; this stroke is used to spread the lubricant over the part being treated.

13. Each stroke should start at the joint or just below the joint (unless massage over joints is contraindicated) and finish above the joint so that strokes will overlap.

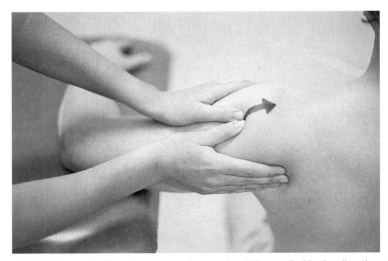

•**Figure 17-2** In the application of massage, forces should be applied in the direction of muscle fibers.

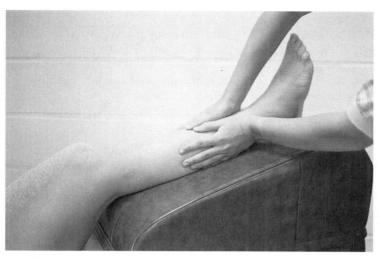

•**Figure 17-3** The part being massaged should be elevated.

14. The pressure should be in line with venous flow followed by a return stroke without pressure. The pressure should be in the centripetal direction (Fig. 17-4).

15. Care should be used over body areas. Hands should be relaxed and pressure adjusted to fit the contour of the area being treated.

16. Bony prominences and painful joints should be avoided if possible.

17. All strokes should be rhythmic. The pressure strokes should end with a swing off, in a small half circle, in order that the rhythm will not be broken by an abrupt reversal.

EQUIPMENT

Table

A firm table, easily accessible from both sides, is most desirable. The height of the table should be reasonably comfortable for the therapist; leaning over or reaching up to perform the required movements should not be necessary. An adjustable table is almost a must in this situation. To facilitate cleaning and disinfecting, a washable plastic surface is much preferred. There should be a storage area close by for linens and lubricant. If the table is not padded, a mattress or foam pad should be used for the comfort of the patient.

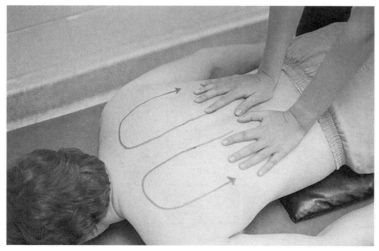

•**Figure 17-4** Massage pressure should be in line of venous flow followed by a return stroke without pressure.

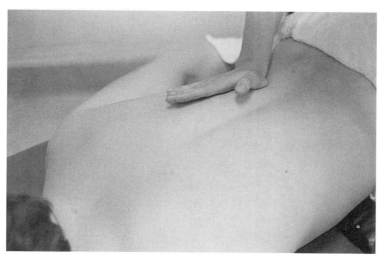

•**Figure 17-22** Superficial friction applied to the back by using the heel of the hand.

the area. She continued the technique on herself, and after 3 months, she had no low back pain and she had restored circulation to her right leg.

Connective tissue massage is a stroking technique carried out in the layers of connective tissue on the body surface.[44] This stimulates the nerve endings of the autonomic nervous system.[34] Afferent impulses travel to the spinal cord and the brain, and this causes a change in reaction susceptibility.[55]

Connective tissue is an organ of metabolism; therefore, abnormal tension in one part of the tissue is reflected in other parts.[34] All pathologic changes involve an inflammatory reaction in the affected part. One of the changes caused by inflammatory reaction is accumulation of fluid in the affected area. The area where these changes can most readily be detected is on the body surface. These changes are often seen as flattened areas or depressed bands that may be surrounded by elevated areas. The flat areas are the areas of main response and the connective tissue is tight, resisting pulling in any direction with movement.

The technique of connective tissue massage is not used as much in the United States as it is in European countries, especially Germany. As more results are seen, especially in the treatment of diseases associated with the pathology of circulation, this technique should become more widely accepted and used in this country.

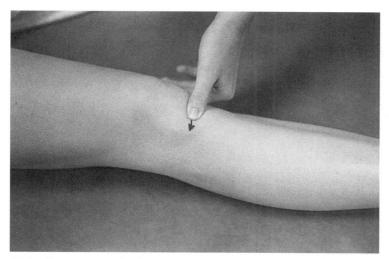

•**Figure 17-23** Transverse tendon friction massage on the patellar tendon.

General Principles of Connective Tissue Massage

Position of the Patient

The patient is usually in the sitting position for a connective tissue massage. Occasionally a patient may be treated in a sidelying or prone position when he or she cannot be treated in a sitting position.

Position of the Therapist

The therapist should be in a position, seated or standing, that provides good body mechanics, is comfortable, and avoids fatigue.

Application Technique

The basic stroke of pulling is performed with the tips, or pads, of the middle and ring fingers of either hand. Fingernails must be very short. The stroking technique is characterized by a tangential pull on the skin and subcutaneous tissues away from the fascia with the fingers. This technique should cause a sharp pain in the tissue. The stroke is a pull, not a push of the tissue. No lubricant is used. All treatments are started by the basic strokes from the coccyx to the first lumbar vertebra. Treatments last about 15–25 minutes. After 15 treatments, which are carried out two to three times per week, there should be a rest period of at least 4 weeks.

Other Considerations

Before any logical plan for treatment can be made, it is important to determine where any alterations in the optimum function of connective tissue have taken place, where the changes started, and, if possible, the cause of the alteration.

Evaluation is a most important part of an effective connective tissue massage program. The technique of stroking with two fingers of one hand along each side of the vertebral column will give much information about the sensory changes that are caused by alterations in the tension of surface tissues.

Indications and Contraindications

There are numerous arterial and venous disorders that may respond to connective tissue massage. Specific disabilities include (1) scars on the skin; (2) fractures and arthritis in the bones and joints; (3) lower back pain and torticollis in the muscles; (4) varicose symptoms, thrombophlebitis (subacute), hemorrhoids, and edema in the blood and lymph; and (5) Raynaud's disease, intermittent claudication, frostbite, and trophic changes in the circulatory system. Connective tissue massage can also be used for myocardial dysfunctions, respiratory disturbances, intestinal disorders, ulcers, hepatitis, infections of the ovaries and uterus (subacute), amenorrhea, dysmenorrhea, genital infantilism, multiple sclerosis, Parkinson's disease, headaches, migraines, and allergies. Connective tissue massage is recommended to help in the process of revascularization following orthopedic complications such as fractures, dislocations, and sprains.

Contraindications to connective tissue massage include tuberculosis, tumors, and mental illnesses that result from psychologic dependence.

Connective tissue massage must be learned and performed initially under the direct supervision of someone who has been taught these highly specialized techniques. More detailed information about connective tissue massage can be found listed in the references.[24,49,70]

ACUPRESSURE AND TRIGGER POINT MASSAGE

acupressure The technique of using finger pressure over acupuncture points to decrease pain.

Acupressure is a type of massage based on the ancient Chinese art of acupuncture. Acupuncture, along with herbal medicine, composes traditional Chinese medicine. Only recently has the amount of research, publication, and interest in acupuncture in Western medical literature increased dramatically.

The Chinese make no distinction between arteries, veins, or nerves when explaining the functions of the body.[50] They concentrate instead on an elaborate system of forces whose interplay is thought to regulate all bodily functions. The traditional, philosophical

Chinese explanation has little correlation with the more scientifically oriented Western concepts of medicine, which rely heavily on anatomic and physiologic principles. Consequently, utilization of acupuncture as a therapeutic technique in Western medical practice has encountered considerable skepticism.

The Chinese believe that an essential life force known as Qi (pronounced che) exists in everyone and controls all aspects of life. Qi is governed by the interplay of two opposing forces, the yang (positive) forces and the yin (negative) forces. Disease and pain result from some imbalance between the two.[51] The yin and yang flow through passageways or lines within the body called jing by the Chinese and known as meridians in the west. The 12 meridians within the body are named according to the part of the body with which they are associated. The meridians on one side of the body are duplicated by those on the other; however, two additional meridians exist that cannot be paired.[52]

1. Lung (L)
2. Large intestine (LI)
3. Stomach (ST)
4. Spleen (SP)
5. Heart (H)
6. Small intestine (SI)
7. Urinary bladder (UB)
8. Kidney (K)
9. Pericardium (P)
10. Triple warmet (TW)
11. Gall bladder (GB)
12. Liver (LIV)
13. Governing vessel (GV) (not paired)
14. Conception vessel (CV) (not paired)

Along these meridians lie the acupuncture points that are associated with each particular meridian. These points are named according to the meridian on which they lie. Whenever there is pain or illness, certain points on the surface of the body become tender.[52] When pain is eliminated or the disease is cured, these tender points seem to disappear.[3] According to acupuncture theory, stimulation of specific points through needling can dramatically reduce pain in areas of the body known to be associated with a particular point. Thousands of acupuncture points have been identified by the Chinese. In the *Nei Ching*, a classical text on Chinese medicine, 365 points that lie on the meridians have been enumerated.[37] Additional acupuncture points have been identified on the auricle as well as the hand.

There is some evidence for the actual physical existence of these points.[74] The electrical resistance of the skin at certain points corresponding to the acupuncture points is lower than that of the surrounding skin, especially when a disease state is present. Examining acupuncture points by sectioning indicated increased nerve endings at these points. Russian investigators have reportedly discovered differences in skin temperature at these points. Despite this evidence, there is no definite physical attribute of all acupuncture points nor is there a thoroughly demonstrated mode of action for the technique. Whatever the explanation, it appears that the locations and effects of stimulating specific acupuncture points for the relief of pain were determined empirically.[42]

Myofascial Trigger Points

In Western medicine, the counterpart of the acupuncture point is the **trigger point**. A **myofascial trigger point** is a hyperirritable locus within a taut band of skeletal muscle, in tendons, myofascia, ligaments and capsules surrounding joints, periosteum, in the skin.[64] Trigger points may activate and become painful because of some trauma to the muscle occurring either from direct trauma or from overuse that result in some inflammatory response.[72] Like acupuncture points, pain is usually referred to areas that follow as specific pattern associated with a particular point. Stimulation of these points has also been demonstrated to result in the relief of pain.[27] Trigger points are classified as being latent or active depending on their clinical characteristics.[62] A latent trigger point does not cause spontaneous pain but may restrict movement or cause muscle weakness.[62] The patient presenting with muscle restrictions or weakness may become aware of pain originating from a latent trigger point only when pressure is applied directly over the point. An active trigger point causes pain at rest. It is tender to palpation with a referred pain pattern that is similar to the patient's pain complaint. This referred pain is felt not at the site of the trigger-point origin, but remote from it. The pain is often described as spreading or radiating. Referred pain is an important characteristic of a trigger point. It differentiates a trigger point from a tender point, which is associated with pain at the site of palpation only. They are palpable within muscles as cord-like bands within a sharply circumscribed area of extreme tenderness. Trigger points are found most commonly in muscles involved in postural support.[35] Acute trauma or repetitive microtrauma may lead to the development of stress on muscle fibers and the formation of trigger points.

Accurate identification of true, *active* trigger points is essential for satisfactory outcomes. Look for these clinical characteristics:

- Patients may have regional, persistent pain resulting in a decreased range of motion in the affected muscles. These include muscles used to maintain body posture, such as those in the neck, shoulders, and pelvic girdle.
- Palpation of a hypersensitive bundle or nodule of muscle fiber of harder than normal consistency is the physical finding typically associated with a trigger point. Palpation of the trigger point will elicit pain directly over the affected area and/or cause radiation of pain toward a zone of reference and a local twitch response.[35]
- Contracting the muscle against fixed resistance significantly increases pain.
- Firm pressure applied over the point usually elicits a "jump sign," with the patient crying out, wincing, or withdrawing from the stimulus.[72]
- One or several fasciculations, called the local twitch response, may be observed when firm pressure is applied over the point.

Acupuncture and trigger points are not necessarily one and the same. However, a study by Melzack, Fox, and Stillwell attempted to develop a correlation coefficient between acupuncture and trigger points on the basis of two criteria: spatial distribution and associated pain patterns.[54] They found a remarkably high correlation coefficient of 0.84, which suggested that acupuncture and trigger points used for pain relief, although discovered independently, labeled by totally different methods, and derived from such historically different concepts of medicine, represent a similar phenomenon and may be explained by the same underlying neural mechanisms.[54]

Physiologic explanations of the effectiveness of acupressure massage may likely be attributed to some interaction of the various mechanisms of pain modulation discussed in Chapter 3.[2] There is considerable evidence that intense, low-frequency stimulation of these points triggers the release of β-endorphin.[60,63,70]

Acupressure Massage Techniques

By using acupuncture charts (Fig. 17-24) or trigger point charts specific points are selected, which are described in the literature as having some relationship to the area of pain.[72] The charts provide the therapist with a general idea of where these points are located. Two techniques may be used to specifically locate acupressure and trigger points. Because it is known that electrical impedance is reduced at these points, an ohmmeter may be used to locate the points. Perhaps the easiest technique is simply to palpate the area until either a small fibrous nodule or a strip of tense muscle tissue that is tender to the touch is felt.[11,15,18]

Once the point is located, massage is begun using the index or middle fingers, the thumb, or perhaps the elbow. Small friction-like circular motions are used on the point. The amount of pressure applied to these acupressure points should be determined by patient tolerance; however, it must be intense and will likely be painful to the patient. Generally, the more pressure the patient can tolerate, the more effective the treatment.

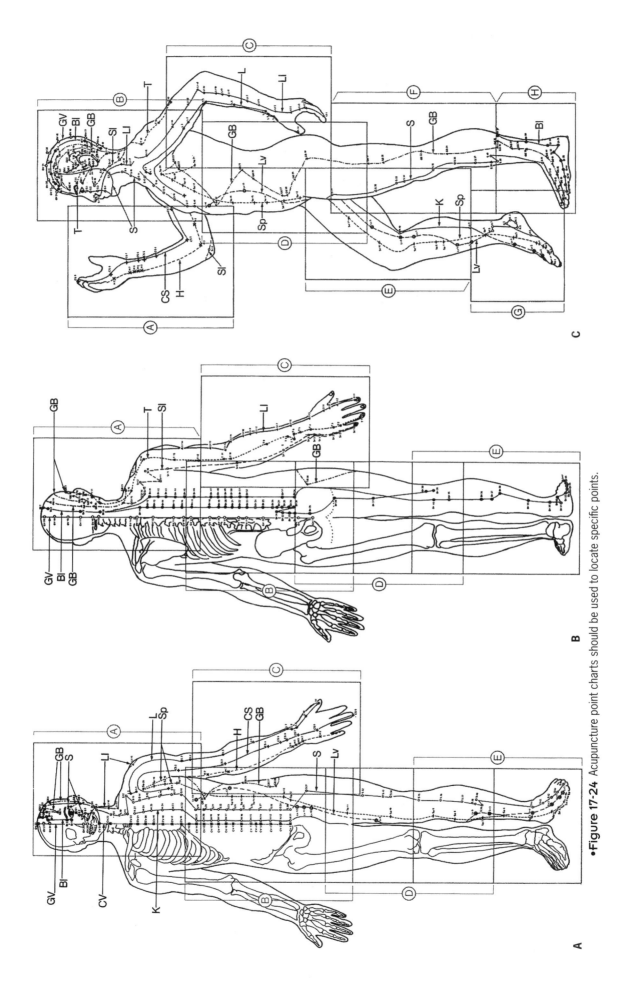

•Figure 17-24 Acupuncture point charts should be used to locate specific points.

Effective treatment times range from 1 to 5 minutes at a single point per treatment. It may be necessary to massage several points during the treatment to obtain the greatest effects. If this is the case, it is best to work distal points first and to move proximally.

During the massage, the patient will report a dulling or numbing effect and will frequently indicate that the pain diminishes or subsides totally during the massage. The lingering effects of acupressure massage vary tremendously from patient to patient. The effects may last for only a few minutes in some but may persist in others for several hours.

MYOFASCIAL RELEASE

Myofascial release is a term that refers to a group of techniques used for the purpose of relieving soft tissue from the abnormal grip of tight fascia.[39] It is essentially a form of stretching that has been reported to have significant impact in treating a variety of conditions.[64] Some specialized training is necessary for the therapist to understand specific techniques of myofascial release, in addition to an in-depth understanding of the fascial system.[4]

Fascia is a type of connective tissue that surrounds muscles, tendons, nerves, bones, and organs. It is essentially continuous from head to toe and is interconnected in various sheaths or planes. Fascia is composed primarily of collagen along with some elastic fibers. During movement the fascia must stretch and move freely. If there is damage to the fascia owing to injury, disease, or inflammation, it will not only affect local adjacent structures but may also affect areas far removed from the site of the injury.[64] Thus it may be necessary to release tightness in both the area of injury as well as in distant areas.[39] It will tend to soften and release inresponse to gentle pressure over a relatively long period of time.[39]

Myofascial release has also been referred to as soft-tissue mobilization, although technically all forms of massage involve mobilization of soft tissue.[55] Soft-tissue mobilization should not be confused with joint mobilization, although it must be emphasized that the two are closely related. Joint mobilization is used to restore normal joint arthrokinematics, and specific rules exist regarding direction of movement and joint position based on the shape of the articulating surfaces. Myofascial restrictions are considerably more unpredictable and may occur in many different planes and directions. Myofascial treatment is based on localizing the restriction and moving into the direction of the restriction regardless of whether that follows the arthrokinematics of a nearby joint.[14] Thus, myofascial manipulation is considerably more subjective and relies heavily on the experience of the clinician.

Myofascial manipulation focuses on large treatment areas, whereas joint mobilization focuses on a specific joint. Releasing myofascial restrictions over a large treatment area can have significant impact on joint mobility.[28] Once a myofascial restriction is located, the massage should be directly through the restriction. The progression of the technique is from superficial to deep. Once more superficial restrictions are released, the deep restrictions can be located and released without causing any damage to superficial tissues. Joint mobilization should follow myofascial release and will likely be more effective once soft-tissue restrictions are eliminated.

As the extensibility is improved in the myofascia, elongation and stretching of the musculotendinous unit should be incorporated.[56] In addition, strengthening exercises are recommended to enhance neuromuscular reeducation, which helps promote new, more efficient movement patterns. As freedom of movement improves, postural reeducation may help to ensure the maintenance of the less restricted movement patterns.

Generally, acute cases tend to resolve in just a few treatments. The longer a condition has been present, the longer it will take to resolve. Occasionally dramatic results will occur immediately after treatment. It is usually recommended that treatment should be performed at least three times per week.[19]

Treatment Considerations

Protecting the Hands

The hands are the primary treatment modality in all forms of massage. Certainly, in myofascial release they are constantly subjected to stress and strain and consideration

myofascial release A group of techniques used for the purpose of relieving soft tissue from the abnormal grip of tight fascia.

Treatment Tip
To treat a myofascial trigger point, a therapist could try several different techniques that have proven to be effective including circular pressure massage, a spray and stretch technique, or a combination of ultrasound and electrical stimulation.

Hands are the most important tool in massage.

must be given to protection of the therapist hands. It is essential to avoid constant hyperextension or hyperflexion of any joints, which may lead to hypermobility. If it is necessary to work in deeper tissues where more force is necessary, then the fist or elbow may be substituted for the thumb and fingers.[14]

Use of Lubricant

It is necessary to use a small amount of lubricant, particularly if large areas are to be treated using long stroking movements. Enough lubricant should be used to allow for traction while reducing painful friction without allowing slipping of the hands on the skin.[14]

Positioning of the Patient

As with the other forms of massage, it is critical to appropriately position the patient such that the effects of the treatment may be maximized. Pillows or towel rolls may be a great aid in establishing and effective treatment position even before the hands contact the patient (Fig. 17-25). The therapist should make certain that good body mechanics and positioning are considered to protect the therapist as well as the patient.

STRAIN/COUNTERSTRAIN

Strain/counterstrain is an approach to decreasing muscle tension and guarding that may be used to normalize muscle function. It is a passive technique that places the body in a position of greatest comfort, thereby relieving pain.[38]

In this technique, the physical therapist locates a trigger point on the patient's body that corresponds to areas of dysfunction in specific joints or muscles that are in need of treatment. These tender points are not located in or just beneath the skin as are many acupuncture points, but deeper in muscle, tendon, ligament, or fascia. They are characterized by tense, tender, edematous sports on the body; they are 1 cm or less in diameter, with the most acute point 3 mm in diameter, although they may be a few centimeters long within a muscle; there may be multiple points for one specific joint dysfunction; they may be arranged in a chain; and points are often found in a painless area opposite the site of pain and/or weakness.[38]

The physical therapist monitors the tension and level of pain elicited by the tender point as he or she moves the patient into a position of ease or comfort. This is accomplished by markedly shortening the muscle. When this position of ease is found, the

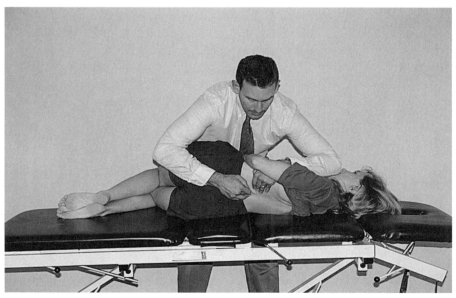

•**Figure 17-25** Myofascial release is a mild combination of pressure and stretch used to free soft-tissue restrictions.

tender point is no longer tense or tender. When this position is maintained for a minimum of 90 seconds, the tension in the tender point and in the corresponding joint or muscle is reduced or cleared. By slowly returning to a neutral position, the tender point and the corresponding joint or muscle remain pain free with normal tension. For example, with neck pain and/or tension headaches, the tender points may be found on either the front or back of the patient's neck and shoulders.[32] The physical therapist will have the patient lay on his or her back and will gently and slowly bend the patient's neck until that tender point is no longer tender (Fig. 17-26). After holding that position for 90 seconds, the physical therapist gently and slowly returns the patient's neck to its resting position. Upon pressing that tender point again, the patient should notice a significant decrease in pain at that tender point.[1,32]

The physiologic rationale for the effectiveness of the strain-counterstrain technique can be explained by the stretch reflex. When a muscle is placed in a stretched position, impulses from the muscle spindles create a reflex contraction of the muscle in response to stretch. With strain/counterstrain, the joint or muscle is not placed in a position of stretch but rather a slack position. Thus muscle spindle input is reduced and the muscle is relaxed, allowing for a decrease in tension and pain.[32]

POSITIONAL RELEASE THERAPY

Positional release therapy (PRT) is based on the strain/counterstrain technique. The primary difference between the two is the use of a facilitating force (compression) to enhance the effect of the positioning.[16,17] Like strain/counterstrain, PRT is an osteopathic mobilization technique in which the body is brought into a position of greatest relaxation.[21] The physical therapist finds the position of greatest comfort and muscle relaxation for each joint with the help of movement tests and diagnostic tender points. Once located, the tender point is maintained with the palpating finger at a subthreshold pressure. The patient is then passively placed in a position that reduces the tension under the palpating finger and causes a subjective reduction in tenderness as reported by the patient. This specific position is adjusted throughout the 90-second treatment period. It has been suggested that maintaining contact with the tender point during the treatment period exerts a therapeutic effect.[16,17] This technique is one of the most effective and most gentle methods for the treatment of acute and chronic musculoskeletal dysfunction (Fig. 17-27).

ACTIVE RELEASE TECHNIQUE

Active release technique (ART) is a relatively new type of manual therapy that has been developed to correct soft-tissue problems in muscle, tendon, and fascia caused by formation of fibrotic adhesions as a result of acute injury, repetitive or overuse injuries, or constant pressure or tension injuries.[45,46] When a muscle, tendon, fascia, or ligament

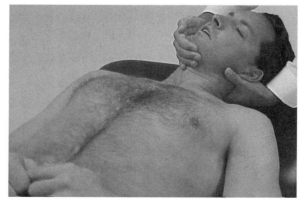

•**Figure 17-26** Strain-counterstrain technique. The body part is placed in a position of comfort for 90 seconds and then slowly moved back to a neutral position.

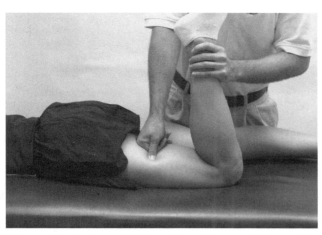

•**Figure 17-27** The positional release technique places the muscle in a position of comfort with the figure or thumb exerting submaximal pressure on a tender point.

is torn (strained or sprained) or a nerve is damaged, the tissues heal with adhesions or scar tissue formation rather than the formation of brand new tissue. Scar tissue is weaker, less elastic, less pliable, and more pain sensitive than healthy tissue. These fibrotic adhesions disrupt the normal muscle function, which in turn affects the biomechanics of the joint complex, and can lead to pain and dysfunction. Active release technique provides a way to diagnose and treat the underlying causes of cumulative trauma disorders that, left uncorrected, can lead to inflammation, adhesions/fibrosis, muscle imbalances resulting in weak and tense tissues, decreased circulation, hypoxia, and symptoms of peripheral nerve entrapment including numbness, tingling, burning, and aching.[45,46]

Active release technique is a deep tissue technique used for breaking down scar tissue/adhesions and restoring function and movement. In the active release technique, the physical therapist should first locate through palpation, those adhesions in the muscle, tendon, or fascia that are causing the problem. Once located the physical therapist then traps the affected muscle by applying pressure or tension with the thumb or finger over these lesions in the direction of the fibers (Fig. 17-28). Then the patient is asked to actively move the body part such that the musculature is elongated from a shortened position while the physical therapist continues to apply tension to the lesion. This should be repeated three to five times per treatment session. By breaking up the adhesions, the patient's condition will steadily improve by softening and stretching the scar tissue, resulting in increased range of motion, increased strength, and improved circulation which optimizes healing. Treatments tend to be uncomfortable during the movement phases as the scar tissue or adhesions tear apart. This is temporary and subsides almost immediately after the treatment. An important part of

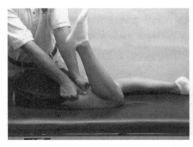 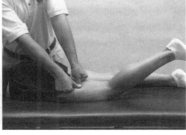

•**Figure 17-28** Active release technique. The muscle is elongated from a shortened position while static pressure is applied to the tender point.

active release technique is for the patient to heed the physical therapist's recommendations regarding activity modification, stretching, and exercise.[12,45,46]

ROLFING

Rolfing, also referred to as structural integration, is a system devised by Ida Rolf that is used to correct inefficient structure or to "integrate structure."[7] The goal of this technique is to balance to body within a gravitational field through a technique involving manual soft-tissue manipulation.[14] The basic principle of treatment is that if balanced movement is essential at a particular joint yet nearby tissue is restrained, both the tissue and the joint will relocate to a position that accomplishes a more appropriate equilibrium.[40,61]

Rolfing A system devised to correct inefficient structure by balancing the body within a gravitational field through a technique involving manual soft-tissue manipulation.

Rolfing is a standardized approach that is administered without regard to symptoms or specific pathologies. The technique involves 10 hour-long sessions, each of which emphasizes some aspect of posture with the massage directed toward the myofascia. The 10 sessions include the following.

1. Respiration
2. Balance under the body (legs and feet)
3. Sagittal plane balance: lateral line from front to back
4. Balance left to right: base of body to midline
5. Pelvic balance: rectus abdominis and psoas
6. Weight transfer from head to feet: sacrum
7. Relationship of head to rest of body: occiput and atlas
8. **and 9.** Upper half of the body to lower half of the body relationship
10. Balance throughout the system

Once these 10 treatments are completed, advanced sessions may be performed in addition to periodic "tune-up" sessions.

A major aspect of this treatment approach is to integrate the structural with the psychologic. An emotional state may be seen as the projection of structural imbalances. The easiest and most efficient method for changing the physical body is through direct intervention in the body. Changing the structural imbalances can alter the psychologic component.[61]

TRAGER

Trager A technique that attempts to establish neuromuscular control so that more normal movement patterns can be routinely performed.

Developed by Milton Trager, **Tragering** combines mechanical soft-tissue mobilization and neurophysiologic reeducation.[71] Unlike Rolfing, Trager has no standardized protocols or procedures. The Trager system uses gentle, passive, rocking oscillations of a body part. This is essentially a mobilization technique emphasizing traction and rotation as a relaxation technique to encourage the patient to relinquish control. This relaxation technique is followed by a series of active movements designed to alter the patient's neurophysiologic control of movement, thus providing a basis for maintaining these changes. This technique does not attempt to make mechanical changes in the soft tissues but rather to establish neuromuscular control, so that more normal movement patterns can be routinely performed. Essentially it uses the nervous system to make changes rather than making mechanical changes in the tissues themselves.[71]

Indications and Contraindications for Massage

The areas of treatment that we most often see patients for are muscle, tendon, and joint conditions. Adhesions, muscle spasm, myositis, bursitis, fibrositis, tendinitis or tenosynovitis, and postural strain of the back all generally fall into this category.

Areas of concern that indicate that you should not treat a patient with massage include arteriosclerosis, thrombosis or embolism, severe varicose veins, acute phlebitis, cellulitis, synovitis, abscesses, skin injections, cancers, and pregnancy. Acute inflammatory conditions of the skin, soft tissues, or joints are also contraindications.

THE CURRENT ROLE OF MASSAGE IN PHYSICAL THERAPY

Therapeutic massage is a skill that has flourished in the "alternative health care" community. Physical therapists at one point in the evolution of the profession seemed to feel that massage was perhaps beneath their level of professional skill requirements and should be delegated to those with lesser skills and more time to spend in patient treatment. Consequently, with the understanding and demand for alternative therapy, massage has made a great comeback in therapeutic use, and most practicing therapists have been outpaced by massage therapists or their former aides. The problem today in choosing massage as a form of intervention is that third-party payers often do not recognize it as the standard of care anymore for some musculoskeletal interventions and will not pay for its selection. This means patients have to go to massage therapists and pay out-of-pocket for this modality.

SUMMARY

1. Massage, as we know it today, is an improved and more scientific version of the various procedures that go back thousands of years to the Greeks, Egyptians, and others.

2. Massage is the mechanical stimulation of tissue by means of rhythmically applied pressure and stretching. It allows the therapist, as a health care provider, to assist a patient to overcome pain and to relax through the application of the therapeutic massage techniques.

3. Massage has effects on the circulation, the lymphatic system, the nervous system, the muscles, myofascia, the skin, scar tissue, psychologic responses, relaxation feelings, and pain.

4. Hoffa massage is the classic form of massage and uses strokes that include effleurage, petrissage, percussion, or tapotement, and vibration.

5. Friction massage is used to increase the inflammatory response, particularly in cases of chronic tendinitis or tenosynovitis.

6. Massage of acupuncture and trigger points is used to reduce pain and irritation in anatomic areas known to be associated with specific points.

7. Connective tissue massage is a reflex zone massage. It is a relatively new form of treatment in this country and has its best effects on circulatory pathologies.

8. Myofascial release is a massage technique used for the purpose of relieving soft tissue from the abnormal grip of tight fascia.

9. Rolfing is a system devised to correct inefficient structure by balancing the body within a gravitational field through a technique involving manual soft tissue manipulation.

10. Trager attempts to establish neuromuscular control so that more normal movement patterns can be routinely performed.

REVIEW QUESTIONS

1. Discuss the evolution of massage as a treatment modality.
2. What are the physiologic effects of massage?
3. What are the reflexive effects of massage on pain, circulation, and metabolism?
4. What are the mechanical effects of massage on muscle and skin?

Indications and Contraindications for Therapeutic Sports Massage

Indications
- Increase coordination
- Decrease pain
- Decrease neuromuscular excitibility
- Stimulate circulation
- Facilitate healing
- Restore joint mobility
- Remove lactic acid
- Alleviate muscle cramps
- Increase blood flow
- Increase venous return
- Retard muscle atrophy
- Increase range of motion
- Edema
- Myofascial trigger points
- Stretching scar tissue
- Adhesions
- Muscle spasm
- Myositis
- Bursitis
- Fibrositis
- Tendinitis
- Revascularization
- Raynaud's disease
- Intermittent claudication
- Dysmenorrhea
- Headaches
- Migraines

Contraindications
- Arteriosclerosis
- Thrombosis
- Embolism
- Severe varicose veins
- Acute phlebitis
- Cellulitis
- Synovitis
- Abscesses
- Skin infections
- Cancers
- Acute inflammatory conditions

5. What psychologic benefits can come with massage?

6. What are the various considerations for setting up equipment and preparing a patient for massage?

7. What are the various stroking techniques used in traditional Hoffa massage?

8. What are the clinical applications for using friction massage?

9. What is connective tissue massage most often used for?

10. What is the difference between acupuncture points and myofascial trigger points?

11. How can myofascial release be used to restore normal functional movement patterns?

REFERENCES

1. Alexander, K.M.: Use of strain-counterstrain as an adjunct for treatment of chronic lower abdominal pain, Phys. Ther. Case Rep. 2(5):205–208, 1999.

2. Archer, P.A.: Massage for sports health care professionals, Champaign, IL, Human Kinetics, 1999.

3. Archer, P.A.: Three clinical sports massage approaches for treating injured athletes, Athl. Ther. Today 6(3):14–20, 36–37, 60, 2001.

4. Barnes, J.: Five years of myofascial release, Phys. Ther. Forum 6(37):12–14, 1987.

5. Barr, J., Taslitz, N.: Influence of back massage on autonomic functions, Phys. Ther. 50:1679–1691, 1970.

6. Bell, G.W.: Aquatic sports massage therapy, Clin. Sports Med. 18(2):427–435, 1999.

7. Bernau-Eigen, M.: Rolfing: a somatic approach to the integration of human structures, Nurse Pract. Forum 9(4): 235–242, 1998.

8. Birukov, A.: Training massage during contemporary sports loads, Soviet Sports Rev. 22:42–44, 1987.

9. Boone, T., Cooper, R., and Thompson, W.: A physiologic evaluation of the sports massage, Athl. Train. 26(1):51–54, 1991.

10. Braverman, D.L., Schulman, R.A.: Massage techniques in rehabilitation medicine, Phys. Med. Rehabil. Clin. North Am. 10(3):631–649, 1999.

11. Brickey, R., Yao, J.: Acupuncture and transcutaneous electrical stimulation techniques, Course manual in acutherapy post graduate seminars, Raleigh, NC, 1978.

12. Buchberger, D.: Use of active release techniques in the post operative shoulder, J. Sports Chiropr. Rehabil. 2(6):60–65, 1999.

13. Cafarelli, E.: Vibratory massage and short-term recovery from muscular fatigue, Int. J. Sports Med. 11:474, 1990.

14. Cantu, R., Grodin, A.: Myofascial manipulation: theory and clinical applications, Gaithersburg, MD, 1992, Aspen.

15. Castel, J.: Pain management with acupuncture and transcutaneous electrical nerve stimulation techniques and photo stimulation (Laser), course manual, 1982.

16. Chaitlow, L.: Positional release techniques (advanced soft tissue techniques), Philadelphia, PA, 1996, Churchill Livingstone.

17. Chaitow, L.: Positional release techniques in the treatment of muscle and joint dysfunction, Clin. Bull. Myofascial Ther. 3(1):25–35, 1998.

18. Cheng, R., Pomerantz, B.: Electroacupuncture analgesia could be mediated by at least two pain relieving mechanisms: endorphin and non-endorphin systems, Life Sci. 25:1957–1962, 1979.

19. Crosman, L., Chateauvert, S., and Weisberg, J.: The effects of massage to the hamstring muscle group on range of motion, J. Orthop. Sport Phys. Ther. 6:168, 1984.

20. Cyriax, J., Russell, G.: Textbook of orthopedic medicine, vol. II., ed. 10, Baltimore, MD, 1980, Williams & Wilkins.

21. D'Ambrogio, K., Roth, G.: Positional release therapy: assessment and treatment of musculoskeletal dysfunction, St. Louis, MO, 1996, Mosby-Yearbook.

22. Dubrovsky V.: Changes in muscle and venous blood flow after massage, Soviet Sports Rev. 18:134–135, 1983.

23. Ebel, A., Wisham, L.: Effect of massage on muscle temperature and radiosodium clearance, Arch. Phys. Med. 33:399–405, 1952.

24. Ebner, M.: Connective tissue manipulations, Malibar, FL, 1985, R.E. Krieger.

25. Elkins, E.: Effects of various procedures on flow of lymph, Arch. Phys. Med. 34:31–39, 1953.

26. Ernst, E.: Does post-exercise massage treatment reduce delayed onset muscle soreness? A systematic review, Br. J. Sports Med. 32(3):212–214, 1998.

27. Fox, E., Melzack, R.: Transcutaneous electrical stimulation and acupuncture: comparison of treatment for low back pain, Pain 2:357–373, 1976.

28. Gordon, P.: Myofascial reorganization, Brookline, MA, 1988, The Gordon Group.

29. Harmer, P.: The effect of preperformance massage on stide frequency in sprinters, Athl. Train. 26(1):55–59, 1991.

30. Head, H.: Die Sensibilitatssstsstorungen der Haut bei viszeral Erkran Kungen, Berlin, 1898.

31. Heller, M.: Low-force manual adjusting. "Strain-counter-Strain." Dyn. Chiropr. 221(12):16, 18, 2003.

32. Hemmings, B., Smith, M., Graydon, J., and Dyson, R.: Effects of massage on physiological restoration, perceived recovery, and repeated sports performance, Br. J. Sports Med. 34(2): 109–114, 2000.

33. Hoffa, A.: Technik der massage, ed. 14, Stuttgart, 1900, Ferdinand Enke.

34. Holey, E.A.: Connective tissue massage: a bridge between complementary and orthodox approaches, Bodywork Mov. Ther. 4(1):72–80, 2000.

35. Hou, C.: Immediate effects of various physical therapeutic modalities on cervical myofascial pain and trigger-point sensitivity, Arch. Phys. Med. Rehabil. 83(10):1406–1414, 2002.

36. Hungerford, M., Bornstein, R.: Sports massage, Sports Medm. Guide 4:4–6, 1985.

37. Hwang Ti Nei Ching (translation), Berkeley, CA, 1973, University of California Press.

38. Jones, L.: Strain-counterstrain, Boise, ID, 1995, Jones Strain-Counterstrain.

39. Juett, T.: Myofascial release—an introduction for the patient, Phys. Ther. Forum 7(41):7–8, 1988.

40. Kallen, B.: Deep impact: rolfing is deeper than the deepest massage—and sometimes more painful. Some athletes swear by it anyway, Men's Fit. 16(7):96–99, 2000.

41. King, R.: Performance massage, Champaign, IL, 1993, Human Kinetics.

42. Kopysov, V.: Use of vibrational massage in regulating the pre-competition condition of weight lifters, Soviet Sports Rev. 14:82–84, 1979.

43. Kuprian, W.: Massage. In Kuprian, W., editor. Physical therapy for sports, Philadelphia, PA, 1981, W.B. Saunders.

44. Latz, J.: Key elements of connective tissue massage, J. Massage Ther. 41(4): 44–45, 46–50, 52–53, 2003.

45. Leahy, M.: Active release techniques soft tissue management system, manual, Colorado Springs, CO, 1996, Active release Techniques, LLP.

46. Leahy, M.: Improved Treatments for carpal tunnel and related syndromes, Chiropr. Sports Med. 9(1):6–9, 1995.

47. Lewis, C.: The use of strain-counterstrain in the treatment of patients with low back pain, J. Man. Manipulative Ther. 9(2):92–98, 2001.

48. Longworth, J.: Psychophysiological effects of slow stroke back massage in normotensive females, Adv. Nurs. Sci. 10:44–61, 1982.

49. Licht, S.: Massage, manipulation and traction, New Haven, CT, 1960, Elizabeth Licht.

50. Man, P., Chen, C.: Acupuncture aesthesia—a new theory and clinical study, Curr. Ther. Res. 14:390–394, 1972.

51. Manaka, Y.: On certain electrical phenomena for the interpretation of Chi in Chinese literature, Am. J. Chin. Med. 3:71–74, 1975.

52. Mann, F.: Acupuncture: the ancient Chinese art of healing and how it works scientifically, New York, 1973, Random House.

53. Martin, N.A., Zoeller, R.F., and Robertson, R.J.: The comparative effect of sports massage, active recovery, and rest on promoting blood lactate clearing after supramaximal leg exercise, J. Athl. Train. 33(1):30–35, 1998.

54. Melzack, R., Stillwell, D., and Fox, E.: Trigger points and acupuncture points for pain: correlations and implications, Pain 3:3–23, 1977.

55. Mennell, J.: Physical treatment, ed. 5, Philadelphia, PA, 1968, Blakiston.

56. Mock, L.E.: Myofascial release treatment of specific muscles of the upper extremity (levels 3 and 4): part 4, Clin. Bull. Myofascial Ther. 3(1):71–93, 1998.

57. Morelli, M., Seaborne, P.T., and Sullivan, S.J.: Changes in H-reflex amplitude during massage of triceps surae in healthy subjects, J. Orthop. Sports Phys. Ther. 12(2):55–59, 1990.

58. Patino, O., Novick, C., Merlo, A., and Benaim, F.: Massage in hypertrophic scars, J. Burn Care Rehabil. 20(3):268–271, 1999.

59. Pemberton, R.: The physiologic influence of massage. In Mock, H.E., Pemberton, R., and Coulter, J.S., editors. Principles and practices of physical therapy, vol. I, Hagerstown, MD, 1939, W.F. Prior.

60. Prentice, W.: The use of electroacutherapy in the treatment of inversion ankle sprains, J. Nat. Athl. Train. Assoc. 17(1):15–21, 1982.

61. Rolf, I.: Rolfing: the integration of human structures, Rochester, VT, 1977, Healing Arts Press.

62. Simons, D.G.: Understanding effective treatments of myofascial trigger points, J. Bodywork Mov. Ther. 6(2):81–88, 2002.

63. Sjolund, B., Eriksson, M.: Electroacupuncture and endogenous morphines, Lancet 2:1085, 1976.

64. Stone, J.A.: Myofascial release, Athl. Ther. Today 5(4):34–35, 2000.

65. Stone, J.A.: Prevention and rehabilitation. Myofascial techniques: trigger-point therapy, Athl. Ther. Today 5(3): 54–55, 2000.

66. Stone, J.A.: Massage as a therapeutic modality—technique, Athl. Ther. Today 4(5):51–52, 1999.

67. Stone, J.A.: Prevention and rehabilitation. The rationale for therapeutic massage, Athl. Ther. Today, 4(4):26, 1999.

68. Sullivan, S.: Effects of massage on alpha motorneuron excitability, Phys. Ther. 71:555, 1991.

69. Suskind, M., Hajek, N., and Hinds, H.: Effects of massage on denervated muscle, Arch. Phys. Med. 27:133–135, 1946.

70. Tappan, F.: Healing massage techniques: holistic, classic, and emerging methods, East Norwalk, CT, 1988, Appleton & Lange.

71. Trager, M.: Trager psychophysical integration and mentastics, Trager J. 5:10, 1982.

72. Travell, J., Simons, D.: Myofascial pain and dysfunction: the trigger point manual, Baltimore, MD, 1983, Williams & Wilkins.

73. Vaughn, B., Miller, K., and Fink, D.: Massage for sports health care, Champaign, IL, Human Kinetics, 1998.

74. Wei, L.: Scientific advances in Chinese medicine, Am. J. Chin. Med. 7:53–75, 1979.

75. Wood, E., Becker, P.: Beard's massage, Philadelphia, PA, 1981, W.B. Saunders.

76. Wyper, D., McNiven, D.: Effects of some physiotherapeutic agents on skeletal muscle blood flow, Phys. Ther. 62:83–85, 1976.

SUGGESTED READINGS

Barnes, M., Personius, W., and Gronlund, R.: An efficacy study on the effect on myofascial release treatment technique on obtaining pelvic symmetry, Phys. Ther. 19(1):56, 1994.

Bean, B., Henderson, H., and Martinsen, M.: Massage: how to do it and what it can do for you, Scholast. Coach 52(5):10–11, 1982.

Beard, G., Wood, E.: Massage: principles and techniques, Philadelphia, PA, 1964, W.B. Saunders.

Beard, G.: A history of massage technique, Phys. Ther. Rev. 32:613–624, 1952.

Beck, M.: Theory and practice of therapeutic massage, Albany, NY, 1994, Malidy.

Breakey, B.: An overlooked therapy you can use ad lib, RN 45:7, 1982.

Chamberlain, G.: Cyriax's friction massage: a review, J. Orthop. Sports Phys. Ther. 4(1):16–22, 1982.

Cyriax, J.: Textbook of orthopedic medicine, vol. I, ed. 8, New York, 1982, Macmillan.

Day, J., Mason, P., and Chesrow, S.: Effect of massage on serom level of β-endorphin and β-lipotrophin in healthy adults, Phys. Ther. 67:926–930, 1987.

Ebner, M.: Connective tissue massage, Physiotherapy 64:208–210, 1978.

Ehrett, S.: Craniosacral therapy and myofascial release in entry-level physical therapy curricula, Phys. Ther. 68(4):534–540, 1988.

Ernst, E., Matra, A., and Magyarosy, I.: Massages cause changes in blood fluidity, Physiotherapy 73:43–45, 1987.

Fritz, S.: Fundamentals of therapeutic massage, St. Louis, MD, 1995, Mosby.

Goats, G.: Massage: the scientific basis of an ancient art: Part 1. The techniques, Br. J. Sports Med. 28(3):149–152, 1994.

Goldberg, J., Seaborne, D., and Sullivan, S.: The effect of therapeutic massage on H-reflex amplitude in persons with a spinal cord injury, Phys. Ther. 74(8):728–737, 1994.

Hall, D.: A practical guide to the art of massage, Runner's World 14(10):58–59, 1979.

Hammer, W.: The use of transverse friction massage in the management of chronic bursitis of the hip or shoulder, J. Man. Physiol. Ther. 16(2):107–111, 1993.

Hanten, W., Chandler, S.: Effects of myofascial release leg pull and sagittal plane isometric contract-relax techniques on passive straight-leg raise angle, JOSPT 20(3):138–144, 1994.

Hilbert, J.E.: The effects of massage on delayed onset muscle soreness, Br. J. Sports Med. 37(1):72–75, 2003.

Hollis, M.: Massage for therapists, Oxford, England, 1987, Blackwell Scientific.

Hovind, H., Neilson, S.: Effect of massage on blood flow in skeletal muscle, Scand. J. Rehabil. Med. 6:74–77, 1974.

Kewley, M.: What you should know about massage, Int. Swim. September:29–30, 1982.

Kirshbaum, M.: Using massage in the relief of lymphoedema, Prof. Nurse 11(4):230–232, 1996.

Malkin, K.: Use of massage in clinical practice, Br. J. Nurs. 3(6):292–294, 1994.

Manheim, C., Lavett, D.: The myofascial release manual, Thorofare, NJ, 1989, Slack.

Martin, D.: Massage, Jogger 10(5):8–15, 1978.

McConnell, A.: Practical massage, Nurs. Times. 91(36):S2–14, 1995.

McGillicuddy, M.: Sports massage: three key principles of sports massage, Massage Today 3(5):10, 2003.

McKeechie, A.A.: Anxiety states; a preliminary report on the value of connective tissue massage, J. Psychosomat. Res. 27(2): 125–129, 1983.

Meagher, J., Boughton, P.: Sportsmassage, New York, 1980, Doubleday & Co.

Morelli, M., Seaborne, D., and Sullivan, S.: H-reflex modulation during manual muscle massage of human triceps surae, Arch. Phys. Med. Rehabil. 72(11):915–999, 1991.

Morelli, M., Seaborne, P.T., and Sullivan, S.J.: H-reflex modulation during massage of triceps surae in healthy subjects, Arch. Phys. Med. Rehabil. 72:915, 1991.

Newman, T., Martin, D., and Wilson, L.: Massage effects on muscular endurance, J. Athl. Train. 31(Suppl.):S-18, 1996.

Pellecchia, G., Hamel, H., and Behnke, P.: Treatment of infrapatellar tendinitis: a combination of modalities and transverse friction massage versus iontophoresis, J. Sport Rehabil. 3(2): 135–145, 1994.

Phaigh, R., Perry, P.: Athletic massage, New York, 1984, Simon & Schuster.

Pope, M., Phillips, R., and Haugh, L.: A prospective randomized three-week trial of spinal manipulation, transcutaneous muscle stimulation, massage and corset in the treatment of subacute low back pain, Spine 19(22):2571–2577, 1994.

Rogoff, J.: Manipulation, traction and massage, ed. 2, Baltimore, MD, 1980, Williams & Wilkins.

Ryan, J.: The neglected art of massage, Phys. Sports Med. 18(12):25, 1980.

Smith, L., Keating, M., and Holbert, D.: The effects of athletic massage on delayed onset muscle soreness, creatine kinase, and neutrophil count: a preliminary report, JOSPT 19(2):93–99, 1994.

Stamford, B.: Massage for patients, Phys. Sports Med. 13(10):178, 1985.

Steward, B., Woodman, R., and Hurlburt, D.: Fabricating a splint for deep friction massage, JOSPT 21(3):172–175, 1995.

Stone, J.A.: Prevention and rehabilitation. Strain—counterstrain, Athl. Ther. Today 5(6):30–31, 2000.

Sucher, B.: Myofascial manipulative release of carpal tunnel syndrome: documentation with magnetic resonance imaging, J. Am. Osteopath. Assn. 93(12):1273–1278, 1993.

Sucher, B.: Myofascial release of carpal tunnel syndrome, J. Am. Osteopath. Assn. 93(1):92–94, 100–101, 1993.

Tappan, F.: Healing massage techniques: a study of eastern and western methods, Reston, VA, 1978, Reston Publishing.

Tiidus, P., Shoemaker, J.: Effleurage massage, muscle blood flow and long-term post-exercise strength recovery, Int. J. Sports Med. 16(7):478–483, 1995.

Trevelyan, J.: Massage, Nurs. Times 89(19):45–47, 1993.

van Schie, T.: Connective tissue massage for reflex sympathetic dystrophy: a case study, N.Z. J. Physiother. 21(2):26, 1993.

Wakim, K.G., Martin, G.M., and Terrier, J.C.: The effects of massage in normal and paralyzed extremities, Arch. Phys. Med. 30:135–144, 1949.

Weber, M., Servedio, F., and Woodall, W.: The effects of three modalities on delayed onset muscle soreness, JOSPT 20(5): 236–242, 1994.

Whitehill, W.: Massage and skin conditions: indications and contraindications, Athl. Ther. Today 7(3):24–28, 2002.

Wiktorrson-Moeller, M., Oberg, B., and Ekstrand, J.: Effects of warming up, massage and stretching on range of motion and muscle strength in the lower extremity, Am. J. Sports Med. 11:249–251, 1983.

Yates, J.: Physiological effects of therapeutic massage and their application to treatment, British Columbia, 1989, Massage Therapists Association.

GLOSSARY

acupressure The technique of using finger pressure over acupuncture points to decrease pain.

Bindegewebsmassage Reflex zone massage; uses a pulling stroke across connective tissue to effect change.

effleurage To stroke; any stroke that glides over the skin without attempting to move the deep muscle masses. The hand is molded to the part, stroking with more or less constant pressure, usually upward. Any degree of pressure may be applied, varying from the lightest possible touch to very deep pressure.

friction massage A technique that affects fibrositic adhesions in tendon, muscle, or ligament. It is performed by small circular movements that penetrate into the depth of a muscle, not by moving the finger on the skin, but by moving the tissues under the skin.

massage The act of rubbing, kneading, or stroking the superficial parts of the body with the hand or with an instrument for the purpose of modifying nutrition, restoring power of movement, or breaking up adhesions.

myofascial release A group of techniques used for the purpose of relieving soft tissue from the abnormal grip of tight fascia.

petrissage Massage technique that is a kneading manipulation. Consists of repeatedly grasping and releasing the tissue with one or both hands or parts thereof, in a lifting, rolling, or pressing movement. The outside characteristic of this movement as contrasted to stroking movements is that the pressure is applied intermittently.

Rolfing A system devised to correct inefficient structure by balancing the body within a gravitational field through a technique involving manual soft tissue manipulation.

tapotement A percussion massage; any series of brisk blows following each other in a rapid alternating fashion: hacking, cupping, slapping, beating, tapping, and pinchment. It is used when stimulation is the objective.

Trager A technique that attempts to establish neuromuscular control so that more normal movement patterns can be routinely performed.

vibration A shaking massage technique; a fine tremulous movement made by the hand or fingers placed firmly against a part that will cause the part to vibrate. Often used for a soothing effect; may be stimulating when more energy is applied.

LAB ACTIVITY

MASSAGE

DESCRIPTION

Massage is most likely the oldest form of mechanical therapy for injury. Even very small children know that rubbing an injured area tends to diminish the pain. As with essentially all physical agents, the massage itself does not produce healing, but the therapeutic effects can assist during the healing process.

There are many types of massage, each with proponents and detractors. The different types of massage have different proposed physiologic and therapeutic effects, although there is a great deal of overlap. In essence, all forms of massage involve the application of mechanical force to various tissues of the body, usually with the therapist's hands. Massage may exert an influence on the injured or dysfunctional tissue via either via a direct mechanical action or neurologic reflexes.

PHYSIOLOGIC EFFECTS

Increase in large-diameter afferent neural input
Increase in venous outflow
Increase in lymph outflow

THERAPEUTIC EFFECTS

Decreased pain
Decreased soft tissue swelling and congestion
Remodeling of collagen

INDICATIONS

The indications for massage vary depending on the type of massage used. In general, pain, swelling, and connective tissue contracture are the indications for massage.

CONTRAINDICATIONS

There are probably no absolute contraindications to massage. Obviously, precautions should be used in the case of fractures, open wounds, and severe pain. The amount of pressure applied can be regulated based on the irritability of the tissue and the desired effect.

MASSAGE

PROCEDURE	EVALUATION		
	1	2	3
1. Check supplies.			
a. Obtain sheet or towels for draping.			
b. Obtain lubricant as indicated.			
2. Question patient.			
a. Verify identity of patient (if not already verified).			
b. Verify the absence of contraindications.			
c. Ask about previous massage treatments, check treatment notes.			

PROCEDURE	EVALUATION		
	1	2	3
3. Position patient.			
a. Place patient in a well-supported, comfortable position. Positioning is particularly crucial for massage.			
b. Expose body part to be treated.			
c. Drape patient to preserve patient's modesty, protect clothing, but allow access to body part.			
4. Inspect body part to be treated.			
a. Check light touch perception.			
b. Check circulatory status (pulses, capillary refill).			
c. Verify that there are no open wounds or rashes.			
d. Assess function of body part (e.g., ROM, irritability).			
5a. Apply Hoffa massage			
a. After applying lubricant, effleurage is applied with a stroking motion from distal to proximal with light to moderate pressure; the deeper tissue is not moved. The initial strokes serve to distribute the lubricant over the treatment area.			
b. Petrissage is a kneading type motion, where the muscles are lifted and rolled.			
c. Tapotement is a series of percussion movements with the tips of the fingers, the ulnar border of the hands, the heel of the hands, or cupped hands.			
d. Vibration is a rapid oscillation or tremor of the hands when they are in firm contact with the skin.			
5b. Apply transverse friction massage.			
a. No lubricant is used.			
b. The tendon or ligament is placed on a slight stretch.			
c. Using deep pressure, such that the skin and thumb or finger, move together over the deeper tissue, apply a back-and-forth motion perpendicular to the fibers of the tendon or ligament.			
d. The duration of the massage should be up to 10 minutes, or as tolerated by the patient.			
5c. Apply connective tissue massage (Bindegewebsmassage).			
a. No lubricant is used.			
b. Using the tips of the third and fourth digits, the skin and subcutaneous tissues are pulled away from the fascia.			
c. The massage extends from the coccyx to the upper lumbar area, and each pulling stroke should produce a transient, sharp pain.			
d. Duration of treatment should be 15–25 minutes or as tolerated by the patient.			
5d. Acupressure/Trigger Point Massage.			
a. No lubricant is used.			
b. Technique is similar to transverse friction massage, but is applied to a trigger or acupuncture point (found using a chart, or by palpation). Trigger points usually are nodular-like lumps in a muscle, and often feel gritty.			
c. Using the tip of any digit, or even the olecranon process, the skin is moved on the trigger point; no motion should take place between the therapist and the patient's skin. The motion is circular, and is confined to the point.			
d. Pressure will be painful, and as hard as the patient can tolerate. The pressure may produce pain radiating to distant areas.			
e. Duration of the massage is between 1 and 5 minutes per point.			

PROCEDURE	EVALUATION		
	1	2	3
6. Complete treatment.			
a. On completion of the massage, remove any lubricant with a towel.			
b. Remove material used for draping, assist the patient in dressing as needed.			
c. Have the patient perform appropriate therapeutic exercise indicated.			
d. Clean the treatment area and equipment according to normal protocol.			
7. Assess treatment efficacy.			
a. Ask the patient how the treated area feels.			
b. Visually inspect the treated area for any adverse reactions.			
c. Perform functional tests as indicated.			

CHAPTER 18 EIGHTEEN

EXTRACORPOREAL SHOCK WAVE THERAPY

CHARLES THIGPEN

OBJECTIVES

Following completion of this chapter, the student therapist will be able to:
- ✓ Describe the mechanical characteristics of extracorporeal shock waves.
- ✓ Identify musculoskeletal pathologies that may benefit from extracorporeal shock wave therapy (ESWT).
- ✓ Discuss the cellular effects of extracorporeal shock wave therapy on bone and tendons.
- ✓ Discuss why these effects may be beneficial to these tissues.

HISTORY OF ESWT

Therapeutic shock waves were first introduced into medicine over 20 years ago for the treatment of kidney stones. Shock waves have since become the primary treatment choice for urinary, biliary, and salivary calculi. More recently, extracorporeal shock wave therapy has been used to treat musculoskeletal conditions such as lateral epicondylitis and plantar fasciitis in the United States.[25] This is especially important considering the difficulty in the treatment of chronic tendinopathies. It is becoming clear that "chronic inflammation" is not present and regeneration of tendocytes is needed to facilitate healing.[1] The biologic effects of ESWT have shown to be effective in stimulating growth of these collagen building cells.[29, 43] Furthermore, other musculoskeletal disorders have been treated in Europe including pseudoarthrosis, nonunion fractures, and during total joint revisions. This chapter will clarify the terminology and principles of shock wave therapy, discuss the potential biologic effects of shock waves, and review the current use of ESWT in the treatment of musculoskeletal conditions. Finally, evidence-based clinical guidelines for use of ESWT will be presented.

ESWT will continue to be used more especially in the treatment that has traditionally been referred to as chronic tendonitis. It is important to discuss this topic briefly before we begin. Traditionally, therapists and physicians have concluded that long-standing symptoms of tendonitis were the result of the healing process being "stuck" in the inflammatory phase. However, it is becoming clear that this is not the mechanism underlying this chronic condition. Current recommendations include a

CASE STUDY 18-1
EXTRACORPOREAL SHOCK WAVE THERAPY (ESWT)

Background: A 22-year-old male presented with a 6-month history of bilateral heel pain (R > L). He noted that his symptoms started approximately 2 weeks after beginning his new job working at a machine shop where he stands 8 or more hours per day on a concrete floor in stiff-soled safety shoes. The patient relates a history of the gradual onset of dull pain in his feet at the end of the work day that he initially attempted to treat with self-administered over-the-counter anti-inflammatories and some shoe inserts he purchased at a local store. He then noticed sharp, stabbing pains through his heels and feet when first standing in the morning and sought the care of his family physician. Currently the patient is taking prescription-strength NSAID and has been referred for further conservative care. On examination the patient was noted to exhibit a pes cavus foot, restricted passive dorsiflexion of the ankle (0°) secondary to tight gastrocsoleus-achilles complex, and point tenderness bilaterally just proximal to the calcaneal insertion of the plantar fascia.

Impression: Bilateral plantar fasciitis (R > L), chronic.

Treatment Plan: The patient was advised to continue his medication regimen. He was fitted with gel heel cushions for continuous wear while ambulatory and assigned light duty at work which reduced his standing time to 4 h/day. He underwent a 1x/week ESWT treatment of his right foot with a medium intensity (0.28 J/mm²) series of shock waves. This was followed by low-intensity prolonged static stretching exercise of the gastrocsoleus-achilles complex and completed with static icing to control transient, localized soft-tissue swelling which accompanies the treatment.

Response: The patient's symptoms diminished (pain decreased from 7/10 to 2/10 on VAS) in the right foot over the course of 6 weeks. Following successful intervention with the right foot, a course of treatment was undertaken for the left foot with similar outcomes. The patient was able to return to full duty without restrictions following a regimen of graduated standing time.

Discussion Questions

- What tissues were injured or affected?
- What symptoms were present?
- What phase of the injury-healing continuum did the patient present for care in?
- What are the physical agent modality's biophysical effects (direct, indirect, depth, and tissue affinity)?
- What are the physical agent modality's indications and contraindications?
- What are the parameters of the physical agent modality's application, dosage, duration, and frequency in this case study?
- What other physical agent modalities could be used to treat this injury or condition? Why? How?
- What is the significance of a positive Tinel sign?
- Would compression over the tarsal tunnel reproduce the symptoms?
- Why does the patient experience sharp, piercing pain with his first steps of the day and dull pain after prolonged standing?
- Is there another potential source of the patient's symptoms?

The rehabilitation professional employs physical agent modalities to create an optimum environment for tissue healing while minimizing the symptoms associated with the trauma or condition.

period of rest, followed by aggressive eccentric exercise to stimulate tendon regeneration.[1,12,20,29,40–43] ESWT's demonstrated biologic effects of decreasing pain and promoting tissue regeneration make it an ideal adjunct to the rehabilitation process. This chapter explores ESWT and its potential benefits in musculoskeletal rehabilitation.

PHYSICAL CHARACTERISTICS OF EXTRACORPOREAL SHOCK WAVE

To understand the potential biologic effects of the mechanical energy of shock waves, it is helpful to understand their physical properties. A shock wave is a sonic pulse that is characterized by the following physical parameters: a high peak pressure (sometimes as high as 100 MPa, but usually around 50–80 MPa), a fast initial rise in pressure (less than

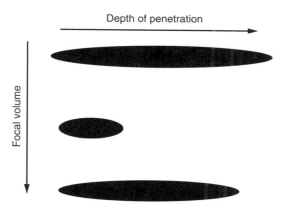

Depth of penetration

Focal volume

•**Figure 18-1** Two-dimensional comparison of shock waves from different sources.

10 nsec), a low tensile amplitude, a short life cycle (usually less than 10 μsec), and a broad frequency spectrum (16–20 Hz).[6,25] These characteristics are in contrast to ultrasound waves whose peak pressure is much lower with frequencies in the range of 1–3 MHz. Additionally, velocity of an ultrasound wave is in the 1400–1600 m/sec where shock wave velocities are greater than 350 m/sec but less than 1000 m/sec. The high peak pressure of a shock wave is the result of the combination of the velocity and frequency of the shock wave. The very high velocities of these wavelets when passed through a medium generate what is essentially a controlled explosion due to the pressure differential from the wavelets (Fig. 18-1). This energy is then dissipated and reflected at tissue interfaces according to the mechanical properties of the tissues through which it passes.[6,25]

The shock wave's pressure disturbance is propagated three-dimensionally due to the sudden rise in ambient pressure of the cell relative to the maximum pressure of the wave. This sudden rise in cell pressure causes an expansion and contraction within the medium causing tensile, compression, and shear stresses within the cell membrane. These stresses are usually in the direction of wave propagation but the impedance and dampening at tissue boundaries reflect and refract within tissues causing steepening and attenuation of the wave. The drastic changes in pressure within the cell cause cavitation within the cells. The resulting collapsing of the cavitating bubbles yields water jets that are proposed to cause cellular level tissue damage.[33]

The impedance and dampening of the acoustic energy is similar to ultrasound waves. The attenuation of shock waves in air is 1000 times more than through water because the attenuation is dependent on the velocity of the wave and density of the tissue. Shock waves are generated within a water medium and applied through water-based coupling gel based on the assumption that the human body's makeup is similar to water (Fig. 18-2). Therefore, the amount of attenuation and steepening that occurs at the tissue boundaries

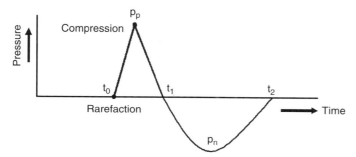

•**Figure 18-2** Two-dimensional graph of positive and negative pressures generated within biologic tissues by shock waves. p_p—maximum positive pressure (MPa), p_n—maximum negative pressure (MPa), t_0—beginning of shock wave, t_1—rarefaction begins causing negative pressure initiating cavitation, and t_2—end of 1 shock wave cycle.

accounts for most of the loss of energy. It has been suggested that the increased efficiency relative to ultrasound allows for more focused and well-controlled energy to be applied to the biologic tissues. Even with this control, biologic tissues respond differently to the same energy based on differences in structural makeup. Keeping in mind these differences in tissue structure is important when applying therapeutic shock waves.[6,26,36]

SHOCK WAVE GENERATION

There are three methods of shock wave generation currently in use in the United States—electrohydraulic, electromagnetic, and piezoelectric. Each of these techniques converts electrical energy into a mechanical shock wave. Currently, electrohydraulic and electromagnetic techniques are both being studied by the Food and Drug Administration (FDA). Each method generates shock waves with different volumes and amounts of energy penetrating to variable tissue depths (Table 18-1).[26]

Electrohydraulic shock wave devices create a spark that discharges rapidly into the water, and vaporizes the surrounding water creating a gas bubble filled with the water vapor. The gas bubble produces a sonic pulse and the subsequent implosion and a reverse pulse that causes another shock wave. The expanding shock waves are reflected by the surface of the ellipsoid and refocused into the focal point. Electrohydraulic shock wave devices are usually characterized by high-energy waves in focal volumes with fairly large axial diameters.[26]

Electromagnetic devices use a metal membrane and an opposing electromagnetic coil. An electric current is passed through the coil producing a strong magnetic field. The resulting variable magnetic field forces the metal membrane away compressing the surrounding fluid medium and creating a shock wave. The wave is passed through a lens to focus it at the desired target tissue. Electromagnetic shock wave devices tend to be used to create low-energy waves.[6,25]

Piezoelectric shock wave devices pass electrical current through large numbers of piezocrystals mounted on the inside of a sphere. The resulting expansion and contraction of the piezocrystals create a shock wave. The piezocrystals are arranged in the sphere so that the resulting shock wave is very focused allowing for a high-energy density within a defined focal volume.[26]

PHYSICAL PARAMETERS OF SHOCK WAVES

Physical parameters used to describe shock waves are **focal volume, pressure field, total acoustical energy, energy flux,** and **energy flux density.** It is not clear which of these parameters are most important for therapeutic effectiveness. It has been suggested, however, that pressure field distribution, energy density, and total acoustical energy are the most important.[26] The focal volume is manipulated to ensure that the target tissue is

TABLE 18-1	Comparison of Physical Parameters for Shock Wave Devices		
HMT Parameter	Dornier Ossatron	Siemens Epos Ultra	Sonocur Basic
Positive peak pressure in MPa	40.6–71.9	7.3–80.4	5.5–25.6
Focal area in mm (maximum dimensions from lowest to highest energy level settings)	$6.6 \times 6.8 \times 67.6$	$7.7 \times 7.7 \times 20.0$	$6.0 \times 6.0 \times 58$
Positive energy flux density in mJ/mm²	0.09–0.34	0.03–0.98	0.016–0.22
Total energy flux density in mJ/mm²	0.12–0.40	0.13–1.70	0.04–0.56

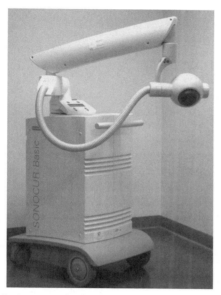

•**Figure 18-3** Sonocur electromagnetic shock wave device.

treated. This is similar to choosing the frequency of ultrasound before treatment to achieve the desired depth of penetration. This is most commonly controlled by feedback from the patient, termed **clinical focusing,** while several studies have used ultrasound and fluoroscopic imaging to locate the treatment site.[6] The pressure field is measured in MPa as a function of time. The pressure field varies across the focal volume and is greatest at the focal center (Fig. 18-3). It is reflective of the maximum amount of acoustical energy within the field. The focal region is defined about three axes to describe the focal volume. The amount of acoustical energy within the focal volume is referred to as **energy flux density** and is calculated as the area below the squared pressure versus time curve. It is a measure of energy per square area for each sonic pulse and expressed in mJ/mm^2. Energy flux density is considered when calculating the threshold values for biologic tissues.[6,26] The most effective energy flux density is not known; however, Rompe et al.[29] have suggested a classification of energy flux density defined as low <0.08 mJ/mm^2, medium 0.08–0.28 mJ/mm^2, and high >0.28 mJ/mm^2. This classification system is based on the response of tendons to shock wave treatment and seems to be an excellent guideline for treatment of bone and tendons. The peak pulse energy (MPa) is determined from a pressure profile and is important when considering the maximum amount of pressure generated by a shock wave within a tissue. The pressure field distribution is the energy flux concentrated within the focal area. When ultrasound wave physics are considered, the focal area may be expanded to a larger wave volume where the peak pressure is half its original value. The biologic effects of the energy within the wave volume should be considered when treating each specific tissue. The total acoustical energy is the energy summed for the entire beam and describes the energy per shock wave. It has been suggested that total acoustical energy is the most important of the physical parameters when treating biologic tissues. Consideration of the potential biologic effects of shock waves will enable the most appropriate acoustical energy to be applied.[6,25,36]

BIOLOGIC EFFECTS

The direct and indirect stresses of shock waves on biologic tissues should be considered. Tensile and shear stresses are created in the direction of shock wave propagation in biologic tissues. The tensile forces are greater than the tensile strength of the water and generate bubbles (cavitation). Oscillations of the bubble diameters increase and decrease the volume of the bubble. Bubbles will fail dependent on the viscosity of the fluid and the pressure of the wave. The more viscous the fluid, the less the oscillation, and therefore the less the pressure.

The collapse of the bubbles creates microscopic high-energy water jets. This indirect effect can cause an increase in tissue temperature and damage cells.[26,29,43] The impact of cavitation and the water jets has been reported to depend strongly on the water content of the tissue and time between shock wave applications; however, no recommendations on appropriate hydration or time intervals have been made.[37] The microjets from the reflected shock waves occurring at tissue boundary areas are where the most biologic effects are expected.[26]

BONE

The effect of shock waves on bony tissue is thought to occur primarily at the interface between cortical and cancellous bone. It is thought that acoustic streaming causes cavitation and increases cell permeability allowing increased vascularity and bony regeneration. More specifically, an increase in stromal cells seems to allow osteogenesis.[43] Additionally, the increase in osteoprogenitor cells coupled with local increases in growth factor, neovascularization, and protein synthesis suggest that shock waves can improve the tissue environment for healing to occur.[20,40-43] However, results from both Rompe. et al.[29] and Wang et al.[43] suggest that it is possible for too much damage to occur and the resulting cellular activity is unable to overcome the damage. This is in contrast to inducing an amount of damage that allows for increases in vascularity and osteogenesis in bone that is not appropriately healed. To prevent cell damage from the short-time effect of high-energy shock wave dosages it has been suggested that less than 2000 pulses are needed to safely stimulate bone remodeling.[20] The use of high-energy devices has been reported in the literature in the treatment of nonunions and pseudoarthrosis.[6] It has been suggested that osteocyte damage and growth plate dysplasia resulting from the use of high-energy shock wave devices (>0.28 mJ/mm^2) may delay fracture healing and mechanical instability.[29] Durst et al.[7] is the only documented case identified in the literature that reported these suggested adverse effects of ESWT. Humeral head osteonecrosis was confirmed by magnetic resonance imaging (MRI) and x-ray 3 years after treatment for calcific tendonitis. The dosage was 1600–1700 pulses at 12–13 kV for three treatments over a month. Given the nonstandard values reported, it is unclear whether the energy density was high, medium, or low. Additionally, most other studies utilized shock wave devices designed specifically for orthopedic use and not a lithotripser. Insufficient detail was given about the device used to compare between studies. However, osteonecrosis may be a complication based on reports in the literature seen in urologic cases.[6,25]

TENDON

The suggested mechanisms for biologic effects of shock waves on tendons are the same as bone. Direct mechanical stresses cause tensile and shear failure within the cellular matrix of the tendon. The resulting cavitation and indirect microjets cause the most damage at the interface of the tendon and bone.[26] Rompe et al.[29] is the only study identified in the literature comparing the effects of shock waves on tendons. Based on their results they have suggested that doses over 0.28 mJ/mm^2 are harmful to the musculotendinous complex and may place the complex at risk for rupture (Table 18-2). No complications have been published in the literature in the treatment of musculotendinous complexes.

TABLE 18-2	Dose Related Effects of Shock Waves[29]	
Amount of Energy (J/mm^2)	Effect on Tendon	Proposed Classification
0.08	No effect seen	Low
0.28	Transient swelling	Medium
0.60	Para-tendinous inflammation and increase in diameter of tendon	High*

*Levels above 0.28 J/mm^2 are not recommended in the treatment of tendons.

CLINICAL APPLICATIONS

FRACTURES

Clinical success has been reported by several authors in the treatment of nonunion,[18,30,34] pseudarthorses,[11,19] acute fractures of the tibia,[38,39] femoral head necrosis,[22] and total hip revisions.[14] Through the aforementioned biologic mechanisms, extracorporeal shock waves are applied at high-energy doses to stimulate bone remodeling. Success rates range from 62 to 83 percent for nonunions and pseudarthroses.[25] Limited results are reported in the literature on the effectiveness for acute fractures, femoral head necrosis, and total hip revisions. Each of these conditions have been reported to be successfully treated when traditional treatments failed, but it is unclear at this time if shock wave therapy should be considered as an initial treatment. Kuderna and Schaden[18] have suggested the cost per injury to be 4–5× less and recovery on average 2 months faster for tibial nonunion fractures treated acutely with high-energy extracorporeal shock waves when compared to traditional surgical intervention.

PLANTAR FASCIITIS

The most studied use of extracorporeal shock wave therapy has been for the treatment of plantar fasciitis (Fig. 18-4). Use of low-energy shock waves have been approved by the FDA for use in the United States.[3] Success rates range from 56 to 75 percent depending on the number of pulses applied, exact tissue treated, and previous treatment received by the patient.[6] There did not seem to be a pattern with any of these variables that would predict successful outcomes in these studies.[3,6,24,32] Success rates were based on pain at the initial treatment time and 6–12 months after treatment.

Several randomized controlled trials have reported positive results suggesting promise that shock wave therapy may be a viable option in the treatment of plantar fasciitis.[3,5,24,32] Boddeker et al.[2] concluded after a biometric review of the literature that effectiveness of shock wave therapy could be neither confirmed nor denied due to the 21 studies reviewed not meeting all of the guidelines for a biometric review. Buchbinder et al.'s[3] results from a randomized control trial also did not support the use of shock wave therapy when compared to a placebo ultrasound treatment for pain, function, and quality of life at 6 and 12 weeks posttreatment. The conclusions of these authors are in contrast to others who have supported the use of shock wave therapy in the treatment of plantar fasciitis.[5,24,29] Differences in authors' conclusions likely owe to several factors including method of patient selection, focusing of the shock wave, and definition of plantar fasciitis. Studies that have randomly assigned patients to treatment groups with only a diagnosis of plantar fasciitis do not reflect actual clinical application of this device. Patients with a well-defined area of heel pain seem to respond better

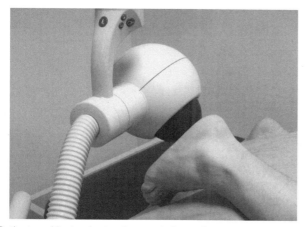

•**Figure 18-4** Patient positioning for treatment of plantar fasciitis.

than those who are diagnosed with "plantar fasciitis." Differing methods of choosing the area to be treated have likely influenced these outcomes. Studies using clinical focusing where the most painful area is treated versus using a radiologic guide to apply the shock wave appear to achieve different results. Reviewed literature seems to support clinical focusing suggesting that reduction of pain is the primary benefit of shock wave therapy. The definition of plantar fasciitis was either not stated or differed between studies ultimately meaning that the comparisons between the studies are limited.

MEDIAL/LATERAL EPICONDYLITIS

Use of the low-energy extracorporeal shock waves in the treatment of lateral epicondylitis has been approved by the FDA (Fig. 18-5). Success rates for shock wave therapy of tendinitis of the elbow are good for lateral epicondylitis ranging from 47 to 81 percent, but poor for a small sample of patients with medial epicondylitis.[6] Relief of pain and assessment of function have been used as outcome measures with all studies reviewed reporting significant improvement in the groups treated with extracorporeal shock wave therapy when compared to conventional treatments.[15,17,23,27,28] Similar to plantar fasciitis, the design of studies has limited broad generalizations to the population. Even so, it seems that low-energy extracorporeal shock wave therapy is a viable modality in the treatment of lateral epicondylitis. More studies should be done before any conclusions can be drawn about the treatment of medial epicondylitis or the treatment of tendinopathies in general.

CALCIFIC TENDINITIS OF THE SHOULDER

Treatment of calcific tendinitis of the shoulder with extracorporeal shock waves has been widely used in Europe and Canada with positive outcomes reported in the literature.[4,8–10,31,35] Success rates range from 60 to 85 percent using pain, function, and size of calcific deposits as outcome measures. When ultrasound or fluoroscopy has been used to focus the shock waves on the calcification, outcomes have improved by over 80 percent.[4] Rompe et al.[31] treated noncalcific rotator cuff tendonitis with extracorporeal shock waves, and while there was an improvement it was not more than the placebo effect. Haake et al.[10] have reported similar outcomes when comparing surgical intervention and ESWT for analogous shoulder tendinopathies. However, reported total cost was 93 percent less for those patients treated with ESWT. The majority (65%) of this difference in total cost was accounted for, attributable to the productivity losses in the workplace. Similar to the differences in outcomes in the treatment of plantar fasciitis, these studies vary according to patient selection criteria, application of

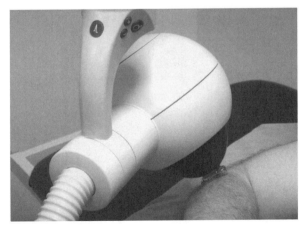

•Figure 18-5 Patient is positioned with adequate coupling gel in an appropriate position to treat lateral epicondylitis. Attenuation of the shock wave is minimized by ensuring contact of the transmitting source with the coupling gel similar to ultrasound application.

ESWT, and randomization. On the whole, the literature suggests that use of shock wave therapy for treatment of calcific tendonitis is useful and is improved when focused by an imaging technique.

EVALUATION OF ESWT LITERATURE FOR EVIDENCE-BASED PRACTICE

It is important to understand several concepts regarding ESWT in an evaluation of the literature regarding ESWT. The parameters and criteria are outlined below:

1. *The difference in tendonitis/fasciitis and tendinosis/fasciosis in regards to pathophysiology and the implications in patient selection.*[13,16,21]

   a. This frames the rationale in choosing treatments which are likely to be effective on a scientific basis. It is not an accident that the patients who seem to respond to ESWT clearly have [developed a chronic tendinosis of fasciosis] (i.e., duration of at least 6 months and failure of other conservative measures, especially nonsteroidal anti-inflammatory drugs (NSAID) and/or steroid injection). Observations that those who respond best have failed steroid injection and other conservative therapies likely indicate a better selection of those patients who have no inflammatory component to their condition.

2. *The success of ESWT treatment appears to be dependent upon delivery of sufficient shock wave energy within a specific time frame.*[29,33,43]

   a. The amount of delivered energy in both intensity and total volume must be great enough to effect the structural and physiologic changes that result in relief of symptoms (pain) and healing (heralded by neovascularity). This appears to require both a direct shock wave effect and cavitation events.

   b. Shock wave energy must be delivered within a relatively short time frame to be effective.

3. *The success or failure of shock wave therapy should be assessed at a point in time after completion of the last ESWT application which allows for the effects of the shock waves to become clinically manifest with regards to symptoms.* At least 12 weeks is suggested by animal studies.[43]

4. *The success of ESWT appears to be dependent upon accurate focusing of the shock wave energy to the precise area of tendinosis/fasciosis pathology.* Studies which have used imaging to select the treatment area have been less effective than those which use pain-guided "clinical focusing."[3,6,23,28,31]

   a. Only clinical focusing using patient feedback can consistently accomplish accurate targeting.

   b. X-ray, fluoroscopy, and ultrasound are of minimal value since one cannot "see" pain with these devices.

ACKNOWLEDGMENTS

We would like to acknowledge the consultation and guidance provided by Dr. Dan Myers, President, and Dr. Bill Jordan, CEO of Sonorex-USA, in the preparation of this chapter. Their generosity and support for the use of the Sonocur device by the University of North Carolina Sports Medicine is greatly appreciated. Finally, their expertise and practical advice concerning the evaluation of the literature has added an important perspective in the use of this technology.

SUMMARY

1. Early studies seem to suggest moderate to good success; lack of consistency in the number of pulses, number of treatments, amount of energy, and application technique limits the ability to compare these studies.

2. ESWT appears to impact biologic tissues in a way that is beneficial for chronic, poorly healing musculoskeletal conditions.

3. As with any treatment, patient selection is paramount. Development of evidence-based criteria to guide treatment is needed.

4. Current evidence suggests location of pain, poor treatment progression greater than 3 months, and significant pain reduction upon initial treatment can be used to guide treatment at this time.

5. The noninvasive nature, lack of adverse side effects, possible decrease in cost, and treatment effectiveness reported support the use of ESWT in the treatment of chronic tendinopathies and nonunion fractures.

REVIEW QUESTIONS

1. List and define the five major mechanical characteristics of extracorporeal shock waves.
2. How do shock waves stimulate tissue healing?
3. Describe the characteristics of pathologies that may benefit from ESWT.
4. List three criteria when selecting patients for ESWT use.
5. What are the suggested dose parameters for treatment of tendonopathies?
6. Describe the four criteria when evaluating and applying ESWT evidence.

REFERENCES

1. Almekinders, L.C., Temple, J.D.: Etiology, diagnosis, and treatment of tendonitis: an analysis of the literature, Med. Sci. Sports Exerc. 30:1183–1190, 1998.
2. Boddeker, I.R., Schafer, H., and Haake, M.: Extracorporeal shockwave therapy in the treatment of plantar fasciitis—a biometrical review, Clin. Rheumatol. 20:324–330, 2001.
3. Buchbinder, R., Ptasznik, R., Gordon, J., Buchanan, J., Prabaharan, V., and Forbes, A.: Ultrasound-guided extracorporeal shock wave therapy for plantar fasciitis, JAMA 288:1364–1372, 2002.
4. Charrin, J.E., Noel, E.R.: Shockwave therapy under ultrasonographic guidance in rotator cuff calcific tendinitis, Joint Bone Spine 68:241–244, 2001.
5. Chen, H.S., Chen, L.M., and Huang. T.W.: Treatment of painful heel syndrome with shock waves, Clin. Orth. Rel. Res. 387:41–46, 2001.
6. Chung, B., Wiley, P.: Extracorporeal shockwave therapy: a review, Sports Med. 34:851–865, 2002.
7. Durst, H.B., Blatter, G., and Kuster, M.S.: Osteonecrosis of the humeral head after extracorporeal shock-wave lithotripsy, J. Bone Joint Surg. (Br.) 84:744–746, 2002.
8. Grob, M.W., Sattler, A., Haake, M., Schmitt, J., Hildebrandt, R., Muller, H.H., and Engenhart-Cabillic, R.: The value of radiotherapy in comparsion with extracorporeal shockwave therapy for supraspinatus tendinitis, Strahlenther. Onkol. 178:314–320, 2002.
9. Haake, M., Deike, B., Thon, A., and Schmitt, J.: Exact focusing of extracorporeal shock wave therapy for calcifying tendinopathy, Clin. Orth. Rel. Res. 397:323–331, 2002.
10. Haake, M., Rautmann, M., and Wirth, T.: Extracorporeal shock wave therapy vs. surgical treatment in calcifying tendinitis and noncalcifying tendinitis of the supraspinatus muscle, Eur. J. Orthop. Surg. Traumatol. 11:21–24, 2001.
11. Haupt, G.: Use of extracoporeal shock waves in the treatment of pseudoarthorsis, tendinopathy, and other orthopedic diseases, J. Urol. 158:4–11, 1997.
12. Hsu, R.W.W., Hsu, W.H., Tai, C.L., and Lee, K.F.: Effect of shock-wave therapy on patellar tendinopathy in a rabbit model, J. Orthop. Res. 22:221–227, 2004.
13. Kahn, K., Cook, J., Taunton, J., and Bonar, F.: Overuse tendinosis, not tendonitis: part I: a new paradigm for a difficult clinical problem, Phys. Sportsmed. 28, 2000.
14. Karpman, R.R., Magee, F.P., Gruen, T.W.S., and Mobley, T.: The lithotriptor and its potential use in the revision of total hip arthroplatsty, Clin. Orth. Rel. Res. 387:4–7, 2001.
15. Ko, J.Y., Chen, H.S., and Chen. L.M.: Treatment of lateral epicondylitis of the elbow with shock waves, Clin. Orth. Rel. Res. 387:60–67, 2001.
16. Kraushaar, B., Nirschl, R.: Tendinosis of the elbow (tennis elbow). Clinical features and findings of histological, immuno-chemical and electron microscopy studies, J. Bone Joint Surg. (Am.) 81:259–278, 1999.
17. Krischek, O., Hopf, C., Nafe, B., and Rompe, J.D.: Shock-wave therapy for tennis and golfer's elbow-1 year follow-up, Arch. Orthop. Trauma Surg. 119:62–66, 1999.
18. Kuderna, H., Schaden, W.: Comparison of 30 tibial non-unions: costs of surgical treatment vs costs of ESWT. In 3rd International Congress of the ESWT, Naples, Italy, 2000.

19. Kuner, E.H., Berwarth, H., and Lucke, S.V.: Aseptic pseudoarthrosis: principles of treatment, Orthopade 25:394–404, 1996.

20. Kusnierczak, D., Brocai, D.R.C., Vettel, U., and Loew, M.: The Influence of extracorporeal shock-wave application on the biological behaviour of bone cells in vitro. In 3rd International Congress of the ESMST, Naples, Italy, 2000.

21. Lemont, H., Ammirati, B., and Usen, N., Plantar Fascitis: A degenerative process (fasciosis) without inflammation, J. Am. Podiatric Soc. 93:234–237, 2003.

22. Ludwig, J., Lauber, S., Lauber, H.J., Dreisilker, U., Raedel, R., and Hotzinger, H.: High-energy shock wave treatment of femoral head necrosis in adults, Clin. Orth. Rel. Res. 387: 119–126, 2001.

23. Maier, M., Steinborn, M., Schmitz, C., Stabler, A., Kohler, S., Veihelmann, A., Pfahler, M., and Refior, H.J.: Extracorporeal shock-wave therapy for chronic lateral tennis elbow-prediction of outcome by imaging, Arch. Orthop. Trauma Surg. 121: 379–384, 2001.

24. Ogden, J.A., Alvarez, R., Levitt, R., Cross, G.L., and Marlow, M.: Shock wave therapy for chronic proximal plantar fasciitis, Clin. Orth. Rel. Res. 387:47–59, 2001.

25. Ogden, J.A., Alvarez, R.G., Levitt, R., and Marlow, M.: Shock wave therapy (orthotripsy) in musculoskeletal disorders, Clin. Orth. Rel. Res. 387:22–40, 2001.

26. Ogden, J.A., Kischkat, A.T., and Schultheiss, R.: Principles of shock wave therapy, Clin. Orth. Rel. Res. 387:8–17, 2001.

27. Rompe, J.D., Hopf, C., Kullmer, K., Heine, J., and Burger, R.: Analgesic effect of extracorporeal shock-wave therapy on chronic tennis elbow, J. Bone Joint Surg. (Br.) 78:233–237, 1996.

28. Rompe, J.D., Hopf, C., Kullmer, K., Heine, J., Burger, R., and Nafe, B.: Low-energy extracorpal shock wave therapy for persistent tennis elbow, Int. Orthop. 20:23–27, 1996.

29. Rompe, J.D., Kirkpatrick, C.J., Kullmer, K., Schwitalle, M., and Krischek, O.: Dose-related effects of shock waves on rabbit tendo Achillis, J. Bone Joint Surg. (Br.) 80:546–552, 1998.

30. Rompe, J.D., Rosendahl, T., Schollner, C., and Theis, C.: High-energy extracorporeal shock wave treatment of nonunions, Clin. Orth. Rel. Res. 387:102–111, 2001.

31. Rompe, J.D., Rumler, F., Hopf, C., Nafe, B., and Heine, J.: Extracorporal shock wave therapy for calcifying tendinitis of the shoulder, Clin. Orth. Rel. Res. 321:196–201, 1995.

32. Rompe, J.D., Schoellner, C., and Nafe, B.: Evaluation of low-energy extracorporeal shock-wave application for treatment of chronic plantar fasciitis, JBJS 84:335–341, 2002.

33. Russo, S., Galasso, O., Marlinghaus, E., Hagelauer, U., and Mayer, J.: The in-vivo cavatation measurement. In 2nd International Congress of the ESMST, London, 1999.

34. Schaden, W., Fischer, A., and Sailler, A.: Extracoporeal shock wave therapy of nonunion or delayed osseous union, Clin. Orthop. Relat. Res. 387:90–94, 2001.

35. Speed, C.A., Richards, C., Nichols, D., Burnet, S., Wies, J.T., Humphreys, H., and Hazleman, B.L.: Extracoporeal shock-wave therapy for tendonitis of the rotator cuff, JBJS 84:509–512, 2001.

36. Thiel, M.: Application of shock waves in medicine, Clin. Orthop. Rel. Res. 387:18–21, 2001.

37. Vara, F.: Treatment of the troncanteric bursitis with local application of extracorporeal shock wave. In 2nd International Congress of the ESMS, London, 1999.

38. Wang, C.J., Chen, H.S., Chen, C.E., and Yang, K.D.: Treatment of nonunions of long bone fractures with shock waves, Clin. Orthop. Rel. Res. 387:95–101, 2001.

39. Wang, C.J., Huang, H.Y., Chen, H.H., Pai, C.H., and Yang, K.D.: Effect of shock wave therapy on acute fractures of the tibia, Clin. Orth. Rel. Res. 387:112–118, 2001.

40. Wang, C.J., Wang, F.S., Yang, K.D., Weng, L.H., Hsu, C.C., Huang, C.S., and Yang, L.C.: Shock wave therapy induces neovascularization at the tendon-bone junction: a study in rabbits, J. Orthop. Res. 21:984–989, 2003.

41. Wang, F.S., Wang, C.J., Huang, H.J., Chung, H., Chen, R.F., and Yang, K.D.: Physical shock wave mediates membrane hyperpolarization and ras activation for osteogenesis in human bone marrow stromal cells, Biochem. Biophys. Res. Commun. 287:648–655, 2001.

42. Wang, F.S., Yang, K.D., Wang, C.J., Huang, H.C., Chio, C.C., Hsu, T.-Y., and Ou, C.-Y.: Shockwave stimulates oxygen radical-mediated osteogenesis of the mesenschymal cells from human umbilical cord blood, J. Bone Mine. Res. 19:973–982, 2004.

43. Wang, F.S., Yang, R.F., Chen, R.F., Wang, C.J., and Sheen-Chen, S.M.: Extracorporeal shock wave promotes growth and differentiation of bone-marrow stromal cells towards osteoprogenitors associated with induciton of TGF-B1, J. Bone Joint Surg. (Br.) 84:457–461, 2002.

GLOSSARY

Clinical focusing Applying the shock wave over the area that causes the most pain as opposed to the area of tissue disruption.

Energy flux Measure of the peak pulse energy within a focal volume.

Energy flux density Measure of the energy flux per square area (usually mm^2).

Focal volume The amount of space over which the shock wave will have a therapeutic effect.

Pressure field A function of time and space and is a reflection of the effect of energy over the focal volume.

Total acoustical energy The amount of acoustical energy delivered in one shock wave pulse.

PART 7 SEVEN

SUMMARY

CHAPTER 19 NINETEEN

THE PHYSIOLOGIC EFFECTS OF THERAPEUTIC MODALITY INTERVENTION ON THE BODY SYSTEMS

ERIC SHAMUS*

STANLEY H. WILSON

OBJECTIVES

Following completion of this chapter, the student therapist will be able to:

✓ Incorporate a scientific approach in the use and application of therapeutic modality interventions.
✓ Analyze injury by understanding the resulting pathophysiology of that injury.
✓ Know the physiologic benefits of interventions.
✓ Use a systems approach in choosing the most appropriate intervention that best counteracts the pathologic effects of a specific injury.

Health insurers and consumers are challenging physical therapists to provide reasonable justification for intervention use. It is not clear that physical therapists are always using a scientific approach in the use and application of interventions. Past decision making on intervention uses focused on habit, manufacturers' claims, or sometimes guesswork. Justification for intervention use based on physiology provides a much more solid foundation.

A component of injury analysis occurs by understanding the resulting pathophysiology of that injury. By knowing the physiologic benefits of interventions, the most appropriate intervention can be chosen to counteract the pathologic effects of that injury.

*We would like to acknowledge Ms. Cheryl Hill, PT, Ph.D. (c), Director of the Physical Therapy Program at Nova Southeastern University, and Dr. Raul Cuadrado, Dean of the College of Allied Health, for their academic support. We would also like to acknowledge the invaluable contribution of the students of Nova Southeastern's physical therapy program to the research on the information provided on the various systems.

SYSTEMS APPROACH

The systems approach serves as an efficient and effective analytical tool for that purpose. The systems approach to physical therapy interventions incorporates the American Physical Therapy Association (APTA) Guide to Physical Therapist Practice.[4] The approach offers a concise, but in-depth look at the physiologic effects of physical therapy interventions on seven body systems. These systems are the following:

- Cardiopulmonary system
- Endocrine system
- Gastrointestinal (GI), genitourinary (GU), OB/GYN systems
- Integumentary system
- Musculoskeletal system
- Neuromuscular system
- Peripheral vascular/lymph systems

Four major purposes are served by the adoption of the systems approach:

- To provide clinicians with an effective and efficient way of choosing interventions commonly used by physical therapists in the treatment of impairments, functional limitations, and disability-related dysfunction.
- To provide clinicians with an enhanced decision-making process when choosing interventions.
- To provide educators with another viable teaching method to guide students in making appropriate choices of interventions based on the physiologic effects on body systems.
- To document general intervention effects. It is best applied, however, in the context of each patient, because the intervention effects may vary from one patient to another.

The purpose of this chapter is to utilize the system approach in the selection of modalities. In the following sections, the theoretical basis of each modality is presented, followed by a brief description of the modality's effects on each of the seven body systems.

ELECTRICAL STIMULATING CURRENTS

Theoretical Basis

As electricity moves through the body's conductive medium, changes in the physiologic functioning can occur at various systems. The electric current creates an electrical field in biologic tissues that stimulates or alters the healing process and creates muscle contraction through nerve or muscle stimulation. Additionally, the current stimulates sensory nerves to help in treating pain and creates an electrical field on the skin surface to transfer ions beneficial to the healing process into or through the skin.

Electrical stimulation (e-stim) has been shown to accelerate and enhance healing by retarding bacterial growth, increasing local circulation, and enhancing the natural process of tissue repair.[27] The following section will provide information on the effects of the different forms of electrical stimulation on the seven body systems. The contraindications are similar for all forms of electrical stimulation when used for the purposes of analgesia, muscle reeducation, and muscle strengthening (see Chapter 5).

INTERFERENTIAL CURRENT (IFC)

Cardiopulmonary System

With the application of IFC, the cardiopulmonary system effects are a result of the muscle pumping action, which increases local blood flow and creates an increased demand on cardiac output.[19] IFC may cause an irregular cardiac rhythm in patients with pacemakers or in those who are at risk because of impaired cardiac function.

Endocrine System

IFC stimulates the release of endogenous opiates such as beta-endorphins that are released for their analgesic effects. IFC may also stimulate the hypothalamus by releasing factors that stimulate the anterior and intermediate lobes of glands.[15,18]

GI, GU, OB/GYN Systems

IFC is contraindicated in cases of pregnancy, but may be used to assist with strengthening pelvic floor muscles after pregnancy and in cases of urinary incontinence.[6]

Integumentary System

When applying the electrodes for IFC, the skin must be clean and intact, and must possess normal sensation. The skin can have erythematous patches under the electrodes after treatment. This should resolve quickly. Skin irritation may result in patients with oily skin or with allergic reactions to the electrodes.

Musculoskeletal System

Frequencies of 0–10 pulses per second (pps) can be used to produce small pulsating contractions of innervated muscle. Frequencies of 20–50 pps should be high enough to produce tetanic contractions of innervated muscle.

Neuromuscular System

IFC is less effective than other forms of e-stim with higher pulse rates, different waveforms, and greater intensities for such goals as muscle reeducation and facilitation retarding disuse atrophy, reducing spasticity, or tissue repair. IFC activates the larger-diameter peripheral nerve fibers to subsequently neuromodulate pain through a spinal gating mechanism. Analgesic effects can be explained through the following theories:

- Gate control theory (GCT). Pain is caused by sensory stimulation of the large diameter (A-beta) afferent fibers. This causes T-cells in the dorsal horn of lamina I and II to activate the substantia gelatinosa (SG). SG activity may block the synaptic transmission of the small-diameter A-delta and type C nerve fibers into the spinal cord, decreasing the perception of pain.[8]
- Central biasing theory (CBT). Intense e-stim of the small C fibers (pain fibers) at trigger point sites for short periods of time causes stimulation of descending neurons, which then affect the transmission of pain information by closing the gate at the spinal cord level.[15]
- Opiate control theory (OPCT). E-stim of sensory nerves may stimulate the release of enkephalin from local sites throughout the central nervous system and the release of B-endorphin from the pituitary gland into the cerebral spinal fluid.[15]

Peripheral Vascular/Lymph Systems

IFC improves muscle pumping action to facilitate the movement of lymph fluid through the lymphatic system, as well as increasing the venous return of blood.[19]

NEUROMUSCULAR ELECTRICAL STIMULATION (NMES)

Cardiopulmonary System

NMES elicits muscle contractions, which stimulate circulation by pumping fluid and blood through venous and lymphatic channels back into the heart, increasing the cardiac output demand. NMES facilitates increases in muscle oxidative enzymes. It is accompanied by an increase in content of the oxygen transport, protein, myoglobin, and a rise in the number of capillaries bringing oxygen to the muscles. Muscle contractions in the lower extremities force fluids out of the interstitial spaces to help with venous and lymphatic return to the heart. This can help reduce the incidence of deep vein thrombosis.[19]

Endocrine System

NMES of sensory nerves may stimulate release of enkephalin from local sites throughout the CNS and the release of endorphins from the pituitary gland. Muscle contractions cause a decrease in pressure that causes an increase in venous and lymphatic return and improves circulation to the area. Muscle contractions also facilitate the transport of hormones throughout the circulatory system.[15]

GI, GU, OB/GYN Systems

NMES can enhance a voluntary exercise program for the pelvic floor muscles. It can assist in strengthening pelvic floor musculature in patients with urinary incontinence and for muscle weakness following pregnancy.[19]

Integumentary System

Low-intensity direct current can assist in the treatment of wounds by creating a positive charge at the wound site to increase the natural healing process. NMES increases skin blood flow and improves skin perfusion when applied to muscles of the lower extremities in patients with spinal cord injuries. The skin has different layers that vary in water content, and offers the primary resistance to current flow.[13]

Musculoskeletal System/Neuromuscular System

NMES facilitates muscle action and reeducates a muscle toward normal function. It can be used for early active range of motion (AROM) in postsurgical and cast-immobilized limbs. It strengthens muscles by activating motor units that induce action potentials in the motor nerve. An intact motor nerve is a prerequisite for activating a muscle when using NMES. The flow of electrons from the stimulator is converted to a flow of ions in the motor nerve. If the stimulus is adequate to depolarize the motor end plate, the sarcoplasmic reticulum becomes depolarized, and consequently Ca^+ is released. This allows crossbridge cycling between the actin and myosin filaments of the muscle, which results in an overlap of the sliding filaments. Muscle recruitment tends to occur from largest to smallest motor units, with activation of fast glycolytic fatigable (FGF) motor units first, followed by fast-twitch, fatigue-resistant units, and ending with slow-twitch, fatigue-resistant units. Following denervation, muscle fibers experience a number of progressive anatomic, biochemical, and physiologic changes that lead to a decrease in the size of the individual muscle fiber. NMES minimizes the extent of atrophy, while the nerve is regenerating. NMES provides proprioceptive, kinesthetic, and sensory input directly to the muscle when peripheral nerves are not functioning.[6,57]

Peripheral Vascular/Lymph Systems

NMES may provide an effective increase in venous or lymphatic drainage when voluntary exercise cannot be performed or when insufficient muscle contraction is available to increase arterial blood flow to the target area. When an electrical field is introduced into an area with edema, it facilitates the movement of charged proteins into the lymphatic channels, and as volume increases, the contraction rate of the lymphatic flow increases.[19]

TRANSCUTANEOUS ELECTRICAL NERVE STIMULATION (TENS)

Cardiopulmonary System

TENS stimulates a muscle pumping action, thereby increasing venous return and lymph flow to heart.[19] Cardiac output and stroke volume demands are therefore subsequently increased.

Endocrine System

TENS inhibits secretion of substance P (pain) from T-cells and allows the release of endorphins and/or enkephalins to counteract substance P in the body.[15]

GI, GU, OB/GYN Systems

TENS can be used to counteract visceral pain. It is effective in stimulation of peristaltic activity in the GI tract and as a noninvasive method that can limit and treat paralytic ileus. Conventional TENS can be used in the treatment of bladder problems (urinary incontinence), secondary to conditions of prostatic hypertrophy, neurologic urinary retention, and interstitial cystitis. TENS can be effective in reducing pain from cervical dilatation and in the treatment of acute pain from dysmenorrhea.[8]

Integumentary System

TENS increases blood flow to the layers of skin. It may be used successfully when electrodes are placed over the site of pain in relation to a dermatome-using trigger, acupuncture, or motor points.[15] Skin irritation may result from sensitivity from the electrode placement.

Musculoskeletal System

TENS reproduces the physical and chemical events associated with normal voluntary muscle contraction (using low-rate TENS set between 20 and 40 pps. TENS stimulates type II (fast-twitch) fiber contraction first, followed by type I (unlike voluntary contraction, where type I contracts first followed by type II).

Neuromuscular System

TENS activate large-diameter A-beta fibers that inhibit the interneurons (substantia gelatinosa) of the spinal cord. This in turn produces inhibition of smaller A-delta and C fibers (pain fibers), along with presynaptic inhibition of the T-cells to close the "gate" and modulate pain. A noxious stimulus generates endorphin production from the pituitary gland. Endogenous opiate-rich nuclei and periaqueductal gray matter in the midbrain and thalamus are also activated by strong stimuli, which signal to the spinal cord to presynaptically inhibit the release of substance P from the A-delta and C fibers.

IONTOPHORESIS

Theoretical Basis

Iontophoresis is the introduction of various ions into the skin by means of a direct electric current for the purpose of transporting chemicals across the membrane. It is used clinically in treatment of inflammatory musculoskeletal conditions, for analgesic effects, scar modification, wound healing, and in treating edema, calcium deposits, and hyperhidrosis. In vivo studies have reported penetration of ions to at least 1 cm into the gluteal muscles. Lidocaine ion penetration was found with a current of 4 mA applied for 10 minutes with a 4 percent lidocaine solution.[20] The effectiveness of iontophoresis is directly related to the medication administered or the solution used for ion transfer. Each medication has its own effect, regardless of the method of application. For example, a corticosteriod inhibits the inflammatory process by reducing the migration of neutrophils and monocytes into the inflamed area and reducing the activity of these white blood cells.[64] Lidocaine, however, causes dilation of blood vessels and a topical anesthesia of the skin.[20]

Cardiopulmonary System

Cardiopulmonary effects are directly related to the medication that is administered. For example, lidocaine produces dilation of blood vessels whereas epinephrine causes vasoconstriction. Epinephrine acts on alpha- and beta-adrenergic receptors throughout the body, producing sympathomimetic effects like cardiovascular stimulation, elevations in blood glucose, and dilation of bronchioles.[62] The use of iontophoresis is contraindicated in patients who have nonshielded pacemakers.

Endocrine System

The redness of the skin that occurs after treatment is probably mediated by histamine release.[54]

GI, GU, OB/GYN Systems

The use of iontophoresis is contraindicated in cases of pregnancy, as noted in Chapter 6.

Integumentary System

The skin is considered isoelectric (no charge). The migration of ions from the continuous direct electrical current changes the normal pH level of the skin, which is normally between 3 and 4. With an acidic reaction, the pH falls below 3; in an alkaline reaction, the pH is greater than 5. Chemical burns may occur under each electrode. It is more common at the cathode, where there is an accumulation of sodium hydroxide. Skin redness can occur at the conclusion of treatment. The alkaline reaction usually causes sclerolysis. Changes in the pH level can also be responsible for the discomfort and skin irritation sometimes associated with iontophoresis.[54]

Peripheral Vascular/Lymph Systems

Unlike systemic concentration, iontophoresis is directed at large quantities of ions into a localized treatment region. The localized ions minimize the systemic concentration caused by circulatory removal of the material from the area.

BIOFEEDBACK

Theoretical Basis

Biofeedback emits electromyographic electrical signals of motor unit action potentials (MUAP) that are picked up, amplified, and translated into audible sounds and/or visible readings. The visual or auditory feedback that is provided to a patient encourages active self-control over a function that is being monitored. The feedback also allows a patient to gain control over physiologic functions of which he or she might otherwise be unaware.[56]

Cardiopulmonary System

There is no direct effect of biofeedback use on the cardiopulmonary system; however, there can be demands on the system with its use in tasks designed to achieve optimal performance. For example, cardiopulmonary precautions should be adhered to during isometric exercise use with biofeedback. When biofeedback is used for relaxation purposes, it can facilitate relaxation of the inspiratory muscles.[5] Accordingly, with decreased muscle tension and stress, there is a decrease in resting heart rate, blood pressure (BP), and respiratory rate. With a decrease in heart rate during treatment, there is a decrease in blood flow to the area being treated, and therefore a decrease in oxygen and nutrient supply to the muscle.

Endocrine System

Biofeedback can possibly help in decreasing anxiety with relaxation techniques.

GI, GU, OB/GYN Systems

Biofeedback can help facilitate pelvic floor muscle contractions that will help limit urinary incontinence. It also helps facilitate sphincter muscle contraction to help prevent fecal incontinence.[58]

Integumentary System

Shearing forces from adhesive tape of the electrodes can cause skin irritation. Allergic reactions of the skin to the electrodes, gel, or tape can be a common response.

Musculoskeletal System

Biofeedback can be used for muscle reeducation by providing feedback that will reestablish neuromuscular control or promote the ability of a muscle or group of muscles to contract. It may also be used to regain normal agonist/antagonist muscle action and for postural control retraining. Biofeedback can also be used to indicate the electrical activity associated with that muscle contraction. Muscle relaxation is enhanced by relaxation techniques in combinations with biofeedback in order to decrease muscle spasms/guarding.[56]

Neuromuscular System

The use of biofeedback shapes the response that enables the CNS to reestablish sensory-motor loops that have been "forgotten" by the patient. Upon reaching the brain, afferent stimuli, in this case sound or visual cues, stimulate cerebral areas that normally receive proprioceptive information. These artificial signals, combined with the visual cue of actually watching the muscle contract, assist in opening a neural loop that sends efferent signals to the appropriate muscle(s). Biofeedback increases neuromuscular control that results in increased firing rate and motor unit recruitment to the target muscle rather than attempting to reestablish neural loops; these pathways are inhibited. The goal of relaxation therapy is to decrease the number of motor impulses being relayed to the spasming muscle.[5]

Peripheral Vascular/Lymph Systems

During muscle relaxation, there should be an increase in blood flow to the target area that will help supply more nutrients, leukocytes, and O_2 and flush out bradykinin, prostaglandins, and acids that are stimulating nociceptors and other free nerve endings. This will also facilitate more ATP production for the type I muscle fibers so they do not run out of ATP or become unable to break their cross-links. By stimulating muscle contractions with biofeedback, lymphatic ducts will be opened with the movement, and unwanted fluid will diffuse into the lymphatic vessels and then be forced up through the lymphatic vessels by the muscle contraction.

CRYOTHERAPY TECHNIQUES

Theoretical Basis

The theoretical basis for the use of cryotherapy is based on the physiologic responses to a decrease in tissue temperature. When cold is applied to a body part, there is a decrease in blood flow and tissue metabolism.[34] As a result, bleeding and the effects of acute inflammation such as pain and edema are greatly reduced.[44] Additionally, it decreases the nerve conduction velocity (NCV), thereby raising the pain threshold.[21]

Cardiopulmonary System

Cryotherapy application results in a transient increase in systolic and diastolic blood pressure as a result of an increase in the total peripheral resistance of the circulatory vessel walls.[37] Decreases in heart and respiratory rate can also result from cryotherapy application.

Endocrine System

When cryotherapy is applied, there is a decrease in the production and release of vasodilator mediators such as histamines and prostaglandins. There is also a decrease in the body's metabolic rate, which leads to a decrease in the production of metabolites and metabolic heat.[37] Cold may inhibit the release of histamine, while others believe that vasoconstriction is part of the initial reaction of the body to maintain core temperature (autonomic neural response).[61] Sympathetic constriction of the blood vessels is mediated chemically through neural transmitters. Both norepinephrine and epinephrine are secreted into the blood vessels and induce vessel constriction.[27]

into the deep channels allowing valves to regulate the flow of lymph out of the interstitial space. Severe edema can lead to sensory disturbances (paresthesias). By decreasing edema, an improvement in cutaneous sensation may be seen.

Musculoskeletal System

Compression stimulates proteoglycan synthesis in cartilage. The increase in circulation stimulated by compression provides nutrients to soft tissue, while the decrease in edema allows for an increase in range of motion (ROM).[38]

Neuromuscular System

The use of compression as a physical therapy intervention can have both positive and negative effects on the neuromuscular system. The appropriate amount of compression decreases swelling with an accompanying decrease in nerve compression and increase in flow of nutrients to nerve tissue. Conversely, however, too much compression can have negative effects by cutting off blood flow, resulting in numbness and tingling in an area.[3] It can assist with alleviating pain by decreasing pressure in the nerve endings through the gate control theory and by the removal of plasma proteins and waste through the lymph system.

Peripheral Vascular/Lymph Systems

Intermittent compression pumps can be effective in aiding venous return and the pressure gradient. Support stockings can minimize dependent edema. Compression increases the hydrostatic pressure of the tissues, which allows the absorption of interstitial fluids into the lymphatic vessels and venous end capillaries. Compression promotes homeostasis of osmotic and hydrostatic pressure in capillaries by an increase in lymphatic and venous return. There is an allowance for endothelial cells to separate, creating an opening in the lymphatics for the entry of interstitial fluids, cellular waste, large protein molecules, plasma proteins, extracellular particles, and cells into the lymphatic channels. The opening of the pores allows the movement of plasma protein out of the intercellular space.

MASSAGE

Theoretical Basis

Massage is a mechanical stimulation of the tissues by means of rhythmically applied pressure and stretching.[51] The pressure compresses the soft tissues and distorts the nerve-ending networks of receptors. Stretching applies tension to soft tissues, and it also distorts the nerve-ending plexuses of the receptors. The use of these two forces can, by changing the lumen of blood vessels and lymph vessel spaces, affect capillary, venous, arterial, and lymphatic circulation.[52,65]

Cardiopulmonary System

The effect of massage on the circulation of the blood takes place through a reflex influence on blood vessels from a sympathetic division in the nervous system.[48] Deep stroking improves circulation by mechanically assisting venous flow back to the heart. It stimulates tissue release of histamines and acetylcholine. Blood pressure is temporarily decreased by dilation of the capillaries, affecting the permeability of the capillary walls. It also temporarily decreases systolic stroke volume, decreasing heart rate through decreased stimulation of the SNS. It slows down the rate of respiration by the reduced stimulation of the parasympathetic nervous system. By freeing tight respiratory muscles and fascia, massage can be used to increase vital capacity and pulmonary function.

Endocrine System

Massage causes presynaptic inhibition with the neurotransmitter, endorphins that may stop the release of pain transmission substances.

GI, GU, OB/GYN Systems

Massage promotes excitation of peristaltic activity in the large intestines, helping to relieve colic and intestinal gas. It can promote movement within the colon, thus relieving constipation. It promotes stimulation of the parasympathetic system, which stimulates digestion.

Integumentary System

Massage stimulates the sebaceous glands of the skin, causing an increase in sebum production. This added sebum improves the skin's condition, texture, and tone. Friction massage creates heat that leads to perspiration derived from a stimulation of the sudoriferous glands located in the skin.[53] The skin may become hyperemic as superficial blood vessels dilate and may feel warm to touch. The skin also carries out a certain amount of respiration and can be assisted by massaging the part that has been in a cast where the normal functioning of the skin has been inhibited. Friction massage can usually be used to mechanically loosen adhesions and to soften scar tissue by flattening out adipose globules under the skin and make the skin smoother. Massage on the surface of the skin can assist in the removal of dead cells that result from prolonged casting.

Musculoskeletal System

Massage increases the retention of nutrients such as nitrogen, sulfur, and phosphorus in bones. It can make the body more mobile by reducing thickening of connective tissue and freeing fascial restrictions. It also relieves muscular restrictions, tightness, stiffness, and spasms. These effects are achieved by direct pressure on the spasm by manipulating the tissue that sends messages of length to the CNS. Results are more flexible, supple, and resilient muscle tissue. It also increases O_2 to muscles, thereby reducing fatigue and postexercise soreness. It improves muscular nutrition. It promotes rapid disposal of waste products and replenishment of nutritive materials through increased circulation. Massage can also interrupt the pain cycle by relieving muscle spasms.

Neuromuscular System

Massage activates sensory receptors. Slow movements are relaxing to the nervous system, while vigorous movements stimulate the nervous system. Massage decreases pain by the release of beta-endorphins, enkephalins, and other pain-reducing neurochemicals. Massage can mechanically stretch tissue. These changes are detected by mechanoreceptors (GTO) and reflexively alter the contraction signal. Muscle spindle activity is increased during abrupt massage strokes. Massage also increases delta wave activity and reduces norepinephrine and cortisol levels by activation of the relaxation response.

Peripheral Vascular/Lymph Systems

Very light effleurage produces reactions through transient dilation of lymphatic and small capillaries. Deeper pressure leads to prolonged dilation. It also increases the number of red and white corpuscles in the blood and elevates the blood platelet count.[23]

REFERENCES

1. Abramson, D., et al.: Effect of paraffin bath and hot fomentation on local tissue temperature, Arch. Phys. Med. Rehabil. 45:87, 1965.
2. Abramson, D., Tuck, S., Lee, S., Richardson, G., et al.: Comparison of wet and dry heat in raising temperature of tissues, Arch. Phys. Med. Rehabil. 48:654–661, 1967.
3. Airaksinen, O.: Intermittent pneumatic compression therapy in post-traumatic lower limb edema: computed tomography and clinical measurement, Arch. Phys. Med. Rehabil. 72:667–670, 1991.
4. American Physical Therapy Association: Guide to physical therapist practice, Phys. Ther. 77(11):1997.
5. Basmajian, J.: Biofeedback: principles and practice for clinicians, Baltimore, MD, 1989, Williams & Wilkins.
6. Benton, L., Baker, L., and Bowman, B.: Functional electrical stimulation: a practical clinical guide, Downey, CA, 1980, Rancho Los Amigos Hospital.
7. Bisgard, J., Nye, D.: Influence of hot and cold application upon gastric and intestinal motor activity, Surg. Gynecol. Obstet. 71:172–180, 1940.

8. Bishop, B.: Pain: its physiology and rationale for management, Phys. Ther. 60:13–37, 1980.

9. Borrell, R., Henley, E., and Purvis, H.: Fluidotherapy: evaluation of a new heat modality, Arch. Phys. Med. Rehabil. 58:69, 1977.

10. Burns, S., Conin, T.: The use of paraffin wax in the treatment of burns, Physiother. Can. 39:258, 1987.

11. Burton, A., Edhold, O.: Man in cold environment, London, 1955, Edward Arnold.

12. Cameron, M.: Physical agents in rehabilitation, Philadelphia, PA, 1999, W.B. Saunders.

13. Carley, P., Wainapel, S.: Electrotherapy for acceleration of wound healing: low-intensity direct current, Arch. Phys. Med. Rehabil. 66:443–446, 1985.

14. Castel, J.: Pain management with acupuncture and transcutaneous electrical nerve stimulation techniques and photo simulation, Symposium on Pain Management, Walter Reed Army Medical Center, Nov. 13, 1982.

15. Castel, J.: Therapeutic ultrasound, Rehabil. Ther. Prod. Rev. Jan/Feb:22–32, 1993.

16. Chamberg, R.: Clinical uses of cryotherapy, Phys. Ther. 49(3):145–149, 1969.

17. Clark, R., Lepherdt, S., and Baker, C.: Cryotherapy and compression treatment protocols in the prevention of delayed onset muscle soreness, J. Athl. Train. 31(2):S33, 1996.

18. Clement-Jones, V.: Increased beta-endorphin but not metenkephalin levels in human cerebrospinal fluid after acupuncture for recurrent pain, Lancet 8:946–948, 1980.

19. Cook, H., et al.: Effect of electrical stimulation on lymphatic flow and limb volume in the rat, Phys. Ther. 74:1040–1046, 1994.

20. Costello, C.: Optimization of drug delivery with iontophoresis, Houston, TX, 1993, Texas Women's University, dissertation.

21. Dejong, R., Hershey, W., and Wagman, I.: Nerve conduction velocity during hypothermia in man, Anesthesiology 27:805–810, 1966.

22. Dyson, M., Luke, D.: Induction of mast cell degranulation in skin by ultrasound, IEEE Trans. Ultraso. Ferroelectr. Freq. Control UFFC 33:194, 1986.

23. Ebel, A., Wishamn, L.: Effect of massage on muscle temperature and radiosodium clearance, Arch. Phys. Med. 33:399–405, 1952.

24. Eldred, E., Lindsley, D., and Buckwald, J.: The effect of cooking on mammalian muscle spindles, Exp. Neurol. 2:144–157, 1960.

25. Evans, P.: The healing process at the cellular level: a review, Physiotherapy 66:256–259, 1980.

26. Griffin, J., Karsalis, T.: Physical agents for physical therapists, ed. 3, Springfield, IL, 1987, Charles C Thomas.

27. Guyton, A.: Textbook of medical physiology, ed. 10, Philadelphia, PA, 2000, W.B. Saunders.

28. Hardy, J.: Spectral transmittance and reflectance of excised human skin, J. Appl. Physiol. 9:257–264, 1956.

29. Hayes, K.: Manual for physical agents, ed. 4, Norwalk, CT, 1999, Appleton & Lange.

30. Hecox, B., Mehreteab, T., and Weisberg, J.: Physical agents: a comprehensive text for physical therapists, Norwalk, CT, 1994, Appleton & Lange.

31. Henley, E.: Engineering and medicine—fluidotherapy, Chemtech April 1982, 215–220.

32. Henry, J., Windos, T.: Compensation of arterial insufficiency by augmenting the circulation with intermittent compression of the limbs, Am. Heart J. 70(1):77–88, 1965.

33. Hensel, H.: Thermal sensations and thermoreceptors in man, Springfield, IL, 1982, Charles C Thomas.

34. Hocutt, J., Jaffe, R., and Rylander, L.: Cryotherapy in ankle sprains, Am. J. Sports Med. 10(3):316–319, 1992.

35. Knight, K.: Cryotherapy in sports injury management, Champaign, IL, 1995, Human Kinetics.

36. Kramer, J.: Ultrasound: evaluation of its mechanical and thermal effects, Arch. Phys. Med. Rehabil. 65:223–227, 1984.

37. Krusen, F.: Handbook of physical medicine and rehab, ed. 2, Philadelphia, PA, 1971, W.B. Saunders.

38. Lafeber, F.: Intermittent hydrostatic compressive force stimulates exclusively the proteoglycan synthesis of osteoarthritic human cartilage, Br. J. Rheumatol. 31(7):437–442, 1992.

39. Lehmann, J., Warren, J., and Scham, S.: Therapeutic heat and cold, J. Clin. Orthop. Rel. Res. 99:207–245, 1974.

40. Lemke, E.: The influence of UV irradiation on vitamin D metabolism in children with chronic renal diseases, Int. Urol. Nephrol. 25(6):595–601, 1993.

41. Licht, S.: Therapeutic heat, New Haven, CT, 1965, Elizabeth Licht.

42. Mathews, J.: The effect of spinal traction, Physiotherapy 58:64–66, 1972.

43. Matson, F., Questa, K., and Matson, A.: The effect of local cooling on post fracture swelling, Clin. Orthop. Rel. Res. 109:201–206, 1975.

44. McMaster, W.: A literary review on ice therapy injuries, Am. J. Sports Med. 5(30):124–126, 1977.

45. Michlovitz, S.: Thermal agents in rehabilitation, ed. 3, Philadelphia, PA 1996, F.A. Davis.

46. O'Donoghue, D.: Treatment of injuries to patients, ed. 3, Philadelphia, PA, 1978, W.B. Saunders.

47. Parrish, J.: UV-A biological effects of ultraviolet radiation, New York, 1979, Plenum.

48. Patrick, M.: Applications of pulsed therapeutic ultrasound, Physiotherapy 64(4):3–104, 1978.

49. Pemberton, R.: The physiologic influence of massage. In Mock, H., Pemberton, R., and Coulter, J., editors. Principles and practices of physical therapy, vol. I, Hagerstown, MD, 1939, W.B. Saunders.

50. Pilla, A., Figueiredo, M., Nasser, P., et al.: Non-invasive low intensity pulsed ultrasound: a potent accelerator of bone repair, Proceedings of the 36th Annual Meeting, Orthopedic Research Society, New Orleans, 1990.

51. Prentice, W.: Therapeutic modalities for allied health professionals, New York, 1998, McGraw-Hill.

52. Prentice, W.: Therapeutic modalities in sports medicine, St. Louis, MO, 1990, Mosby.

53. Salvo, S.: Massage therapy: principles and practice, Philadelphia, PA, 1999, W.B. Saunders.

54. Sanderson, J., DeRiel, S., and Dixon, R.: Iontophoretic delivery of non-peptide drugs: formulation optimization for maximum skin permeability, J. Pharm. Sci. 78:361–364, 1989.

55. Saunders, D.: Use of spinal traction in the treatment of neck and back conditions, Clin. Orthop. 179:31–38, 1983.

56. Schwartz, M.: Biofeedback: a practitioner's guide, New York, 1987, Guyford Press.

57. Stiff, M.: Appliances of electrostimulation in physical conditioning: a review, J. Appl. Sport Sci. Res. 4:20–26, 1990.

58. Sugar E., Firlit, C.: Urodynamic feedback: a new therapeutic approach for childhood incontinence/infection, J. Urol. 128:1253, 1982.

59. Ter Haar, C.: Basic physics of therapeutic ultrasound, Physiotherapy 73(3):110–113, 1987.

60. Urbach, F.: The biological effects of ultraviolet radiation, London, 1969, Pergamon.

61. Vanhoutte, P., Leusen, I.: Vasodilatation, New York, 1981, Raven Press.

62. Weiner, N.: Norepinephrine, epinephrine, sympopathomimetic amines. In Gilman, A., Goodman, L., Rall, T., and Murad, F., editors. Goodman and Gilman's the pharmacological basis of therapeutics, ed. 7, New York, 1985, McMillan.

63. Williams, A., McHale, I., and Bowditchm, M.: Effects of MHz ultrasound on electrical pain threshold perception in humans, Ultrasound Med. Biol. 13:249, 1987.

64. Wingard, L., Brody, T., Larner, J., and Schwartz, A.: Glucocorticoids and other adrenal steroids. In Human pharmacology, St. Louis, MO, 1991, Mosby Yearbook.

65. Wood, E., Becker, P.: Beard's massage, ed. 4, Philadelphia, PA, 1997, W.B. Saunders.

APPENDICES

APPENDIX A-1

LOCATIONS OF THE MOTOR POINTS

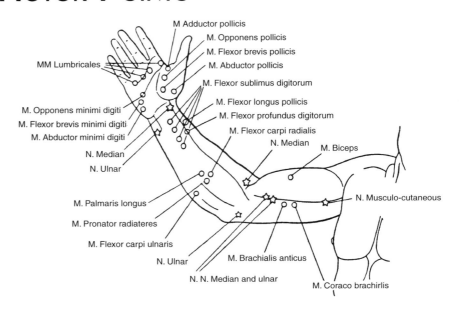

M Adductor pollicis
M. Opponens pollicis
M. Flexor brevis pollicis
M. Abductor pollicis
M. Flexor sublimus digitorum
M. Flexor longus pollicis
M. Flexor profundus digitorum
M. Flexor carpi radialis
N. Median
M. Biceps
N. Musculo-cutaneous

MM Lumbricales

M. Opponens minimi digiti
M. Flexor brevis minimi digiti
M. Abductor minimi digiti
N. Median
N. Ulnar

M. Palmaris longus
M. Pronator radiateres
M. Flexor carpi ulnaris
N. Ulnar
N. N. Median and ulnar
M. Brachialis anticus
M. Coraco brachirlis

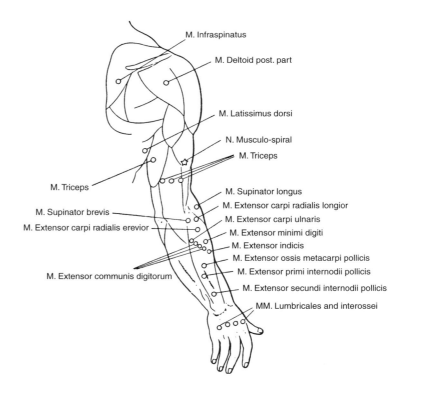

M. Infraspinatus
M. Deltoid post. part
M. Latissimus dorsi
N. Musculo-spiral
M. Triceps

M. Triceps

M. Supinator brevis
M. Extensor carpi radialis erevior

M. Supinator longus
M. Extensor carpi radialis longior
M. Extensor carpi ulnaris
M. Extensor minimi digiti
M. Extensor indicis
M. Extensor ossis metacarpi pollicis
M. Extensor primi internodii pollicis
M. Extensor secundi internodii pollicis
MM. Lumbricales and interossei

M. Extensor communis digitorum

570

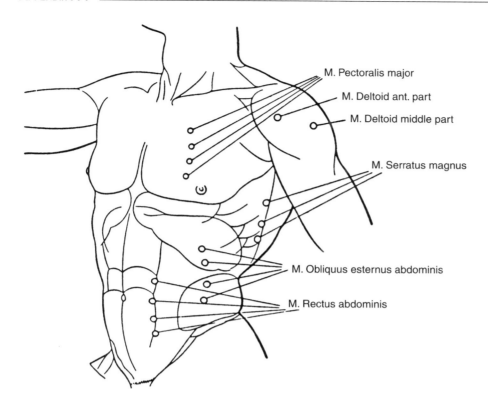

M. Pectoralis major

M. Deltoid ant. part

M. Deltoid middle part

M. Serratus magnus

M. Obliquus esternus abdominis

M. Rectus abdominis

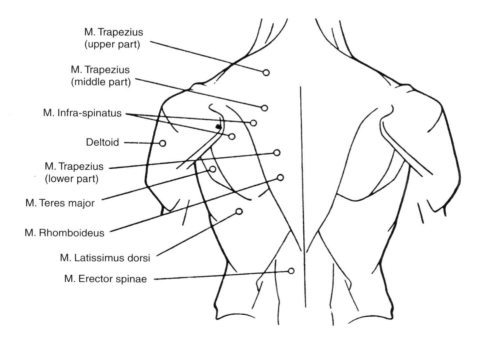

M. Trapezius
(upper part)

M. Trapezius
(middle part)

M. Infra-spinatus

Deltoid

M. Trapezius
(lower part)

M. Teres major

M. Rhomboideus

M. Latissimus dorsi

M. Erector spinae

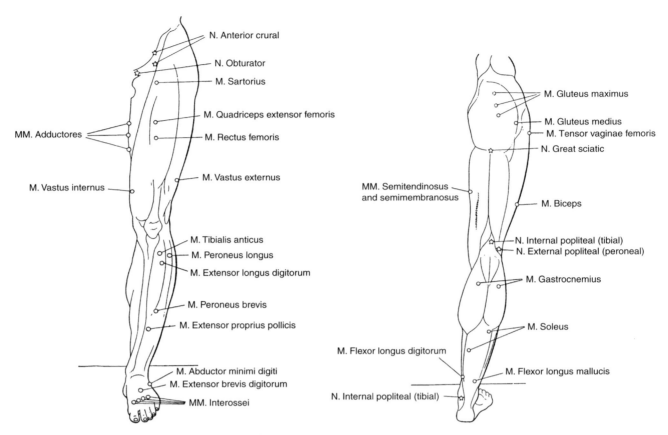

N. Anterior crural

N. Obturator

M. Sartorius

M. Quadriceps extensor femoris

M. Rectus femoris

MM. Adductores

M. Vastus externus

M. Vastus internus

M. Tibialis anticus

M. Peroneus longus

M. Extensor longus digitorum

M. Peroneus brevis

M. Extensor proprius pollicis

M. Abductor minimi digiti

M. Extensor brevis digitorum

MM. Interossei

M. Gluteus maximus

M. Gluteus medius

M. Tensor vaginae femoris

N. Great sciatic

MM. Semitendinosus
and semimembranosus

M. Biceps

N. Internal popliteal (tibial)

N. External popliteal (peroneal)

M. Gastrocnemius

M. Soleus

M. Flexor longus digitorum

M. Flexor longus mallucis

N. Internal popliteal (tibial)

M = Muscle
N = Nerves

APPENDIX A-2

UNITS OF MEASURE

Milliseconds (msec)	$= \frac{1}{1000}$ of a second
Microseconds (μsec)	$= \frac{1}{1,000,000}$ of a second
Nanosecond (nsec)	$= \frac{1}{1,000,000,000}$ of a second
Milliamp (mA)	$= \frac{1}{1000}$ of an ampere
Microamp (μA)	$= \frac{1}{1,000,000}$ of an ampere
Angstrom (Å)	$= \frac{1}{10,000,000,000}$ of a meter
Nanometer (nm)	$= \frac{1}{1,000,000,000}$ of a meter
Hertz (Hz)	$= 1$ cycle per second
Kilohertz (KHz)	$= 1000$ cycles per second
Megahertz (MHz)	$= 1,000,000$ cycles per second

INDEX

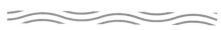

Note: Page numbers followed by italic *f* or *t* denote figures or tables, respectively.

A

A-alpha fibers, 68*t*
A-beta fibers, 68*t*, 71–72, 71*f*
A-delta fibers, 68*t*, 69
Absolute refractory period, 108, 157
Absorption
    definition, 6, 6*f*, 13
    Law of Grotthus-Draper, 7, 7*f*
AC. *See* Alternating current
Accommodation, 66, 79, 90–90, 102
Acetylcholine (ACh), 214
Acidic reaction, 166, 175, 179
Acoustic energy. *See also* Extracorporeal shock
    wave therapy; Ultrasound
    characteristics, 11
    vs. electromagnetic energy, 11
    transmission in biologic tissues, 361–363
Acoustic impedance, 363, 363*t*, 403
Acoustic microstreaming, 375, 376*f*, 403
Acoustic spectrum, 3, 13
ACTH. *See* Adrenocorticotropic hormone
Action potential
    definition, 107, 157
    elicitation in electrophysiologic testing,
        210–211
Active electrode, 157
Active release technique, 526–527, 527*f*
Activity Pattern Indicators Pain Profile, 63
Acupressure, 520–524, 523*f*, 533
Acute injury
    bioelectric field changes in response to, 118–119
    definition, 27
    edema formation, 486–489
    initial treatment, 21–23, 22*t*
    therapeutic modality selection, 22*t*, 25*t*
Acute pain, 61, 70. *See also* Pain
Adrenocorticotropic hormone (ACTH), 73, 79
Afferent, 66, 79, 250
Afferent nerve fibers, 66*t*, 67*f*, 68*t*
Age
    electrophysiologic testing and, 216
    wound healing and, 21
Air space plate, 264–265, 265*f*, 266*f*, 286
Alkaline reaction, 167, 175, 179
All-or-none response, 111, 157
Alpha motor neuron, 214
Alternating current (AC), 89*f*, 102. *See also*
    Biphasic current
Ampere, 84, 102
Amplifier, 204
Amplitude
    compound motor action potential, 224*f*, 225
    definition, 250, 372, 403
    sensory nerve action potential, 218–219, 218*f*

Analgesia, 70–75, 334. *See also* Pain control
Analgesic creams, 380, 380*f*
Anesthesia, 334
Ankle sprain, 488
Annulus fibrosus, 456, 481
Anode, 107, 157
Anoxia, 481
Anterior primary rami, 215, 250
Antidromic, 250
Applicator, 286
Arndt-Schultz principle, 6–7, 13
Atrophy, 20, 129–131
Attenuation, 362–363, 403
Average current, 102
Avulsion fracture, 65, 79
Axon(s), 213–214
Axonopathy, 213, 250

B

Bandwidth, 198
Beam nonuniformity ratio (BNR), 369–370, 371*f*,
    403
Beat, 145, 157
Beat modulation, 92
Beta-endorphins, 69, 73–74, 74*f*, 79, 136
Bindegewebsmassage, 518–520, 533
Bioelectromagnetics, 118–120, 157
Biofeedback
    electromyographic. *See* Electromyographic
        biofeedback
    instrumentation
        finger phototransmission, 184
        peripheral skin temperature, 183–184
        skin conductance activity, 184
    for postimmobilization loss of motion, 184
    role of, 183
Biphasic action potential, 218, 250
Biphasic current. *See also* Alternating current
    definition, 91, 102
    vs. monophasic, for electrical stimulation, 121
    waveforms, 87, 88*f*
Bipolar arrangement, 198
BNR. *See* Beam nonuniformity ratio
Bone healing. *See also* Fracture(s)
    extracorporeal shock wave therapy, 541
    laser therapy, 423
    traction, 454
    ultrasound, 387–388
Bradykinin, 79
Bursts, 92, 93*f*, 102

C

C fibers, 68*t*, 69
Cable electrodes, 267, 268*f*, 286

Calcium deposits, 388
Camphor, 324
Capacitor electrodes, 263–266, 264*f*, 286
Capsaicin, 324
Carbon arc lamp, 439
Cardiopulmonary system
    effects of biofeedback, 556
    effects of compression devices, 564
    effects of cryotherapy, 557
    effects of electrical stimulation, 552, 553, 554
    effects of iontophoresis, 555
    effects of massage, 565
    effects of thermotherapy, 559
    effects of traction, 563
    effects of ultrasound, 561
    effects of ultraviolet therapy, 562
Carpal tunnel syndrome
    electrophysiologic testing, 206–207
    nerve conduction studies, 230–231
Cathode, 107, 157
Cavitation, 375, 376*f*, 403
Cell membrane, response to electrical current,
        111–113, 112*f*
Central biasing theory
    definition, 72, 79, 157
    electrical stimulation and, 136, 553
Central conduction study, 229
Cervical radiculopathy, 208
Cervical traction
    manual, 475–476, 475*f*, 476*f*
    mechanical, 476–478, 477*f*
Chronaxie, 110*f*, 111, 157
Chronic injury, 21, 27. *See also* Chronic wounds
Chronic pain. *See also* Pain
    definition, 61, 80
    electrical stimulation, 76
Chronic venous insufficiency
    characteristics, 45, 46*f*
    compression therapy, 42, 44
Chronic wounds
    compression therapy, 44
    cryotherapy, 28–29
    electric stimulation, 30–37, 33*f*, 34*f*, 35*f*, 36*f*
    hydrotherapy, 29–30, 30
    laser therapy, 39–41, 40*f*
    therapeutic modality selection, 44–48, 50–52,
        51*f*
    thermotherapy, 29
    ultrasound, 35–37, 38*f*
Circuit. *See* Electrical circuit
Circulation
    effects of massage, 505
    effects of tissue temperature change, 292–293
Clinical focusing, 541, 547

Clot formation, 16–17
CMAP. *See* Compound motor action potential
CMMR. *See* Common mode rejection ratio
Coherence, 30, 411
Cold hydrocollator packs, 301–302, 301*f*, 338–339
Cold spray, 306–308, 307*f*, 344–345
Cold whirlpool, 303–306, 304*f*, 342–343
Collagen, 17
Collimated beam
   laser, 411–412, 412*f*, 430
   ultrasound, 369, 403
Common mode rejection ratio (CMRR), 186, 198
Complex regional pain syndrome, 310
Compound motor action potential (CMAP)
   amplitude, 224*f*
   definition, 223, 250
   latency, 224*f*
   setup, 223, 224*f*, 225*f*
   shape, 224*f*
Compression therapy
   case studies, 488, 492
   clinical applications
      acute injury, 22
      ankle sprain, 488
      chronic wounds, 44
      inflammation, 23
      lymphedema, 492
      wound healing, 23
   clinical procedures, 492–494, 493*f*, 494*f*, 499–500
   cold and, 494
   contraindications, 496, 499
   electrical stimulation and, 495, 495*f*
   equipment, 490*f*, 492–494, 493*f*, 494*f*
   indications, 496, 499
   lab activity, 499–500
   parameters
      inflation pressure, 490–491
      on-off time sequence, 491
      total treatment time, 490–491, 490*f*
   patient setup and instructions, 492–494, 493*f*, 494*f*, 499–500
   physiologic effects, 499, 564–565
   sequential pumps, 494–495, 495*f*
   theoretical basis, 564
Compressions, 403
Conductance, 84, 102
Conduction, 290, 291*t*, 334
Conductive garments, 36*f*
Conductors, 84, 102
Congestion, 306, 334
Connective tissue
   massage, 518–520
   stretching, 385–387, 386*f*
Consensual heat vasodilation, 313, 334
Constructive interference, 145, 145*f*, 157
Continuous wave laser, 417, 417*f*, 430. *See also*
      Laser(s); Laser therapy
Continuous wave ultrasound, 371–372, 372*f*, 403.
      See also Ultrasound
Contraction, muscle. *See* Muscle, contraction
Contrast bath
   case study, 310
   clinical procedures, 346–347
   for complex regional pain syndrome, 310
   definition, 334
   lab activity, 346–347
   technique, 308–311, 309*f*
   treatment tip, 296, 309

Contusion
   Cryo-Cuff, 312
   ultrasound, 383–385
Convection, 291*t*, 334
Conversion, 291*t*, 334
Corticosteroids, 20
Cosine law, 7, 7*f*, 13, 274, 442
Coulomb, 102
Counterirritants, 324
Coupling medium, 378–379, 379*f*, 403
Cryo-Cuff, 311, 312, 348–349, 494
Cryokinetics, 311, 334
Cryotherapy
   for acute injury, 21, 28–29
   contraindications, 47–48*t*, 295
   definition, 291, 334
   frostbite risk, 297
   indications, 25*t*, 295
   for inflammation, 23, 29
   physiologic effects, 295–296, 297*t*, 557–558
   precautions, 298
   response to, 297–298
   techniques
      cold hydrocollator packs, 301–302, 301*f*, 338–339
      cold spray, 306–308, 307*f*, 344–345
      cold whirlpool, 303–306, 304*f*, 342–343
      contrast bath, 308–311, 309*f*, 346–347
      Cryo-Cuff, 311, 312, 348–349
      cryokinetics, 311
      ice immersion, 311
      ice massage, 298–301, 298*f*, 299*f*, 336–337
      ice packs, 302–303, 302*f*, 340–341
      patient positioning, 335
   theoretical basis, 557
Current. *See also* Electrical current
   interferential, 145–147, 145*f*, 146*f*, 552–553.
      See also Electrical stimulation
   Russian, 143–144, 143*f*, 144*f*
Current of injury, 118–119, 157
Cycle, 87

D
DC. *See* Direct current
Decay time, 90, 102
Decubitus ulcers. *See* Pressure ulcers
Deflection, 219
Delayed-onset muscle soreness, 295
Demyelination, 213, 250
Denervated muscle, 134, 157
Deoxyribonucleic acid (DNA), 434, 435, 447
Depolarization, 107–109, 157
Destructive interference, 145, 145*f*, 157
Dexamethasone, 389
Diabetes mellitus, 45–46, 46*f*
Diathermy
   contraindications, 275
   definition, 4, 13, 259, 286
   effectiveness, 259–260
   guidelines for safe use, 280
   indications, 275–276
   microwave. *See* Microwave diathermy
   nonthermal effects, 261
   precautions, 276–278
   shortwave. *See* Shortwave diathermy
   thermal effects, 260
Differential amplifier, 186, 198, 250

Diode laser, 412, 414–415, 415*f*, 430. *See also*
      Laser(s); Laser therapy
Dipoles, 157
Direct current (DC). *See also* Monophasic current
   characteristics, 89*f*, 91, 91*f*, 102
   for iontophoresis, 167, 167*f*, 168–169
   treatment tip, 96
Direct effect, 419, 430
Disk
   fluid mechanics, 455, 455*f*
   herniation, 455*f*, 456, 481
   material, 481
   nucleus, 456, 481
   protrusion, 455, 481
Distal motor latency (DML), 223, 224*f*, 225*f*, 250
Distal sensory latency (DSL), 220, 221*f*, 250
Divergence, 412, 430
DNA. *See* Deoxyribonucleic acid
Drum electrodes, 268–269, 268*f*, 286
Duration
   compound motor action potential, 226
   definition, 91, 102, 250
Duty cycle, 371, 372*f*, 403
Dynorphin, 69, 79

E
EBS. *See* Electrical bone growth stimulator
Eddy currents, 266, 267*f*, 286
Edema, 486
   characteristics, 484
   definition, 20, 334, 498
   negative effects, 489
   pathophysiology, 486–487
   treatment
      elevation, 489, 489*f*
      external pressure, 490
      intermittent compression. *See* Compression therapy
      laser therapy, 425
      muscle contraction, 489–490
      thermotherapy, 313
      ultrasound, 384
      weight-bearing activities, 490
Effective radiating area (ERA), 365–367, 366*f*, 367*f*, 403
Efferent, 72, 79, 250
Efferent nerve fibers, 66
Effleurage, 512, 513*f*, 533
Elastin, 17
Electrets, 117, 157
Electrical bone growth stimulator (EBS), 387
Electrical circuit, 94, 102. *See also* Parallel circuit; Series circuit
Electrical current
   compared to water flow, 85*t*
   components, 84–85
   definition, 102
   density, 122–123, 122*f*, 123*f*, 157
   flow, 85, 85*t*, 96
   measurement, 84
   modulation, 92, 93*f*
   physiologic responses, 96–97, 105–106
   total, 90, 90*f*
Electrical field, 263, 264*f*, 286
Electrical impedance, 84, 102
Electrical potential, 84, 84*f*, 102
Electrical safety, 97–99, 98*f*, 99*f*
Electrical shock, 97–98, 98*t*

Electrical stimulation. *See also* High-voltage
  pulsed galvanic current (HVPC)
  case studies
    control of swelling, 130
    muscle reeducation, 114, 115
    muscle strengthening, 113, 116
    pain control, 130, 137
    wound healing, 52
  characteristics, 9
  circuits, 95–96, 95*f*
  clinical applications
    acute injury, 22
    atrophy retardation, 129–131
    in denervated muscle, 134–135
    edema, 132, 134, 494
    fibroblastic-repair phase, 23
    fracture healing, 142
    increased range of motion, 131–132, 133*f*
    inflammation, 23
    maturation-remodeling phase, 24
    muscle pump contractions, 129
    muscle reeducation, 114, 115, 128–129
    muscle strengthening, 113, 116, 131
    pain control, 130, 135–138, 141
    swelling, 130, 144
    tendon and ligament healing, 142–143
    wound healing, 52, 141–142
  clinical procedures
    muscle reeducation, 161–162
    muscle strengthening, 163–164
    pain control, 158–160
  clinical research evidence, 49
  compression therapy and, 495, 495*f*
  contraindications/precautions, 47–48*t*
  currents
    biphasic vs. monophasic, 121–122
    generators, 86–87
    types, 85–86, 86*f*
  equipment, 133*f*
  functional, 139–140
  indications, 25*t*
  interferential current, 145–147, 145*f*, 146*f*
  lab activities
    muscle reeducation, 161–162
    muscle strengthening, 163–164
    pain control, 158–160
  low-intensity, 140–143
  low-voltage continuous direct current, 138–139
  mechanisms of action, 30–32, 552
  noncontractile, 132, 134
  parameters
    chemical effects, 125
    current density, 122–123, 122*f*, 123*f*
    current flow direction, 126, 127*f*
    duration, 124–125
    ease of excitation, 126
    electrode placement, 126–127, 127*f*
    frequency, 123–124
    intensity, 124, 125*f*
    monophasic vs. biphasic current, 121–122,
      122*f*
    polarity, 125
    tissue impedance, 122
  physiologic responses
    by body system, 552–555
    cell and tissue, 120–121
    cell membrane, 111–113, 112*f*
    depolarization, 107–109, 108*f*

    intercellular structures, 114–115
    muscle, 111, 553, 554, 555
    nerve, 106–107, 553, 554, 555
    normal bioelectric fields, 117–120,
      118*f*, 119*f*
    strain-related potentials, 117, 117*f*
    tissue electrical circuits, 115–116
  placebo effect, 138
  Russian currents, 143–144, 143*f*, 144*f*
  theoretical basis, 552
  ultrasound and, 392–393, 392*f*
Electrode(s)
  active, 107, 167, 170, 179, 190, 198
  cable, 267, 268*f*, 286
  capacitor, 263–266, 264*f*, 286
  dispersive, 170
  drum, 268–269, 268*f*, 286
  for electromyographic biofeedback, 189
  for electromyography, 219
  for electrophysiologic testing, 203–204, 205*f*
  indifferent, 107, 157
  induction, 286
  pad, 265–266, 266*f*, 267*f*, 286
  placement, 126–127, 127*f*
  reference, 186, 198
Electrolytes, 166, 179
Electromagnetic energy
  vs. acoustic energy, 11
  Arndt-Schultz principle, 6–7
  characteristics, 4–5, 5*f*
  contact with tissue, 6*f*
  cosine law, 7, 7*f*
  inverse square law, 8, 8*f*
  Law of Grotthus-Draper, 7
  modalities using, 8–10. *See also specific*
    modalities
Electromagnetic spectrum
  definition, 3, 13
  regions, 5*f*
  visible light, 4*f*
Electromyographic biofeedback. *See also*
    Biofeedback
  audio feedback, 191–192
  case study, 191
  characteristics, 9
  clinical applications, 192–193
  clinical procedures, 199–200
  contraindications, 189
  converting activity to meaningful data,
    188–189, 188*f*
  definition, 182, 185, 198
  electrical activity measurement, 186
  electrode placement, 190, 190*f*
  electrodes, 189
  equipment, 186, 187*f*
  indications, 189, 192–193
  information display, 190
  lab activity, 199–200
  motor unit recruitment, 185–186
  physiology, 185, 185*f*, 556–557
  separation and magnification of electromyo-
    graphic activity, 186–188, 187*f*
  signal processing, 189
  signal sensitivity, 192
  skin preparation, 189–190
  theoretical basis, 556
  treatment tips, 186, 192, 193
  visual feedback, 190–191

Electromyography (EMG). *See also* Electrophysio-
    logic testing
  action potential elicitation, 211
  for cervical radiculopathy, 208
  clinical procedures
    amplitude, 238
    contraction level, 239–240, 239*f*
    duration, 238
    fibrillation potentials, 234, 234*f*, 235
    insertion, 233–234
    myotonic discharges, 235
    other potentials, 235
    positive sharp waves, 234*f*, 235
    rest, 235–236
    shape, 236–238, 237*f*
    sound, 238–239
    voluntary activity, 236
  definition, 182, 250
  electrodes, 204
  indications, 244
  limitations, 241
  purpose, 202
  rationale, 232–233
  sensitivity and specificity, 240–241
  setup, 231–232, 231*f*
Electron
  definition, 84, 102
  excited state, 410, 410*f*, 411*f*, 430
  flow, 84–85, 85*t*. *See also* Electrical current
Electrophoresis, 166, 179
Electrophysiologic testing. *See also* Electromyogra-
    phy; Nerve conduction study; Somatosen-
    sory evoked potential (SEP) testing
  action potential elicitation, 210–211
  age considerations, 216
  auditory feedback, 207
  case studies, 206–207, 208, 209
  characteristics, 202
  clinical applications
    axonopathy, 209
    carpal tunnel syndrome, 206–207
    radiculopathy, 208
  clinical procedures, 252–255
  electrodes, 203–204, 205*f*
  equipment, 204*f*
  lab activity, 252–255
  limb temperature considerations, 216
  record generation, 211
  sequence, 215–216
  visual feedback, 207
Electropiezo activity, 117, 157
Electrotherapeutic devices. *See also specific devices*
    and modalities
  circuits, 95–96, 95*f*
  electrical safety, 97–99, 98*f*, 99*f*
  generators, 85–87, 86*f*
Emission, 430
Endocrine system
  effects of biofeedback, 556
  effects of compression devices, 564
  effects of cryotherapy, 557
  effects of electrical stimulation,
    553, 554
  effects of iontophoresis, 556
  effects of massage, 565
  effects of thermotherapy, 559
  effects of ultrasound, 561
  effects of ultraviolet therapy, 562

Endogenous opioids, 69, 72, 79
Endorphins, 73, 79
Endothelial cells, 485–486, 498
Endothelial-derived relaxing factor, 490, 498
Energy flux, 547
Energy flux density, 541, 547
Enkephalin, 69, 79
Enkephalinergic interneurons, 72, 73, 79
Enterococcus faecalis, 41
Epicondylitis, 544, 544*f*
Epithelial cells, 31
ERA. *See* Effective radiating area
Erb's point, 250
Erythema, 299, 334, 435, 447. *See also* Minimal
    erythemal dose
ESWT. *See* Extracorporeal shock wave therapy
Exercise
    in inflammatory-response phase, 23
    in maturation-remodeling phase, 24
    for pain control, 76–77
Extracellular matrix, 17
Extracorporeal shock wave therapy (ESWT)
    case study, 538
    characteristics, 11–12
    clinical applications
        calcific shoulder tendinitis, 544–545
        fractures, 543
        medial/lateral epicondylitis, 544
        plantar fasciitis, 538, 543–544, 543*f*
    evidence-based practice, 545
    history, 537–538
    physiologic effects, 541, 541*t*
    shock waves in
        characteristics, 538–540, 539*f*
        generation, 540
        parameters, 540–541, 540*t*

F
F-wave, 229, 250
Facet joints, 456, 481
Faradic current, 102
Fasciculation potential, 236, 250
Federal Communications Commission (FCC),
    261, 286
Fiber-optics, 413–414, 430
Fibril, 485, 498
Fibrillation potentials, 234, 234*f*, 235, 250
Fibrin, 16
Fibrinogen, 16
Fibroblastic-repair phase of healing
    pathophysiology, 17, 18*f*
    therapeutic modalities, 22*t*, 23
    ultrasound effects, 36–37
Fibroplasia, 17, 27
Fibrosis, 481
Filter, 87, 102, 198
Fluidotherapy
    clinical procedures, 322–323, 322*f*,
        358–359
    definition, 334
    physiologic effects, 322, 561
    theoretical basis, 561
Fluorescence, 444, 447
Fluorescent ultraviolet lamp, 439
Fluori-Methane, 306–308, 307*f*
Focal volume, 540–541, 547
Focusing, 79
Foramen opening, unilateral, 458, 481

Fracture(s). *See also* Bone healing
    nonunion
        extracorporeal shock wave therapy, 543
        low-intensity stimulation, 142
        postimmobilization pain and loss of motion
            cold whirlpool treatment, 305
            ice massage, 300
            ultrasound, 370
            warm hydrocollator packs, 317
    stress, ultrasound in assessment, 388
Free nerve endings. *See* Nociceptors
Frequency
    definition, 6, 13, 102, 430
    in electrical stimulation therapy, 123–124
    pulse, 91
    units of measure, 86
    window selectivity, 157
Friction massage, 518, 518*f*, 519*f*, 533
Frostbite, 297
Functional electrical stimulation, 139–140, 157

G
Gain, 207
Gallium arsenide (GaAs) lasers, 414–415, 418*t*,
    419, 419*f*. *See also* Laser(s); Laser therapy
Gap junctions, 116, 157
Gastrointestinal system
    effects of cryotherapy, 557
    effects of massage, 566
    effects of thermotherapy, 559
    effects of ultraviolet therapy, 562
Gate control theory, 71–73, 71*f*, 72*f*, 135–135, 553
Genitourinary system
    effects of biofeedback, 556
    effects of electrical stimulation, 553, 554, 555
    effects of traction, 563
    effects of ultrasound, 561
    effects of ultraviolet therapy, 562
GFI. *See* Ground-fault interruptor
Glycosaminoglycans, 17
Golgi tendon organs, 66, 66*t*
Granulation tissue, 17
Grotthus-Draper, Law of, 7, 13
Ground, 97, 102
Ground-fault interruptor (GFI), 98, 102
Ground state, 410, 410*f*, 411*f*, 430
Ground substance, 17

H
H-wave. *See* Hoffman's reflex
Harness, traction, 467, 467*f*, 468*f*, 469*f*
Healing process
    factors impeding, 20–21
    fibroblastic-repair phase, 17, 18*f*
    inflammatory-response phase, 15–17, 16*f*
    maturation-remodeling phase, 19–20, 19*f*
Heat transfer, 290–291, 291*t*. *See also*
    Cryotherapy; Thermotherapy
Helium neon (HeNe) lasers, 413–414, 418*t*.
    See also Laser(s); Laser therapy
Hemorrhage, 20
Henneman size principle, 210
Heterodynes, 146, 146*f*, 157
High-voltage current, 84, 102
High-voltage pulsed galvanic current (HVPC)
    application techniques, 31–35, 33*f*, 34*f*, 35*f*
    mechanisms of action, 31–32
    waveform, 35*f*

Histamine, 15
Hoffman's reflex, 229–230, 250
Hot packs. *See* Warm hydrocollator packs
Hot spots, 363, 403
Humidity, in wound healing, 21
Hunting response, 296, 334
HVPC. *See* High-voltage pulsed galvanic current
Hybrid currents, 157
Hydrocollator, 334
Hydrocollator packs
    cold. *See* Cold hydrocollator packs
    warm. *See* Warm hydrocollator packs
Hydrocortisone, 389
Hydrogel sheets, ultrasound treatment and, 379
Hydrotherapy. *See also* Cryotherapy;
    Thermotherapy; Whirlpool
    for chronic wounds, 29–30, 50
    clinical research evidence, 50
    definition, 291, 334
Hyperalgesia, 69
Hyperemia, 313, 334
Hyperplasia, 435, 447
Hypertrophic scars, 20

I
Ice immersion, 311
Ice massage, 298–301, 298*f*, 299*f*, 336–337
Ice packs
    clinical procedures, 302–303, 302*f*, 340–341
    ultrasound and, 391, 392*f*
Impedance, 122, 157, 363
Indication, 334
Indifferent electrode, 107, 157
Indirect effect, 419, 430
Induction electrodes, 266–269, 267*f*, 268*f*, 286
Inflammation
    chemical mediators, 15
    chronic, 17, 387
    clinical procedures
        compressive therapy, 22*t*, 23
        cryotherapy, 22*t*, 23
        electrical stimulation, 21, 22*t*, 23
        laser therapy, 22*t*, 23, 39, 422, 425
        transverse friction massage, 518, 519*f*
        ultrasound, 22*t*, 35–36, 383–384
        ultraviolet radiation, 435–436
    definition, 334
    pathophysiology, 15, 16*f*
    responses to, 15
Infrared radiation
    characteristics, 4*f*, 5*f*
    definition, 4, 13, 290, 334, 430
Infrared therapy. *See also* Cryotherapy;
    Thermotherapy
    lamps, 320–321, 321*f*, 356–357
    modalities, 9–10, 291
    patient positioning, 335
    physiologic effects, 560
    theoretical basis, 560
Injury(ies)
    acute. *See* Acute injury
    bioelectric field changes in response to,
        118–119, 119*f*
    chronic. *See* Chronic injury
    edema formation, 486–489
Insulators, 84, 102
Integration, 198
Integumentary system. *See* Skin

Intensity
    definition, 403
    electrical stimulus, 124, 125*f*
    ultrasound, 373, 373*t*
Intercellular structures, electrical current effects, 114–115
Interference
    constructive, 145, 157
    destructive, 145, 157
    in electrical stimulation therapy, 145–147, 145*f*, 146*f*
Intermittent compression. *See* Compression therapy
Intermolecular vibration, 266, 286
Interneurons, 72, 79
Interphase interval, 87, 89*f*
Interpulse interval, 89, 89*f*, 102
Intervertebral foramen, 458, 459*f*
Inverse square law, 8, 8*f*, 13, 441–442
Inversion traction, 461–462, 461*f*, 462*f*
Ion transfer, 179. *See also* Iontophoresis
Ionization, 166, 179
Ions
    definition, 84, 102, 179
    for iontophoresis, 172*t*, 173*t*
    movements in solution, 166
    movements in tissue, 166–168
    sensitivity to, 175
Iontophoresis
    burns from, 175
    case studies, 168, 174
    clinical procedures, 180–181
    contraindications, 171
    current, 168–169, 169*f*
    definition, 102, 165, 179
    electrodes, 170–171, 171*f*
    generators, 167, 167*f*, 168–169
    indications, 171, 172, 173*t*
    ion selection, 171, 172*t*, 173*t*
    lab activity, 180–181
    mechanisms of action, 166–168, 555
    medication dosage, 170
    vs. phonophoresis, 165
    physiologic effects, 555–556
    precautions, 174–175
    theoretical basis, 555
    treatment duration, 170
    treatment tips, 175

J
Joint capsule, 65, 79
Joint contracture
    ultrasound effects, 385
Joint swelling, 498

K
Kehr's sign, 61
Keloids, 20
Keratin, 434, 447
Keratinocytes, 434, 447
Knee arthroplasty, 315
Krause's end bulbs, 65, 66*t*

L
Lambert-Eaton syndrome, 230
Laser(s)
    definition, 409, 430
    generators

    characteristics, 413
    gallium arsenide, 414–415
    helium neon, 413–414
    physics, 410–412, 410*f*, 411*f*, 412*f*
    types, 412–413
Laser therapy
    characteristics, 10
    clinical applications
        acute injury, 23
        bone response, 423
        edema, 425
        immunologic responses, 421
        indications, 25*t*, 431
        inflammation, 23, 39, 422, 425
        pain, 422–423, 424
        scar tissue, 422, 425
        wound healing, 39–40, 420–421, 424–425, 424*t*
        wound tensile strength, 421
    clinical procedures, 423–425, 424*f*, 431–432
    clinical research evidence, 50
    contraindications, 47–48*t*, 426, 431
    depth of penetration, 419, 419*f*
    dosage, 417–418, 417*f*
    lab activity, 431–432
    precautions, 40, 47–48*t*, 426
    safety considerations, 425–426
    techniques, 40–41, 40*f*, 415–417, 416*f*
    treatment times, 418, 418*t*
Latency
    compound motor action potential, 224*f*, 225
    definition, 250
    vs. nerve conduction velocity, 228–229
    sensory nerve action potential, 218*f*, 220
Lateral epicondylitis, 544, 544*f*
Lateral spinothalamic tract, 67*f*
Law of Grotthus-Draper, 7, 13
Leucotaxin, 15
Leukocytes
    in chronic inflammation, 17
    in inflammatory-response phase of healing, 15
    laser effects, 39
LIDC. *See* Low intensity direct current (LIDC)
Lidocaine, 389
Ligament(s)
    deformation, 454, 481
    effects of traction, 454–455
    low-intensity stimulation for injuries, 142–143
Limb temperature, in electrophysiologic testing, 216
LLLT. *See* Low level laser therapy (LLLT)
Longitudinal waves, 361, 403
Low back pain
    lumbar positional traction, 458–461, 459*f*, 460*f*
    shortwave diathermy, 269
    treatment tip, 9
Low intensity direct current (LIDC), 32
Low-intensity stimulators (LIS), 140–143
Low level laser therapy (LLLT), 413. *See also* Laser therapy
Low-voltage current, 84, 102, 138–139
Lumbar traction
    manual, 462–465, 463*f*, 464*f*, 465*f*
    mechanical
        body position, 468–471, 469*f*, 470*f*, 471*f*
        intermittent vs. sustained, 472–473
        patient setup and equipment, 465–467, 467*f*, 468*f*, 469*f*

        progressive and regressive steps, 473–474, 474*f*
        traction force, 471–472, 472*f*
        treatment duration, 473
    positional, 458–461, 459*f*, 460*f*
Lymph, 485, 486, 498
Lymphatic system
    anatomy, 485
    effects of biofeedback, 556
    effects of cryotherapy, 557
    effects of electrical stimulation, 553, 554
    effects of iontophoresis, 556
    effects of massage, 566
    effects of ultrasound, 562
    peripheral, 485–486, 485*f*, 486*f*
    purposes, 485
Lymphedema
    case study, 492
    definition, 484, 498
    formation, 487–488
Lymphocytes, 17

M
M-wave, 229
Macrophages, 17
Macroshock, 97, 98*t*, 102
Macrotears, 20, 27
Magnetic field, 263, 286
Manual traction. *See also* Spinal traction
    cervical, 475–476, 475*f*, 476*f*
    lumbar, 462–465, 463*f*, 464*f*, 465*f*
Mark:space ratio, 372. *See also* Duty cycle
Massage
    clinical procedures, 510–511, 510*f*, 511*f*, 512*f*, 534–536
    contraindications, 525, 528–529, 534
    definition, 504, 533
    equipment, 509–510
    friction, 533
    history, 503–504
    indications, 525, 528, 534
    lab activity, 534–536
    lubricants, 510, 511*f*
    mechanical effects, 505–507
    patient preparation, 510–511, 510*f*, 511*f*, 512*f*
    physiologic effects, 504–507, 534, 565–566
    positioning, 507, 508*f*, 509*f*, 511*f*, 512*f*
    psychologic effects, 507
    reflexive effects, 504–505
    techniques
        active release, 526–527, 527*f*
        acupressure, 520–524, 523*f*
        connective tissue, 518–520
        effleurage, 512, 513*f*
        friction, 518, 518*f*, 519*f*
        Hoffa massage, 512–517
        myofascial release, 524–525, 525*f*
        myofascial trigger points, 521–522
        percussion, 514, 515*f*, 516*f*, 517*f*
        petrissage, 514, 514*f*, 515*f*
        positional release, 526, 527*f*
        Rolfing, 528
        routine, 517
        strain/counterstrain, 525–526, 526*f*
        Tragering, 528
        vibration, 514, 517, 517*f*
    theoretical basis, 565
    treatment considerations, 507–509, 508*f*, 509*f*

Maturation-remodeling phase of healing
    pathophysiology, 18–19, 19f
    progressive controlled mobility in, 24
    therapeutic modalities, 22t, 24
Maximum voluntary isometric contraction, 157
McGill Pain Questionnaire, 63, 64f
Mechanical traction. *See also* Spinal traction
    cervical, 476–478, 477f
    lab activity, 482–483
    lumbar. *See* Lumbar traction, mechanical
Mechanoreceptors, 66t, 68t
Medial epicondylitis, 544, 544f
Median nerve
    distal motor latency study, 224f, 225, 225f
    nerve conduction study, 252–254
    nerve conduction velocity study, 226, 227f
Medical galvanism, 102, 138–139
Meissner's corpuscles, 65, 66t
Melanin, 436, 437, 447
Meniscoid structures, 456, 481
MENS. *See* Microcurrent electrical nerve
    stimulator
Menthol, 324
Mercury arc lamp, 439, 440f
Meridians, acupressure, 521
Merkel's corpuscles, 65, 66t
Metabolites, 334
Methyl salicylate, 324
Microcurrent electrical nerve stimulator (MENS),
    86, 102. *See also* Low-intensity stimulators
Microshock, 97, 98t, 102
Microstreaming. *See* Acoustic microstreaming
Microtears, 20, 27
Microwave diathermy
    applicators, 273, 274f
    characteristics, 5f, 9
    contraindications, 275
    equipment components, 273, 273f, 274f
    generators, 273
    indications, 25t, 275–276
    precautions, 276–278
    pregnancy risk, 276
    principles, 272–273
    vs. shortwave diathermy, 275
    technique, 274
    treatment tip, 10
Minimal erythemal dose, 440–441, 441f, 447
Modulation
    beat, 92
    burst, 92, 93f
    current, 92, 93f
    definition, 102
    ramping, 93
Monochromaticity, 412, 430
Monophasic current. *See also* Direct current
    vs. biphasic, for electrical stimulation, 121, 122f
    definition, 102
    waveforms, 87, 88f
Motor nerves, nerve conduction study. *See* Nerve
    conduction study, motor nerves
Motor points, 570–572f
Motor unit action potential (MUAP), 236–238,
    237f. *See also* Electromyography
MUAP. *See* Motor unit action potential
Muscle. *See also* Musculoskeletal system
    contraction by electrical stimulation
        for circulation enhancement, 129
        current intensity, 96

    in denervated muscle, 134–135
    for increased range of motion, 131–132, 133f
    for reeducation, 114, 115, 128–129
    for strengthening, 113, 116, 131
    denervated, 134, 157
    fibers, 214
    guarding, 193, 198
    maximum voluntary isometric contraction, 157
    reeducation
        electrical stimulation, 114, 115, 128–129,
            163–164
        electromyographic biofeedback, 192–193
    relaxation of guarding, electromyographic
        biofeedback, 193
    spasm, 20
        effect of tissue temperature change, 293–294
        massage, 506
    spindles, 66t
    strengthening, electrical stimulation, 113, 116,
        131, 163–164
    twitch, 109, 157
Musculoskeletal system. *See also* Muscle
    effects of biofeedback, 556
    effects of compression devices, 565
    effects of cryotherapy, 557
    effects of electrical stimulation, 553, 554, 555
    effects of massage, 505–506, 566
    effects of thermotherapy, 559
    effects of traction, 456, 564
    effects of ultrasound, 561–562
    effects of ultraviolet therapy, 563
Myasthenia gravis, 230
Myofascial pain, 295, 334
Myofascial release, 524–525, 525f, 533
Myofascial trigger points. *See also* Trigger points
    characteristics, 521–522
    laser therapy, 416, 424, 424t
Myopathic, 250
Myotonic discharges, 235, 250

N
Near field, 368f, 369
Necrosin, 15
Nerve cells. *See also* Neuromuscular system
    depolarization, 107–109, 108f
    excitation time, 109, 110f
Nerve conduction study (NCS). *See also*
    Electrophysiologic testing
    definition, 250
    indications, 244
    limitations, 241
    motor nerves
        advanced techniques, 230
        amplitude, 225
        central conduction studies, 229
        clinical procedure, 252–253
        duration, 226
        Hoffman's reflex, 229–230
        latency, 224f, 225
        nerve conduction velocity, 226, 227f, 228
        principles, 223–224
        repetitive nerve stimulation, 230
        rise time, 225–226
        vs. sensory nerves, 222–223
        setup, 223, 224f, 225f
        shape, 224f, 226
    purpose, 202
    sensitivity and specificity, 240–241

    sensory nerves
        amplitude, 218–219, 218f
        clinical procedure, 254–255
        latency, 218f, 220, 221f
        nerve conduction velocity, 220, 222
        setup, 217–218, 217f
        shape, 218f, 219–220
        variations, 222
    tests performed, 216
    upper extremity, 230–231
Nerve conduction velocity (NCV)
    definition, 250
    electrodes, 203
    vs. latency, 228–229
    motor nerves, 226, 227f, 228
    sensory nerves, 220, 222
Nerve impulse, propagation, 108, 108f
Nerve root impingement, 456–457, 466, 481
Neuromuscular electrical stimulator (NMES), 86,
    102
Neuromuscular junction, 214, 250
Neuromuscular system
    effects of biofeedback, 556
    effects of compression devices, 565
    effects of electrical stimulation, 553, 554, 555
    effects of massage, 566
    effects of thermotherapy, 559
    effects of traction, 456–457, 564
    effects of ultrasound, 562
Neurotransmitter, 67, 79, 108–109, 109f
NMES. *See* Neuromuscular electrical stimulator
Nociception, 65, 69–70, 79
Nociceptors, 65, 66t, 68t
Noise, 186, 198
Norepinephrine, 67, 79
Normative values, 250
Nucleus pulposus, 455
Numeric pain scales, 63–64
Nutrients, 344
Nutrition, wound healing and, 21

O
Occlusive dressings, wound healing and, 21
Ohm, 84, 102
Ohm's law
    definition, 85, 102
    in electrophysiologic testing, 210
Opiate pain control theory, 136–137, 553
Opiate receptors, 79
Orthodromic, 217, 250
Oscillator, 87, 102
Oscilloscope, 207
Output amplifier, 87, 102
Oxygen tension, in wound healing, 21

P
Pacinian corpuscles, 65, 66t
Pad electrodes, 265–266, 266f, 267f, 286
Pain
    central biasing theory, 72, 79, 136, 157, 553
    cognitive influences, 74–75
    definition, 60
    gate control theory, 71–73, 71f, 72f, 135–136,
        553
    neural transmission, 66–70
    opiate control theory, 136–137, 553
    sensory receptors, 65–66, 66t
    types, 61, 69

Pain assessment
    Activity Pattern Indicators Pain Profile, 63
    documentation, 65
    McGill Pain Questionnaire, 63, 63*f*
    numeric pain scales, 63–64
    pain charts, 63, 63*f*
    visual analog scales, 62, 62*f*
Pain control
    approach to, 75–77
    clinical procedures
        cold application, 70
        electrical stimulation, 76, 130, 137, 141,
            158–160
        electromyographic biofeedback, 193
        laser therapy, 422–423, 424
        massage, 505
        ultrasound, 388
    goals, 65
    neurophysiologic mechanisms, 70–75
Paraffin bath
    clinical procedures, 318–320, 319*f*, 354–355
    definition, 335
    physiologic effects, 560
    theoretical basis, 560
Parallel circuit, 94–95, 95*f*, 102
PEMF. *See* Pulsating electromagnetic field
Percussion, 514, 515*f*, 516*f*, 517*f*
Periaqueductal gray, 72, 79
Periosteum, 65, 79
Peripheral nervous system, 211–213, 212*f*
Peripheral vascular system
    effects of biofeedback, 556
    effects of compression devices, 565
    effects of cryotherapy, 557
    effects of electrical stimulation, 553, 554
    effects of iontophoresis, 556
    effects of paraffin bath, 560
    effects of thermotherapy, 559–560
    effects of traction, 564
    effects of ultraviolet therapy, 563
Permeability, voltage-sensitive, 157
Persistent pain, 61
Petrissage, 514, 514*f*, 515*f*, 533
Phagocytic cells, 15
Phases, 87, 102
Phonophoresis
    clinical procedure, 406
    definition, 403
    vs. iontophoresis, 165
    media, 390*t*
    medications delivered by, 389–391
Photokeratitis, 437, 447
Photon, 410, 430
Photosensitization, 435, 447
Piezoelectric activity, 117, 157
Piezoelectric effect, 365, 366*f*, 403
Pitting edema
    appearance, 487*f*
    definition, 498
    formation, 487
    ultrasound, 384
Plantar fasciitis, 538, 543–544, 543*f*
Plantar warts, 388
Plasma cells, 17
Platelets, 15
Pneumatic compression therapy. *See* Compression
    therapy
Polarity, electrical stimulus, 125

Polymodal nociceptors, 79
Polyneuropathy, 251
Polyphasic current, 103
Population inversion, 411, 411*f*, 430
Positional lumbar traction, 458–461, 459*f*, 460*f*.
    See also Spinal traction
Positional release therapy, 526, 527*f*
Positive sharp waves, 234*f*, 235, 251
Posterior primary rami, 215, 251
Potential difference, 84*f*
Power, 373, 403
Pressure field, 541, 547
Pressure ulcers
    characteristics, 45*f*
    electrical stimulation, 52
    pathophysiology, 44–45
    ultraviolet therapy, 443, 444
Proprioceptive nervous system, 455, 481
Proprioceptors, 66, 66*t*
Prostaglandins, 79
Proteoglycans, 17
Prothrombin, 17
Psoriasis, 436, 438, 442–443
Pulsatile current, 87, 89*f*
Pulsating electromagnetic field (PEMF), 387
Pulse, 87, 103
Pulse amplitude, 89–90, 89*f*
Pulse charge, 90, 103
Pulse duration, 91
Pulse frequency, 91
Pulse period, 91, 103
Pulsed electromagnetic energy (PEME).
    See Pulsed shortwave diathermy
Pulsed electromagnetic energy treatment
    (PEMET). *See* Pulsed shortwave diathermy
Pulsed electromagnetic field (PEMF).
    See Pulsed shortwave diathermy
Pulsed lavage, 30
Pulsed shortwave diathermy. *See also* Shortwave
    diathermy
    generators, 270, 271*f*
    precautions, 277
    principles, 269–270, 269*f*
    treatment time, 271–272
    treatment tips, 261, 269
Pulsed ultrasound, 371–372, 372*f*, 403. *See also*
    Ultrasound

Q
Qi, 521

R
Radial nerve, nerve conduction study, 221*f*
Radiant energy, 3–4
Radiation, 3, 13, 291*t*, 335
Radiculopathy, 251
Ramping, 93, 103
Range of motion, electrical stimulation, 131–132,
    133*f*
Raphe nucleus, 72, 79
Rarefactions, 361, 403
Rate of rise, 90, 91, 103
Raw activity, 188, 198
Rectification, 103, 198
Referred pain, 61, 79
Reflection, 6, 6*f*, 13
Refraction, 6, 6*f*, 13
Regulator, 87, 103

Repetitive nerve stimulation, 230, 251
Resistance, 84, 103
Resting potential, 107, 107*f*, 157
Reticular formation, 79
Rheobase, 109, 110, 110*f*, 157
Ribonucleic acid (RNA), 434, 435, 447
Rise time, 225–226
RNA. *See* Ribonucleic acid
Rolfing, 528, 533
Ruffini corpuscles, 65, 66*t*
Russian current, 143–144, 143*f*, 144*f*, 157

S
Salicylates, 389
SAR. *See* specific absorption rate
SATP intensity. *See* Spatial-averaged temporal
    peak (SATP) intensity
Scar formation
    effects of laser, 422, 425
    effects of ultrasound, 37, 385
Scars, hypertrophic, 20
Sclerotome, 61, 79
Sensitivity, 240, 251
Sensitization, 79
Sensory nerve action potential (SNAP), 218–222,
    218*f*, 221*f*, 251
Sensory receptors, 213–214, 293
Sensory stimulation, for pain relief, 72
SEP. *See* Somatosensory evoked potential (SEP)
    testing
Series circuit, 94, 94*f*, 103
Serotonin, 67, 69, 80
SG. *See* Substantia gelatinosa
Shape
    compound motor action potential, 224*f*, 226
    sensory nerve action potential, 218*f*, 219–220
Shock waves
    characteristics, 538–540, 539*f*
    generation, 540
    parameters, 540–541, 540*t*
Shortwave diathermy
    capacitor electrodes, 263–266
    case studies, 269, 272
    characteristics, 5*f*, 9
    clinical procedures, 287–289
    contraindications, 47–48*t*, 275
    equipment components, 261*f*, 262*f*
    generators, 261–263
    indications, 25*t*, 275–276
    induction electrodes, 266–269, 267*f*, 268*f*
    lab activity, 287–289
    vs. microwave diathermy, 275
    precautions, 47–48*t*
    pregnancy risk, 276
    pulsed. *See* Pulsed shortwave diathermy
    treatment tip, 261
    vs. ultrasound, 278–280, 278*f*, 279*f*, 385
Shoulder, calcific tendinitis, 544–545
Signal gain, 191, 198
Skin
    anatomy, 435*f*
    effects of biofeedback, 556
    effects of compression devices, 565
    effects of cryotherapy, 557
    effects of electrical stimulation, 553, 554, 555
    effects of infrared therapy, 560
    effects of iontophoresis, 556
    effects of massage, 506–507, 566

Skin (*Cont.*):
  effects of paraffin bath, 560
  effects of thermotherapy, 559
  effects of traction, 564
  effects of ultrasound, 561
  effects of ultraviolet radiation, 434–437
  effects of ultraviolet therapy, 562–563
Skin lesions
  ultraviolet radiation for diagnosis, 444
  ultraviolet therapy, 10, 436, 438, 442–443
Smoothing, 198
SNAP. *See* Sensory nerve action potential
Soft-tissue healing
  traction, 457
  ultrasound, 383–385
Somatosensory evoked potential (SEP) testing
    See also Electrophysiologic testing
  principles, 242–243
  purpose, 203
SPA. *See* Stimulus-produced analgesia
Spatial-average intensity, 373
Spatial-averaged temporal peak (SATP) intensity, 373
Spatial peak intensity, 373
Specific absorption rate (SAR), 262, 286
Specificity, 240, 251
SPF. *See* Sun protection factor
Spinal nerve(s), 211–215, 212*f*
Spinal traction
  case studies, 457, 466, 478
  clinical procedures, 482–483
  contraindications, 478–479, 482
  definition, 481
  indications, 478–479, 482
  inversion, 461–462, 461*f*, 462*f*
  lab activity, 482–483
  lumbar positional, 458–461, 459*f*, 460*f*
  manual cervical, 475–476, 475*f*, 476*f*
  manual lumbar, 462–465, 463*f*, 464*f*, 465*f*
  mechanical cervical, 476–478, 477*f*
  mechanical lumbar
    body position, 468–471, 469*f*, 470*f*, 471*f*
    intermittent vs. sustained, 472–473
    patient setup and equipment, 465–467, 467*f*, 468*f*, 469*f*
    progressive and regressive steps, 473–474, 474*f*
    traction force, 471–472, 472*f*
    treatment duration, 473
  physiologic effects
    articular facet joints, 456
    bone, 454
    cardiopulmonary, 563
    entire body part, 457
    genitourinary, 563
    ligaments, 454–455
    muscles, 456, 563
    nerves, 456–457, 563
    peripheral vascular, 563
    skin, 563
    spinal movement, 453–454, 454*f*
  theoretical basis, 563
Spondylolisthesis, 481
Spontaneous activity, 235–236, 251
Spontaneous emission, 410, 410*f*, 430
Sprain, compression therapy, 488
Standing wave, 363, 403

Staphylococcus aureus, 41
Stereodynamic interference current, 147, 157
Sterilization, 444
Stimulated emission, 410–411, 430
Stimulus-produced analgesia (SPA), 80
Strain/counterstrain, 525–526, 526*f*
Strain-related potentials, 117, 117*f*, 157
Strength-duration curve, 109, 109*f*, 110–111, 110*f*, 157
Stress fractures, 388
Stretching window, 385, 403
Substance P, 69, 80
Substantia gelatinosa (SG), 69, 72, 80
Summation of contractions, 124, 124*f*, 157
Sun protection factor (SPF), 447
Synaptic transmission, 67–70
Synovial fringes, 481

T
T cell, 80
Tanning, 436–437
Tapotement, 514, 515*f*, 516*f*, 517*f*, 533
Temporal-averaged intensity, 372*f*, 373
Temporal peak intensity, 372*f*, 373
Tendon(s)
  extracorporeal shock wave therapy, 541, 541*t*
  low-intensity stimulation, 142–143
TENS. *See* Transcutaneous electrical nerve stimulator
Tetanization, 124, 124*f*, 157
Tetany, 103
Therapeutic massage. *See* Massage
Therapeutic ultrasound. *See* Ultrasound
ThermaCare wraps, 323, 323*f*
Thermal, 335
Thermopane, 304, 335
Thermoreceptors, 66*t*, 68*t*
Thermotherapy
  clinical procedures
    counterirritants, 324
    fluidotherapy, 322–323, 322*f*, 358–359, 561
    infrared lamps, 320–321, 321*f*, 356–357
    paraffin bath, 318–320, 319*f*, 354–355, 560
    patient positioning, 335
    ThermaCare wraps, 323, 323*f*
    warm hydrocollator packs, 316–318, 316*f*, 318*f*, 352–353, 558–560
    warm whirlpool, 314–316, 314*f*, 350–351
  clinical research evidence, 50
  contraindications/precautions, 47–48*t*, 314
  definition, 291, 335
  in fibroblastic-repair phase, 23
  indications, 25*t*, 314
  in inflammatory-response phase, 23
  in maturation-remodeling phase, 24, 29
  physiologic effects, 297*t*, 312–313, 559–561
    on circulation, 292–293
    on muscle spasm, 293–294
    on performance, 294–295
  theoretical basis, 558–559
  treatment tips, 293, 314
Thrombin, 17
Thromboplastin, 16–17
Tissue sensitivity, 65
Tissue separation, 20
Total acoustical energy, 541, 547
Total current, 90, 90*f*

Traction, spinal. *See* Spinal traction
Trager, 528, 533
Transcutaneous electrical nerve stimulator (TENS), 86, 103, 554–555. *See also* Electrical stimulation
Transcutaneous electrical stimulator, 86, 103
Transformer, 87
Transmission, 6, 13
Transmitter substance, 108–109, 109*f*
Transverse friction massage, 518, 519*f*
Transverse waves, 361, 403
Trigger points, 61, 80, 521. *See also* Myofascial trigger points
Twitch muscle contraction, 157

U
Ultrasound
  absorption in tissues, 362–363, 363*t*
  advantages, 361
  amplitude, 372
  beam, 369–370
  case study, 370
  characteristics, 11
  clinical applications
    acute injury, 22–23
    bone healing, 387–388
    calcium deposits, 388
    connective tissue stretching, 368*f*, 385–386
    inflammation, 35–36, 50, 383, 387
    maturation-remodeling phase, 24
    pain control, 388
    plantar warts, 388
    pressure ulcers, 37, 38*f*
    scar tissue and joint contracture, 385
    soft-tissue healing and repair, 383–385
    stress fracture assessment, 388
  clinical procedures
    bladder coupling, 381, 382*f*, 405
    coupling methods, 378–379, 379*f*
    direct coupling, 379–380, 380*f*, 405
    duration of treatment, 377–378, 378*f*
    immersion, 381, 381*f*, 406
  clinical research evidence, 49
  cold packs and, 391, 392*f*
  continuous wave, 371–372, 372*f*, 403
  contraindications, 47–48*t*, 393, 404
  definition, 13
  electrical stimulation and, 392–393, 392*f*
  equipment
    generators, 363–365, 364*f*
    guidelines for safe use, 393–394
    ideal characteristics, 365*t*
    transducers, 364*f*, 365–367, 366*f*, 367*f*
  hot packs and, 391
  ice packs and, 391, 392*f*
  indications, 386, 404
  intensity, 373, 373*t*
  lab activity, 404–406
  nonthermal effects, 375–376, 376*f*, 404
  penetration in tissues, 362–363, 363*t*
  physiologic effects, 374–376, 404, 561–562
  placebo effects, 388
  power, 373
  precautions, 47–48*t*, 393
  pulsed, 371–372, 372*f*, 403
  reflection, 363, 363*t*
  vs. shortwave diathermy, 278–280, 278*f*, 279*f*, 385

theoretical basis, 561
thermal effects, 374–375, 404
as thermal modality, 361
transducer movement, 381–383
transmission in tissues, 361–363, 362f, 363t
treatment frequency, 367–369, 368f, 377
treatment records, 383
Ultraviolet light-C (UVC), 41. *See also* Ultraviolet
    therapy
Ultraviolet radiation. *See also* Ultraviolet therapy
    carcinogenic effects, 42, 437
    characteristics, 5f, 10, 433–434
    definition, 4, 4f, 13
    for diagnostic procedures, 444
    generators, 438–439
    physiologic effects
        cells, 434
        eyes, 437
        skin, 434–437, 562–563
    for sterilization, 444
    systemic effects, 438
    types, 41
Ultraviolet therapy. *See also* Ultraviolet radiation
    case studies, 436, 438, 443
    clinical applications
        calcium and phosphorus malabsorption, 443
        indications, 442
        pressure sore, 443, 444
        procedure, 448–450
        psoriasis, 436, 438, 442–443
        sterilization, 444
    clinical procedures, 41–42, 42f, 43f, 440–442,
        448–450
    clinical research evidence, 49
    contraindications, 443
    lab activity, 448–450

lamp positioning, 441–442
minimal erythemal dose determination,
    440–441, 441f
physiologic effects, 562–563
precautions, 42
theoretical basis, 562
treatment tip, 10
Unilateral foramen opening, 458, 481
Units of measure, 573
UVC. *See* Ultraviolet light-C

V
Vascular reaction, 15
Vascular supply, 20
Vasoconstriction, 295, 335
Vasodilation, 335
Velocity, sound waves, 6, 362
Vibration, 266, 286, 533
Viscoelastic properties, 454, 481
Visible light, 4f, 5f
Visual analog scales, 62, 62f
Vitamin D deficiency, 443
Volt, 84, 103
Voltage, 84, 103
Voltage sensitive permeability, 106, 157
Voluntary activity, 236, 251

W
Warm hydrocollator packs
    case study, 317
    clinical procedures, 316–318, 316f, 318f
    physiologic effects, 559–560
    theoretical basis, 558–559
    ultrasound and, 391
Warm whirlpool
    case study, 315

clinical procedures, 314–316, 314f, 350–351
physiologic effects, 558–560
Watt, 85, 103
Wave(s)
    longitudinal, 361, 403
    standing, 363, 403
    transmission frequency, 361–362
    transverse, 361, 403
Waveform
    current flow direction, 87
    definition, 103
    pulses vs. phases, 87
    shape, 87, 88f, 90f
Wavelength, 6, 13, 430
Whirlpool. *See also* Hydrotherapy
    cold, 303–306, 304f, 342–343
    electrical safety and, 98, 98f
    maintenance, 306, 316
    warm, 314–316, 314f, 350–351, 558–560
Wolff's law, 24, 454, 481
Wound(s)
    bioelectric activity, 118
    debridement, hydrotherapy, 29, 50
    healing
        laser therapy, 420–421, 424–425, 424t
        low-intensity stimulation, 142
    infection
        hydrotherapy, 30
        therapeutic modality selection, 50–51
        ultraviolet light therapy, 41
    tensile strength, laser therapy, 421
Wrist, nerve conduction studies, 217, 217f,
    221f

X
Xenon compact arc lamp, 439